Florence Nightingale and Hospital Reform

Volume 16
of the Collected Works of
Florence Nightingale

The Collected Works of Florence Nightingale

List of Volumes

Note: Short title denoted by bold.
Edited by Lynn McDonald, except as indicated.

Volume **1**	Florence Nightingale: An Introduction to Her **Life and Family**, **2001**
Volume **2**	Florence Nightingale's **Spiritual Journey**: Biblical Annotations, Sermons and Journal Notes, **2001**
Volume **3**	Florence Nightingale's **Theology**: Essays, Letters and Journal Notes, **2002**
Volume **4**	Florence Nightingale on **Mysticism and Eastern Religions**, ed. Gérard Vallée, **2003**
Volume **5**	Florence Nightingale on **Society and Politics**, Philosophy, Science, Education and Literature, **2003**
Volume **6**	Florence Nightingale on **Public Health Care**, **2004**
Volume **7**	Florence Nightingale's **European Travels**, **2004**
Volume **8**	Florence Nightingale on **Women**, Medicine, Midwifery and Prostitution, **2005**
Volume **9**	Florence Nightingale on **Health in India**, ed. Gérard Vallée, **2006**
Volume **10**	Florence Nightingale on **Social Change in India**, ed. Gérard Vallée, **2007**
Volume **11**	Florence Nightingale's ***Suggestions for Thought***, **2008**
Volume **12**	Florence Nightingale: **The Nightingale School**, **2009**
Volume **13**	Florence Nightingale: **Extending Nursing**, **2009**
Volume **14**	Florence Nightingale: The **Crimean War**, **2010**
Volume **15**	Florence Nightingale on **Wars and the War Office**, **2011**
Volume **16**	Florence Nightingale and **Hospital Reform**, **2012**

Florence Nightingale and Hospital Reform

Lynn McDonald, editor

Volume 16
of the Collected Works of
Florence Nightingale

Wilfrid Laurier University Press
www.wlupress.wlu.ca

We acknowledge the financial support of the Government of Canada through the Book Publishing Industry Development Program for our publishing activities.

Library and Archives Canada Cataloguing in Publication

Nightingale, Florence, 1820–1910

Florence Nightingale and hospital reform / Lynn McDonald, editor.

(Collected works of Florence Nightingale ; v. 16)
Includes bibliographical references and index.
Issued also in electronic format.
ISBN 978-0-88920-471-3

1. Hospital buildings — Great Britain — Design and construction — History — 19th century. 2. Public hospitals — Great Britain — Design and construction — History — 19th century. 3. Military hospitals — Great Britain — Design and construction — History — 19th century. 4. Nurses — Health and hygiene — Great Britain — History — 19th century. 5. Health care reform — Great Britain — History — 19th century. 6. Crimean War, 1853–1856 — Hospitals. 7. Crimean War, 1853–1856 — Influence. I. McDonald, Lynn, 1940– II. Title. III. Series: Nightingale, Florence, 1820–1910. Collected works of Florence Nightingale ; v. 16.

RA986.N54 2012 725′.51094109034 C2012-904266-8

Electronic monograph.
Issued also in print format.
ISBN 978-1-55458-288-4 (PDF)

1. Hospital buildings — Great Britain — Design and construction — History — 19th century. 2. Public hospitals — Great Britain — Design and construction — History — 19th century. 3. Military hospitals — Great Britain — Design and construction — History — 19th century. 4. Nurses — Health and hygiene — Great Britain — History — 19th century. 5. Health care reform — Great Britain — History — 19th century. 6. Crimean War, 1853–1856 — Hospitals. 7. Crimean War, 1853–1856 — Influence. I. McDonald, Lynn, 1940– II. Title. III. Series: Nightingale, Florence, 1820–1910. Collected works of Florence Nightingale (Online) ; v. 16.

RA986.N54 2012 725′.51094109034 C2012-904267-6

Cover design by Leslie Macredie. Front cover image: St Thomas' Hospital as it was soon after its opening in 1871, courtesy of Wellcome Trust Library. Front flap: Nightingale statue in the main lobby of the Glasgow Royal Infirmary, with a bronze relief of Lord Lister, courtesy of NHS Greater Glasgow and Clyde Archives. Back flap: Stained glass window depicting Nightingale at the Barrack Hospital, Scutari, courtesy of Iain Campbell. Back cover: Nightingale statue with hospital equipment at the Glasgow Royal Infirmary, courtesy of Sandra Hunter.

♾ Printed in Canada

Wilfrid Laurier University Press
Waterloo, Ontario, Canada N2L 3C5
E-mail: press@wlu.ca
Web: www.wlupress.wlu.ca

Collected Works of Florence Nightingale website:
www.sociology.uoguelph.ca/fnightingale

Contents

Military Hospitals: Letters, Notes, Articles and Reports

Civil Hospitals: Letters and Notes

Appendix

Acknowledgments

As this last volume in the *Collected Works of Florence Nightingale* goes to press, I am very aware of the debt I owe to so many people for assistance at various stages from finding long-buried letters to their transcription and verification. As usual, thanks are due to the Henry Bonham Carter Will Trust for permission to publish Nightingale original manuscripts, and indeed for treating Nightingale material as public domain. To the owners of Nightingale manuscripts thanks are due for their important role in conserving, while permitting scholarly access, and for providing copies for the *Collected Works.*

Many people worked on the preparation of the texts, many as volunteers. Thanks go to transcribers Gwyneth Watkins and Victoria Rea; assistants with proofreading, Patricia Warwick, Antonia Butler, Mary Boyce, Arun Dhanota and the late Cherry Ambrose; for assistance with French translations, Dr Gérard Vallée. For assistance with sources on Montreal hospitals, thanks to Annmarie Adams and David Theodore, for assistance with hospital site visits in England to Dr Eileen Magnello and Pat Smedley.

Archivists and librarians around the world provided skilled assistance, often beyond the call of duty. New material appeared by e-mail thanks to alert archivists and researchers in several countries.

At Wilfrid Laurier University Press thanks are due to Dr Brian Henderson, director; Rob Kohlmeier, managing editor; Doreen Armbruster, typesetter; Leslie Macreadie and Penelope Grows, marketing; Lisa Quinn, peer review; Steve Izma, technical support; and Heather Blain-Yanke, production manager. Thanks are due to the anonymous peer reviewers for helpful comments. The copy editing was done by Kristen Peterson Chew.

In spite of the assistance of so many people errors undoubtedly remain, which are the responsibility of the editor. I would be grateful for notification of any errors, and for information on missing identifications. Corrections will be made in the electronic text and any later print publication.

Lynn McDonald
5 November 2012

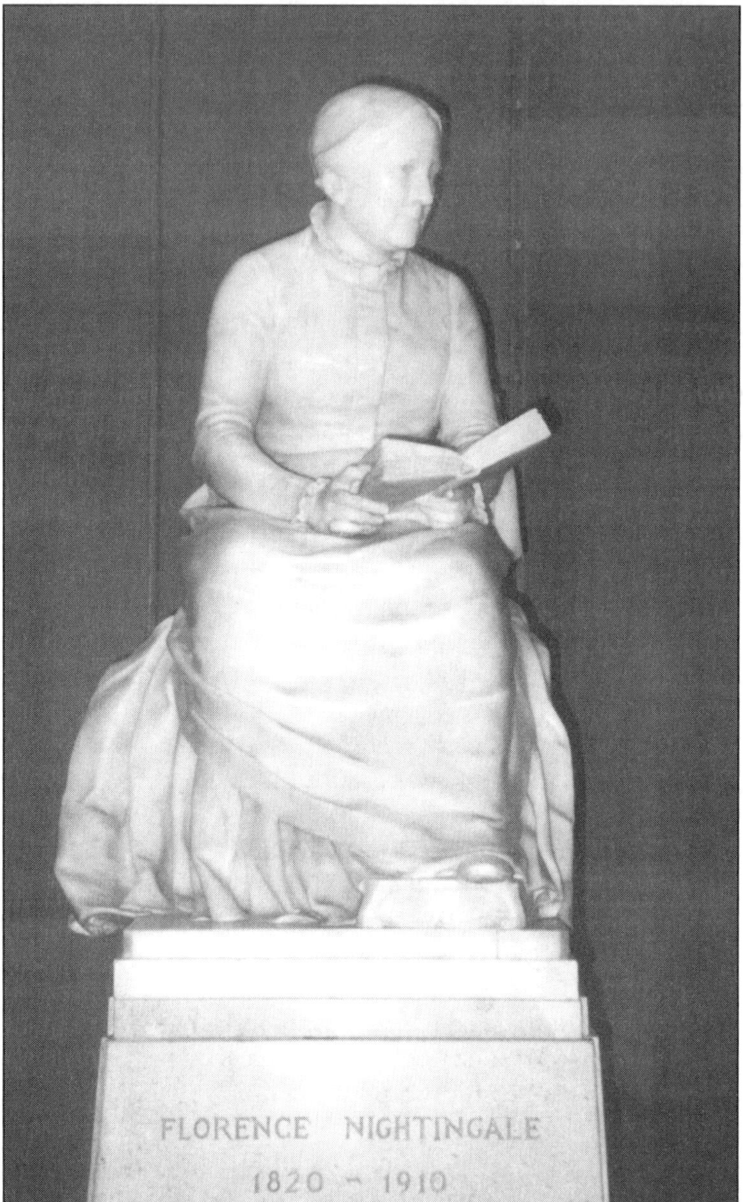

Marble statue of Nightingale by an unknown sculptor, Glasgow Royal Infirmary. Photograph courtesy of Sandra Hunter.

Dramatis Personae

Frances Nightingale (1788-1880), mother
William Edward Nightingale (1794-1874), father
Parthenope (Nightingale), Lady Verney (1819-90), sister
Samuel Smith (1794-1880), uncle
(Sir) Harry Verney (1801-94), brother-in-law, MP
(Sir) Douglas Galton (1822-99), Royal Engineer, hospital expert
Henry Bonham Carter (1827-1921), cousin, secretary, Nightingale Fund

T. Graham Balfour (1813-91), army statistician
(Lord) de Grey (1827-1909), secretary for war
(Dr) William Farr (1807-83), superintendent of statistics
George Godwin (1815-88), architect, editor, *The Builder*
(Sir) William Heathcote (1801-81), building committee, Winchester
Sidney Herbert (1810-61), Lord Herbert of Lea, secretary for war
(Sir) Joshua Jebb (1793-1863), prison reformer, Nightingale Fund
(Sir) John McNeill (1795-1883), doctor, Nightingale Fund
William Rathbone (1819-1902), philanthropist, Nightingale Fund
(Lord) Panmure (1801-74), secretary of state for war
William Rawlinson (1810-98), civil engineer, collaborator
(Dr) John Sutherland (1808-91), sanitary expert, collaborator
Victoria (1840-1901), crown princess of Prussia
Sarah E. Wardroper (1813-92), superintendent, Nightingale School

List of Illustrations

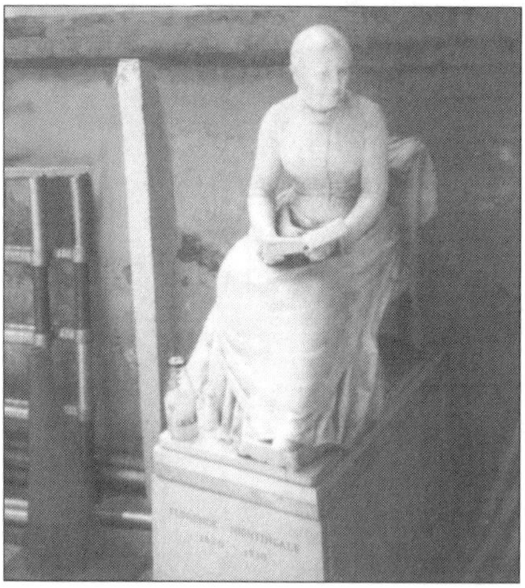

Marble statue of Nightingale in a storage area of the Glasgow Royal Infirmary, where it was in the early days of the Collected Works project. Photograph courtesy of Dr Ross Camidge. The statue was subsequently moved to the main lobby (see pictures on pp viii, 229 and 974).

Florence Nightingale: A Précis of Her Life

Florence Nightingale was born in Florence, Italy, 1820, the second daughter of wealthy English parents taking an extended European wedding trip. She was raised in England at country homes, Lea Hurst, in Derbyshire, and Embley, in Hampshire. She was educated largely by her father, who had studied classics at Trinity College, Cambridge. At age sixteen Nightingale experienced a "call to service," but her family would not permit her to act on it by becoming a nurse, then a lower-class occupation and thoroughly unthinkable for a "lady." Lengthy trips to Rome and Egypt were allowed (1847-48 and 1849-50 respectively). She had earlier (1837-39) been taken on a long trip with her family, mainly to Italy and France. These European trips not only improved her language skills (she was fluent in modern French, German and Italian as well as competent in ancient Latin and Greek), but exposed her to republican politics and Italian independence (she was in Rome and France during the revolts of 1848).

Nightingale was finally permitted to spend three months at the (Protestant) Deaconess Institution in Kaiserswerth, near Düsseldorf, Germany, in 1851 and several weeks with Roman Catholic nursing orders in Paris in 1853. Her father gave her an annuity in 1853 to permit her to become the superintendent of the Establishment for Gentlewomen during Illness, Upper Harley Street, London. She left there in 1854 to lead the first team of British women nurses sent to war. The British Army was poorly prepared for that war and the death rate from preventible disease was seven times that from wounds. The Barrack Hospital at Scutari, where she was stationed, was structurally unfit to be a hospital, had defective drains and had to be re-engineered by a team of visiting experts before the death rate could be brought down.

Nightingale's work as a public health and social reformer effectively began on her return from the Crimean War in 1856. Recognized as a national heroine, she chose to work behind the scenes for structural changes to prevent that war's high death rates from ever recurring. She lobbied to get a royal commission established to investigate the causes of the medical disaster and recommend changes. She herself briefed witnesses, analyzed data and strongly influenced the thrust of the report.

At the same time, at the request of the war minister, Lord Panmure, Nightingale prepared a "précis" on the problems of the war, which was to take six months, but which turned out to be an 853-page report two years later. This she had printed privately and distributed to trusted friends and collaborators. Both the "précis," *Notes on Matters Affecting the Health, Efficiency and Hospital Administration of the British Army Founded Chiefly on the Experience of the Late War*, and the official royal commission report were finished in 1858.

Nightingale fell ill while doing this work, it is thought from the chronic form of brucellosis, the disease from which (again this is conjecture) she nearly died in the war. She spent most of the rest of her life as an invalid, seeing people on a one-to-one basis and making her influence by research and writing. The illness was certainly painful and incapacitating, but Nightingale learned how to work around it, to focus her hours of working time on the most important projects, that is, those with the best prospect of saving lives.

Nightingale was baptized in the Church of England and remained in it for the rest of her life, although often despairing of its paltry role for women, the minimal demands it made of its adherents generally and its social conservatism. Her experience of religious conversion in 1836 and call to service in 1837 (the latter specifically dated 7 February and frequently referred to) were both shaped by reading the work of an American Congregational minister, Jacob Abbott, notably *The Corner-stone.* Her faith was nourished by broad reading, from the medieval mystics, liberal theologians and the German historical school to contemporary sermons, popular devotional books, tracts and religious novels. The family had been largely Unitarian in earlier generations, but her paternal grandmother was evangelical Church of England. Her parents took the family to the Church of England while at Embley, Wesleyan chapels while at Lea Hurst. There are Lutheran influences also on Nightingale from her Kaiserswerth time.

God for Nightingale was a perfect Creator who made and runs the world by *laws*, which human beings can ascertain by rigorous, preferably statistical, study. With the knowledge thus gained we can then intervene for good, thereby becoming God's "co-workers." Ongoing research is required, for human interventions, however well intentioned, may have negative, unintended consequences. This approach appears in all the work Nightingale did, whether in health care or social reform more broadly.

To guide her in doing the research necessary to discover "God's laws" Nightingale developed an effective methodological approach. Her sources were L.A.J. Quetelet, a Belgian statistics expert, on the conduct of research, and J.S. Mill on the philosophical grounding.

Nightingale's ardent and consistent liberal politics are another theme informing her social reform work. Her family (and the Verney family, into which her sister married) were strong Liberal supporters. Her brother-in-law, Sir Harry Verney, was a Liberal MP, as were cousins and family friends. She herself gave money to the Liberal Party and even wrote campaign letters for (a small number) of suitably progressive Liberal candidates. At a time of considerable political flux Nightingale's politics were consistent: she was a thorough "small l" liberal in her ideas, a supporter of free inquiry and expression and religious toleration. The Liberal Party seemed to be the best political manifestation of these goals. Again, as with the Church of England, the Liberal governments often failed to live up to their principles—she desperately wanted them to be liberal on India.

For most of her long working life Nightingale was confined to her room, describing herself variously as "a prisoner to my room" or even "a prisoner to my bed." Some days she could not see anybody, but usually she had interviews, sometimes several and sometimes lengthy ones, with nursing leaders, probationers, medical experts, politicians and Indian officials. Many people who requested interviews with her were turned down. Time with family and friends was fitted in around this "business," God's business in her understanding, saving lives. People who did not get interviews, however, normally got letters in reply, often long and careful explanations, and offers of assistance.

Nightingale added to her network as newer, younger experts, MPS and officials came into office. She always worked collectively, seeking advice from experts, nursing, medical or statistical. Her own articles and reports she had vetted by appropriate experts. When she could not aid the cause for someone, she suggested someone who could.

Nightingale continued to produce papers and reports of various kinds well into her seventies. She did not do any serious writing in her eighties, when blindness and failing mental faculties gradually stopped her. There are brief messages only from 1902 on. She was given honours in her last years—notably the Order of Merit in 1907. She died at age ninety and was buried in the churchyard of St Margaret's, Wellow, the family's parish church. Consistent with her wishes, the family declined an offer of burial at Westminster Abbey.

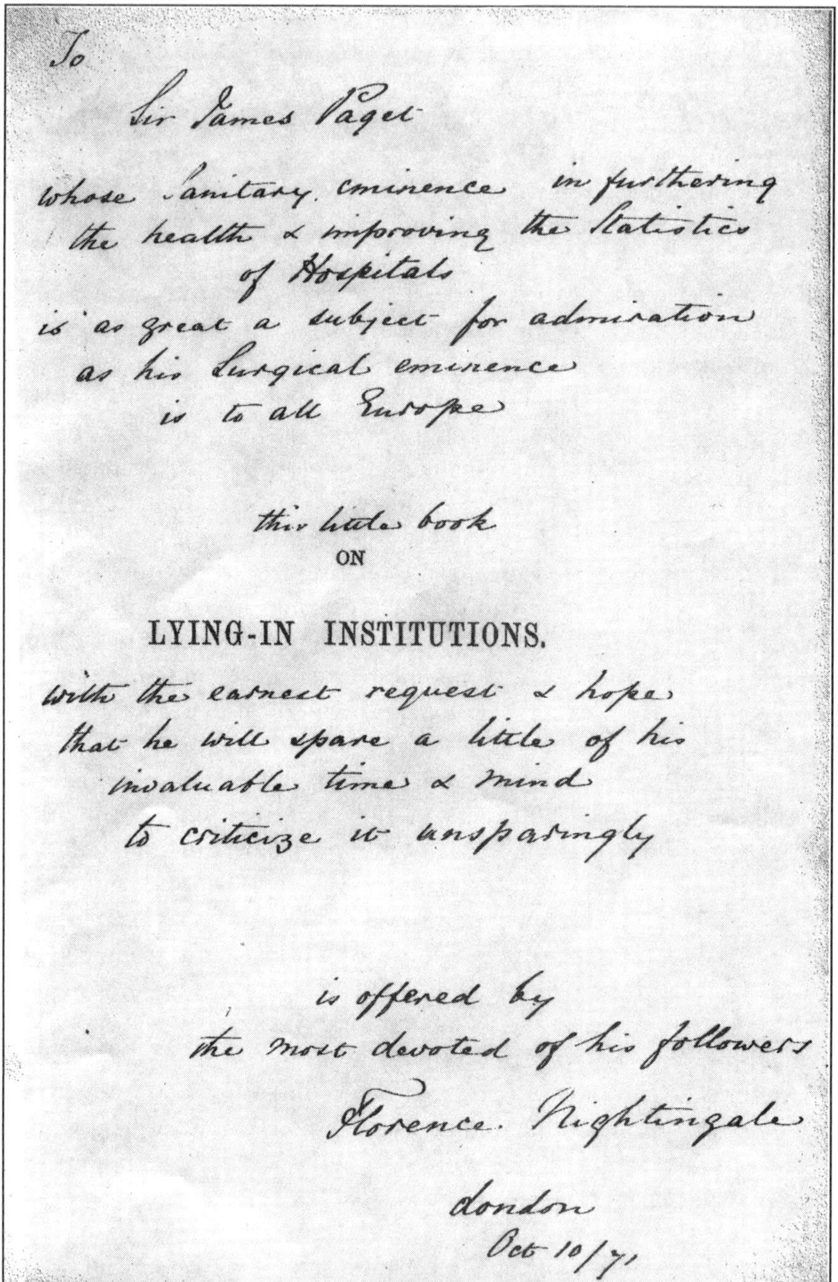

To

Sir James Paget

whose Sanitary eminence in furthering
the health & improving the Statistics
of Hospitals
is as great a subject for admiration
as his Surgical eminence
is to all Europe

this little book
ON
LYING-IN INSTITUTIONS.
with the earnest request & hope
that he will spare a little of his
invaluable time & mind
to criticize it unsparingly

is offered by
the most devoted of his followers
Florence Nightingale

London
Oct 10/71

Dedication page of Nightingale's *Notes on Lying-in Institutions*, for Sir James Paget, a close colleague on hospital statistics. Courtesy Royal Society of Medicine website.

An Introduction to Volume 16

Hospital Reform completes the sixteen volumes in *The Collected Works of Florence Nightingale* with material that permits an overview of such a central concern of Nightingale's working life as hospital reform. Subjects range from her early work on army hospitals and her far larger output on civil hospitals to her use of statistics and other research on the health of the population at large.

The first volumes in the *Collected Works* introduce Nightingale's family and background: *Life and Family* (vol. 1) and *European Travels* (vol. 7). Four volumes relate the influence of her faith: *Spiritual Journey, Theology* and *Mysticism and Eastern Religions* (vols. 2, 3 and 4) and *Suggestions for Thought* (vol. 11). *Public Health Care* (vol. 6) is the first of four that deal with hospital and nursing concerns; it includes her *Notes on Nursing for the Labouring Classes* and much on workhouse infirmaries; *The Nightingale School* (vol. 12) reports the foundation and work of her school at St Thomas' Hospital, and *Extending Nursing* (vol. 13) relates its extension throughout Britain, Europe and much of the world. *Women* (vol. 8) includes her work on maternal health (with *Introductory Notes on Lying-in Institutions*), prostitution, women in medicine and letters to many women correspondents. The present volume, *Hospital Reform*, completes the sub-set, with its focus on hospital design and construction.

Two volumes report Nightingale's massive work on India: *Health in India* (vol. 9) and *Social Change in India* (vol. 10). Two report her work on wars: *The Crimean War* (vol. 14) and *Wars and the War Office* (vol. 15), which takes up the implementation of War Office reforms post-Crimea and reports all her work on later wars.

Hospital Reform has its roots in *The Crimean War*, notably in Nightingale's pioneering analysis of what went wrong in the war hospitals to result in such high death rates. The same year that her main reports on that war appeared—1858—she sent her first paper to the National

Association for the Promotion of Social Science, "Notes on Hospitals," which she then expanded for separate publication in 1859. These two papers have been published together here as a critical edition, followed by her greatly enlarged and revised 1863 *Notes on Hospitals*.

Hospital Reform also reprints Nightingale's 1859 short paper, *A Contribution to the Sanitary History of the British Army*, which permits a revisiting and rethinking of some of the Crimean War hospital material. This fine piece of analysis constitutes Nightingale's last crack at the subject of what went wrong, and also serves, as does all of her analytical material, to introduce remedies to avoid such mistakes in the future.

Two sections of correspondence and short publications follow the major published works: the first on military hospitals (including barracks and camps), the second and longer on civil hospitals (including some material on schools and towns). The links between the two sections are significant, for hospitals have common characteristics and risks, whether their patients are soldiers or civilians. Nightingale's publications too go back and forth between the two types of patient, but it makes sense to have some demarcation, given the differences in administrative procedures and legal framework between civil and military institutions and their staffs.

The military section contains much material on the building of two great military hospitals, the Royal Victoria Hospital, Netley, and the Herbert Hospital, Woolwich: the bad and good examples, respectively, of hospital construction. Some further excerpts from Nightingale's "confidential report," *Notes on the Health of the British Army*, are included here, as not all of this 853-page report could be included in *The Crimean War* volume.

The material on civil hospitals ranges over subjects from general hospitals to workhouse infirmaries, convalescent and cottage hospitals, children's hospitals and midwifery institutions. Much of it was written in answer to specific requests for help and advice. For some hospitals there is ample documentation of what Nightingale did or tried to do. For many there are only occasional references in correspondence, with any actual letters to the architect or hospital officials having gone missing. Nightingale often wrote her comments directly on hospital plans, but none of these annotated plans has survived.

Nightingale, throughout her life, placed a high value on the importance of architecture. During her European travels as an adolescent and young woman, she had a privileged look at the finest European cathedrals, basilicas, hospitals, public buildings and monuments. She considered architecture to be humanity's "fittest homage" and its "worthiest tribute" to God. Michelangelo to her was "the Archangel Michael," for his great St Peter's Basilica in Rome.[1]

Upon embarking on her work as a hospital reformer, Nightingale went so far as to contend, in 1858, that the "public hospitals of a country" could be taken as "a standard of the knowledge" of its government, and even as the standard "of civilization amongst a people" (see p 307 below). She did not continue making such grand claims regarding the natures of architecture, but she did continue to argue for better housing as a necessary condition for a high standard of moral conduct, as well as for people's physical health. In one of her 1858 articles in *The Builder*, she issued a challenge: "Let us reform our hospitals now, and as we improve our cities and towns, they will be less required" (see p 307 below). In 1872, Nightingale told her colleague Dr Sutherland that "to make people's dwellings fit for sick, or rather such as will not make sickness," was "our first duty" (see p 769 below).

It must be understood that Nightingale's approach to health care was always holistic: it was best to build health and prevent disease, through such measures as decent housing and nutrition, clean air and water. When sickness occurred, the preferred response was home visits by a doctor and nurse: hospitals were always only a last resort, as a "hard necessity of an inferior, imperfect civilization" (see p 764 below). This view of hospitals as a last resort was one she often repeated, with slightly different wordings.

Nightingale's own hospital experience was limited. She headed a small charitable hospital, the Establishment for Gentlewomen during Illness, in Harley St., for a year and a half, the same length of time she spent as superintendent of nursing at the British war hospitals in the Crimean War. She never had a post at a regular civil hospital, although she had accepted one, at King's College Hospital, London, just before she left for the Crimean War.

A little known, and very brief, part of Nightingale's hospital experience was her voluntary work at the Middlesex Hospital during the London cholera epidemic of 1854. Some 53 percent of cases admitted (June-November 1854) died, yet only two nurses and a scrubber contracted the disease. A history of the hospital concludes that "such comparative immunity was in all probability due to the care taken by

---

1 *European Travels* (7:100 and 278-80).

the hospital of its nurses, and also to the presence beneath its roof for a short time of Miss Florence Nightingale." She is said, moreover, to have acquired much of the experience she used at Scutari at the Middlesex, a plausible point, for her position at the time was head of the genteel Harley St. institution. At the Middlesex, Nightingale undertook "the superintendence of the cholera patients ... brought in every half hour from the Soho district, Broad Street, etc."[2]

Nightingale has been criticized for not acting promptly after the Crimean War to establish her nurse training school with the funds raised in her honour during that war. The reason for this delay was her concern over hospital safety. Her calling was to save lives, for which trained nursing was a means, but not the end. Faulty hospital construction, from bad design and building materials to an unhealthy site, caused deaths—not only to patients but also to nurses, doctors and other hospital staff. It is telling that Nightingale added a note about nurse mortality to the 1859 edition of *Notes on Hospitals*, specifically mentioning that 54 percent of nurse deaths were from preventible causes (see p 516 below). In that note she also asserted that "nothing gives such a really good criterion of the sanitary (or non-sanitary) construction of hospitals" as "the mortality of nurses" (see p 516 below).

Not one to mince words on the dangers of poor hospital design, Nightingale said: "I know of no class of murderers who have killed so many people as hospital architects" (see p 823 below). This was in 1877, when many improved hospitals had, in fact, already been built. Similarly, the unnecessarily high death rate at the (old) Winchester Infirmary constituted for Nightingale a "hospital massacre" like that at Scutari. Moreover, while the unnecessary deaths at Scutari lasted only "a short period," mistakes made in regular civil hospitals lasted a long time (see p 595 below).

It is thus no coincidence that Nightingale published a massive amount of material on hospital construction, sites and materials before she turned to nursing proper. Her lengthy *Notes on the Health of the British Army* (at 853 pages) and her first (short) paper, "Notes on Hospitals," came out in 1858, her first edition of *Notes on Nursing* two years later, in 1860.

Nightingale wanted value for money in hospital construction, and no frills. She did not like extravagance and sometimes protested the

---

2 Hilary St George Saunders, *The Middlesex Hospital 1745-1948* 38.

amount of space given to administration, although she also was vigorous in promoting measures to protect administrative employees from disease. More often, however, she called for greater expenditures. She learned to be wary of half measures and argued "it is always cheaper to build a good hospital than a bad one" (see p 649 below). What is bad ultimately costs more, she had found, while "what is good is cheap in the end," and said that even the French military found out "that good beds are the cheapest" (see p 654 below). In *Notes on Hospitals*, she stated, "it so happens that the safest for the sick is in reality the most economical mode of construction" (see p 126 below).

Late in her life, in connection with fundraising for St Thomas' Hospital in 1895, Nightingale had occasion to ask rhetorically, "As science goes on, do not hospitals become more expensive?" Doctors ordered more expensive food and appliances: "everything is supplied; nothing is spared," while "no one asks where the funds come from." Yet she was not disapproving—it would be a pity to let hospitals "be starved" when things had been worked up to this level (12:463).

Throughout her long life, Nightingale would make time to examine and criticize plans for new hospitals and for major renovations and extensions. Typically this entailed sending her initial comments and the plans to public health expert Dr John Sutherland and/or to Royal Engineer Douglas Galton for another opinion. Sometimes Nightingale needed only confirmation on some points she wanted to raise; at other times she sought comprehensive advice. Certainly she wanted to make sure that they did not contradict each other.

Nightingale was frequently asked to endorse a hospital's building plans, as attaching her name to a project would aid in raising funds for it. She agreed only when the plans and site met a high standard. When she considered a project to be sound, which might be after considerable changes, she would make her own financial contribution. Sometimes she wrote a letter of support to be read out at a public meeting or sent to the local newspaper (or both); sometimes she would dangle bribes before planning committees to entice them to make crucial changes. The conditions might be as onerous as their entirely ditching a plan to rebuild on the same site and purchasing a new site and commissioning radically improved plans. In the case of the Winchester Infirmary, Nightingale went so far as to induce a prominent member of the nobility, who happened to be both a diplomat and a local landowner, to make his contribution contingent on a new building at a different site rather than merely renovating the old building (see p 587 below).

Nightingale's contributions were sizable for her income, but hardly the most generous. They were usually £50 or £100, with apologies that she could not give ten times more. She also had cause to complain that people identified her by name as a supporter of their projects when they had rejected her advice. For example, in September 1860 Nightingale said that since the publication of her evidence to the royal commission on the Crimean War in 1858, she had been sent the plans for "some dozen" hospitals "purporting to be constructed" on her principles (see p 624 below), but which were far off what she advocated. In 1863, she said that there was not one large civil hospital in England that could be called a "model." The Herbert Hospital was a model for a military hospital (see p 582 below) but even it was a disappointment, for the hospital was overbuilt and for years had empty wards.

Much of the material in this volume is obsolete in the sense of its having no relevance to contemporary hospital practice. Ward size—such a major concern both in Nightingale's publications and correspondence—is perhaps the most obvious, now obsolete, issue. Modern best practice has moved to the use of single rooms rather than wards in hospitals as the most effective way to avoid hospital-acquired infections. In Nightingale's day, before the availability of bells and telephones, let alone equipment for electronic monitoring, multiple-person wards were necessary, as the nurse had to be able to see all patients. As Nightingale explained in 1862, whether a ward be for "four or forty," a trained nurse was required (see p 631 below).

Her advocacy of pavilion-type hospitals is similarly dated, yet they were the great reform of the day, facilitating good ventilation and light, and minimizing the chances of cross-infection. Each pavilion was, in effect, a small hospital of its own. Many pavilion-style hospitals were built in Britain over the course of time covered in this volume. Nightingale not only was a major influence in these developments in Britain but soon also in Continental Europe, the United States and Canada. Pioneering pavilion hospitals on which she contributed to the design include the City Hospital of Berlin (Städtisches Krankenhaus, Friedrichshain), which influenced the next German and Austrian hospitals, Johns Hopkins University Hospital in Baltimore and the Royal Victoria Hospital, Montreal. Nightingale was the "single greatest influence" on hospital architecture for a century.[3]

---

3 Margaret A. Williams, "Design for Therapeutic Outcomes," in Sara O. Marberry, ed., *Innovations in Healthcare Design* 106.

Staff sizes at hospitals were much lower in Nightingale's day. In *Notes on Hospitals* (1863), a ratio of 150 staff to 500 patients is given as standard practice. When well-trained nurses were scarce, Nightingale preferred fewer and better nurses to a larger number of inept, gossipy or otherwise unreliable nurses—a lesson she had learned during the Crimean War.

Nurses' homes are no longer used in many countries, notably where nurse training is given in universities or colleges. For all of Nightingale's lifetime they were a logical part of the system, and so receive a lot of her attention in this volume. Nurses in training, and the vast majority later employed in hospitals, would be single women. Long hours were the norm for virtually all paid employment, and Nightingale never contested this matter. Instead, she strove to make working and living conditions for nurses the best possible, to make the long hours bearable. Labour-saving devices, good design, adequate time off, generous holidays and good meals were deemed necessary to keep up the health of hospital nurses and probationers.

At this time, before the availability of take-away food, frozen dinners and home deliveries, and such conveniences as central heating, refrigerators, freezers and microwaves, a nurses' home made sense. It provided a separate room to each nurse or pupil, along with a communal lounge and dining room. The Nightingale Home at St Thomas' Hospital was of a particularly high standard for hygiene and comfort, and American visitors remarked on how pleasant and welcoming it was.

The ward system as Nightingale conceived it required a high level of dedication on the part of the ward sister, and effectively assumed that she had neither husband nor children. As late as 1896 Nightingale told nurses, "While you have a ward, it must be your *home* and its inmates must be your children. Don't be like water turned on from a cock, and turned off again."[4] Her object of keeping matron and nurse teams who trained together is another obsolete goal of Nightingale's, or certainly an impossible expectation given current mobility patterns.

Technological advances have ensured that numerous other urgent concerns of Nightingale's day no longer exist, such as the need to place toilets externally to the main building, cut off from the wards by

4 Supplementary remarks in Mrs Roundell, *Agnes Jones, or She Hath Done What She Could.*

a lobby, and ventilated with windows on both sides. Kitchens, similarly, need not be in separate buildings—to prevent fumes and damp from entering the wards. Again, the important reasons for keeping the laundry distant from wards—to avoid contamination from soiled sheets and dressings—are no longer relevant.

British hospitals, or at least large ones, had chapels and chaplains in Nightingale's day. In Church of England hospitals, prayers from the Book of Common Prayer were read in the wards regularly. Prayers for healing were not then used and there seems to have been no suggestion that such prayers might actually promote recovery. Nightingale herself seems to have believed that illness could serve to make the sick reflect critically on their lives. This is apparent on the occasions when she was asked to advise on hospital prayers (see p 773 below).

The reform of workhouse infirmaries was always a high priority for Nightingale for these institutions treated the poorest of society, those destitute of any means of support. They were the main hospitals used by the poor, treating more than five patients for every one in the regular civil hospitals. Nightingale worked both on the introduction of nursing into these institutions (reported in *Public Health Care* and *Extending Nursing*, volumes 6 and 13) and improvements in their design and construction, the subject of this volume. The two went together, as the introduction of trained nurses called for a new building, or at least a nurses' home, such as a whole new building for the Highgate Infirmary and a nurses' home at St Marylebone Workhouse Infirmary.

Nightingale took particular pleasure in the building of pavilion workhouse infirmaries, the first of which was Chorlton, near Manchester, which opened in 1866. She was particularly pleased that it turned out to be not only the best, but the cheapest hospital built, for that meant its example would then be followed (see p 732 below). The gradual upgrading of the workhouse infirmaries into regular hospitals is another important development in this volume. Without the radical reform of the workhouse infirmaries, the launching of the National Health Service in 1948 would have been unimaginable.

The volume ends with biographical sketches of the two engineers with whom Nightingale worked so much on hospital reform, and a list of architects on whose plans she worked. A final appendix gives "bons mots" or succinct remarks about hospitals—variously their faults, an alternative vision or actual reforms—ranging from the sober and realistic to the sardonic and witty.

The Need for Hospital Reform

The backward state of hospitals, even leading teaching hospitals, when Nightingale undertook the project of hospital reform, has to be understood from the beginning. An excellent example is that of the famous St Bartholomew's Hospital, London, founded in 1553. By Nightingale's day, it had a highly reputable medical school and a number of eminent physicians and surgeons on its staff. However, correspondence between Elizabeth Herbert and Nightingale in 1854 reveals both "jobbery," or corrupt practices in staff appointments or contracts, and abysmal living conditions endured by nurses. Writing to Nightingale, then at the Harley St. hospital, Herbert drew her attention to these problems:

> Sidney has begged me to write and ask you whether you can give him any facts in writing as to abuses which exist in St Bartholomew's Hospital? They are making a stir about it owing to the shameful system of jobbing going on to obtain appointments of different kinds in the hospital and Sidney says if he could get some authentic information on the subject of the nurses, their bad pay and worse lodgings, he could get the evil more or less remedied and public attention, at any rate, turned that way.

Nightingale, in reply, said some improvements had been made in nurses' conditions in that the night nurses had rooms allotted to them at the top of the house, but the day nurses still slept in wooden cages on the landings.[5]

When Nightingale took on civil hospital reform post-Crimea, the scholarly literature[6] on defects was scarce, and scarcer still was informa-

---

5 E. Herbert letter 29 May [1854], Claydon House Bundle 300/301, reply in *Women* (8:654-55).

6 For general background on hospital reform in the period see: Brian Abel-Smith, *The Hospitals 1800-1948: A Study in Social Administration in England and Wales*; Jeremy Taylor, *Hospital and Asylum Architecture in England 1840-1914: Building for Health Care*; Geoffrey Rivett, *The Development of the London Hospital System 1823-1982*; Christine Stevenson, *Medicine and Magnificence: British Hospital and Asylum Architecture, 1660-1815*; Harriet Richardson, ed., *English Hospitals 1660-1948: A Survey of Their Architecture and Design*; John D. Thompson and Grace Goldin, *The Hospital: A Social and Architectural History*; Gwendoline M. Ayers, *England's First State Hospitals and the Metropolitan Asylums Board 1867-1930*; J.H. Woodward, *"To Do the Sick No Harm": A Study of the British Voluntary Hospital System until 1875*; F.N.L. Poynter, ed., *The Evolution of Hospitals in Britain*; Lavinia Mitton, *The Victorian Hospital.*

tion on what might be done to correct them. The pioneer advocate for safer, pavilion-style hospitals was a French doctor, Jacques René Tenon 1724-1816), who published in book form his five critical "memoirs" on hospitals (his book was to raise money for hospitals) in 1788.[7] It seems that Nightingale did not know that work directly, but she did know John Pringle's even earlier exposé of the problems of military hospitals, *Observations on the Diseases of the Army in Camp and Garrison* (1752), and John Howard's reports on European hospitals, *An Account of the Principal Lazarettos in Europe* (1789). Tenon did not live to see most of his advice acted upon, but a number of pavilion hospitals, with ample grounds, began to appear: the small Beaujon in Paris, small pavilion hospitals in Brussels and Bordeaux and in 1853 the large Paris pavilion hospital, Lariboisière, which so much impressed Nightingale. When I made my own pilgrimage to the Lariboisière in May 2012, the pavilions were all still there, but modified on the inside.

There are early English pavilion hospitals, which Tenon had seen on a trip to England: the Royal Naval Hospital, Plymouth, built 1856-64 by architect Alexander Rovehead and the Royal Hospital, Haslar, at Portsmouth, built 1746-61 by Theodore Jacobsen. Christopher Wren's splendid Royal Marine Hospital at Greenwich, built 1696-1712, was constructed with extensive gardens and a fine site, although for reasons of grand appearance rather than hygienic standards. The English editor of Tenon's *Memoirs* commented that the origins of the pavilion plan remained a mystery, as did the reason why English naval surgeons isolated themselves and their architectural plans.[8] There is no direct evidence of designers considering the actual effects of the new design on hospital stays or death rates.

Through her family connections, Nightingale knew the renowned prison reformer Joshua Jebb (1793-1863), who had brought sanitary principles into prison construction.[9] He is likely to have been a helpful early source for her on hospitals, but direct correspondence on the subject is missing (Jebb was a member of the original Nightingale Fund Council and correspondence between the two is available on nursing). A Nightingale letter to her brother-in-law, Sir Harry Verney, in 1867 refers to Jebb having shown her plans for a convict hospital.[10]

---

7 Jacques Tenon, *Mémoires sur les hôpitaux de Paris*, available in English translation by Dora B. Weiner, ed., *Memoirs on Paris Hospitals*; see her Introduction xxiv-xxv.

8 Weiner, Introduction, in *Memoirs on Paris Hospitals* xxv.

9 See, for example, his *Modern Prisons: Their Construction and Ventilation*, 1844.

10 Letter 11 March [1867], Wellcome (Claydon copy) Ms 9002/115.

The first British doctor to take up the cause of reformed hospital construction was John Roberton (1797-1876), who was also a vice-president of the Manchester Statistical Society. He began to publish on safer hospitals in 1856, based on his own informal observations. Nightingale was then still at Scutari, acquiring her much more extensive experience of unsafe hospitals. George Godwin (1815-88), architect and editor of *The Builder*, also took up the issue in 1856, citing Roberton and, soon, Nightingale.

Following French leadership on hospital reform led to complications for Nightingale and colleagues. The French clearly were the first to publish on hospital design for health reasons, and to design hospitals deliberately on the pavilion principle to that end; they had also been the pioneers of military medicine. For all these developments, however, French hospitals, both military and civil, still had high death rates. Lariboisière was "one of the best hospitals in existence" in its plans, but it nonetheless produced "one of the highest rates of mortality," on this account, Nightingale thought, of its use of artificial ventilation (see p 156 below).

The same dilemma would appear somewhat later in Nightingale's work on maternity hospitals. When the midwifery nurse training program began at King's College Hospital, Nightingale did not know of Tenon's devastating revelations, in his fourth memoir, about the high French maternal mortality rates, knowledge that would have been enormously useful in the King's experiment. In that memoir he observed that puerperal fever never seemed to affect women who gave birth at home, however bare their abode, a point that Nightingale found still held.

Nightingale was aware, from numerous informal sources, that the French superiority in military medicine in the first year of the Crimean War did not last. French mortality rates in the second year of that war were much higher than those of the British, mainly on account of the radical reforms the British made. Nightingale, however, did not know the actual numbers of French Crimean War deaths, for they were not published until after she had finished her own analysis. Deaths per troop numbers in the first winter was 23 percent for the British, but only 11 percent for the French. In the second winter, the British lowered their death rate to 2.5 percent, while the French nearly doubled theirs to 20 percent,[11] despite all the experience from

11 Jean Charles Chenu, *De la mortalité dans l'armée et des moyens d'économiser la vie humaine, extraits des statistiques médico-chirurgicales* 131.

the first winter, the building of a railway to bring in supplies and the end of active fighting. Nightingale's early great enthusiasm for French hospitals would be replaced with greater caution.

Roberton reported[12] having visited the great European hospitals in Brussels, Bordeaux and Paris, most notably the pavilion-style Lariboisière, which he described as "truly a palace for the sick" (137). The "novel" Bordeaux Hospital, with its thirty-eight-bed pavilions, received a glowing description, including the grounds, windows opposite each bed, the absence of bed curtains, the placement of nurses' rooms, bathrooms and toilets, and entrance from the outside.

> It follows, of course, that each ward is itself *a separate hospital*, having no communication with the other wards, so that if we were to suppose one of these to be crowded with the worst kind of surgical maladies for causing foulness, the foul air could not find a passage into any other ward—a hospital atmosphere would be impossible (139).

In this influential paper he further argued that hospitals had to have "excess air," more than merely sufficient amounts to sustain life. Roberton held that it was "well known" to doctors that "most of our hospitals" were at times unhealthy, and that patients, instead of being cured, grew worse, and sometimes died rapidly in "considerable numbers" of "an infectious malady known by the name of hospital gangrene." Yet, while cubic space was "highly important," it was a "secondary consideration to the getting rid of fetid and pestiferous exhalations." A "continual renewal" of the atmosphere was needed in hospitals, while "ample air space is all that is required" for well people, and the space provided in provincial hospitals was not half what it ought to be. He recommended no less than 2000 cubic ft. per bed, and reported visiting one hospital with only 715 cubic ft. (137). He was decidedly in advance of medical opinion in advocating so much cubic space. Nightingale herself did not go to that level for some time.

Roberton's paper stated that it had long been "a painful conclusion of experience that the larger the hospital the higher the rate of mortality" (142). The Middlesex Hospital in London was a model for its ventilation, but he complained that the building plan allowed the generation of a "hospital atmosphere" (143). Still, he did not feel

---

12 John Roberton, "On the Defects, with Reference to the Plan of Construction and Ventilation, of Most of Our Hospitals for the Reception of the Sick and Wounded," *Transactions of the Manchester Statistical Society* (1855-56):133-48.

that there was any need to limit the size of the hospital or number of patients, so long as the pavilion principle was observed. The windows should be tall, reaching nearly to the ceiling, and the flow of air imperceptible. Nightingale would repeat all those points for years, as well as the opinion that "artificial ventilation" was "injurious" (146). In his second paper, published in 1858, two years after the end of the Crimean War, Roberton quoted with approval Nightingale's evidence to the royal commission on the war. He was pleased that she cited his paper in her first "Notes on Hospitals" paper.[13]

The Pavilion Principle

Nightingale probably never read the great French source on pavilion hospitals, Tenon's 1788 *Memoirs on Paris Hospitals.* She certainly never referred to it by name, but became familiar with its ideas through later writers, and of course through the actual French and Belgian hospitals constructed in the early nineteenth century based on Tenon's work. Interestingly, while British reformers cited French hospitals for their advances, Tenon himself credited British hospitals with some of his inspiration. He praised British naval hospitals for the use of the pavilion style, and St Bartholomew's Hospital for at least its partial use.

In due course, reform-minded British doctors and architects would make pilgrimages to France and Belgium to see the first, purpose-built pavilion hospitals. Yet, while British reformers continued to credit the French with superior hospital design, they found decided French faults and British superiority on ventilation. Nightingale, in 1861, went so far as to state:

> You may poison a patient through his wound just as well as you may poison him by foul air. And this the French are constantly doing. And all the fresh air in the world will not save him from being poisoned thus—in the finest pavilion palace in the world. [See p 535 below.]

The pavilion principle facilitated cross-ventilation, with windows facing each other across a relatively narrow ward. Nightingale clearly felt that to interrupt this natural flow of fresh air by artificial ventilation meant wasted opportunity for the best ventilation possible.

---

13 John Roberton, "Additional Suggestions, with a View to the Improvement of Hospitals for the Sick and Wounded," *Transactions of the Manchester Statistical Society* (Manchester: John Harrison 1858, session 1857-58):38.

The proper (or improper) maintenance of adequate air, measured in cubic feet per person or bed, is a recurring issue in this volume. Early concerns focus on establishing a basic minimum, with negative examples given of hospitals with less. Army hospitals typically had only 500-700 cu. ft. (when navy hospitals had 1200-1500 cu. ft.). Having a high ceiling to achieve greater cubic feet did not work, however, for the air close to the ceiling was effectively wasted. Nightingale indeed often stressed that superficial area was of even greater importance than cubic feet, for ease of nursing care and for hygiene itself.

Nightingale's early statements on minimum cubic space give 1500 cu. ft., with 2000 cu. ft. necessary for hospitals in crowded urban centres. In 1861 she stipulated 1500 cu. ft. for a provincial hospital in an "open situation," and 2000 cu. ft. in London. But, as she put it, if the situation was such as to need 2000 cu. ft., the hospital "had better not be there at all" (see p 603 below). She repeated this point the following year (see p 631 below). In 1861, 2000 cu. ft. was a "useless expense" for a provincial hospital, for which 1500 would be adequate. By the time of the building of the Liverpool Royal Infirmary in the 1880s, however, Nightingale was calling for a minimum 2000 cu. ft. for all regular hospitals (see p 877 below).

Pavilions should run north-south, Nightingale maintained, to ensure that the sun shone in from both east and west, so that there would be sun "on both sides during the day" (see p 701 below). This arrangement was not possible if the pavilions were arranged in a square. For the same reason, there had to be adequate space between the pavilions. In Edinburgh, when a new Royal Infirmary was opened in 1879, the pavilions were too close to each other and Nightingale lamented the loss of light.

Adequate light appears frequently as a concern in the pavilion model. There are comments in Nightingale's writings for windows to be placed so as to ensure ventilation, but also for patient comfort, most notably to permit reading. Patients over the acute stage of a disease needed variety of scene. Adequate lighting at night was important, also, to prevent mistakes. Sinks had to be lighted to make sure that vessels were not emptied into the wrong one, such as bedpans into the sinks for teacups and plates. In *Notes on Nursing* Nightingale devoted a full chapter to light, right after the chapter on ventilation; her priorities for nursing echoing her views on hospital design. Adequate ventilation got more lines of writing from her, as a more obvious life-and-death factor, but the necessity of sunlight appears frequently.

In 1862, before the Herbert Hospital was completed, the model British pavilion hospital was the military hospital at the Cavalry Barrack, York, which Nightingale described as "the best hospital in Europe at present existing" (see p 631 below). When the workhouse Highgate Infirmary was opened in 1870, it became the cheapest example of a pavilion hospital, and one with "admirable" sanitary results (see p 747 below). The French Lariboisière, so much praised in her earlier work, was left behind.

In defence of the pavilion model, Nightingale pointed out that the sick at the Herbert Hospital remained in hospital one third the time they had at the old, badly ventilated corridor-style hospital which it replaced (see p 699 below). Moreover, this reduction occurred on top of the improvements in health produced by new sanitary measures brought in by the royal commission on the Crimean War. There were 579 constantly sick at the old Woolwich Hospital, Nightingale noted, compared with about 200 at the Herbert Hospital, where they stayed one third the time.

Nightingale felt that pavilion hospitals were often unjustly criticized for their cost. The first English pavilion infirmary planned, at Blackburn in 1858 (but not built until later), was "of a monstrous and useless cost," thanks to its having eight eight-bed wards or pavilions. However, the fault here lay not in the pavilion model, but in the choice of small wards. Since a nurse could supervise twenty-eight or even forty patients, and a nurse was needed for each ward, possibly a night nurse, too, smaller wards meant significantly higher ongoing staff costs.

Nightingale's influence on the acceptance and spread of the pavilion style has been well recognized in the later scholarly literature as well as by experts of her day. According to Cor Wagenaar, in a paper largely on European hospital design, "The tremendous success of the pavilion type was further enhanced by the work of Florence Nightingale."[14] This was "The first revolution: a victory of science, philosphy and technology." The paper then describes the building of the first non-French pavilion hospital, in Berlin, and its influence in later building in Germany and Austria.

Determining the best size for a ward, whether in a pavilion or block hospital, is a constant issue in this volume. Nightingale frequently

14 Cor Wagenaar, "Five Revolutions: A Short History of Hospital Architecture," in Cor Wagenaar, ed., *The Architecture of Hospitals* 26.

specified from twenty-eight to forty beds, maintaining that a good trained nurse could observe forty beds as easily as thirty. For "sanitary well-being," however, twenty-four, twenty-eight or thirty-two beds, "not more," were "the best number" (see p 631 below). The necessity for wards (as opposed to single rooms) lay in the need of the nurse to be able to see all her patients at once, a serious consideration when there were no electric bells or telephones, let alone equipment for electronic monitoring.

With wards being a necessity for adequate patient care, privacy had to be sacrificed accordingly. Presumably it was less of an issue then for most people, and certainly so for ordinary soldiers and working-class people at the time, who would have been accustomed to crowded conditions. In any event, as Nightingale observed, "Privacy does not extend beyond the bed on each side the patient." If someone had one bed on each side, "there might as well as be ten" (see p 583 below). The grouping of such numbers of patients—in turn—required careful attention to the adequacy of ward ventilation, yet another reason for preferring the pavilion model.

The mortuary, or "deadhouse," had to be well segregated from wards and living space, and autopsies were not to be performed, ever, in an operating theatre. Nightingale further noted that it was dangerous to build a hospital too near to a graveyard. In all these points she revealed an understanding of disease as caused by or spread by some substance to be found in the remains of the dead, in reality bacteria, although she did not know that then and would likely have used the term "miasma." She also protested the location of the mortuary at one hospital, even though it was to be in a separate building, for its closeness to the kitchen and washhouse, as it would have a bad effect on all "the imaginations and the gossip" of patients and others who would have to pass it routinely (see p 554 below). In the case of the new children's hospital in Lisbon, Nightingale argued for a separate entrance to the "deadhouse" to the dissecting room for relatives of deceased children (see p 530 below).

The management of laundry was important, for inadequate separation resulted in hospital diseases. Chutes for dirty linen had to work efficiently and be conveniently located, or dirty linen would be haphazardly stored and not promptly sent out for washing. Nightingale discovered that the "foul linen" chutes at St Thomas' did not work properly, so that dirty linen was removed only four times a week. She asked Douglas Galton how the chutes worked at the model Herbert

Hospital (see p 467 below). Dirty linen should not be "treasured up in any ward, scullery or closet" in the hospital, she wryly commented: the sooner it was sent away and washed the better. Chutes in a large hospital should be built into the wall, of glazed, impervious, earthenware. The laundry should be in a separate building, better off the site of the hospital itself. If on-site, it should be at the furthest distance possible from the wards.

Finding an adequate site for a hospital was a major requirement, for a poor site could cause unnecessary deaths, no matter how advanced the construction and how excellent the medical and nursing care. The hospital at Netley was seriously defective, Nightingale (and others) thought, simply because of its location next to an unsewered town and tidal estuary. Its size, length of corridors and lack of ventilation were at least remediable, if with massive rethinking. However, its situation on a muddy estuary that had sewage flowing into it from a town then of some 30,000 made it liable to disease, or so Nightingale thought. She wanted hospitals to be built on high ground, with cleansing winds.

For London and other large cities, the dilemma of choosing an appropriate site was obvious. Such populations called for a large, general hospital, but cities were notorious for their polluted air. Nightingale's proposed solution was to keep only accident and emergency patients in the downtown core, and to build the main hospital out in the suburbs in a healthier environment.[15] When she did not succeed in getting general hospitals to do so, she retreated to arguing for the establishment of a convalescent branch outside the city.

Hospital site selection would be a matter of major consideration in the correspondence on the Winchester Infirmary (its existing hospital had an unconscionably high death rate) and St Thomas' Hospital in London, where Nightingale (unsuccessfully) opposed the site on the Thames River.

Nightingale became an advocate for temporary buildings, especially of iron, for reasons similar to those for her preference for the pavilion type of building. During the Crimean War, she had become convinced of the safer conditions afforded by the temporary civil hospital at Renkioi, built by the great engineer I.K. Brunel, which avoided the great death rates of the hospitals based in old barracks

---

15 Many doctors took this position also. See "M Lévy on Hospitals," *Medical Times and Gazette* 19 April 1862:407-09.

and hospitals. She was proud that the death rate among men housed in huts in the last six months of the Crimean War was less than that of men living in English barracks during peacetime (see p 56 below). She remained convinced throughout her life of the utility of such temporary buildings, although the idea was in fact not taken up either by civil or military authorities. In 1862 Nightingale tried, unsuccessfully, to persuade St Thomas' Hospital authorities to move the hospital into huts as temporary quarters while the new hospital was being built (see p 776 below).

One of Nightingale's undated notes mused about saving lives by making hospitals "iron villages" of cottages, with one or two patients in each room, the cottages taken down and rebuilt every few years (see p 833 below). In 1888 Nightingale was still saying that huts were more healthy than a two- or three-storey building (see p 892 below). She imagined hospitals, "instead of being crowded palaces with layers of sick, as being iron villages of cottages, with one or at most two patients" each, the structures taken down every few years (see p 833 below).

Nurses' Working and Living Conditions

The low status of nurses when Nightingale began her work on hospital reform raised many problems. In the large homes of the wealthy, maids' rooms were typically relegated to attics and basements. It would be a lifelong struggle of Nightingale to get nurses out of the category of domestic servant, and literally out of basements and attics. Nurses were junior to doctors in rank and salary, as they were in education and responsibility. Nonetheless, Nightingale saw nurses as professional people deserving of respect and autonomy, a status which should be reflected in the accommodation accorded them.

Nightingale made many pleas to hospital officials: "do not pinch up the head nurses' rooms," reminding them that their "room is their only home," and so ought to have "space and comfort" (see p 664 below). For the team sent to Montreal in 1876, she specified that every nurse should have a separate room and a large window to herself. By the 1880s, she was stipulating that sleeping rooms for nurses had to have fireplaces. For the nurses in Syndey, Australia, she had to argue against putting their rooms in the basement, even in "the beautiful climate of Sydney" (see p 740 below). They could put "stores, dining rooms, boardrooms" in a basement, "but nothing else" (see p 740 below).

Nurses needed privacy, comfort, warmth and light; they should have private washing facilities, and adequate (shared) baths and toilets nearby. Bathing facilities should be sufficient for nurses to be able to take a bath once every twenty-four hours (see p 905 below). The point of assuring a sufficient number of separate toilets and baths for nurses would be made time after time to hospital building committees, which obviously had not provided adequate facilities. In 1889, for example, Nightingale was still insisting that partitions for nurses' rooms go up to the ceiling for a hospital in Montreal, and that each room had to have its own washbasin (see p 905 below). Nurses should not have to use patients' toilets, especially those of smallpox and fever patients (see p 815 below), concerns which evidently were for both health and privacy.

It is not surprising, then, that the fight for decent working conditions for nurses is a major theme of this volume, showing up both in Nightingale's letters and publications. Good-quality nursing was jeopardized by bad physical conditions, both in the hospital itself and the nurses' living quarters. The first trained nurses at the Edinburgh Royal Infirmary were housed in the old fever house. Nurses at the Sydney Infirmary, Australia, and at the Montreal General Hospital were also badly housed; illness resulted and one of the first six nurses sent to Montreal died.

Similar points regarding the establishment of comfortable space for matrons also appear. Nightingale insisted on adequate, private space for the matron, in addition to office space. A matron needed her own separate bedroom and sitting room, both of which had to be physically separate from her office, which should be in a highly accessible place.

Nightingale advised that nurses also had to have a convenient, airy, comfortable scullery, later known as a duty room, by their wards. Such a room had to be large enough to serve as a day room, where nurses could make tea, take a break and have their meals brought in when necessary. A size of 12 ft. × 12 ft. is specified for one hospital (see p 331 below). Nurses had to be able to take a brief break at a time of their own choosing, Nightingale believed, and they could be trusted to choose when that would not jeopardize patient care. It seems that one hospital at least deliberately chose not to provide a place for nurses to sit down to ensure that they stayed on the job. A miffed Nightingale pointed out that the nurses were conscientious and often stayed longer in their wards than their stated hours required (see p 897 below).

Hospitals also had to provide adequate cleaning staff. Nurses were to be responsible for ensuring ward cleanliness, but they were not to do the cleaning themselves. As Nightingale said in *Notes on Hospitals*, "A nurse must not be a scrubber. And a scrubber cannot be a nurse" (see p 123 below).

Hospitals were known to be dangerous places for women. Nightingale never used the terms "rape" or "sexual assault," but it is quite clear that she was thinking of such risks. Wherever possible, she wanted men's and women's ward to be placed on different floors. When this was not possible, she advised that the women's ward be cut off by a swing door, with a lock and key, always to be kept locked at night (see p 653 below). Other recommendations include night nurses not going back and forth between men's and women's wards. Separate night nurses should be provided for those wards. Quarters for female and male staff should be separate and distinct. "Holes and corners" were inherently dangerous places, to be avoided in hospital construction. This point seems to have been missed by many secondary authors, who have interpreted this concern as unwarranted monitoring of nurses' personal lives.[16]

Care in design for safety appears often in Nightingale's work. Fire hydrants and fire escapes are specified and staircases had to be of stone, or underlaid by stone, as a safety measure against fire. The need to provide constant oversight for potentially suicidal patients is explained. Storage arrangements had to be safe, minimize opportunities for pilfering by staff and patients, and prevent (as much as possible) the entry of contraband liquor and forbidden foods for patients into the hospital.

Requests for the best labour-saving devices appear frequently. Nightingale wanted hot and cold water to be provided everywhere, so that it did not have to be carried. Lifts (elevators) are frequently called for and devices for lifting patients are noted. When dealing with hospitals in hot climates, she recommended hollow walls and double ceilings to promote air circulation and cooling. Measures for energy efficiency appear, namely, a proposal to re-use steam generated for washing and heating to power mangles and wringers (see p 243 below).

By the time Nightingale started work on hospital reform, she had been appointed life governor to two leading London hospitals: to the

16 Catherine Judd, *Bedside Seductions: Nursing and the Victorian Imagination, 1830-1880* 39.

London (later the Royal London) Hospital, Whitechapel, in March 1856, and to St Mary's, Paddington, in the same year.[17] She used the connections she made in both cases to press for reforms in nursing and hospital statistics.

Nightingale visited the London Hospital on 1 December 1856, a few months after her return from the Crimean War. She was given a tour and she signed the visitors' book. After the visit she wrote a doctor there for information on the use of Parian cement, a fine non-porous cement and hence the best material for hospital walls. He in turn made inquiries and wrote back with details. The objections he found to it concerned its cost and colour, but he was generally positive about it and also suggested that Parian cement might have improved since the building of the London.[18]

Nightingale evidently had earlier considered the location of St Mary's, Paddington, to be good, for she asked in a letter in 1853, when a new building was needed for the Establishment for Gentlewomen during Illness, "Could we take a wing of the magnificent new hotel building opposite the Paddington Station?"[19] To Douglas Galton, probably, she referred to a steward at St Mary's, Paddington, "who has fitted up the ventilation of his sinks and water closets there with great success. When we get so far as fittings, I should take his advice" (see p 249 below).

Nightingale declined the honour of being named a life governor for other hospitals. For example, in 1867, she was elected an honorary governor of the Clinical Hospital and Dispensary for Children, Park Place, Cheetham Hill Rd. A draft reply by Dr Sutherland thanked the hospital for the honour, but explained that she was too much occupied to accept.[20]

The differences between regular civil hospitals and workhouse infirmaries appear at many times both in correspondence and in publications in this volume. As background, notes Nightingale wrote on the contrasts are given below.

---

17 Letter from Robert J. Newman, secretary, St Mary's Hospital, Paddington, 17 December 1856, Add Mss 45796 f113.

18 Nightingale's letter to W.J. Little is not extant; his reply is dated 11 December 1856, Add Mss 45796 ff108-09. "Parian" refers to the island of Paros, the source of the cement material.

19 Letter to Lady Canning [1853], Add Mss 45796 f33.

20 Letter 12 July 1867, with draft reply, Florence Nightingale Museum (LMA) H1/ST/NC2/V25/67.

Hospital

1. Acute medical and surgical cases
   Accidents
   Operations
   No infirm
   No incurables
   No consumption
   Few chronic cases
2. Admissions by night of accidents and even acute cases
3. Medical school
   Resident and house medical officers, sleeping in the hospital
   Operating theatres
   Training school for nurses

Infirmary (Parish)

1. Few *acute* cases of any kind
2. *No* accidents, except by chance
   Scarcely any operations, none of an instant nature
3. No medical school
   One (resident) medical superintendent and his assistant
   No house surgeons or physicians, no resident medical officers besides superintendent. No theatres.
4. No training school for nurses, except in the very largest infirmaries, and even there not at all the same proportion of probationers.

Consequences necessitating or producing in Hospital

1. Emergency or emergencies *by night* and even by day, for which extra nurses have to be put on. Sister has to sleep off her ward. Night nurse never to be left alone without *instant* help at hand. Day nurses *are* never alone. There is a crowd of M.O.s. Even thus, sudden delirium necessitates the provision by which instant further help may be summoned by night. By day, students in wards besides residents, dressers, clinical clerks, necessitating constant control of ward by head nurse. She must be constantly on the spot, except for recreation.

2. By night, house doctors are frequently summoned. Minor operations frequently performed by night, and even capital ones (such as tracheotomy in diphtheria) to save life. Sister summoned for accident and operations. Sisters and nurses have operating theatre work.

4. Training of probationers by head nurse in the ward.

Infirmary

1. Few or no emergencies. Head nurses may sleep and "meal" away from their wards. Nursing staff smaller in proportion. Night superintendent in her rounds enough to help and supervise night nurses. Rarely any but chronic delirium, easily provided for beforehand.

2. and 3. Rare for medical officer to be summoned at night, or head nurse. No students. . . .

4. None to train, except in a few infirmaries.[21]

21 Undated notes, ADD MSS 45820 ff170-71.

The contrasts between regular civil hospitals and army hospitals were similarly great, but for different reasons. The main cause lay in an army regulation requiring any soldier not fit for active duty to go to hospital, while a civilian with a minor illness would stay home and go to bed. Army hospitals, accordingly, mainly held light cases. What would be considered "severe" case in an army hospital would be a "light" case in a regular hospital, consequently, army hospitals simply did not have enough serious cases to be useful for training.[22]

Germ Theory, Contagion and Infection

Nightingale's views on germ theory, and the proliferation of misinformation on it, have already been described in earlier volumes of the *Collected Works*.[23] The issue comes up again in correspondence and publications on hospital design. Nightingale's much-noted preference for miasma theory over germ theory was not at all exceptional for the time, 1858, when she was writing, and did not in any way result in bad practice. Her insistence on diligence in cleanliness and ventilation served to eradicate the causes of disease whatever called.

In the 1850s, it was not known that germs were distinct, living organisms, and many doctors as well as Nightingale referred to "poisonous" substances as causes for disease. She, like doctors of the time, considered that something in the miasms caused disease. She referred to "enteric fever poison" as the disease-causing agent, when in fact the cause was not a chemical, but a bacillus that had not yet been discovered. Her references to "organic matter," made as early as 1858, can be seen as a nod in the right direction, for the word "organic" implied something living.

Nightingale's objections to "contagion theory" seem to have been partially founded on a strictly etymological approach, the term being based on the word for touch. It followed, she thought, that adherence to germ theory would jeopardize patient care, and even to patients being feared and abandoned by their caregivers, as happened to victims of leprosy and plague. It logically followed, she said in 1867, that the "germ hypothesis must stop all human contact," on pain of risk of

---

22 Note, Add Mss 45825 f74.

23 See *Health in India* (9:862-65) and *Nightingale School* (12:13-21). For general background, see Michael Worboys, *Spreading Germs: Disease Theories and Medical Practice in Britain, 1865-1900.*

disease or death (see p 696 below). She strenuously opposed the quarantine of ships, a measure that impeded trade without, she thought, achieving any good end.

Nightingale was careful to contrast "contagion" with the notion of "infection," which was a fact, not a hypothesis. In 1858, there was "no such thing" as contagion, and no such thing as "inevitable infection" (see p 53 below). Infection could be the product of emanations from sewage. Still, Nightingale felt, the fault for its existence lay in those in charge of the disease, not the disease itself, or any inevitable result of the conditions. So then could infection come from steam generated in the laundry, a point she made from the earliest version of "Notes on Hospitals" in 1858 to the last in 1863. There was "*no* inevitable infection in infectious laundry, unless small, dark, wet, unventilated and overcrowded—and full of steam loaded with organic (see p 69 below) matter" (see p 924 below). Fundamentally, Nightingale opposed the "doctrine" of contagion out of concern for its being used as "an adequate excuse for non-exertion to prevent" the recurrence of disease (see p 51 below). At that early date, 1858, she acknowledged only smallpox and cowpox as diseases with specific causes, otherwise preferring the generalized "miasma" theory.

In 1861, Nightingale told William Farr:

> I never saw a fact adduced in favour of contagion which would bear scientific inquiry. And I could name to you men whom *you* would acknowledge as scientific who place "contagion" on the same footing as witchcraft and other superstitions.[24]

She repeated the "witchcraft" term again in 1867, when she wrote some "remarks" supporting a pamphlet on infection (see p 696 below). Here she reiterated her position that the germ hypothesis was "at variance" with the results of sanitary experience, resulting from the application of public health laws. With the benefit of hindsight one might say that the public health laws removing filth were effective because they removed or killed germs. Nightingale would use the "witchcraft" association again in 1873, calling contagionists the "witch finders of the nineteenth century."[25]

---

24 In *Health in India* (9:867); on Farr, see the biographical sketch in *Society and Politics* (5:831-32).

25 *Social Change in India* (10:132).

It is quite clear that, whatever she said against "contagion," Nightingale believed in the transmission of disease by fingers as well as by air, blood, excreta, other body fluids and hard surfaces. She discussed precautions to prevent the spread of disease right from the start of her hospital writing, and became only more stringent over time. An instance is evident as early as 1853 when, as superintendent at the Harley St. institution, she ordered "gutta percha rings," rubber-based devices used before the invention of protective gloves. The letter discussing this order was written to Lady Canning (1817-61), who was, in effect, Nightingale's superior as head of the ladies' committee, and who continued to work with Nightingale on nursing matters during the Crimean War.

> Not having heard anything of your gutta percha rings, I went out *foraging*, and finding their companions at the gutta percha place in Bond St., I took the liberty of inquiring whether any such had been sent to your house in Grosvenor Sq., and finding that 6 dozen had been sent there, and the man of the gutta percha establishment showing me your order in his file, I ventured to desire them to be brought here. I hope I have not taken an impertinent step.
>
> We shall require much more than 5 doz., probably in all 12 doz. I suppose that I had better order the remaining 6 doz. at the same place and the same price? May I?[26]

In a note giving hypothetical rules for a small hospital, also from 1853, Nightingale stated: "No cases refused, not even the infectious and syphilitic—these treated in a ward and by a sister to themselves."[27] When her school opened at St Thomas', she purchased "finger stalls" and "thumb stalls" for nurses and probationers, another early protective device.

In all three editions of *Notes on Hospitals*, from 1858 to 1863, Nightingale opposed the use of separate wards for infectious cases, insisting that, with adequate ventilation and other measures, no such isolation was needed. As a precaution, however, she proposed leaving a bed vacant beside a fever patient. As early as 1858, however, Nightingale argued for separate space for casualty and convalescent cases from ordinary sick (see p 306 below). In 1859, she advised that the post-mortem room and deadhouse should be located out of the hospi-

26 Letter 7 September [1853], Leeds District Archives, Canning 177/2/5.
27 Draft rules, in *Nightingale School* (12:67).

tal building, and that no post-mortems should ever done in an operating theatre (see p 642 below). Clearly the transmission of disease from corpses to living persons is implied. By 1860, she was clear that erysipelas and hospital gangrene cases required segregation (see p 526 below).

The excess in Nightingale's statements against contagion and inevitable infection, when read carefully, is effectively a rejection of the notion of the "inevitability" of infection. In 1858, she asserted explicitly that illnesses acquired in hospital were not inevitable, but the result of "gross carelessness and ignorance," and that as soon as the practical view of the subject was acted upon, "we shall cease to hear of hospital contagions" (see p 54 below). She told James Paget, also in 1861, that she was "very sorry" if she "had said anywhere that ventilation was more than cleanliness or that either would stand up in lieu of efficient drainage" (see p 536 below). This seems to be something of an admission that her earlier argument that infectious patients need not be placed in separate wards was wrong. Here she is clear that not even the best ventilation could ensure the safety of the other patients.

By 1861 Nightingale was urging the careful separation of out-patients' departments from in-patients in hospitals of all kinds. This was not only to prevent the entry of illicit alcohol and other contraband, as all functions, especially toilets and baths, were to be kept separate. By 1862 she stipulated strict separation of wards and administrative offices so that there would be "no community of ventilation," even by a window over a door. Also in 1862, Nightingale told Sir Harry Verney that venereal disease was "*generated* by vice [prostitution], not only *communicated* by infection."[28] This is not a bad description for the time, given that the bacillus that causes syphilis was not identified until 1903. In 1870, her remark that the "Nusterabad nuisance directly produced cholera"[29] is not off the mark, for "nuisance" meant excreta, and cholera bacilli thrive in the bowel.

In 1863 Nightingale said that mixing up patients of any kind with administrative staff exposed sick and well to risk of disease. She advised careful separation of wards from administrative services, especially the laundry. Again, this seems to indicate she was moving, or had moved, away from her initial position against isolating infectious patients. She was unequivocal in 1865 that erysipelas, gangrene and such-like cases

---

28 In *Women* (8:427).
29 In *Health in India* (9:644).

should not be placed in a general ward in a hospital. They should be "placed under complete segregation or removed when, unfortunately, they arise within the hospital to complete segregation in a separate set of wards under a separate head nurse and nurses." The reason for such separation was that "good-natured patients will lend their things, whatever you do to prevent it," so that "no ventilation or construction" could make such cases non-infectious.[30]

Correspondence abounds in this volume on the need to keep infectious wards, their bed linen and food vessels separate from those for non-infectious patients. The staffs should be separate, and if a doctor or nurse had to go between the two, they had to allow time to change clothing and wash. Nightingale clearly changed her mind on the need to isolate infectious patients. Why and how appears in more detail in the reviews of and reaction to the publication of her 1863 *Notes on Hospitals* (see p 226 below).

In 1866, Nightingale pointed out that the "unwashed hands of a stupid doctor or nurse may certainly convey disease to and fro'," such as between lying-in and fever wards (see p 448 below). Hands obviously imply contact, but not inevitable infection—disinfectant washing and the use of protective gloves could prevent the disease from spreading. By 1869 she considered it necessary to move typhus and smallpox cases out of the hospital at once (see p 456 below). In 1882, she said that an isolated room was needed for a sick nurse. By 1891 infectious children in a ward were said to require a separate kitchen and nurses' scullery. Infirmary laundry was not to be washed within the hospital's boundaries.

Nightingale and Sutherland followed the ongoing scientific debates on etiology. For example, Dr Sutherland told her (ca. 1869-70) that he had obtained a copy of botanist Ernst Hallier's instructions for India, but that Hallier's fungus theory of cholera causation had been shown to be "untrue." The fungi Hallier saw were developed in excreta as well as in other media, the suggestion being that they were contemporaneous with the disease, not the cause of it. Nightingale queried Sutherland: "Does that disprove in itself the theory?"[31]

---

30 Letter, in *Women* (8:170).

31 Undated notes [c1870], Add Mss 45754 f77.

In 1877, the "home sister at St Thomas'," Mary Crossland (1837-1914), had occasion to complain to Nightingale about the "disorganized" teaching of an instructor at the Nightingale School, Dr J.S. Bristowe, but Crossland shortly credited him with a "clear lecture" on contagion. While Nightingale had objected to use of the term for its narrow association with transmission of disease by touch, he broadened it to cover moral, physical, parasitical, vegetable, animal, internal and external contagion; the different states of contagion and different ways of imparting it; the mode of its diffusion; how poison multiples in the system and is gotten out of it; the behaviour of contagia external to the body and its nature—whether gas, fluid, organic or inorganic, with "organic" meaning a living entity. Bristowe proved that it was "organic," Crossland stated.[32] Whether or not Nightingale approved of this lecture, we do not know. She did not interfere. The Nightingale School taught a rudimentary understanding of germ theory to probationers as early as 1873.[33]

In 1879, Nightingale described hospital diseases as a consequence of dirty linen (bandages) being left in the hospital too long. When she referred to "enteric fever poison" as a proxy for germs, in 1882, she evidently was still adhering to miasma theory, but was leaning to greater specificity in the causal agent (see p 836 below). In another example of this time, she related typhoid to sub-soil, and referred to a general "fever epidemic" passing into "enteric fever." These statements predate Robert Koch's definitive publication in 1884 on the bacillus that causes cholera, the discovery that prompted Nightingale to accept germ theory. By 1888 Nightingale would stress the need for outpatients' departments to be in physically separate buildings.

In 1889, Nightingale recommended that nurses in infectious wards not go back and forth to the nurses' home, but have sleeping and eating spaces in the infection ward building. In 1891, in reviewing laundry plans for the Derbyshire Royal Infirmary, she called for a distinct laundry for soiled bandages, etc., for infectious patients. Nightingale nonetheless reiterated that there was "*no* inevitable infection in infectious laundry, unless full of steam loaded with organic matter," using "organic matter" to refer to what we would call germs: words she had first used in "Notes on Hospitals." A note in 1893 said, "the thing is

32 Crossland letter 9 November 1877, Add Mss 47738 f73.

33 John Croft, *Notes of Lectures at St Thomas' Hospital*, related in *Nightingale School* (12:16).

to remove the cause": Infection from one patient to another was "not the sole danger, while cause remains."[34] In 1895, she considered a separate "block" for fever patients to be desirable, as St Thomas' had done, and not just have separate wards (see p 938 below).

There is much in her work on the appropriate materials for hospital walls, floors, toilets, basins, baths, storage compartments, garbage and laundry chutes. Nightingale opposed the use of curtains around beds in wards for impeding ventilation, suggesting instead that "low, movable screens" should be used for privacy (see p 579 below). Mattresses made from horsehair were the best because they did not retain miasma. Many technical details in the text appear, such as comparing the exact amount of moisture a brick can hold (12½ oz.), with a piece of cement of the same size (¼ oz.) or 1/25th as much. There are details on keeping water separate for different kinds of washing and the amount of water needed per patient.

Despite the substantial amount of writing Nightingale did on infection control and the unequivocal evidence of her acceptance of germ theory, there is much secondary literature claiming the contrary.[35] F.B. Smith, as well as misrepresenting her views on germ theory generally, made the bizarre claim that she worked "behind the scenes . . . to stop the introduction of carbolic acid antiseptic procedures into hospitals, on the grounds that they made doctors careless and scrubbers lazy."[36] Smith gave no evidence of any such advice—and none has appeared—and ignores her many and detailed admonitions and advice on the use of carbolic acid, including what strength to use for what purposes.[37]

The great attention to detail about fittings at the Herbert Hospital made it exemplary. In 1866, Nightingale wanted the St Thomas' matron and resident medical officer to go over it for examples to be used in the new St Thomas' (see p 790 below).

---

34 Note 15 June 1893, Add Mss 47766 f134.

35 For a refutation of many of F.B. Smith's and others' accusations, see Lynn McDonald, "Florence Nightingale Revealed in Her Own Writings," *Times Literary Supplement* 6 December 2000:14-15; "Appendix B: The Rise and Fall of Florence Nightingale's Reputation," in *Life and Family* (1:843-47), and "Appendix B: Secondary Sources on Nightingale and Women," in *Women* (8:1039-53); and "The Revisionist Literature on Nightingale," in *Extending Nursing* (12:31-36).

36 F.B. Smith, *Florence Nightingale: Reputation and Power* 164.

37 See in particular her advice in her nursing article in Richard Quain, *Dictionary of Medicine*, in *Nightingale School* (12:742-45).

Specialized Hospitals

Specialized hospitals in Britain date from roughly the mid-nineteenth century. The first children's hospital in Britain was built in Liverpool, opening in 1851. The famous Great Ormond St. Hospital for Sick Children opened in 1852, and the first convalescent hospital, at Cranleigh, Surrey dates from 1855.

Nightingale stressed the special needs of children as hospital patients in many places. Children were even more vulnerable to hospital-acquired infections than adults, Nightingale believed; consequently, even more care had to be taken to keep them out of hospital altogether. There are numerous admonitions that children should not be kept a day longer than "absolutely essential" for treatment purposes (see p 170 below). In a note which she did not publish she went even further: "one *must* say . . . keep no child an *hour* longer in hospital than is positively needful."[38] However, in the final edition of *Notes on Hospitals,* Nightingale kept the admonition that "in a child's hospital much more than in others, the patient must not stay a day longer than is absolutely necessary" (see p 528 below).

More attendance was required for children than adults, for children could not be left alone at all. Almost a nurse for each child was necessary, Nightingale suggested. In *Notes on Hospitals,* she gave detailed attention to the necessary administrative structure in a children's hospital, keeping the control in the hands of women and strictly limiting male access.

She gave considerable attention to the safety of children in hospital, to prevent burns, scalding and injuries while they were at play. She mentioned neither sexual assault nor molestation, but that she took care to ensure that male employees and visitors would not have unsupervised access to children suggests that precautions were needed. Nightingale was always a believer in prevention first: it was best that hospitals be constructed without "holes and corners," with adequate locks and keys and suitable rules to ensure the oversight of vulnerable patients and staff.

Nightingale remained wary about children's hospitals, concerned that they had become fashionable but were not better or safer than regular hospitals for treating children. She would have preferred greater attention to be paid to and money spent on removing the

38 Undated note, in *Public Health Care* (6:9).

causes that made children ill in the first place. Prevention and health promotion were always better strategies than cure after the fact.

Nightingale had never worked in a children's ward or a children's hospital, and so had to rely on observations provided for her by ward sisters and matrons who had. She actively sought information and observations on the alternatives from such colleagues. In 1863 Nightingale advised against having children's wards in general hospitals—children should either go to a children's hospital or be mixed up with adults in a general hospital. In 1891, she said that "the only rationale for children's wards" was the care of infants under six months of age (see p 924 below).

When hospitals did establish children's wards, Nightingale said that they should be in a highly frequented area, for the protection of the children. Children depended on adults being aware of anything untoward occurring, for they could not complain themselves, and those children who did complain, Nightingale pointed out, risked reprisals from nurses.

For all her reservations, however, Nightingale did accept when asked to advise on plans for a children's hospital, and would give her carefully considered advice. The first hospital for which she gave detailed advice at all, in 1859, in fact, was for a children's hospital in Lisbon. In 1875, at the request of a prominent Russian pediatrician, she wrote a critique of the Moscow Children's Hospital, then in planning.

Nightingale approved—indeed, strongly advocated—convalescent hospitals in the country and seaside, which would often be small cottage hospitals. In 1863, she wrote that London had too much hospital accommodation, but not enough convalescent. Convalescent hospitals, she felt, should be built by the sea where possible, and should be "in nearly every respect almost the very reverse" of requirements of an acute care hospital (see p 926 below).

Cottage hospitals themselves were not necessarily a good thing, Nightingale thought, as they were not intrinsically safer, and might take patients away from better general hospitals in towns. She was not dogmatic on this point but held, as for a general hospital, that the case would have to be made that any proposed cottage hospital should exist at all. All the same, where the same medical treatment, nursing and medical comforts could be supplied to the sick poor at home, Nightingale argued, "these recover better than in hospitals." She hoped that hospitals would be gradually replaced by "a system of district nursing" (see p 764 below).

Statistics for Safer Hospitals

The key role statistics could and should play in developing safer hospitals appears in many places in this volume. Since the aim of a hospital was to have the sick recover in the shortest time possible, statistics were needed to ascertain what those recovery times were. This faith in statistics is a concomitant of Nightingale's belief in God as the ruler of the universe, and the creator of laws of nature or scientific laws. With adequate statistics, she put forward, people could "administer the laws of health": with certainty even (see p 333 below). Workhouse and hospital statistics were an "unworked mine," she wrote; both types of institution had been "created for the relief of human distress," but "whether they relieve it or not" was not known (see p 643 below).

Army statistics should be thorough, but not try to deal with causation, "hardly a statistical matter," she told army statistician T. Graham Balfour (see p 388 below). Published statistics should not "intermingle causation," but should be "the driest of all reading" (see p 393 below). Nightingale worked hard with Balfour on improving army statistical reports, and congratulated him when improvements appeared. She considered British Army statistics to be the best in the world.

While the end was causal analysis, Nightingale's opinion was that the statistics themselves should be published as they were, without inferences. Great attention had to be paid to aggregation. Nightingale complained of statistics that were overly aggregated, so that trends of particular diseases could not be discerned. Cholera, notably, was so important that cases should be reported separately from dysentery and diarrhea, for its absence was worthy of note (see p 398 below). However, she also complained of inadequate aggregation in army statistics, for example, suggesting, for example, that more totals by disease should be made available.

Nightingale always wanted to get evidence that a proposed reform actually worked before pursuing it in other hospitals. Desirably, a new approach should be tried first in one place, before being generalized. For the Woolwich Female Hospital, for example, she cautioned, "it would be very desirable to put up one hospital first and let us see. Improvements always suggest themselves" (see p 414 below).

From a later, more gender-conscious time, the imbalance in space provided between men and women patients seems remarkable. In the case of the Liverpool Royal Infirmary in 1882, the specifications gave eighteen men's and fourteen women's beds per physician, and thirty-two men's and eighteen women's per surgeon. Imbalances are so common, in fact, that the equal number of beds for convalescent men and women at the Herbert Memorial Home seems exceptional. Nightingale never protested, nor apparently did anyone else. However, as Nightingale was always conscious of the risks to patients entering a hospital, it would not make sense for her to have demanded more beds for women.

Much correspondence on hospital reform is missing sometimes, one suspects, for its incriminating evidence. Nightingale often wrote her remarks directly on the plans, not one of which has survived, yet we often know something of their nature from remarks she passed on variously to Dr Sutherland, Douglas Galton or Henry Bonham Carter. In 1888, Nightingale reminded Galton that the plans of the hospitals of Lincoln, Aylesbury, Blackburn, Swansea and Oldham, and a great many others, "passed through your (and my prentice) hands" (see p 887 below). Of this list, there are detailed remarks only for Aylesbury.

That Nightingale's influence on actual hospital design was enormous can be seen in the naming of what became the standard pavilion ward—long, narrow, with windows on opposite sides—as the "Nightingale ward." From 1861 to the beginning of World War II it was "the dominant accommodation in Britain, indeed very nearly the only available design for a nursing unit."[39] That particular design was excellent in providing ease of supervision for the needs of the time. Technological advances later made other options possible, notably much more efficient means of artificial heating and ventilation and improved means for monitoring patients (electric bells, telephones and later monitoring devices). When antibiotics became available, roughly from the time of World War II, the practice of medicine itself changed and the "Nightingale ward" was no longer needed. Patients could be treated and cured, with a short hospital stay, and without the need for visual observation day and night. Consumer demand, and a greater desire for privacy, both had their impact on ward size and shape. A few observations on these later changes will be made in the Epilogue.

To give an overview of the full range of Nightingale's work, and to relate it to other developments in hospital reform, the following chronology is provided. It includes the names of hospitals on which correspondence shows she worked, but for which direct sources could

---

39 John D. Thompson and Grace Goldin, *The Hospital: A Social and Architectural History* 231.

not be found. For those for which there is a considerable amount of material separate introductions are given.

Chronology of Nightingale's Work on Hospital Reform

Left justified: significant events on hospitals.
Right justified: Nightingale's work on.

1853 Hôpital de Lariboisière, Paris, opens, first large pavilion hospital

1856 George Godwin publishes first articles on pavilion hospitals in *The Builder*; Dr John Roberton gives paper, "On the Defects, with Reference to the Plan of Construction and Ventilation, of Most of Our Hospitals for the Reception of the Sick and Wounded," to the Manchester Statistical Society

late 1856 FN begins work on Netley Hospital (opened in 1863)

1857 FN begins work with Douglas Galton on Herbert Hospital, Woolwich, first large pavilion hospital in England (opened 1865)

1858 Vincennes Military Hospital opens, pavilion style

1858 FN paper "Notes on Hospitals" read to the Liverpool meetings of the National Association for the Promotion of Social Science; publishes three papers on Netley in *The Builder*

1859 FN publishes 2nd ed. of *Notes on Hospitals* and "A Contribution to the Sanitary History of the British Army"

1859 (to 1861) FN works on Glasgow Royal Infirmary (her advice not taken)

1859 (to 1862) FN works on Buckinghamshire Infirmary, Aylesbury (architect David Brandon)

1859 (to 1860) FN works on Lisbon Children's Hospital (architect A.J. Humbert)

1859 (to 1866) FN works on St Thomas' Hospital (opened 1871) (architect Henry Currey)

1861 (to 1864) FN works on Winchester Infirmary (architect William Butterfield)

1861 FN works on Royal Hospital for Incurables

1861 FN works on convalescent hospital for Sellonites, near Ascot

1861 FN works on Royal Hospital Devonport (architect Alfred Norman)

1861 Joseph Adshead advocates for a convalescent hospital for Manchester (not built)

1861 (to 1862) FN works on Leeds Hospital (architect George Gilbert Scott)

1861 FN works on North Staffordshire Infirmary
1862 (to 1865) FN works on Malta hospitals (architect T.H. Wyatt)
1862 York Cavalry Hospital "the best hospital at present in Europe" (plans Douglas Galton)
1862 (to 1863) FN works on Fort Pitt Hospital
1862 FN works on Birkenhead Infirmary (architect Thomas Layland)
1863 FN publishes 3rd ed. of *Notes on Hospitals*
1863 FN works on female hospital plans (with Douglas Galton)
1864 (to 1865) FN works on Swansea Infirmary (architect Alex Graham)
1865 FN corresponds on Chorlton Union Workhouse, first workhouse pavilion hospital (architect Thomas Worthington)
1866 (to 1874) FN works on Sydney Infirmary
1867 FN works on Catherine Hayes Hospital, Sydney (children's hospital, architect John Horbury Hunt)
1867 FN works on Herbert Convalescent Home, model cottages (architect T.H. Wyatt)
1868 FN works on St Pancras Workhouse Infirmary, Highgate (architect John Giles)
1868 FN corresponds on Prestwich Union Workhouse Infirmary (architect Thomas Worthington)
1868 FN works on Städtisches Krankenhaus im Friedrichshain, Berlin (architects Martin Gropius and Heino Schmieden)
1869 FN works on Derby Infirmary (architect Isaac Henry Stevens)
1869 James Y. Simpson publishes *Hospitalism: Its Effects on the Results of Surgical Operations*
1871 FN works on Glamorganshire Convalescent Home
1872 (to 1874) FN works on Wellow School, near Embley, Hampshire
1874 (to 1876) FN works on Montreal General Hospital (architect Alex Graham, but not built)
1874 FN works on Vladimir Children's Hospital, Moscow (with Dr Rauchfuss)
1879 (to 1881) FN works on children's hospital, Heidelberg
1879 Opening of Children's Hospital, Pendlebury, a model children's hospital

1882 (to 1883) FN works on St Marylebone Workhouse Infirmary (supplementary) Nurses' Home (architect Henry Saxon Snell)
1882 FN works on Nurses' Home for Prince Alfred Hospital, Sydney
1882 (to 1885) FN works on Liverpool Royal Infirmary (architect Alfred Waterhouse)
1885 (to 1890) FN works on Gordon Boys' Home (architect William Butterfield)
1885 FN works on Haydock Cottage Hospital
1886 (to 1887) FN works on Carlsruhe Clinique and Training School (architect Professor Weinbrenner)
1888 (to 1889) FN works on Royal Victoria Hospital, Montreal (architect Henry Saxon Snell)
1888 FN works on Women's Hospital, Euston Rd. (architect John Brydon)
1891 (to 1894) FN works on Derbyshire Infirmary Nurses' Home (architect Keith D. Young)

Key to Editing

All the manuscript material in the *Collected Works* has been carefully transcribed and verified (see *Life and Family* Appendix E: Research Methods and Sources for a description of the process of obtaining and processing this information). Illegible words and passages are so indicated, with [illeg] or [?] inserted to indicate our best reading of the word or words in question. Dates for material cited or reproduced are given wherever possible, in square brackets if they are estimates only. The type of material, whether a note, actual letter, draft or copy is given as precisely as possible. Designations of letter/draft/copy signify that the source was Nightingale's own files, given to the British Library or to St Thomas' Hospital, and Library or to St Thomas' Hospital, and probably drafts or copies kept by her. The designation of "letter" is used only when there is good reason to believe that it was actually sent and received (a postmarked envelope, for example, or the archive being other than Nightingale's own files). The electronic I-text (that is, the transcriptions as "input," before editing) gives full information on supporting material (envelopes, postmarks), and whether the piece was in pen, pencil, dictated or typed.

The practice was to use the best source possible, the original letter where available. Where a draft or copy was also available this is noted. Sometimes the original was no longer available and a typed copy in an archive or a published letter had to be used.

All sources indicated as "Add Mss" (Additional Manuscripts) are British Library, the largest source of Nightingale material. The Wellcome Trust History of Medicine Library is abbreviated "Wellcome." Most of those materials are copies of correspondence at Claydon House, indicated as (Claydon copy). If not so indicated they are originals. The designation "from a letter" means that less than the complete letter was used, and the address and ellipses at the beginning and end are omitted. Postscripts that merely repeat points or move on to a completely different subject are omitted without ellipses. Standard letter closings have usually been omitted. For officials or persons making inquiries they are typically:

Believe me to be, Sir,
ever your faithful servant
Florence Nightingale

To Dr Sutherland, Nightingale was usually "yours faithfully," abbreviated "yrs ffly." To family and close friends the typical closing was "ever yours," often with initials. Ending salutations are kept when they are unusual. Postscripts and post-postscripts, usually separated by initials, are common. They are often omitted.

To avoid use of "ibid." and "op. cit.," and to reduce the number of footnotes generally, citations are given at the end of a sequence if the same source is cited more than once. Subsequent citations are noted in the text with the new page or folio number given in parentheses. References to material that appears in earlier volumes of the *Collected Works* are identified by our short title, volume number and page number rather than the archival source.

To make the text as accessible as possible, spelling, punctuation and capitalization have been modernized and standardized, and most abbreviations replaced with full words, e.g., Ms. becomes manuscript. Frequently used abbreviations are kept, such as W.O. for War Office, A.M.D. for Army Medical Department, and A.H.C. for Army Hospital Corps. British spellings have been maintained and standardized (labour, honour). The French spelling for hygiène here becomes hygiene. We have kept Nightingale's old-fashioned ""farther," "bye-word" and "unpractical," and expressions like "out of window," but change "shew" to show, ancle" to ankle, "organise" to organize, "inclose" to enclose, "expence" to expense, "idiosyncracy" to idiosyncrasy, "burthen" to burden and "sate" to sat. 6½ A.M. becomes 6:30 A.M. We change "story" to storey when it refers to a floor, and "preventable" to "preventible." We use modern spellings of words with "ae" and "oe," hence pyemia, septicemia, diarrhea, anesthetic and fetid. Laundry "shoots" become chutes. We change "aseptik" to aseptic. "Diets" are hospital meals, a "nuisance" generally excrement. A "dust" chute is for garbage. A "water closet" or "W.C." is a toilet or a toilet room, while a "lavatory" is strictly for washing, as a bath or "bathing room" is only for baths. An "outdoor" patient is an out-patient. A "separation" ward is an isolation ward. A "lock" ward or hospital is for the compulsory treatment of syphilitic patients, usually prostitutes. "Overlooking" hospital plans means looking over them, not ignoring them.

The nursing hierarchy in Nightingale's time was as follows:

matron or lady superintendent
assistant matron (in larger hospitals)
ward sister (or charge nurse)
head nurse (trained)
assistant nurse (untrained)
probationer (in training)
ward maid (cleaner)

The term "student" always refers to a medical student, never a nurse in training. The Horse Guards refer to the headquarters of the British Army. Blue Books are official government reports.

We have followed the trend to lesser use of capitals, even to kings, queens and bishops.

There is much confusion with hospital names, which themselves changed over time with mergers, and which were often referred to with abbreviations. Sometimes a hospital would be called by the name of the city in which it was located—the Aylesbury Infirmary—although the actual name was that of the county, Buckinghamshire County Infirmary, later the Royal Buckinghamshire Hospital. The "royal" designation normally was late in appearing, so that a hospital's current name might never appear in correspondence here.

Workhouse infirmaries in time disguised their "workhouse" origins and stigma. Printed stationery for the Holborn Union Infirmary, for example, merely says "The Infirmary."[1] The better workhouse infirmaries were later amalgamated with regular hospitals, and a new name given the new institution, for example, the Chorlton Workhouse Union became part of Withington Hospital and the St Marylebone Workhouse Infirmary was merged into St Charles Hospital.

Roman numerals are replaced with Arabic (except for royalty, popes and the citation of classical texts). We have left Nightingale's use of masculine generics as they are, hence "man," "men," "he," etc., referring to human beings generally. Nightingale's "Esq." titles for men have been omitted. Any words the editor has added to make sense (usually in the case of rough notes or faint writing) appear in square brackets. Translated passages are by the editor.

Italics are used to indicate underlining and small capitals for double (or more) underlining. All indications of emphasis in texts are

1 Add Mss 45810 f237.

Nightingale's (or that of her correspondent or source), *never* the editor's. Any use of (sic) also is Nightingale's, *never* the editor's. When taking excerpts from written material Nightingale indicated ellipses with x x and we have kept these. Ellipses for editorial purposes are indicated with ... for skipped material within a sentence .... if to the end of the sentence or more than a sentence has been dropped. Passages that break off abruptly, or in which folios are missing, are so indicated.

We refer to Nightingale, and indeed all adult women, by their surnames, the normal practice for references to men. We note with some dismay the frequent practice in the secondary literature of using first names, even nicknames, for women, reserving surnames, initials and honorifics for the (apparently) superior sex. The use of first names and nicknames for the period in question seems especially inappropriate, even unauthentic as well as sexist, for such names were then strictly limited to immediate family and close, old friends. Nightingale always used women's surnames in referring to nurses, usually with an honorific, "Miss," "Mrs," "Sister" or "Nurse." Women typically signed their letters with their surnames and initials without using first names, let alone nicknames, at all.

Correspondents' full names are given in the source headings, but normally they are referred to by the name Nightingale used: hence Mrs Wardroper, Dr Sutherland, or simply the last name.

Editorial notes appear in footnotes or, if very brief, in square brackets in the text. Articles (the, a, an) and the appropriate form of the verb to be have been supplied to make sense. Persons who changed their names (usually through marriage or the acquisition of a title, sometimes for purposes of inheritance) are referred to by the more commonly used name, cross-referenced in the index to any other used. Dates to identify people are given at the first appropriate moment; italicized entries in the index indicate entries with identifying information. Of course for many people, notably servants and acquaintances, identifying information is not available.

The bibliography provides full information on most books cited. Newspaper sources, government reports and periodical references are given in footnotes only. References to classical and other works available in many editions (now often on the Internet) are by book, chapter, canto, scene, line, etc., as appropriate, and are not repeated in the bibliography.

Notes on Hospitals

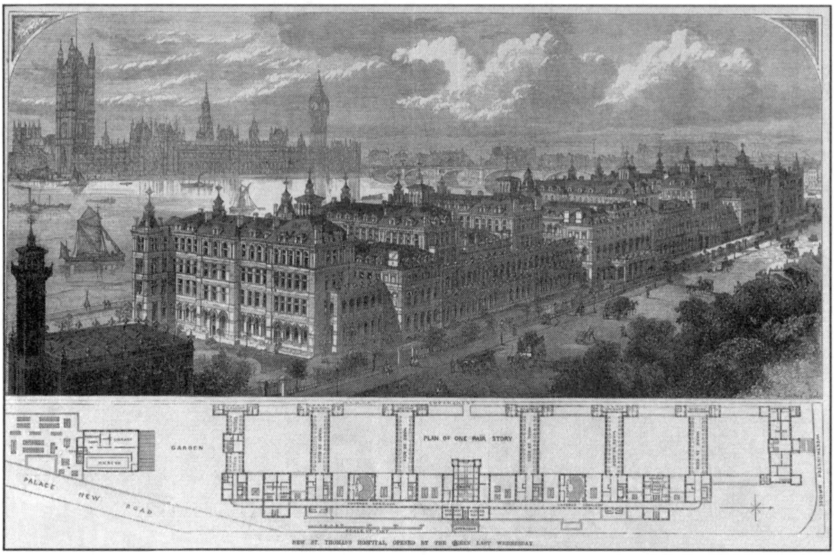

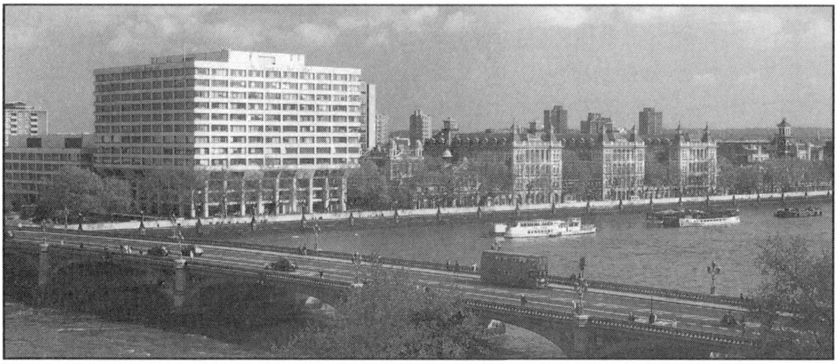

Top: St Thomas' Hospital as it was soon after its opening in 1871, the model (civil) pavilion hospital, designed by Henry Currey. Courtesy of Wellcome Trust Library.

Bottom: Recent photograph of St Thomas' Hospital, showing the new building at the left (post-World War II) and three old pavilions (renovated on the inside) to the right. Photograph courtesy of Gordon Museum, King's College, London.

Notes on Hospitals, 1st and 2nd Editions 1858 and 1859

Notes on Hospitals is Nightingale's first publication to focus on the problems of civil hospitals. Initially given as a paper at the meetings of the National Association for the Promotion of Social Science, in Liverpool in October 1858, it was duly published in the association's *Transactions.* Nightingale then had it printed separately in 1859, with appendixes on her evidence for the royal commission on the Crimean War, and her three articles in *The Builder.*

When she wrote *Notes on Hospitals* in 1858, Nightingale was still working on her massive *Notes on the Health of the British Army.* Civil hospitals get much attention in that report, as they do in her evidence to the royal commission, but the prime focus in them, naturally, was what went wrong in the war hospitals and what to do differently in the future. Here, her focus changes to regular civil hospitals, with Crimean War examples drawn in where a flagrant example served. The commonalities between the two types of institution are obvious as both were buildings whose mortality rates were affected by their design, location and administrative procedures.

In Part 1 of *Notes on Hospitals,* Nightingale set out the problem of high hospital mortality rates. She named four defects of hospital construction: the agglomeration of large numbers under one roof, and defects in cubic space, light and ventilation, although later she noted that she could not determine their relative influences. Part 1 ends with a succinct statement of the principles of the pavilion model.

In Part 2, she specified sixteen sanitary defects usual in ward construction, mainly elaborations of the four defects of Part 1. New sections appear on kitchens, laundry, site and sewers. Further details are given on the materials to be chosen. There is a strong plea for "natural ventilation," meaning open windows and fireplaces, as opposed to "artificial ventilation." That disease is not inevitable but preventible is a major theme in the paper. It was an "all-important question" to determine this for, if inevitable, one would have to consider whether hospitals should exist at all; if preventible, it was "our duty to prevent" the propagation and spread of such diseases (see p 51 below).

Nightingale's campaign against "contagion" as a cause, with inevitable infection its result, drew on her classical knowledge. She quoted from late ancient authors, from those after the time of the "fathers of history and of medicine." That contagion theory was favoured in the "southern and less educated parts of Europe" was a sign to her of decline. The "more intelligent" authors, like Thucydides (c460-399 BCE), from the golden age of classical thought were not "contagionists." Aretaeus, who lived centuries later, around 100 CE, appeared to be the "first medical author who believed in contagion.

The word "infection" was "admissible," Nightingale thought, so long as it did not imply inevitability, for it expressed a "fact," not a mere "hypothesis," such as germ theory. At this time she allowed for specific causes for "two or three diseases," naming smallpox and cowpox. Otherwise she, as doctors of the time, assumed miasms to be the causal agent for infectious diseases. "Noxious gas," "noxious matter" and "noxious effluvia" appear, each relative to a disease-causing substance in the air, a patient's body, or in moisture, respectively (see pp 58, 59 and 64 below).

In this 1858 paper, Nightingale was so confident that "sanitary precautions" could prevent the spread of disease that she thought it unnecessary "to set apart wards" for infectious disease (see p 54 below). She would later abandon that view and, over time, argued for increasingly stringent measures for the isolation of infectious patients. In the 1859 edition, she dropped the contention that it was a "vulgar error" to suppose that epidemics "*spread* disease from person to person, either by infection or contagion." Rather, epidemics did not spread but developed in constitutions "made ripe for them by neglect," or by natural laws.

Nightingale clearly exaggerated the good effects of ventilation at this time. In the 1858 paper, she asserted that "abundance of pure air will prevent infection," a point she said was confirmed by "all my own hospital experience." Today, we would agree with her subsequent point that infection was "preventible," if not that "carelessness" or "ignorance" were always responsible for failure to prevent it.

The section on defective hospital kitchens—Point 11—was mainly a plea for better nutrition for patients. At the time, there was no distinct nutritionist profession. Doctors were responsible for prescribing patients' food, or "diets" as they were called, and patients' drinks, meaning alcoholic "stimulants." Nurses ensured that these orders were carried out. Defective kitchens—with their resulting bad cooking—were the norm, to the extent that, Nightingale thought, they should be listed with other causes of "hospital unhealthiness." The failure of patients to recover and patient relapses were the obvious consequences of these defects. Nightingale advised that kitchens be detached from the main building in all but the smallest hospitals, to keep damp and fumes away from the sick.

Nursing considerations are minor in this 1858 paper, limited to brief references in Point 10 to patient-nurse ratios and the efficient use of time and space.

Defect No. 14 was the building of hospitals in towns, a matter on which Nightingale would campaign for many years. Here, she said flatly, "If the recovery of the sick is to be the object of hospitals, they will not be built in towns." If medical training were the object—an argument often made in favour of hospitals being centrally located—she countered with the benefit of students seeing recovery from sickness, rather than its lingering; moreover, twice the number of cases would be brought to their attention in a hospital with half the hospital stay (see p 70 below).

In Point No. 16, Nightingale noted that, even in pavilion hospitals, ventilation and light would be "seriously interfered with" unless the distance between the pavilions was double the height of the walls. Two storeys were better than three, and one was preferable.

A note added to the printed paper compared the death rate of nurses in metropolitan London hospitals with those of the female population of London. The nurses' rate was 40 percent higher. Moreover, "the loss of a well-trained nurse by preventible disease is a greater loss than is that of a good soldier," for "a good nurse is more difficult to find than a good soldier" (see p 98 below).

When Nightingale had the paper reprinted as a short book in 1859, she added one further paragraph with cautions on the pavilion principle, reflecting very recently gained experience. It warned that it was possible to build a pavilion hospital "with almost as many defects" as advantages. *All* the details had to be respected, especially site and space between buildings, points that will be seen frequently in later correspondence.

A considerable amount of correspondence is available on the presentation of Nightingale's paper to the meetings of the National Association for the Promotion of Social Science at Liverpool, mainly with

William Farr and Edwin Chadwick (1800-90). In September 1858, Dr Farr offered to take her paper to Liverpool, if she would entrust him with it. Evidently she did, for his next letter reports his own "great satisfaction" with it, and asks if she would not go herself.[1] He next reported that her "two papers" (the paper was in two parts) were referred to him and that he recommended that they be read in full, "on the ground of their intrinsic excellence"; they were "capably written and will do much good." He called her language on contagion "strong," but "not too strong about quarantine."[2] After the papers were read (we do not know by whom), Farr reported that they had been read "to a large audience," and were well received. Family friend Charles H. Bracebridge, who with his wife had accompanied Nightingale to the Crimean War, moved to have the papers printed.[3]

Edwin Chadwick wrote Nightingale from Liverpool promptly after the reading of her paper, reporting that it had "just been read with the very best effect." Lord Shaftesbury, Mr Tomlinson and Mr Bracebridge had spoken on it "exceedingly well," and the resolution recommending separate printing and circulation was carried "by acclamation."[4] Nightingale and Chadwick were in correspondence on other hospital subjects at the same time, so points on the meeting appear in those letters (see p 510 below).

After the meetings, Lord Shaftesbury suggested to Nightingale that she give the manuscript to the city of Liverpool, which she duly did, with a covering letter to the mayor that it go to the Free Library (see p 76 below). When this volume was being prepared, the manuscript was housed in the Liverpool Record Office.

The paper, as given in Liverpool, ended by calling on engineers, doctors and hospital committees to find the remedies so urgently needed. Few people had had "so sad or so large an experience" of the results of hospital defects than she. Nightingale regretted that "our England, which ought to take the lead in everything," should be behind a country "where everything is done by a despotic government" (see p 72 below). She meant, but did not name, France under Napoléon III.

The text below combines the original paper, as sent to Liverpool, with the printed editions of 1858 and 1859. Words added in the 1858

1 Farr letters 20 and 29 September 1858, Add Mss 43398 ff79 and 80.

2 Farr letter 5 October 1858, Add Mss 43398 f82.

3 Farr letter 16 October 1858, Add Mss 43398 f83.

4 Chadwick letter Thursday [14 October 1858], Add Mss 45770 f65.

printed text are indicated, followed by those they replaced. It will be obvious that the editing she did for publication was modest. Points 3 and 4 are reversed between 1858 and 1859; she added tables and, most significantly, four plans: two French and two British, one military and one civil one each. The French plans are both good examples of hospital construction, the British both bad.

Source: Florence Nightingale, "Notes on the Sanitary Condition of Hospitals, and on Defects in the Construction of Hospital Wards," paper read at the National Association for the Promotion of Social Science 1858, Liverpool, dated 22 September 1858. Reprinted as *Notes on Hospitals, being Two Papers Read before the National Association for the Promotion of Social Science, at Liverpool, in October 1858, with Evidence Given to the Royal Commissioners on the State of the Army in 1857*, 2nd edition (London: John W. Parker 1859) 1-21

< > indicates added in the printed 1858 articles
[ ] indicates original manuscript, omitted in printed articles
<< >> indicates added to the 1859 edition

Part 1

Feeling very desirous of contributing whatever aid I can to [the subject of] improvement in hospital construction and administration—especially at this time, when several new hospitals are being built—it has occurred to me to transmit a few notes on [their] defects which have come under my own observation in an extended experience of these institutions.

No one, I think, who brings ordinary powers of observation to bear on the sick and maimed can fail to observe a remarkable difference in the aspect of cases, in their duration and in their termination in different hospitals. To the superficial observer there are two things only apparent—the disease and the remedial treatment, medical or surgical. It requires a considerable amount of experience, in hospitals of various constructions and varied administrations, to go beyond this, and to be able to perceive that <conditions arising out of> these have a very powerful effect indeed upon the ultimate issue of cases which pass through the wards.

It is sometimes asserted that there is no such striking difference in the mortality of different hospitals as one would be led to infer from their great apparent difference in sanitary <state> [condition]. There is, undoubtedly, some difficulty in arriving at correct statistical comparison to exhibit this. For, in the first place, different hospitals receive very different proportions of the same class of diseases. The ages in one hospital may differ considerably from the ages in another. And the state of the cases on admission may differ very much in each hospital. These elements, no doubt, affect considerably the results of treatment, altogether apart from the sanitary state of hospitals.

In the next place, accurate hospital statistics are much more rare than is generally imagined, and at the best they only give the mortality which has taken place in the hospital<s>, and take no cognizance of those cases which are discharged in a <hopeless> [dying] condition, to a much greater extent from some <hospitals> than <from> [in] others.

We have known incurable cases discharged from one hospital, to which the deaths ought to have been accounted, and received into another hospital, to die there in a day or two after admission.

Again, the sanitary state of any hospital ought not to be inferred solely from the greater or less mortality. If the function of a hospital were to kill the sick, statistical comparisons of this nature would be admissible. As, however, its proper function is to restore the sick to health as speedily as possible, the elements which really give information as to whether this is done or not are those which show the proportion of sick restored to health, and the average time which has been required for this object; a hospital which restored all its sick to health after an average of six months' treatment could not be considered as by any means so healthy as a hospital which returned all its sick recovered in as many weeks. The proportion of recoveries, the proportion of deaths and the average time in hospital must all be taken into account in discussions of this nature, as well as the character of the cases and the proportion of different ages among the sick.

Hospital mortality statistics [therefore] give little information on the point, because there are elements in existence of which such statistics take no cognizance.

<(In Paris an Annual Report of the Hospitals ("Compte Moral Adminstratif") is published. But the only useful statistical information to be gleaned from it is the number of *sous*[5] each patient has cost. For, although it gives the numbers of adults, male and female, and of children, who have been admitted, and who have died during the year, yet this in itself tells little.

If the hospitals of London and of Paris would give us the information contained under the eight following heads, so important would

5 The French word for pennies.

be the knowledge thereby conveyed that it would be worthwhile to go back for many years to construct such tables and to continue the same forms hereafter.

1. The numbers admitted for each decennial period for each sex per annum.

2. The numbers, similarly arranged, remaining in hospital at the end of the preceding year.

3. The numbers dead for each sex at each decennial period of age per annum.

4. The numbers discharged cured, similarly arranged per annum.

5. The numbers discharged incurable, similarly arranged per annum.

6. The numbers remaining in hospital at the end of the current year, similarly arranged.

7. The *diseases* remaining, admitted, died, cured, discharged incurable and remained, arranged for each sex and each decennial period of age per annum.

8. The duration of cases, similarly arranged).>

In one set of metropolitan hospitals, for example, I find the mortality about two and a half percent upon the cases treated, while in other metropolitan hospitals the deaths reach from about 12 to 16 percent. To judge by the mortality <of> [in] these cases would be most fallacious. Because in the first class of hospitals every ailment, however slight, constitutes a title to hospital admission, while in the latter class of hospitals, special diseases only, at all times accompanied by a high rate of mortality, are admitted. Hence the duration of the cases admitted, and the general course and aspect of disease afford <important criteria> [a much better criterion] whereby to judge of the healthiness or unhealthiness of any hospital, <in addition to that> [than] afforded by the mortality statistics. Besides, careful observers are now generally convinced that the origin and spread of fever in a hospital, or the appearance and spread of hospital gangrene, erysipelas and pyemia generally, are much better <tests> [criteria of] the defective sanitary state of a hospital than its mortality returns. But I would go further and state that, to the experienced eye of a careful observing nurse, the daily, I had almost said hourly, changes which take place in patients, and which changes rarely come under the cognizance of the periodical medical <visitor> [visitant], afford a still more important class of data from which to judge of the general adaptation of a hospital for the reception and treatment of sick.

One insensibly allies together restlessness, languor, feverishness and general *malaise*, with closeness of wards, defective ventilation, defective structure, bad architectural and administrative arrangements, until it is impossible to resist the conviction that the sick are suffering from something quite other than the disease inscribed on their bed ticket, and the inquiry insensibly arises in the mind, what can be the cause? To this query many years' experience of hospitals in <various> [almost all] countries and climates enables me to answer explicitly, as the result of my own [personal] observation, that even admitting to the full extent the great value of the hospital improvements of recent years, a vast deal of the suffering, and some at least of the mortality in these establishments, is avoidable.

What, then, are those defects to which such results are to be attributed? I should state at once that to original defects in the sites and plans of hospitals, and to deficient ventilation and overcrowding accompanying such defects, is to be attributed a [very] large proportion of the evil I have mentioned.

The facts flow almost of necessity from ascertained sanitary experience. But it is not often, excepting perhaps in the case of intelligent house surgeons, that the whole process whereby the sick, who ought to have had rapid recoveries, are retained week after week, or perhaps month after month <in hospital>, is continuously observed. (I have known a case of slight fever received into hospital, <the fever pass off> [where the fever passed off] in less than a week, <and yet> [but] the patient, from the foul state of the wards, [was] not restored to health at the end of eight weeks.)

<The defects to which such occurrences are mainly to be attributed are four> [These are the four radical defects in hospital construction]:

1. The agglomeration of a large number of sick under the same roof.
2. Deficiency of space.
3. Deficiency of ventilation.
4. Deficiency of light.

But on the very threshold of the subject we shall probably be told that, not to these defects, but to "contagion" and "infection," is much of the unhealthy condition of some hospitals attributable, at least so far as concerns the occurrence of zymotic diseases. On the very threshold, therefore, we are obliged to make a digression in order to discuss the meaning of these two familiar words, and to lay these spectres which have terrified almost all ages and nations.

This is the more necessary, because on the exact influence exercised by these two presumed causes of hospital sickness and mortality depends to a great degree the possibility of our introducing efficient hospital attendance and nursing. Unfortunately both nurses and medical men, as well as medical students, have died of zymotic diseases prevailing in hospitals.

<(To show the great importance of this point I give the following tables, kindly prepared by Dr Farr, from returns furnished to me with the greatest readiness by fifteen of the metropolitan hospitals. Table 1 gives the ages of living and dying among the nursing staff. Table 2 gives the mortality from zymotic diseases, and the comparison between the nurses' mortality and the mortality of the female population of London.

Editor: The tables and form are omitted here as they are identical to those in the third edition (see p 97 below).

It is an all-important question to decide whether the propagation of such diseases is inevitable or preventible. If the former, then the whole question must be considered as to whether hospitals, necessarily attended <with> [by] results so fatal, should exist at all. If the latter, then it is our duty to prevent their propagation.

The idea of "contagion," as explaining the spread of disease, appears to have been adopted at a time when, from the neglect of sanitary arrangements, epidemics attacked whole masses of people, and when men had ceased to consider that nature had any laws for her guidance. Beginning with the poets and historians, the word finally made its way into medical nomenclature, where it has remained ever since, affording to certain classes of minds, chiefly in the southern and less educated parts of Europe, a satisfactory explanation for pestilence and an adequate excuse for non-exertion to prevent its recurrence.

<(The history of the doctrine of "contagion" is given by Dr Adams in his very learned translation of the works of Paulus Aegineta, Vol. 1, p 284 (Sydenham Society). He says in his comment:

> The earlier ancient authors appear to have entertained no suspicions of contagion as a cause of febrile or of other complaints. [x x] The works of the fathers of history and of medicine have likewise been ransacked in vain for any traces of the doctrine of contagion.[6]

---

6 A direct quotation from Francis Adams, trans., *The Seven Books of Paulus Aegineta* 1:284, followed by a paraphrase on Thucydides, whose *History of the Peloponnesian Wars* recounts the plague in Athens, which lasted c430-26 BCE and killed many people. Thucydides himself was a victim but recovered to give what is considered a good description of the disease.

Thucydides, and after him several of the Latin poets, describe the plague of Athens, which appears to have been a form of dysentery, as communicable from person to person. The later Greek historians contain allusions to the infectious nature of certain diseases, but Procopius, though cognizant of one of the greatest pestilences on record, was a non-contagionist.

Virgil's allusions to contagious diseases among cattle will be found in Ecl. I Georg. III, 464.[7]

Aretaeus appears to be the first medical author who believed in contagion. Galen seems to have held the doctrine of infection. Of the later Greek and Arabian medical writers, some were contagionists, and others make no allusion to the subject.[8] Dr Adams states in regard to plague, a disease which in later times has been considered as the very type of all "contagious" pestilences:

> The result of our investigations into the opinions of the ancients on this subject leads us to the conclusion that all, or at least the most intelligent of the medical authorities, held that the plague is communicated not by any specific virus, but in consequence of the atmosphere around the sick being contaminated with putrid effluvia.[9]

The obvious practical result of this view of infection is that abundance of pure air will prevent infection. All my own hospital experience confirms this conclusion. If infection exists, it is preventible. If it exists, it is the result of carelessness or of ignorance. "Contagion," as a doctrine on which distinct practical proceedings have been taken, appears to be of very modern invention, but it has been not the less injurious to civilization and humanity, from the loss of life which has from time to time followed from the practices which it inculcates, and from the immense tax which it has entailed upon commerce.)>

And now, what does "contagion" mean? It implies the communication of disease from person to person by *contact.* It presupposes the existence of certain germs like the sporules of fungi, which can be bottled up

---

7 Cited by Nightingale from Adams, trans., *Paulus Aegineta* 1:285. In part 3 of Virgil's poem *The Georgics,* written in 29 BCE, a shepherd is described as killing a listless animal to "check the mischief, 'ere it creep with dire contagion through the unwary herd."

8 Cited from Adams, trans., *Paulus Aegineta* 1:286. Aretaeus of Cappadocia practised in Rome and Alexandria c100 CE; Galen (129-200 CE) of Pergamum, Turkey, a Roman physician of Greek origin.

9 A direct quotation from Adams, trans., *Paulus Aegineta* 1:287. The bacillus that causes plague was finally identified in 1894, by bacteriologist Alexander Yersin.

and conveyed any distance attached to clothing, to merchandise, especially to woollen stuffs, for which it is supposed to have a particular affection, and to feathers, which of all articles it especially loves—so much so, that, according to quarantine laws, a live goose may be safely introduced from a plague country, but if it happen[s] to be eaten on the voyage, its feathers cannot be <admitted> [introduced] without danger to the entire community. There is no end to the absurdities connected with this doctrine. Suffice it to say, that in the ordinary sense of the word, there is no <proof, such as would be admitted in any scientific inquiry, that there is any such thing as "contagion."> [such thing as "contagion."]

There are two or three diseases in which there is a specific virus, which can be seen, tasted, smelt and analyzed, and which in certain constitutions propagates the original disease by inoculation, such as smallpox, cowpox, etc. But these are not "contagions" in the sense supposed.

[With regard to the mysterious imponderable invisible non-entities which make up our current "contagions," they may safely be dismissed into the limbo of extinct superstitions. The word "contagion" is therefore altogether objectionable.] The word "infection" <which is often confounded with "contagion"> expresses a fact and does not involve a hypothesis.

<(Curiously enough, these directly communicable diseases were excluded from the operation of general quarantine law by the International Quarantine Conference of Paris, 1851, which restricted the objects of quarantine to plague, yellow fever and cholera, while it gave a logical *coup de grâce* to the "contagion" hypothesis by abolishing the "suspected bill of health.")>

But just as there is no such thing as "contagion," there is no such thing as *inevitable* "infection." Infection acts through the air. Poison the air breathed by individuals and there is infection. Shut up 150 healthy people in a Black Hole of Calcutta,[10] and in twenty-four hours an infection is produced so intense that it will, in that time, have destroyed nearly the whole of the inmates.

[Norman Chevers, in his *Brief Review*,[11] states that they certainly died by suffocation from mere deprivation of respirable air.]

Sick people are more susceptible than healthy people, and if <they be> [sick people are] shut up together without sufficient space and

10 A reference to a probably exaggerated account of British soldiers dying in a dungeon at Fort William, Calcutta, after being captured when the fort was taken (briefly) in 1756.

11 Norman Chevers, *A Brief Review of the Means of Preserving the Health of European Soldiers in India.*

sufficient fresh air, there will be produced not only fever, but erysipelas, pyemia and the usual tribe of hospital-generated epidemic diseases.

Again, if we have a fever hospital with overcrowded, badly ventilated wards, we are quite certain to have the air become so infected as to poison the blood, not only of the sick, so as to increase their mortality, but also of the medical attendants and nurses, so that they also shall become subjects of fever.

It will be seen at a glance that in every such case and in every such example the "infection" is not inevitable, but simply the result of [gross] carelessness and ignorance. <As soon as this practical view of the subject is admitted and acted upon, we shall cease to hear of hospital contagions.>

In certain hospitals it has been the custom to set apart wards for what are called "infectious" diseases, but in reality there ought to be no diseases so considered. With proper sanitary precautions, diseases reputed to be the most "infectious" may be treated in wards among other sick without any danger. Without proper sanitary arrangements, a number of healthy people may be congregated together so as to become subject to the worst horrors of "infection."

[It is high time that common sense should deal with the question. For there does not seem to be much hope that we shall be delivered out of these superstitions from any other quarter.]

No stronger condemnation of any hospital or ward could be pronounced than the simple fact that any zymotic disease has originated in it, or that such diseases have attacked other patients than those brought in with them. And there can be no stronger condemnation of any town than the outbreak of <fatal> epidemics in it. Infection, and incapable management or bad construction, are, in hospitals as well as in towns, convertible terms.

[It is a vulgar error to suppose that epidemics are occasioned by the *spread* of disease from person to person, either by infection or contagion. Epidemics do not *spread*—they develop themselves in constitutions already made ripe for them by neglect of natural laws. Unless these laws [be] ignored, epidemics, as experience seems to show, will not occur, the epidemic being, in fact, the last or, so to speak, the retributive stage of a succession of antecedent phenomena extending over months or years, and all traceable to the neglect of natural laws. It is worse than folly, after the penalty has been incurred, to cry out "contagion" and call for the establishment of, in the case of nations, quarantine, in the case of hospitals, "infectious" wards, instead of relying on measures of hygiene. Epidemics are lessons to be profited by: they teach not "contagion," nor that "infection" is inevitable, but that unless nature's laws be studied and obeyed, she will infallibly step in and vindicate them sooner or later. In the words of the Registrar-General, which are as applicable to hospitals as to states, "sanitary measures and not quarantines are the real safeguards of nations."]

It was necessary to say thus much to show to what hospital diseases are *not* <necessarily> due. <To the following defects in site, construction and management, as we think, they are mainly to be attributed.> [To defects in site and construction and to defective management, as we think, they are mainly to be attributed.]

1. *The Agglomeration of a Large Number of Sick under one Roof.* It is a well-established fact that, other things being equal, the amount of sickness and mortality on different areas bears a ratio to the degree of density of the population.

Why should undue agglomeration of sick be any exception to this law? Is it not rather to be expected that, the constitutions of sick people being more susceptible than those of healthy people, they should suffer more from this cause?

But if anything were wanting in confirmation of this fact, it would be the enormous mortality in the hospitals which contained perhaps the largest number of sick ever at one time under the same roof, viz., those <at> [of] Scutari. The largest of these too-famous hospitals had at one time 2500 sick and wounded under its roof, and it has happened that <of Scutari patients> [out of these] two out of every five have died. <In the hospital tents of the Crimea, although the sick were almost without shelter, without blankets, without proper food or medicines, the mortality was not above one half <what it was at Scutari>. Nor was it even so high as this in the small Balaclava General Hospital, while in the huts of the Castle Hospital, on the heights above Balaclava, at a subsequent period, the mortality among the wounded did not reach 3 percent.>

[But] It is not to this <however>, that we appeal, as <the only> [a] proof of the danger of surface overcrowding [so much as] it is to the fact of 80 cases of hospital gangrene having been recorded during one month at Scutari (and many, many more, passed unrecorded, to the fact that, out of 44 secondary amputations of the lower extremities consecutively performed, 36 died, and to the cases of fever which broke out in the hospital, not by tens but by hundreds.

All experience tells the same tale, both among sick and well. Men will have a high rate of mortality in large barracks, a low one in separate huts, even with a much less amount of cubic space. (It must never be forgotten that, during the last six months of our occupation <in> [of] the Crimea, the death rate among our men barracked in huts, was <only two thirds of what> [actually less than] it is among the men in barracks at home.)

The example which France and Belgium have lately set us of separating their hospitals into a number of distinct pavilions, containing generally not more than 100 sick each, should be elsewhere <everywhere> imitated. It may be useful, <by way of illustrating good and bad hospital structure, to annex> [by way of illustration, to exhibit] plans of the newest civil and military hospitals constructed in Paris, in contrast with plans of the newest civil and military hospitals constructed in England.

The Lariboisière, as a civil hospital, the Vincennes as a military one, <exhibit> [are both] the latest and the best specimens of hospital construction in Paris <Plans 1 and 3>. King's College as a civil hospital, Netley as a military one, are among the latest—we would we could say the best plans of hospital construction in England <Plans 2 and 4>.

The Lariboisière, as will be seen from the plan, contains <612> [600] beds under six different roofs. In the Vincennes plan the pavilions are end-to-end <two and a half in each wing> [two in each wing and half a one at the end of each wing], and contain about 600 <beds> [patients] in four pavilions and two half pavilions. Netley Hospital is to contain 1000 sick and invalids, under two roofs.

2. *Deficiency of [Cubic] Space:* Wherever cubic space is deficient, ventilation is bad. Cubic space and ventilation will therefore go hand in hand. The law holds good with regard to hospitals, barracks and all inhabited places. Deficiency of cubic space is confounded by unskillful <sanitary> statisticians with surface overcrowding in towns, although the things are quite different and lead to different results. In a recent paper it has been argued that, because the statistics of disease in towns of different densities do not show so large a proportionate mortality from consumption as takes place in the army, *therefore* the allegation that the army mortality is caused by overcrowding and bad ventilation is incorrect. We happen to know that deficient external ventilation and overcrowding in barracks, as [both] regards cubic space, [and surface overcrowding] <stand> [stands] as follows:

The cavalry barracks, as a whole, are <the> least overcrowded [in either sense], and have the freest external movement of air. Next come the infantry, and the most crowded and the least ventilated externally are the Guards' barracks, so that the mortality from consumption which follows the same order of increase in the different arms augments with [the] increase of crowding, and [consequent] difficulty of ventilation.

If overcrowding or its concomitant, bad ventilation, among healthy people, generates disease, it does so to a far greater extent among the sick in hospitals. In civil hospitals the amount of cubic space varies between 600 and 2000 cubic feet per bed. In some military hospitals it is under 300, and from 700 to 800 appear to be considered a somewhat extravagant allowance. The army regulation as to cubic space in hospitals is overcrowding. At Scutari, at one time, not even half the regulation space was given, and the great overcrowding consequent thereupon was one element in the disastrous result which followed. Anyone in the habit of examining hospitals with different relative amounts of cubic space cannot fail to have been struck with the very different appearance of the sick, and with the different state of the ward atmosphere. It is impossible to ventilate a ward in a brick or stone hospital by natural means, when the cubic space is less than a certain amount. Crowded wards, are, in fact, offensive with all the windows open.

In the country, less cubic space is essential than in towns. In detached huts or pavilions, especially if <they> [such people] be <together> [shut up together] but one storey high, less cubic space is necessary than where numbers are massed together.

Under all circumstances, however, <the progress of the cases> [the appearance of patients] (in solidly built hospitals) will betray any curtailment of space much below 1500 cubic feet. In Paris 1700, and in London 2000 and even 2500 cubic feet are now thought advisable.

The master of some large works in London lately mentioned the following fact: he was in the habit of sending those of his workmen who met with accidents to two different metropolitan hospitals. In one> they recovered quickly; in the other they were frequently attacked with erysipelas, and some cases were fatal. On inquiry it appeared that, in the former hospital, a larger amount of cubic space was allowed than in the latter, <which is also so deficient in external ventilation and in construction that nothing but artificial ventilation could effectively change its atmosphere.>

It is no less important to have a sufficient surface area between the adjoining and the opposite beds. *Piling* cubic space above the patient is not all that is wanted. In the lofty corridors of Scutari I have seen two long rows of opposite beds with scarcely three feet from foot to foot. Certainly it cannot be thought too much, under any circumstances, to give to each bed a territory to itself of at least eight feet wide by twelve feet long.

<4> [3]. *Deficiency of Ventilation.* The want of fresh air may be detected in the appearance of patients sooner than any other want. No care or luxury will compensate indeed for its absence. Unless the air *within* the ward can be kept as fresh as it is *without*, the patients had better be away. Except in a few cases well known to physicians, the danger of admitting fresh air directly is very much exaggerated. Patients in bed <are not peculiarly inclined to> [do not] catch cold, and in England, where fuel is cheap, somebody is indeed to blame if the ward cannot be kept warm enough, and if the patients cannot have bedclothing enough, for as much air to be admitted from without as suffices to keep the ward fresh.

<("Catching cold" in bed follows the same law as "catching cold" when up. If the atmosphere is foul, and the lungs and skin cannot therefore relieve the system, then a draught upon the patient may give him cold. But this is the fault of the foul air, not of the fresh.)>

No artificial ventilation will do this. Although in badly constructed hospitals, or in countries where fuel is dear and the winter[s] very cold, artificial ventilation may be necessary, it never can compensate for the want of the open window. The ward is never fresh, and in the best hospitals at Paris, artificially ventilated, it will be found that, till the windows are opened in the morning, the air is close. Natural ventilation, or that by open windows and open fireplaces, is the only efficient means for procuring the life-spring of the sick—fresh air. But to obtain this the ward should be at least sixteen feet high, and the distance between the opposite windows not more than thirty feet.

The amount of fresh air required for ventilation has been hitherto very much underrated, because it has been assumed that the quantity of carbonic acid[12] produced during respiration was the chief noxious gas to be carried off. The total amount of this gas produced by an adult in twenty-four hours is about 40,000 cubic inches, which, in a barrack room, say, containing sixteen men, would give 370 cubic feet per diem. Allowing eight hours for the night occupation of such a room, when the doors and windows may be supposed to be shut, the

12 Carbon dioxide.

product of carbonic acid would be 123 cubic feet, or about fifteen and a half cubic feet per hour. This large quantity, if not speedily carried away, would undoubtedly be injurious to health, but there are other gaseous poisons produced with the carbonic acid which have still greater power to injure. Every adult exhales by the lungs and skin forty-eight ounces, or three pints, of water in twenty-four hours. Sixteen men in a room would therefore exhale in eight hours sixteen pints of water, and 123 cubic feet of carbonic acid into the atmosphere of the room. With the watery vapour there is also exhaled a large quantity of organic matter, ready to enter into the putrefactive condition. This is especially the case during the hours of sleep, and as it is a vital law that all excretions are injurious to health if reintroduced into the system, it is easy to understand how the breathing of damp foul air of this kind, and the consequent reintroduction of excrementitious matter into the blood through the function of respiration, will tend to produce disease.

If this be so for the well, how much more will it be so for the sick? for the sick, the exhalations from whom are always highly morbid and dangerous, as they are one of nature's methods of eliminating noxious matter from the body, in order that it may recover health.

One would think that the first and last idea in constructing hospitals would be to contrive such means of ventilation as would be perpetually and instantly carrying off these morbid emanations. One would think that it would be the first thing taught to the attendants to manage such means of ventilation. Often, however, it is *not even* the *last* thing taught to them.

A much larger mass of air is required to dilute and carry away these emanations than is generally supposed, and the whole art of ventilation resolves itself into applying in any specific case the best method of renewing the air sufficiently without producing draughts or occasioning excessive varieties in temperature. Trifling varieties are rather beneficial than otherwise in most cases. A cooler atmosphere at night acts like a tonic.

<3> [4]. *Deficiency of Light.* What is the proportionate influence of the four defects enumerated in delaying recovery I am not competent to determine.

Second only to fresh air, however, I should be inclined to rank light in importance for the sick. Direct sunlight, not only daylight, is necessary for speedy recovery, except, perhaps, in ophthalmic and a small number of other cases. Instances could be given, almost endless, where, in dark wards or in wards with a northern aspect, even when thoroughly warmed, or in wards with borrowed light, even when thoroughly ventilated, the sick could not by any means be made speedily to recover. The effect of light on health and disease has been ably discussed in an article on light in the August number, <1858>, of the *North British Review*. Its importance has been long recognized, in the medical profession, as may be learned from the writings of Sir Andrew Wylie, Dr Milne Edwards and Mr Ward. Dark barrack rooms, and barrack rooms with northern aspects, will furnish a larger amount of sickness than light and sunny rooms.

Among kindred effects of light I may mention, from experience, as quite perceptible in promoting recovery, the being able to see out of <a> window, instead of looking against a dead wall, the bright colours of flowers, the being able to read in bed by the light of a window close to the bedhead. It is generally said that the effect is upon the mind. Perhaps so, but it is no less so upon the body on that account.

All hospital buildings in this climate should be erected so that as great a surface as possible should receive direct sunlight—a rule which has been observed in several of our best hospitals, but I am sorry to say passed over in some of <those> [our] most recently constructed [hospitals]. Window blinds can always moderate the light of a light ward, but the gloom of a dark ward is irremediable.

The axis of a ward should be as nearly as possible north and south, the windows on both sides, so that the sun shall shine in (from the time he rises till the time he sets) at one side or the other. There should be a window to at least every two beds, as is the case now in our best hospitals. Some foreign hospitals, in countries where the light is far more intense than in England, give one window to every bed. The window space should be one third of the wall space. The windows should reach from two or three feet of the floor to one foot of the ceiling. The escape of heat may be diminished by plate or double glass. But while we *can* generate warmth, we cannot generate daylight, or the purifying and curative effect of the sun's rays.

Part 2 [Sixteen Sanitary Defects in the Construction of Hospital Wards]

Considering, then, that the conditions essential to the health of hospitals are principally these: (1) fresh air, (2) light, (3) ample space, [and] (4) subdivision of sick into separate buildings or pavilions. Let us examine the causes in the usual ward construction which prevent us from obtaining these <and other necessary> conditions. The principal causes are as follow, <viz.>:

1. Defective means of natural ventilation and warming;
2. Defective height of wards;
3. Excessive width of wards between the opposite windows;
4. Arranging the beds along the dead walls;
5. Having more than two rows of beds between the <opposite> windows;
6. Having windows only on one side or having a closed corridor connecting the wards;
7. Using absorbent materials for walls and ceilings and washing floors of hospitals;
8. Defective condition of water closets;
9. Defective ward furniture;
10. Defective accommodation for nursing and discipline;
11. Defective hospital kitchens;
12. Defective hospital laundries;
13. Selection of bad sites and bad local climates for hospitals;
14. Erecting hospitals in towns;
15. Defects of [drainage] <sewerage>;
16. Construction of hospitals without free circulation of external air.

1. [Then] *Defective Means of Ventilation and Warming*. When the question of ventilation first assumed a practical shape in this country, it was supposed that 600 cubic feet of air per hour were sufficient for a healthy adult, in a room where a number of people are congregated together. Subsequent experience, however, has shown that this is by no means enough. As much as 1000 cubic feet have been found insufficient to keep the air free from closeness and smell, and it is highly probable that the actual quantity required will ultimately be found to be at least 1500 cubic feet per hour per man.

In sick wards we have more positive experience as to the quantity of air required to keep them sweet and healthy. It has been found in certain Parisian hospitals, in which the ventilating arrangements were deficient, that pyemia and hospital gangrene had appeared among the patients. These diseases disappeared on the introduction of ventilating arrangements whereby 2500 cubic feet of air per bed per hour were supplied to the wards. Notwithstanding this large quantity, however, the ward atmosphere was found not to be sufficiently pure. In other wards the quantity of air was increased to as much as 4000 or 5000 cubic feet per bed per hour—an amount which keeps the wards perfectly sweet. But again we say do not trust to artificial means; without natural ventilation the air will never be *fresh.*

In this country, have no other than the open fireplace. It is the safest warmer and ventilator. Heated air from metal surfaces is especially to be avoided. It seems likely that we shall soon be enabled to have open fireplaces in the middle of wards, the draught being carried under the floor. It is obvious that fireplaces in the side walls are in the wrong place. There is great loss and unequal distribution of heat in consequence.

2. *Defective Height of Wards.* It is not possible to ventilate sufficiently a ward of ten or twelve feet high. And again, it is not possible to ventilate a ward where there is a great height above the windows. A ward of thirty beds can be well ventilated with a height of about <sixteen or> seventeen feet, provided the windows reach to within one foot of the ceiling. Otherwise, the top of the ward becomes a reservoir for foul air.

3. *Too Great Width of Wards between the Opposite Windows.* It does not appear as if the air could be thoroughly changed, if a distance of more than thirty feet intervenes between the opposite windows, if, in other words, the ward is more than thirty feet wide. This is the true starting point from which to determine the size of your ward and the number of beds you will have in it. If you make your length too great in proportion to this width, your ward becomes a tunnel—a form fatal to good ventilation. This was the case with the great corridor wards at Scutari.

If, on the other hand, you make your wards too short in proportion to this width, you multiply corners in a greater ratio than you multiply sick. And direct experiment has shown that the movement of the air in the centre of a ward is three or four times as great as it is at the corners. The movement of the air in a hospital ward should always be slightly perceptible over the face and hands, and yet there should be no draughts.

4. *Arranging the Beds along the Dead Walls.* This deprives the patient of the amount of light and air necessary to his recovery, and has, besides, the disadvantage that when the windows are opened the effluvia must blow over all the intervening beds before escaping. This arrangement is to be seen at Portsmouth Military Hospital, Chatham Garrison Hospital, in the new part of <the> Edinburgh Infirmary, and is proposed at Netley Hospital.

5. *Having more than Two Rows of Beds between the Windows.* In the double wards, or wards back to back, of the new part of Guy's, of King's College [St Mary's, London], and <of> the fever hospitals, this arrange-

ment is seen. It is objectionable on every account. These double wards are <from twelve to> nearly twenty feet wider than they ought to be between the opposite windows for thorough ventilation. The partition down the middle with apertures makes matters rather worse; complaint has been made that it beats down the draught on the heads of the inner rows of patients. It also prevents the head nurse from having that view of her whole ward at once, which she ought to have for proper care of it. The only hospital in which this arrangement of four rows of beds could be comparatively unobjectionable would be in a one-storeyed hut hospital, <ventilated through the ceiling> like that of Dr Parkes[13] at Renkioi (on the Dardanelles during the Crimean War), but his were magnificent huts, and the partition was little more than a bulkhead. In the ordinary huts of the Sardinian camp hospitals at Balaclava I have seen this arrangement produce pernicious effects.

6. *Having Windows only on one Side, or having a closed Corridor connecting the Wards.* <As it is a necessity of hospital construction that every ward ought to have direct communication with the external air by means of a sufficient number of windows on its opposite sides, it follows that to have a dead wall on one side, or to cover one of the sides by a corridor, is directly to interfere with the natural ventilation of the ward. To join all the ward doors and windows on one side by means of a corridor is much more objectionable than even to have a dead wall, because the foul air of all the wards must necessarily pass into the corridor, and hence, without extraordinary precautions, such as are not usually nor likely to be bestowed on such matters,> these corridors are the certain means of engendering a hospital atmosphere. If anyone had wished to see the corridor plan in all its horrors, Scutari would have shown them to him on a colossal scale. But <the evils connected with corridors> [they] may be seen on a smaller scale in almost every hospital in London, and Netley also is to have its corridor.

This country is much indebted to Mr Roberton of Manchester, to the medical staff of the Middlesex Hospital, and to the Army Sanitary Commission for their advocacy of the pavilion system of hospital construction, in opposition to the corridor system, as also for their enlightened labours in the cause of good hospital construction generally.

7. <*Using*> *Absorbent Materials for Floors, Walls and Ceilings of Hospitals, and Washing Floors.* The amount of organic matter given off by res-

---

13 Edmund Alexander Parkes (1819-76), at the civil hospital at Renkioi, later professor of military hygiene at Netley and an ally.

piration and in other ways from the sick is such that the floors, walls and ceilings of hospital wards—if not of impervious materials—become [most] dangerous absorbents.

The boards are in time saturated with organic matter, and only require moisture to give off noxious effluvia. When the floors are being washed, the smell of something quite other than soap and water is perfectly perceptible, and there cannot be a doubt that washing <floors> is one [main] cause of erysipelas, etc., in some hospitals.

In Scutari, where the wards were overcrowded, the cases offensive and the floors ill-laid, rotten and dirty, the accumulated saturations of weeks and months were such that the floors could not be scoured without [literally] poisoning the patients.

There is no remedy for this but filling up the grain of the wood (which ought to be oak) with beeswax and turpentine, like the French *parquet*, or oiling and *lacquering*, i.e., saturating the floor with linseed oil, and then rubbing it over with a peculiar *lacque* varnish, and polishing it so as to resemble French polish, like the Berlin hospital floors. Both processes render the floor non-absorbent—both processes do away with the necessity of scouring altogether. The French floor *stands* the most wear and tear, but must be cleaned by a *frotteur*,[14] which cleaning is more laborious than scrubbing, and does not remove the dust. The Prussian floor requires repreparing every three years. But the wet and dry rubbing, or process of cleaning, is far less laborious than either *frottage* or scrubbing, and completely removes the dust, and freshens the ward in the morning. By either process the sick would gain much in England. The Berlin flooring is by no means perfect, on account of this deficient durability of surface, and might be improved.

As to the walls and ceilings of wards, plaster or brick whitewashed are equally objectionable. Pure, white, polished, non-absorbent cement is the only material fit for hospital walls. If anyone [here] has inhabited the wards of war hospitals, after several weeks or months of constant occupation by sick and wounded, where little or no attempt had been made to limewash the uneven dirty plaster walls saturated with organic matter, he will not wonder at the stress which is here laid upon the importance of impervious walls.

8. *Defective Condition of Water Closets.* It is hardly necessary to say more than this: there can be no safety for the sick if any but water

14 A frotteur is a floor polisher; frottage is the polishing.

closets of the best construction are used, as also if they are not built *externally* to the main building, and cut off by a lobby, separately lighted and ventilated, from the ward. The same thing may be said of sinks. I have known outbreaks of fever even among the <healthy> [well] from an ill-constructed and ill-placed sink in this country.

The smell of latrines which are not water closets, as used in French hospitals, although externally built, is quite perceptible at the end of the ward nearest to them.

9. *Defective Ward Furniture.* Hospital bedsteads should always be of iron, the rest of the furniture of oak. Hair[15] is the only material yet discovered fit for hospital mattresses. It is not hard nor cold. It is easily washed. It does not retain miasma. Straw has the advantage of being easily renewed, but it is not desirable. It is too hard and too cold not to render necessary the use of a blanket *under* the patient, which use is likely to encourage bedsores. I speak from actual experience of the fatal effect of using the paillasse with patients much reduced. It may lower their vital energy beyond repair.

For all eating, drinking and washing vessels, and for other utensils, the use of glass or earthenware is superior to that of tin or any other metal, on account of its greater cleanliness. Notwithstanding the greater amount of breakage and of expense, glass or earthenware is therefore best wherever possible. Some kinds of tin vessels cannot by any amount of cleaning be freed from an unclean smell.

10. *Defective Accommodation for Nursing and Discipline.* Simplicity of construction in hospitals is essential to discipline. Effectual and easy supervision is essential to proper care and nursing.

Every *unneeded* closet, scullery, sink, lobby and staircase represents both a place which must be cleaned [and] which must take hands and time to clean, and a hiding or skulking place for patients or servants disposed to do wrong. And of such no hospital will ever be free. Every five minutes wasted upon cleaning what had better not have been there to be cleaned is something taken from and lost by the sick.

In considering the pavilion plan to be in future received as the sanitary necessity for hospital construction, we must look upon it as susceptible of many modifications. <In deciding which of these shall be adopted,> there are four essentials to be considered as regards the head of nursing and discipline: (1) economy of attendance, (2) ease

---

15 Clarified as horse hair (see p 141 below).

of supervision, (3) convenience as to number of sick in the same ward and on the same floor, so as to save extra attendants and unnecessary waste of time and strength on the stairs, [and] (4) efficiency as to accommodation for nurses so as to overlook their wards.

First. *Economy as to Attendance.* I <would> [had] rather not enumerate the instances where I have seen that, often from the most various causes, one result arises, viz., that more time and care are given to passages, stairs, etc., than to the sick. Extreme simplicity of construction and of detail is essential to obviate this. A convenient arrangement of lifts, and the laying of hot and cold water all over the building, [economizes] attendance—certainly as much as one attendant to every thirty sick.

Secondly. *Ease of Supervision.* The system of scouts, watch, alarm, is well understood in many wards where patients would be puzzled to give the things names. Some patients will know both things and names. Attendants require inspection as well as patients. Whatever system of hospital construction is adopted should provide for easy supervision at unexpected times. The Vincennes plan is better adapted for this than the Lariboisière plan, inasmuch as there <is> [are] a greater number of patients on the same level, and stairs are spared.

Third and Fourth. *Distribution of Sick in Convenient Numbers for Attendance, and Position of Nurses' Rooms.* Four wards of ten patients <of> each, taking the average of patients as in London, cannot be efficiently overlooked by one head nurse. Forty patients in one ward can be fully overlooked by one head nurse. She ought to have her room so placed that she can command her whole ward, day and night, from a window looking into the ward. This cannot be the case if she has four wards. If she has two, they ought to be built end to end, with her room placed between and looking into both wards.

Four wards of ten patients of each cannot be attended by one night nurse, taking the average of London cases. Forty patients in one ward can be fully attended by one night nurse. Small wards are indeed objectionable in working a hospital.

If we are to be guided, however, by the results of recent experience in hospital building, we shall probably come to the conclusion that, taking sanitary and administrative reasons together, thirty-two patients is a good ward unit.

Let us see what we do in our military hospitals at home. The first thing <that> [which] will strike anyone in most of our regimental hospitals is the extraordinary number of wards and of holes and corners in comparison with the number of sick. In a hospital for a battalion

500 or 600 strong, you find eight or ten little bedrooms, miscalled wards, a little kitchen, everything in fact on little scale, like a collapsed French hospital. How much more sensible would it be to have one, or at most two large wards for thirty sick each, with a small "casualty" ward [and an itch ward!]. How much less the expense of erection and administration, how much easier the discipline and oversight, how much better the ventilation!

To return to large general hospitals. These "casualty" wards, as they are called, for noisy or offensive cases are much better placed apart, with a completely appointed staff of their own, than attached one small ward to each larger one. Patients requiring much attention, whose condition fits them the most for the small wards, cannot be put there, because either they are more or less neglected or they unduly monopolize the service of the ward attendants. If convalescent patients are put into them, they are comparatively removed from inspection, and often play tricks there. If <separate> "casualty" wards are provided, as they ought to be, the small ward (often seen in French hospitals), at the end of the larger ward, is only an incubus.[16]

11. *Defective Hospital Kitchens.* Two facts every careful [experienced] observer [of the sick] can establish from experience.

1. The necessity <for> [of] variety in food, as an essential element of health, owing to the number of materials required to preserve the human frame. In sickness it is still more important because, the frame being in a morbid state, it is scarcely possible to prescribe beforehand with certainty what it will be able to digest and assimilate. The so-called "fancies" of disease are in many cases valuable indications.

2. The importance of cooking so as to secure the greatest digestibility and the greatest economy in nutritive value of food.

Yet so little was either of these elements of health understood in the late Crimean War, <so little is either understood> [is understood] up to this hour in the diets, rations and cooking of either sick or well in the army, that we still see the everlasting sameness of ration, the eternal boiled meat of the "full," "half" and "low" diet of the hospital kitchen. As the present quartermaster general says, "the men live upon boiled meat for twenty-one years."

In the war hospitals of the East, it was practically learnt, though never theoretically acknowledged, that in order to make the patient

16 A type of minor demon.

eat at all, he must not be fed on this hard-boiled, never-varying meat of "full" or "half" diet. Hence the wasteful and violent expenditure of "extras," as they are called, which, in the hands of inexperienced surgeons, left to their own unassisted inventions, often laid them open to criticism. But no attempt was made to compose a better or more varied diet, hardly any, till the arrival of Soyer,[17] to improve the system of cooking.

Some few improvements have lately been made in the hospital kitchens of the army at home; what variety of cooking there is even now in the barracks is often done at the expense of, and by the men themselves. A proper system of hospital diets will 'ere long be introduced in the army hospitals. I have often been surprised by the primitive kitchens of some of our civil hospitals, with which little variety of cooking is possible.

These things show how little diet and cooking are even yet thought of as sanitary and curative agents. There still exists a confusion of ideas about "spoiling" the sick, about "too much indulgence" of the patients, and even yet comparatively little is practically known as to what is, and what is not, essential for restoration to the utmost vigour.

12. *Defective Hospital Laundries.* It is hardly necessary to go back to the time in the Crimean War when, in a Scutari hospital, six shirts were washed in a month for a number of 2000 patients, which was constantly changing, when the number per man per month of all articles of all descriptions washed was less than three. The pestilential filth of that time is known now to all. But it is not so well known that, even now, there is scarcely an army hospital which has such a thing as a laundry. The bedding is generally washed by the barrack department; no one appears to know how. It is done by contract. And the body linen is generally washed, if such a term ought to be used, in a small washhouse or lean-to shed, with or without a boiler, and without any means for drying, getting up or airing linen. The linen is taken out of the damp washhouse, possibly into the damp air and there hung up for a longer or a shorter time; and if the "orderly" be careful of his patients, he will complete the process by drying the linen before it is put on in front of the ward fire.

A great deal has been said about the communication of "infectious" disease, both in civil and military hospitals, from patients' linen

17 Alexis Benoit Soyer (1809-58), chef at the Reform Club who, as a volunteer, revolutionized army cooking during the Crimean War.

to washerwomen. The usual conclusion arrived at <on such occasions> [when this takes place] is that such and such a disease is "very infectious." E.g., I was lately told in a civil hospital that the washerwomen became infected with fever from the patients' linen. Have those who put forward this doctrine of inevitable "infection" among washerwomen ever examined the process of washing, the appliances by which it is done, and the place where the women wash? If they will do so, they will very generally find a small, dark, wet, unventilated and overcrowded little room or shed, in which there is hardly space to turn about—so full of steam loaded with organic matter that it is hardly possible to see across the room.

Is it surprising that the linen is badly washed, that it is imperfectly dried and that the washerwomen are poisoned by inhaling organic matter and foul air? An ordinary hospital washhouse is a very likely place indeed to contract disease in, but it supplies equal reason for demurring *in toto* to the doctrine that the occurrence is inevitable, or that the disease is to blame. Ignorance and mismanagement lie at the root of all such presumed cases of "infection." And it would better serve the cause of humanity if, instead of citing such facts—if they be facts—as illustrations that such and such a disease is infectious, people would reform these washing establishments and convert them into proper laundries, from which properly cleansed and prepared linen could be supplied to the sick, and in which the health of the servants could be preserved from injury.

Let laundries be constructed with sufficient area and cubic space for each washer, with abundance of water, with proper means of drainage, and of ventilation for removing the vapour, and with properly constructed drying and ironing rooms, and we shall cease to hear of washerwomen "catching" fever.

13. *Selection of Bad Sites and Bad Local Climates for Hospitals.* As the object to be attained in hospital construction is to have pure dry air for the sick, it will be evident that this condition cannot be fulfilled if a damp climate be selected. It is a well-known fact, e.g., that in the more damp localities of the south of England, certain classes of sick and of invalids linger, and do not recover their health. Again, retentive clay subsoils keep the air over entire districts of the country always more or less damp. And soils of this character should not be selected as sites for hospitals. Self-draining, gravelly or sandy subsoils are best. River banks, estuary shores, valleys, marshy or muddy ground ought to be avoided. It <may> [might] seem superfluous to state that a hos-

pital should not be built over <an old graveyard or on other ground charged with organic matter> [an old dung heap or over a crowded graveyard],[18] [did we not know that such things were being done at the present moment]. Although hospitals are intended for the recovery of health, people are very apt to forget this, and to be guided in the selection of sites by other considerations—such as cheapness, convenience and the like—whereas the professed object in view being to secure the recovery of the sick in the shortest time, and to obtain the smallest mortality, that object should be distinctly kept in view as one which must take precedence of all others.

A doctrine has recently been promulgated in a government report that we are only to consider what is best for the *majority* of the sick in a hospital. If we cannot do the best possible for *all* the sick, by all means let us leave the rest at home. In practice a hospital may be found <only> to benefit a majority, and to inflict suffering on the remainder. Let us use our intelligence to see whether we cannot have hospitals constructed so as to be <of> [an] equal benefit to all.

14. *Erecting Hospitals in Towns.* Nearly all that has been said under the last head, mutatis mutandis [with appropriate changes], may be repeated here. If the recovery of the sick is to be the object of hospitals, they will not be built in towns. If medical schools are the object, surely it is more instructive for students to watch the recovery from, rather than <the lingering in> [long duration of] sickness. Twice the number of cases would be brought under their notice in a hospital in which the sick recovered in half the time necessary in another.

According to all analogy, the duration of cases, the chances against complete recovery, the rate of mortality, must be greater in town than in country hospitals. Land in towns is too expensive for hospitals to be so built as to secure the conditions of ventilation and of light and of spreading the inmates over a large surface area, instead of piling them up three or four storeys high—conditions now known to be essential to recovery.

15. *Defects in Drainage.* Sewers may become cesspools of the most dangerous description, if improperly made and placed. At Scutari, if the wind changed so as to blow up the open mouths of the sewers,

---

18 The point was made again in the third edition, but again without naming the hospital, presumably King's College Hospital, which was rebuilt on the graveyard of St Clement Dane's Church, and named in a letter to Dr Bowman (see p 503 below).

such change was frequently marked by outbreaks of fever among the patients, and by relapses among the convalescents from fever. Where there are no means for externally ventilating the sewers, no means for cleansing or flushing them, and where the bottoms are rough and uneven, such occurrences cannot fail to take place. The emanations from the deposits in the sewers were blown back through the pipe drains into the privies, and thence into the corridors and wards where the sick were lying. Where sewers pass close to or under occupied rooms, the walls or covers being defective, exhalations will infallibly escape into those rooms. Such could be distinctly perceived in Scutari hospitals, and cases of cholera distinctly traced to such a cause.

Not very long ago, five fatal cases of fever occurred in rapid succession <among the nurses> in one of our [best] civil hospitals, which were traced to a defective drain. Where a main sewer is too large, as is the case at Netley Hospital, mischief may also ensue.

16. *Construction of Hospitals without Free Circulation of External Air.* To build a hospital with one closed court with high walls, or, what is worse, with two closed courts, is to stagnate the air even before it reaches the wards.

All closed corners stagnate the air, even where the building forms but three sides of a square, unless the wings are so short that they can hardly be called wings. The only safe plan is to leave the corners entirely open, as at Vincennes, where they are connected only by an arcade on the ground floor.

Even in the pavilion structure, unless the distance between the pavilions <be> [is] double the height of the walls, the ventilation and light are seriously interfered with. For this, among other reasons, two storeys are better than three, and one is preferable to two, provided it be erected <upon> <on> an arched basement.

To build a hospital in the midst of a crowded neighbourhood of narrow streets and high houses, [as is now being done in the case of a well-known London hospital,] is to insure a stagnation of the air without which no ventilation within, no cubic space, however ample, will be able to remedy.

I have here given the defects; few have had so sad or so large an experience of their results as I have had. I appeal to those who are wiser, and have more practical power than I have, for the remedies: [to] architects, [to] hospital committees, to civil and royal engineers, to medical officers, to officers of health, to all the men of science and benevolence of whom our country is so justly proud. It is hard that in a country where everything is done by a despotic government,[19] such advances in the sanitary construction of hospitals should have been made, and that our England, which ought to take the lead in everything good, should be left behind.

<Note on the Hospital Plans

These four plans, two English and two French, may be taken as representing the degree of constructive ability directed to the planning of hospitals in the two countries. The contrast presented by them is certainly very striking.

Compare, for example, the extreme simplicity of the plan of the Military Hospital at Vincennes with the great complication of that at Netley. The former consists of a centre and two wings, detached but connected by a corridor one storey high running along the basement. The centre contains the offices, and the wards are in the wings. Each wing consists of two pavilions for sick soldiers, and one small pavilion for sick officers. The pavilions are completely cut off from each other by a large, specially ventilated staircase, carried above the roof. Each ward has a profusion of windows opposite each other, abundance of light and of ventilation, quite independent of the ventilation of the adjoining pavilions. The wards, moreover, run nearly north and south, and receive the sunlight freely throughout the day.

Netley Hospital, on the other hand, presents a perfect rabble of wards and offices, thrown together as if by accident. All the sick wards in each flat have their ventilation connected by a corridor running along and covering the whole southwest face of the building, as if designed to obstruct natural ventilation, to keep out sunlight and to ensure the equal diffusion of a hospital atmosphere throughout the entire line of wards. It is true that a complicated system of ventilation is proposed to remove this latter defect, but there should have been no such defect to remove. It will also be seen that the only ward windows opening to the external air are on the northeast and coldest side of the building.

Netley may be fairly described as a hospital without sufficient sunlight or natural ventilation. The Vincennes Hospital has an obvious defect in the position of part of the administrative offices, but even in this respect it is better than Netley, while in all that pertains to the welfare of the sick it is very greatly superior.

---

19 A reference to France under Napoléon III.

Let us next compare the civil hospital plans.

One of these is that of an unfinished metropolitan hospital, the other is the plan of the noble Lariboisière at Paris. The English hospital plan presents an epitome of almost every defect in hospital construction. It is an involved Netley plan, with sick in the corridors, for not only have the wards windows only on one side, but there are four rows of beds between the opposite windows. Moreover, the arrangement of wards, corridors, chapel, etc., seems as if intended to stagnate the air outside. All is complicated, and there is a want of that simplicity of plan which is essential to the free circulation of air, without as well as within the sick wards.

Turn next to the Lariboisière. The corridor running round the central garden is only one storey high, so as not to impede the free flow of the air and sunlight. The sick pavilions are all detached from each other. They are, in fact, separate hospitals, with only one hundred sick under one roof. Like the Vincennes pavilions, they have a profusion of windows, and abundant means of natural ventilation within as well as without. In the much brighter and hotter, as well as colder, climate of Paris, a large proportion of the hospital wall is glass, and the sick are ranged between the windows, so that the ward effluvia can readily escape.

The English plans, on the contrary, show that in our duller and milder climate, in both senses, our hospital architects do their best to shut out our rare and imperfect sunlight, and to keep pure air out of the wards as much as possible, while they provide for the sick being so arranged that the effluvia must pass over a succession of beds before escaping.

Anyone making even a cursory examination of these four plans can hardly fail to arrive at the conclusion that the French plans, with certain obvious defects, show a high appreciation of the importance of hospital hygiene, while the English plans, on the contrary, prove that we have hardly yet begun even to study this branch of knowledge.>

<<It is one thing, however, to lay down correct principles of construction, but it is quite another thing to realize them in practice. It is quite possible to build a pavilion hospital with almost as many defects as the principle presents advantages and it is in this way that good principles are confounded with bad ones. For example, if a piece of ground be selected for a pavilion hospital, which, from its size or shape or exposure, necessitates the giving up of any one of those details, the aggregate of which constitutes what is called the pavilion principle of construction, you can no longer obtain the advantages of the princi-

ple. Suppose your area is so contracted that you cannot place your pavilions at their proper distance from each other, namely, double their height, and you nevertheless persist in building a pavilion hospital, do not blame the principle because your wards are gloomy or even dark. Study the principle, therefore, in all its bearings, before you begin to build, and you will in this way avoid errors of application.>>

Source: From a dictated letter, signed by Nightingale, to W.H. Brace, Wellcome Ms 5482/32

Great Malvern
15 January 1859

Sir, Messrs Harrison, Printers, have forwarded to me your letter of the 12th instant [this month] relative to a report of mine upon hospitals. The report in question was prepared by order of the secretary of state for war and is a private document. It is therefore out of my power, as you will readily understand, to comply with your request for a copy.

I will gladly send you a paper of mine upon hospitals that was read at Liverpool, as soon as it is printed, although I fear it will not be of the use to you which you indicate.

Source: From a dictated letter, signed by Nightingale, to A.H. Clough,[20] Balliol College 305/8

Great Malvern
28 January 1859

Dear Mr Clough, Do you think that you would be so good as to send "the old plans, with Sutherland's insertions" to Dr Sutherland, 41 Finchley New Road, N.W., the day you receive this, if possible. There are a few odd mistakes in the proofs you were so good as to send me and I am sending them to him. He will correct them better if he has the old ones.

The "successful crystal poetess"[21] told me she was anxious to have the volume of transactions out by the end of this month and I am anxious not to be the one to delay it.

---

20 Arthur Hugh Clough (1819-61), poet, husband of cousin, and secretary to the Nightingale Fund Council.

21 Isa Craig (1831-1903), later Craig-Knox, assistant secretary to the National Association for the Promotion of Social Science. She won a prize for her Burns centenary poem, awarded at the Crystal Palace in 1858.

Source: From a dictated letter to Isa Craig, signed by Nightingale, Florence Nightingale Museum LDFNM 0867

Great Malvern
1 February 1859

My dear Madam

I beg to re-enclose to you the proofs, *corrected*, of the hospital plans for my paper, also the manuscript of an "explanation" of the plans, which ought to come at the end of the paper and before the plans. If you think that I ought to see the revises, I will trouble you to send them to me, otherwise not. I am very sorry to have given you so much trouble as it is.

I hope you will allow me to congratulate you on your poetical success. It gave me very great pleasure and I hope it did so to you, because it was so well deserved. Like Petrarch,[22] whose sonnets were the only embroidery of his life, while his serious occupation was something widely different, I think you succeed so well in poetry for the same reason.

Source: From a letter to William Farr, Wellcome Ms 5474/8

Highgate
13 June 1859

I have never thanked you for the corrected Crimean tables, including the deaths in battle.

I sent two copies of my *Notes on Hospitals* for Messrs Clode and Hammick to the General Registrar Office. Would you express to them my gratitude for the *nurse* tables, of which the fruits are there, as you will perhaps point out to them. And should anybody else at your office have contributed to that labour, would you kindly tell me, as the least I can do is to send them copies to show that the labour has not been quite wasted.

Perhaps, too, again I am reckoning on 11bienfaits futurs" [future benefits] as p 2 of the same book records (in a note) our want of hospital forms.

Dr Aitken[23] has told me of three hospitals in Scotland where they would gladly accept and *use* them: Glasgow, Edinburgh and Dundee, if the forms were sent to them. . . .

I have had the erring page 30 reprinted. It is a curious specimen of printers' corrections (?). Both the first proof and the revise were right,

22 Francesco Petrarch (1304-74), Italian poet.

23 William Aitken (1825-92), later Sir, member of the pathology commission in the Crimean War.

as I find on reference. The printers put in the error of their own heads from the "press" copies.

Editor: George Godwin, editor of *The Builder,* described the 1859 publication of *Notes on Hospitals* as a "separate and inexpensive" form of her papers given at Liverpool, which "we strongly advise all architects obtain . . . and master."[24] As the next letter explains, Nightingale sent the original manuscript to the mayor of Liverpool, William Preston, for deposit at the Free Library of Liverpool.

Source: From a letter to William Preston, Liverpool Record Office

13 September 1859

I was happy to accede to the request conveyed to me by Lord Shaftesbury that the manuscript to which you refer in your most kind letter of 22 August should be placed at the disposal of the council. If any value attaches to the written copy, I shall be very glad that it shall remain in the Free Library of Liverpool—a town to which I, of all others, owe the most grateful admiration, as out of her has come, as I have always considered, sanitary salvation to the army of the Crimea and to all England, more or less.

I venture to send the published copy of the same manuscript and two others on the same subject, hoping that you will do me the honour to add them to the same Free Library.

I regret that my increasing ill health has delayed so long my grateful reply to your kind letter.

Editor: Nightingale sent a copy of the 1859 edition of *Notes on Hospitals* to Theodor Fliedner at Kaiserswerth, with an inscription: "Pastor Fliedner, in remembrance of her 'education' at Kaiserswerth, Florence Nightingale, September 1860."[25]

The work for a new edition began in 1862 and went well into 1863.

---

24 "Hospital Construction: The Hospital of Lariboisière," *The Builder* 17,855 (25 June 1859):417.

25 Theodor Fliedner (1800-64). This copy belongs to the Kaiserswerth Diakoniewerk Archives.

Source: From a letter to William Farr, Wellcome Ms 5474/57, typed copy Add Mss 43399 f90

15 November 1862

I am (sadly and unwillingly) doing a third edition of my *Notes on Hospitals* for Parkers, which was promised eighteen months ago, before my misfortunes.[26]

In the weekly for 21 February 1852, you gave a table of the mortality of the London hospitals. Could you give us such a table for such a number of years as would enable a general *life table* of the London hospitals to be calculated (excluding the question of age, of course). It would tell very much if we could show that each hospital has its own *life risk*, and would add another argument to the case against those hospitals.

Could a similar case be made for a few of the best country hospitals in open districts? This would be very useful in the comparison. But at all events the London table would tell its own tale. I need hardly say that I would gladly pay (for any such information) a fee, such as would be given to any less celebrated actuary.

Source: From a letter to John Clark-Kennedy,[27] Wellcome RAMC 801/9/19/4

14 July 1863

I have been bound to the publishers of my *Notes on Hospitals* for two years to prepare them a third edition of it, but have never fairly begun it till now. My object in this formal announcement is to ask you whether you would be so good as to allow me to print in the Appendix (as enclosed) part of your admirable description of the men's convalescent institution at Vincennes, and to mention in the text from whom I had it, by name, while giving a short account of the object of the institution.

I have had prepared a place, taken from your sketch (by a regular copyist) for the woodcutter. I have never had any account or plan of the institution nearly so instructive as yours. And I have been able to obtain no official account of it—it not being under the Assistance Publique.

---

26 The deaths in August and October 1861, respectively, of Sidney Herbert and Arthur Hugh Clough.

27 John Clark-Kennedy (1817-67), quartermaster general after the Crimean War (see p 168 below).

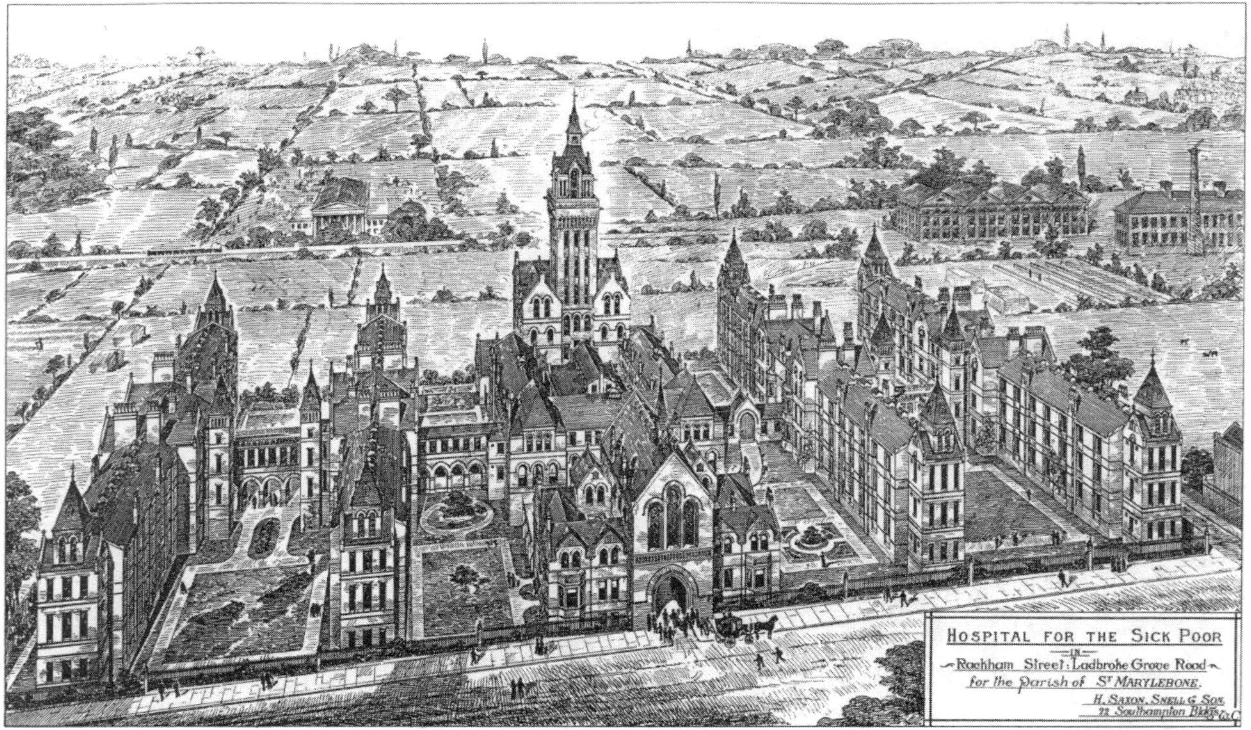

St Marylebone Workhouse Infirmary, new pavilion hospital. From Henry Saxon Snell, *Charitable and Parochial Institutions*, p 11.

Notes on Hospitals, 3RD EDITION 1863

The 1863 edition of *Notes on Hospitals* is so massively augmented and rewritten that it is effectively a new book. As well, Nightingale removed the appendixes of the 1859 edition, which reprinted her "Answers to Written Questions" and her three articles from *The Builder*. A new preface boldly asserts the need for a Hippocratic oath for hospitals akin to that for doctors: that they should "do the sick no harm," even though it was "a strange principle to enunciate as the very first requirement." Nevertheless, Nightingale considered it necessary to state such a principle, especially for hospitals in large crowded cities, which had mortality rates higher than those that occurred for the same class of diseases in patients treated at home.

By 1863 some progress had been made in Britain on Nightingale's ideas of hospital reform. The massive army hospital at Netley opened in 1863, not what it should be, Nightingale thought, but substantially improved from its original plans. The model pavilion hospital for Woolwich, designed by Douglas Galton, with much input from Nightingale, was under way in that same year, to open as the Herbert Hospital in 1865. Designs for civil pavilion hospitals had been drawn up by that time, although none had actually been built. Nightingale was acutely aware of how tough a struggle it was to convince hospital boards of the new ideas, and her correspondence from this period, and for decades following, shows how often basic points had to be remade. The situation at the new hospitals at Winchester and Derby, where Nightingale had strong allies, serve as examples of the tenacity of the old guard, who took much time and effort to be persuaded.

The reason for a new book, as given in the new preface, was not just the need to spread understanding of the progress that had been made since 1858, but also to spread knowledge of those principles that had not yet been established. Nightingale then outlined the five subjects of the book, of which only the first two had been treated in the original 1858 paper: (1) an overview of actual sanitary conditions in hospitals and (2) a list of defects. Nightingale regrouped the sixteen defects of the 1858 paper into ten, but expanded the content considerably. Next came three completely new sections, the first of which put forward (desirable) principles of construction, with examples of improved plans, for both hospitals and convalescent institutions. The second section reported the statistical form adopted by the International Statistical Congress, and the third was a proposed form for recording outcomes for a long list of types of surgery, supplied by surgeons she canvassed.

In the introductory section, Nightingale fleshed out the "four defects" of her original paper. To the first defect—that of large numbers under one roof—she added the dangers of mismanagement and liability to unforeseen events increasing with size. The Scutari Barrack Hospital furnished "confirmation," she said, for it contained "perhaps the largest number of sick ever at one time under the same roof," 2500, where (during its worst time) two out of every five patients died. She added the example of the Hôtel-Dieu in Paris, before its reconstruction, when it held 1200 beds. A major established hospital in peacetime, it housed 2000 and up to 4000 or even 7000 sick, with bed-sharing, and one in four there died.

In the expanded 1863 edition, Nightingale explained that the cost of land was too high in cities and towns to secure adequate light and ventilation for hospitals. Town hospitals were typically three or four storeys high, whereas country hospitals could be spread out over a larger surface area. Desirably, Nightingale always argued, hospitals would be one storey high, at most two. When she could not stop hospitals from building in towns she retreated to urging their pairing with a convalescent institution in the country, moving patients into it as quickly as possible. To her, a central location was needed only for accidents and emergencies.

While only four plans were included in the second edition of *Notes on Hospitals*, as an appendix, the third edition contained eleven full pages of plans, placed in the appropriate section of the book, along with many smaller plans and figures, also placed where they fit in the text. The four provided in the second edition reappear here, namely, the two positive French plans (Lariboisière and Vincennes) and the two negative British plans (Netley and King's College, the latter demoted to a smaller sketch). However, positive British plans (meaning by British architects) appear for the first time in the third edition: the Bucks Infirmary, Herbert Hospital, three Malta hospitals, the Herbert convalescent home and the Lisbon Children's Hospital. A number of bad British examples are represented by small sketches: the Royal Free Hospital (London), Portsmouth Military, Manchester Royal Infirmary, Marine Hospital (Woolwich), St Bartholomew's, a convalescent home (Walton-on-Thames), several Indian military hospitals and native hospitals. The Naval Hospital, Yarmouth, is described as one of the best of the older hospitals. Two further French good examples were added (a maternity hospital, Hôpital de la Clinique, and a convalescent home, Garches).

Whole new chapters are provided in the third edition, on convalescent hospitals, children's hospitals, Indian military hospitals, hospitals for soldiers' wives (all the above with plans) and hospital statistics (with model forms).

The chapter on statistics built on the work Nightingale and her colleagues had done for the International Statistical Congress of 1860. Sample forms are given on hospital admissions and discharges, an annual report (tracking in-patients and out-patients), costs per patient per bed, and "sanitary statistics of wards," with entries required for the dimensions of each ward, its windows, type of ventilation, toilet and bathing facilities. The intent is clear: to make it as easy as possible for hospitals to keep meaningful statistics and learn from them.

In this statistics chapter Nightingale argued for indicators of hospital *success*, in effect—not just mortality rates. "If the function of a hospital were to kill the sick," she drily observed, statistical comparisons of this nature would be "admissible." Their "proper function," however, was "to restore the sick to health as speedily as possible," hence information was required on the proportion of sick restored to health and the average time required (see p 85 below). Judgments of hospitals based solely on mortality, moreover, could be "fallacious," since the proportion of serious cases varied by hospital. Instead, the origin and spread of fever, gangrene, erysipelas and pyemia were "better tests of the defective state" of hospitals than their mortality returns (see p 86 below). Further, "no stronger condemnation of any hospital or ward could be pronounced than the simple fact that any zymotic disease has originated in it, or that such diseases have attacked other patients," in short, to have patients acquiring new diseases while in hospital.

The hospital mortality figures Nightingale used, developed by William Farr, caused much offence as they look abnormally high, a point that shall be returned to (see p 225 below). Briefly, for London hospitals a rate of 90.84 percent appears, meaning that over a year's time 90.84 deaths occurred per 100 beds, not that 90.84 percent of the patients admitted died; deaths per admissions, the more usual rate, would have been lower. The rate per bed per year is a meaningful one for comparative purposes, but it does startle. In the Registrar General's report of these data, a suitable qualification was added, a point omitted in Nightingale's publication.

For cross-references the page numbers in this volume have been substituted for the original.

Source: Florence Nightingale, *Notes on Hospitals*, 3rd edition (London: Longman, Green, Longman, Roberts and Green 1863)

Preface

It may seem a strange principle to enunciate as the very first requirement in a hospital that it should do the sick no harm. It is quite necessary, nevertheless, to lay down such a principle, because the actual mortality *in* hospitals, especially in those of large crowded cities, is very much higher than any calculation founded on the mortality of the same class of diseases among patients treated *out of* hospital would lead us to expect. The knowledge of this fact first induced me to examine into the influence exercised by hospital construction on the duration and death rate of cases received into the wards, and it led me to lay before the Social Science Association a paper reprinted with the present title. Since the publication of the first edition of that paper, great advances have been made in the adoption of sound principles of hospital construction, and there are already a number of examples of new hospitals realizing all, or nearly all, the conditions required for the successful treatment of the sick and maimed poor. Besides this, much additional experience has been obtained in many important points, especially in the details of hospital buildings and fittings.

In order to spread a knowledge of the progress already made, as well as of those principles which may now be considered as established, I have been asked to prepare the present edition. In doing this, it has been necessary to rewrite nearly the whole of it, and to make so many additions to the matter that it is in reality a new book.

F.N.

Notes on Hospitals

It is proposed in the following pages to give, first, a general account of the sanitary condition of existing hospitals; and a statement of those structural defects in hospitals which have influenced the progress of medical and surgical cases while under treatment in them; third, the principles of construction which ought to be kept in view in building new hospitals; fourth, improved plans for hospitals and convalescent institutions; and lastly, certain proposals adopted by the International Statistical Congress for improving the method of tabulating hospital statistics, together with a proposal for a uniform system of registering statistics of surgical operations, their complications and results.

1. Sanitary Condition of Hospitals

No one, I think, who brings ordinary powers of observation to bear on the sick and maimed can fail to observe a remarkable difference in the aspect of cases, in their duration and in their termination in different hospitals. To the superficial observer there are two things only apparent—the disease and the remedial treatment, medical or surgical. It requires a considerable amount of experience, in hospitals of various constructions and varied administrations, to go beyond this, and to be able to perceive that conditions arising out of these elements have a very powerful effect indeed upon the ultimate issue of cases which pass through the wards.

It is sometimes asserted that there is no such striking difference in the mortality of different hospitals as one would be led to infer from their great apparent difference in sanitary condition. There is, undoubtedly, some difficulty in arriving at correct statistical comparison to exhibit this. For, in the first place, different hospitals receive very different proportions of the same class of diseases. The ages in one hospital may differ considerably from the ages in another. And the state of the cases on admission may differ very much in each hospital. These elements affect considerably the results of treatment, altogether apart from the sanitary state of hospitals. But the fact has sometimes been made use of in a way no one could have anticipated. A high and increasing death rate has been actually put forward, not as the result of these causes, but as the result of increasing celebrity, which can have no other practical meaning than this, that a greater number of people go there to die next year, because so many have died there this year, a principle equally applicable in private practice, and according to which the physician or surgeon who loses the largest percentage of cases is the man most worthy of confidence.

In the next place, accurate hospital statistics are much more rare than is generally imagined, and at the best they only give the mortality which has taken place *in* the hospitals, and take no cognizance of those cases which are discharged in a hopeless condition, to die immediately afterwards, a practice which is followed to a much greater extent by some hospitals than by others.

We have known incurable cases discharged from one hospital to which the deaths ought to have been accounted, and received into another hospital, to die there in a day or two after admission, thereby lowering the mortality rate of the first at the expense of the second.

Making every allowance for difficulties attending an inquiry into the comparative mortality of hospitals, there are, nevertheless, certain very startling facts which ought to arrest the attention of everyone interested in the welfare of sick or maimed. The Registrar General, in his last Annual Report, has given a set of Occasional Tables on the Mortality of Public Institutions in England, which contain data of more than usual interest and importance on this subject. Returns were obtained from 106 hospitals, giving the number of inmates in each hospital on 8 April 1861. This number is taken as an approximation to the average of inmates at each establishment. The number of deaths registered in each hospital during the year 1861 is also given—so that, assuming the approximate accuracy of the data, the mortality percent in each hospital can be ascertained for the year. The following classified abstract contains the results of the inquiry, and they are certainly striking enough.

Mortality Percent in the Principal Hospitals of England, 1861

	No. of special inmates on 8 April 1861	Average no. of inmates in each hospital	No. of deaths registered in the year 1861	Mortality percent on inmates
In 106 principal hospitals of England	12,709	120	7,227	56.87
24 London hospitals	4,214	176	3,828	90.84
14 hospitals in large towns	1,870	156	1,555	83.16
25 county and important provincial hospitals	2,248	90	886	39.41
30 other hospitals	1,136	38	457	40.23
13 naval and military hospitals	3,000	231	470	15.67
1 Royal sea bathing infirmary (Margate)	133	133	17	12.78
1 Dane Hill metropolitan infirmary (Margate)	108	108	14	12.96

It will be seen that the hospitals are grouped according to locality. Now let us compare three of these groups with each other. We have twenty-four London hospitals affording a mortality of no less than 90.84 percent, very nearly every bed yielding a death in the course of the year. Next, we have twelve hospitals in large provincial towns, Bristol, Birmingham, Liverpool, Manchester, etc., yielding a death rate of 83.16 percent. And there are twenty-five county hospitals in country towns, the mortality in which is no more than 39.41 percent. Here we have at once a hospital problem demanding solution. However the great differences in the death rates may be explained, it cannot be denied that the most unhealthy hospitals are those situated within the vast circuit of the metropolis, that the next lower death rate takes place in hospitals in densely populated large manufacturing and commercial towns, and that by far the most healthy hospitals are those of the smaller country towns.

These results are quite reliable, and are preferable to those derived from individual hospitals. Otherwise, it might be stated that the death rate of certain hospitals situated in large towns is so enormous that every bed is cleared out in the year, and in some of them once in about nine months.

Facts such as these (and it is not the first time that they have been placed before the public) have sometimes raised grave doubts as to the advantages to be derived from hospitals at all, and have led many a one to think that in all probability a poor sufferer would have a much better chance of recovery if treated at home.

The sanitary state of any hospital ought not, however, to be inferred solely from the greater or less mortality. If the function of a hospital were to kill the sick, statistical comparisons of this nature would be admissible. As, however, its proper function is to restore the sick to health as speedily as possible, the elements which really give information as to whether this is done or not are those which show the proportion of sick restored to health, and the average time which has been required for this object; a hospital which restored all its sick to health after an average of six months' treatment could not be considered as by any means so healthy as a hospital which returned all its sick recovered in as many weeks. The proportion of recoveries, the proportion of deaths and the average time in hospital must all be taken into account in discussions of this nature, as well as the character of the cases and the proportion of different ages among the sick, and this brings me to the great importance of correct hospital statistics as an essential element in hospital administration.

Hospital mortality statistics have hitherto given little information on the efficiency of the hospital, i.e., as to the extent to which it fulfills the purpose it was established for, because there are elements in existence of which such statistics have hitherto taken no cognizance. In one set of hospitals in the table, I find the mortality from 12½ to 15½ percent upon the cases treated, while in other hospitals the deaths reach from 83 to 90½ percent. To judge by the mortality only in these cases would be most fallacious. Because in the first class of hospitals, ailments not of a dangerous nature constitute a title to hospital admission, while in the latter class of hospitals, dangerous and special diseases, at all times accompanied by a high rate of mortality, are largely admitted. Hence the duration of the cases admitted, and the general course and aspect of disease, afford important criteria whereby to judge of the healthiness or unhealthiness of any hospital, in addition to that afforded by the mortality statistics.

Perhaps the most delicate test of sanitary condition in hospitals is afforded by the progress and termination of surgical cases after operation, together with the complications which they present. The statistics of medical cases, although affording important data for our purpose, are of themselves imperfect indices of the healthiness of wards, but it is otherwise with operation cases. In these the constitution gives immediate evidence of suffering from the neglect of hygiene, and many a life is sacrificed from not recognizing this fact. In another section I have dealt with this important subject, and have given the method of keeping the statistics of hospitals proposed by me, and adopted by the International Statistical Congress, and also a proposal for registering surgical operations and their results.

Careful observers are now generally convinced that the origin and spread of fever in a hospital, or the appearance and spread of hospital gangrene, erysipelas and pyemia generally, are much better tests of the defective sanitary state of a hospital than its mortality returns.

(The following suggestive passages from Mr Paget's[1] address delivered before the British Medical Association, 1862, have an important bearing on this subject:

> In every case of erysipelas, pyemia or the like, we ought to work till we can discover its probable origin; we should have the strongest feeling that these diseases are not spontaneous nor inevitable. In

1 James Paget (1814-99), later Sir, surgeon, close ally of Nightingale's.

every case, the hospital, or the house, or our own practice, should be brought to trial—to private trial, if you will, yet a just and true trial—a trial before our own conscience, and if the hospital, the house or the practice be found guilty, let it be condemned and amended.

Of all the remedies I have used or seen in use, I can find but one thing that I can call remedial for the whole disease, pyemia, and that is a profuse supply of fresh air. In the three most remarkable recoveries I have seen, the patients might be said to have lain day and night in the wind—wind blowing all about their rooms.)

But I would go further and state that to the experienced eye of a careful observing nurse, the daily, I had almost said hourly, changes which take place in patients, and which changes rarely come under the cognizance of the periodical medical visitor, afford a still more important class of data from which to judge of the general adaptation of a hospital for the reception and treatment of sick. One insensibly allies together restlessness, languor, feverishness and general *malaise*, with closeness of wards, defective ventilation, defective structure, bad architectural and administrative arrangements, until it is impossible to resist the conviction that the sick are suffering from something quite other than the disease inscribed on their bed ticket, and the inquiry insensibly arises in the mind, what can be the cause? To this query many years' experience of hospitals in various countries and climates enables me to answer explicitly as the result of my own observation that even admitting to the full extent the great value of the hospital improvements of recent years, a vast deal of the suffering, and some at least of the mortality, in these establishments is avoidable.

What, then, are those defects to which such results are to be attributed? I should state at once that to original defects in the sites and plans of hospitals, and to deficient ventilation and overcrowding accompanying such defects, is to be attributed a large proportion of the evil I have mentioned.

The facts flow almost of necessity from ascertained sanitary experience. But it is not often, excepting perhaps in the case of intelligent house surgeons, that the whole process whereby the sick, who ought to have had repaid recoveries, are retained week after week, or perhaps month after month, in hospital, is continuously observed. I have known a case of slight fever received into hospital, the fever pass off in less than a week, and yet the patient, from the foul state of the wards, not restored to health at the end of eight weeks.

I appeal to all careful hospital officers whether each has not known, within his own experience, instances on a large and fatal scale of disease produced in hospital; I myself could fill a book with them. One such may be given. In a small hospital, in one of the healthiest counties in England,[2] in nine months, twenty-four poor creatures ran the gauntlet of their lives from erysipelas alone, of which disease eight died, and most of these after very trifling accidents or operations. None of them ought to have produced erysipelas at all, much less have ended fatally.

But on the very threshold of the subject we shall probably be told that to "contagion" and "infection" is much of the unhealthy condition of some hospitals attributable, at least so far as concerns the occurrence of zymotic diseases. On the very threshold, therefore, we are obliged to make a digression in order to discuss the meaning of these two familiar words, and to lay these spectres which have terrified almost all ages and nations.

This is the more necessary, because on the exact influence exercised by these two presumed causes of hospital sickness and mortality depends to a great degree the possibility of our introducing efficient hospital attendance and nursing. Unfortunately both nurses (see Note A, at the end of this section) and medical men, as well as medical students, have died of zymotic diseases prevailing in hospitals. It is an all-important question to decide whether the propagation of such diseases is inevitable or preventible. If the former, then the whole question must be considered as to whether hospitals necessarily attended with results so fatal should exist at all. If the latter, then it is our duty to prevent their propagation.

The idea of "contagion," as explaining the spread of disease, appears to have been adopted at a time when, from the neglect of sanitary arrangements, epidemics attacked whole masses of people, and when men had ceased to consider that nature had any laws for her guidance. Beginning with the poets and historians, the word finally made its way into medical nomenclature (see Note B, at the end of this section), where it has remained ever since, affording to certain classes of minds, chiefly in the southern and less-educated parts of Europe, a satisfactory reason for pestilence, and an adequate excuse for non-exertion to prevent its recurrence.

And now, what does "contagion" mean? It implies the communication of disease from person to person by *contact.* It presupposes the

2 The Winchester Infirmary, on which there is much correspondence on building a new infirmary on a new site (see p 585 below).

existence of certain germs, like the sporules of fungi, which can be bottled up and conveyed any distance attached to clothing, to merchandise, especially to woollen stuffs, for which it is supposed to have a particular affection, and to feathers, which of all articles it especially loves—so much so, that, according to quarantine laws, a live goose may be safely introduced from a plague country, but if it happen to be eaten on the voyage, its feathers cannot be admitted without danger to the entire community. There is no end to the absurdities connected with this doctrine. Suffice it to say that, in the ordinary sense of the word, there is no proof such as would be admitted in any scientific inquiry that there is any such thing as "contagion."

There are two or three diseases in which there is a specific virus, which can be seen, tasted, smelt and analyzed, and which in certain constitutions propagates the original disease by inoculation, such as smallpox, cowpox, etc. But these are not "contagions" in the sense supposed.

(Curiously enough, these directly communicable diseases were excluded from the operation of general quarantine law by the International Quarantine Conference of Paris, 1851, which restricted the objects of quarantine to plague, yellow fever and cholera, while it gave a logical *coup de grâce* to the "contagion" hypothesis by abolishing the "suspected bill of health.")

The word "infection," which is often confounded with "contagion," expresses a fact, and does not involve a hypothesis. But just as there is no such thing as "contagion," there is no such thing as *inevitable* "infection." Infection acts through the air. Poison the air breathed by individuals, and there is infection. Shut up 150 healthy people in a black hole of Calcutta (see p 53 above), and in twenty-four hours an infection is produced so intense that it will, in that time, have destroyed nearly the whole of the inmates. Sick people are more susceptible than healthy people, and if they be shut up without sufficient space and sufficient fresh air, there will be produced not only fever, but erysipelas, pyemia and the usual tribe of hospital-generated epidemic diseases.

Again, if we have a fever hospital with overcrowded, badly-ventilated wards, we are quite certain to have the air become so infected as to poison the blood, not only of the sick, so as to increase their mortality, but also of the medical attendants and nurses, so that they also shall become subjects of fever.

It will be seen at a glance that, in every such case and in every such example, the "infection" is not inevitable, but simply the result of carelessness and ignorance. As soon as this practical view of the subject is admitted and acted upon, we shall cease to hear of hospital contagions.

In certain hospitals it has been the custom to set apart wards for what are called "infectious" diseases, but in reality there ought to be no diseases so considered. With proper sanitary precautions, diseases reputed to be the most "infectious" may be treated in wards among other sick without any danger. Without proper sanitary arrangements, a number of healthy people may be congregated together so as to become subject to the worst horrors of "infection."

No stronger condemnation of any hospital or ward could be pronounced than the simple fact that any zymotic disease has originated in it, or that such diseases have attacked other patients than those brought in with them. And there can be no stronger condemnation of any town than the outbreak of fatal epidemics in it. Infection, and incapable management, or bad construction, are, in hospitals as well as in towns, convertible terms.

It was necessary to say thus much to show to what hospital diseases are *not* necessarily due. To the following defects in site, construction and management, as we think, they are mainly to be attributed.

1. *The agglomeration of a large number of sick under one roof.* It is a well-established fact that, other things being equal, the amount of sickness and mortality on different areas bears a ratio to the degree of density of the population.

Why should undue agglomeration of sick be any exception to this law? Is it not rather to be expected that, the constitutions of sick people being more susceptible than those of healthy people, they should suffer more from this cause?

There is a reason, of course, for everything, and in the present case the reason why agglomeration of a large number of sick under one roof leads to disaster is the simple fact that agglomeration argues either stern necessities of another kind, or great ignorance and danger of mismanagement, and besides all this, it argues unforeseen events, and altogether such a deficiency in the general administrative arrangements as is sure to be accompanied by want of proper ventilation, want of cleanliness and other sanitary defects.

If anything were wanting in confirmation of this fact, it would be the enormous mortality in the hospitals which contained perhaps the largest number of sick ever at one time under the same roof, viz., those at Scutari. The largest of these too-famous hospitals [the Barrack Hospital] had at one time 2500 sick and wounded under its roof, and it has happened that, of Scutari patients, two out of every five have died. In the hospital tents of the Crimea, although the sick were almost without shelter, without blankets, without proper food or medicines, the mortality was not above one half what it was at Scutari, but these tents had only a few beds in each. Nor was it even so high as this in the small Balaclava General Hospital, which had part of its sick placed in detached wooden huts. While in the well-ventilated detached huts of the Castle Hospital, on the heights above Balaclava, exposed to the sea breeze, at a subsequent period, the mortality among the wounded did not reach three percent. It is not to the comparative healthiness of these small hospitals, however, that we appeal as the only proof of the danger of surface overcrowding. It is to the fact of eighty cases of hospital gangrene having been recorded during one month at Scutari (and many, many more passed unrecorded); to the fact that, out of 44 secondary amputations of the lower extremities consecutively performed, 36 have died; and to the cases of fever which broke out in the hospital, not by tens, but by hundreds.

But by far the most remarkable illustration of the effects produced on the sick and maimed by agglomeration is that afforded by the experience of the Hôtel-Dieu, at the latter end of the last century, and before its reconstruction.

I am indebted to M Husson's *Étude sur les hôpitaux*[3] for a plan (No. 1) of the Hôtel-Dieu, as it then was, showing the relation of all parts of the hospital on the same floor. It will be observed that there was direct atmospheric communication through the entire suite of wards occupied by above 550 beds on a single floor. The whole hospital contained 1200 beds. But the number of beds by no means represented the number of sick, who were sometimes placed in the beds as close together as they could lie. In this way, from 2000 to 5000 or even 7000 sick were sometimes in the hospital at one time. And one out of every four patients used to die.

So late as the year 1788, *each of the beds* in the Hôtel-Dieu was intended to hold either two or four sick. There is an extremely curious notice of this subject in M Husson's *Étude sur les hôpitaux*, given in Note C at the end of this section. From this it appears that, in the sixteenth century, notwithstanding the use of multiple beds, holding, in 1515, from

3 Armand Husson (1809-74), director, Assistance Publique, author, *Étude sur les hôpitaux, considérés sous le rapport de leur construction, de la distribution et de leurs batiments,* 1862.

eight to twelve patients each, the number of sick so far exceeded the bed accommodation that the beds, in 1530, were occupied by relays of patients, and that forms were provided on which the sick whose turn it was to be out of bed could rest in the meantime.

Plan No. 1
Paris: Hotel-Dieu before the Fire of 1772

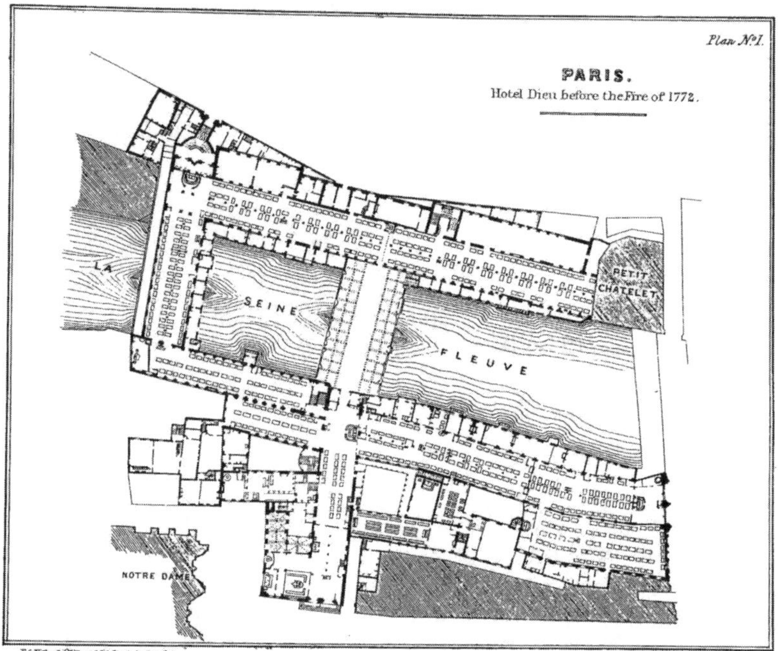

London Longman, Green & Cº

The subject is almost too painful to dwell on, especially as we must take it for granted that the administration of the period acted according to the best of its judgment. Only let the warning be taken. And let us not reproduce, even on a small scale, the same structural defects or mismanagement which led to such terrible loss of life. Fortunately for humanity, every patient has long since acquired the right to his own separate bed.

2. *Deficiency of Space per Bed.* Wherever cubic space is deficient, ventilation is bad. Cubic space and ventilation will therefore go hand in hand. The law holds good with regard to hospitals, barracks and all inhabited places.

If overcrowding, or its concomitant, bad ventilation, among healthy people, generates disease, it does so to a far greater extent among the sick in hospitals. In civil hospitals, the amount of cubic space varies between 600 and 2000 cubic feet per bed. In some military hospitals it used to be under 300, and from 700 to 800 was considered a somewhat extravagant allowance. The old army practice of allotting from 600 to 800 cubic feet per bed in hospitals, under which army hospitals proved to be so unhealthy, *was* overcrowding. At Scutari, at one time not even half the regulation space was given, and the great overcrowding consequent thereupon was one element in the disastrous result which followed.

Anyone in the habit of examining hospitals with different relative amounts of cubic space cannot fail to have been struck with the very different appearance of the sick, and with the different state of the ward atmosphere. Cubic space is an essential element in the question of ventilation. It is impossible, with due regard to warmth, to ventilate a ward in a brick or stone hospital without mechanical means, when the space per bed is less than a certain amount. Crowded wards are, in fact, offensive, with all the windows open.

In airy positions in the country, less cubic space is essential than in closely built towns. In detached huts or pavilions, especially if they be but one storey high, less space is necessary than where numbers are massed together in large buildings, or in more storeys than one.

Under all circumstances, however, the progress of the cases (in solidly built hospitals) will betray any curtailment of space much below 1500 cubic feet. In Paris 1700, and in London 2000 and even 2500 cubic feet are now thought advisable. But, query, should there be a hospital at all in any position which requires such an amount of space? Does not this very fact testify as loudly as it can, this is no fit place for sick?

The master of some large works in London lately mentioned the following fact: he was in the habit of sending those of his workmen who met with accidents to two different metropolitan hospitals. In one they recovered quickly; in the other they were frequently attacked with erysipelas, and some cases were fatal. On inquiry it appeared that in the former hospital a larger amount of space was allowed than in the latter, which is also so deficient in external ventilation and in construction that nothing but artificial ventilation could effectively change its atmosphere.

It is even more important to have a sufficient surface area between the adjoining and the opposite beds. Piling space above the patient is not all that is wanted. In the lofty corridors of Scutari I have seen two long rows of opposite beds with scarcely three feet from foot to foot. Certainly it cannot be thought too much, under any circumstances, to give to each bed a territory to itself of at least eight feet wide by twelve or thirteen feet long.

3. *Deficiency of Ventilation.* The want of fresh air may be detected in the appearance of patients sooner than any other want. No care or luxury will compensate indeed for its absence. Unless the air *within* the ward can be kept as fresh as it is *without*, the patients had better be away. What must then be said when, as in some town situations, the air *without* is not fresh air at all? Except in a few cases, well known to physicians, the danger of admitting fresh air directly is very much exaggerated. Patients in bed are not peculiarly inclined to catch cold, and in England, where fuel is cheap, somebody is indeed to blame if the ward cannot be kept warm enough, and if the patients cannot have bed clothing enough, for as much air to be admitted from without as suffices to keep the ward fresh.

("Catching cold" in bed follows the same law as "catching cold" when up. If the atmosphere is foul, and the lungs and skin cannot therefore relieve the system, then a draught upon the patient may give him cold. But this is the fault of the foul air, not of the fresh.

In the wooden hospital huts before Sebastopol, with their pervious walls and open ridge ventilators, in which the patients sometimes said that they "would get less snow if they were outside," such a thing as "catching cold" was never heard of. The patients were well covered with blankets, and were all the better for the cold air.)

No artificial ventilation will do this. Although in badly constructed hospitals, or in countries where fuel is dear and the winter very cold, artificial ventilation may be necessary, it never can compensate for the want of the open window. The ward is never fresh, and in the best hospitals at Paris, artificially ventilated, it will be found that, till the windows are opened, the air is close. A well-waged controversy has lately been carried upon this very point in Paris. Eminent authorities in England had decried the pavilion system, on the ground that the atmosphere of a certain Paris pavilion hospital was "detestable," not because of the pavilion architecture, but because of its artificial ventilation defying the best pavilion building to ventilate its patients. What is all that luxury of magnificent windows for but to admit fresh air? To shut up your patients tight in artificially warmed air is to bake them in a slow oven. Open the Lariboisière windows, warm it with open fires, drain it properly, and it will be one of the finest hospitals in the world.

Natural ventilation, or that by open windows and open fireplaces, is the only efficient means for procuring the life-spring of the sick—

fresh air. But to obtain this the ward should be at least fifteen to sixteen feet high, and the distance between the opposite windows not more than thirty feet. The amount of fresh air required for ventilation has been hitherto very much underrated, because it has been assumed that the quantity of carbonic acid produced during respiration was the chief noxious gas to be carried off. The total amount of this gas produced by an adult in twenty-four hours is about 40,000 cubic inches, which, in a barrack room, say, containing sixteen men, would give 370 cubic feet *per diem.* Allowing eight hours for the night occupation of such a room, when the doors and windows may be supposed to be shut, the product of carbonic acid would be 123 cubic feet, or about fifteen and a half cubic feet per hour. This large quantity, if not speedily carried away, would undoubtedly be injurious to health, but there are other gaseous poisons produced with the carbonic acid which have still greater power to injure. Every adult exhales by the lungs and skin forty-eight ounces, or three pints of water, in twenty-four hours. Sixteen men in a room would therefore exhale in eight hours sixteen pints of water, and 123 cubic feet of carbonic acid, into the atmosphere of the room. With the watery vapour there is also exhaled a large quantity of organic matter, ready to enter into the putrefactive condition. This is especially the case during the hours of sleep, and as it is a vital law that all excretions are injurious to health if re-introduced into the system, it is easy to understand how the breathing of damp foul air of this kind, and the consequent re-introduction of excrementitious matter into the blood through the function of respiration, will tend to produce disease.

If this be so for the well, how much more will it be so for the sick? For the sick, the exhalations from whom are always highly morbid and dangerous, as they are one of nature's methods of eliminating noxious matter from the body, in order that it may recover health. Indeed this is so well acknowledged that it has given rise to all the doctrine of infection—to a just horror of breathing what comes from the sick, even to the morbid fear of entering a cab in which a case of fever or smallpox has been for half an hour. Nay, we have heard a myth of scarlet fever being "carried in a bedside carpet."

One would think the inference in people's minds from these just (and unjust) terrors would be to remove instantly every hindrance to the foul air being carried off, but instead of that, their inference is to shut it up or to run away from the sick.

One would think that the first and last idea in constructing hospitals would be to contrive such means of ventilation as would be perpetually and instantly carrying off these morbid emanations. One would think that it would be the first thing taught to the attendants to manage such means of ventilation. Often, however, it is *not even* the *last* thing taught to them.

A much larger mass of air is required to dilute and carry away these emanations than is generally supposed, and the whole art of ventilation resolves itself into applying in any specific case the best method of renewing the air sufficiently without producing draughts, or occasioning excessive varieties in temperature. Trifling varieties are rather beneficial than otherwise in most cases. A cooler atmosphere at night acts like a tonic.

4. *Deficiency of Light.* What is the proportionate influence of the four defects enumerated in delaying recovery I am not competent to determine.

Second only to fresh air, however, I should be inclined to rank light in importance for the sick. Direct sunlight, not only daylight, is necessary for speedy recovery, except, perhaps, in certain ophthalmic and a small number of other cases. Instances could be given, almost endless, where, in dark wards or in wards with a northern aspect, even when thoroughly warmed, or in wards with borrowed light, even when thoroughly ventilated, the sick could not by any means be made speedily to recover. The effect of light on health and disease has been long recognized in the medical profession, as may be learned from the writings of Sir Andrew Wylie, Dr Milne-Edwards,[4] and Mr Ward. Dark barrack rooms, and barrack rooms with northern aspects, will furnish a larger amount of sickness than light and sunny rooms.

Among kindred effects of light I may mention, from experience, as quite perceptible in promoting recovery, the being able to see out of a window, instead of looking against a dead wall; the bright colours of flowers; the being able to read in bed by the light of a window close to the bed head. It is generally said that the effect is upon the mind. Perhaps so, but it is no less so upon the body on that account.

All hospital buildings in this climate should be erected so that as great a surface as possible should receive direct sunlight—a rule which has been observed in several of our best hospitals, but, I am sorry to say, passed over in some of those most recently constructed. Window blinds can always moderate the light of a light ward, but the gloom of a dark ward is irremediable.

---

4 Henri Milne-Edwards (1800-85), French zoologist.

The axis of a ward should be as nearly as possible north and south, the windows on both sides, so that the sun shall shine in (from the time he rises till the time he sets) at one side or the other. There should be a window to at least every two beds, as is the case now in our best hospitals. Some foreign hospitals, in countries where the light is far more intense than in England, give one window to every bed. The window space should be one third of the wall space. The windows should reach from two or three feet of the floor to one foot of the ceiling. The escape of heat may be diminished by plate or double glass. But while we *can* generate warmth, we cannot generate daylight, or the purifying and curative effect of the sun's rays.

NOTE A. ON THE MORTALITY OF HOSPITAL NURSES

To show the great importance of this point, I give the following tables, kindly prepared by Dr Farr from returns furnished to me with the greatest readiness by fifteen of the metropolitan hospitals. Table 1 gives the ages of living and dying among the nursing staff. Table 2 gives the mortality from zymotic diseases, and the comparison between the nurses' mortality and that of the female population of London.

TABLE 1

Numbers and Ages of Matrons, Sisters and Nurses (Living and Dying) in Fifteen London Hospitals

(Names of the Hospitals: St. Mary's; St. George's; Westminster; Charing Cross; Middlesex; University College; Royal Free; King's College; St. Bartholomew's; London; Guy's; St. Thomas'; Smallpox; Fever; and Consumption)

Living (1858)

		Total		Specified ages of the living, March 1858											
	Total of all ages	Ages specified	Ages *not* specified	Under 20	20	25	30	35	40	45	50	55	60	65	70 and up
Matrons, sisters and nurses	521	391	130	1	10	45	55	93	64	59	34	18	8	4	--
Matrons and sisters	118	90	28	--	--	4	11	22	16	20	8	5	3	1	--
Nurses	403	301	102	1	10	41	44	71	48	39	26	13	5	3	--

Dying (1848-57)

		Total		Ages of the Dying											
	Total of all ages	Ages specified	Ages *not* specified	Under 20	20	25	30	35	40	45	50	55	60	65	70 and up
Matrons, sisters and nurses	79	79	--	--	--	4	11	8	18	8	10	7	6	2	5
Matrons and sisters (so distinguished)*	19	19	--	--	--	--	2	1	4	--	3	2	1	1	5
Nurses	60	60	--	--	--	4	9	7	14	8	7	5	5	1	--

* In the returns of deaths, four hospitals do not distinguish the matrons and sisters from the nurses, and in this table they are included with the nurses.

Table 2
Mortality of Matrons, Sisters and Nurses, at Different Ages, in Fifteen London Hospitals, Compared with the Mortality of the Female Population of London

	Matrons, sisters and nurses (1848-1857)		Female population of London	
	Annual rate of mortality to 1000 living at the respective ages			
Ages	By *all* returned *diseases*	By *zymotic* diseases	By *zymotic* diseases (1848-57)	By *all* returned *diseases* (1848-54)
25 to 35	15.89	9.53	2.19	9.92
35 to 45	15.80	10.94	2.73	14.65
45 to 55	17.80	11.87	3.17	20.36
55 to 65	46.36	14.26	4.94	36.02

The fatal zymotic diseases included in this table are fever and cholera, and it will be seen that these two diseases occasioned nearly 50 percent of the total mortality among the nursing staff, as against 16 percent among the London female population. This single fact is quite enough to prove the very great importance of hospital hygiene. The calculated total mortality is also very much higher among the nurses, even if we assume that the deaths in the returns are all deaths due to hospital nursing, which is very doubtful. If we assume that the non-zymotic mortality among nurses ought to be the same as it is among the female population, and if to this we add the zymotic deaths among nurses, we find the total mortality among nurses to exceed the total mortality among the female population of the metropolis by about 40 percent. The loss of a well-trained nurse by preventible disease is a greater loss than is that of a good soldier from the same cause. Money cannot replace either, but a good nurse is more difficult to find than a good soldier.

The data from which these tables have been deduced are imperfect, and it would be very desirable if in future all hospitals would keep a register of nurses. The following form would be one well calculated to give the required information. The subject is of additional importance in connection with the proper working of a superannuation fund for nurses:

Form of Register of Sisters and Nurses in _____ Hospital (Commenced from 1 January 1859)

			Date			
No.	Name	Age when first appointed	Of appointment	Dismissal, resignation or superannuation	State of health on leaving the service; and, if ill, the disease, its duration and probable cause	Date of death, cause of death and fatal disease
1	Jane Jones (sister)	25	6 June 1858	Resigned 6 August 1858	In good health	
2	Mary Evans (nurse)	29	2 April 1848			7 July 1854, typhoid fever, after 11 days' illness

NOTE B. ON THE HISTORY OF THE DOCTRINE OF CONTAGION

The history of the doctrine of "contagion" is given by Dr Adams in his translation of the works of Paulus Aegineta, vol. 1, p 284 (Sydenham Society). He says, in his comment, "the earlier ancient authors appear to have entertained no suspicions of contagion as a cause of febrile or of other complaints." "The works of the fathers of history and of medicine have likewise been ransacked in vain for any traces of the doctrine of contagion."

Thucydides, and after him several of the Latin poets, describe the plague of Athens, which appears to have been a form of dysentery, as communicable from person to person.[5] The later Greek historians contain allusions to the infectious nature of certain diseases, but Procopius, though cognizant of one of the greatest pestilences on record, was a non-contagionist.[6] Virgil's allusions to contagious diseases among cattle will be found in Ecl. I Georg. III, 464.

Aretaeus appears to be the first medical author who believed in contagion. Galen seems to have held the doctrine of infection. Of the later Greek and Arabian medical writers, some were contagionists, and others make no allusion to

5 For citations see p 51 above.

6 Procopius (c500-85), Byzantine historian, described a great plague which killed an estimated 100 million people worldwide. He estimated in *The Wars of Justinian* deaths of 10,000 a day in Constantinople, which later historians give as 5000.

the subject. Dr Adams states, in regard to plague, a disease which, in later times, has been considered as the very type of all "contagious" pestilences:

> The result of our investigations into the opinions of the ancients on this subject leads us to the conclusion that all, or at least the most intelligent of the medical authorities, held that the plague was communicated not by any specific virus, but in consequence of the atmosphere around the sick being contaminated by putrid effluvia.[7]

The obvious practical result of this view of infection is that abundance of pure air will prevent infection. All my own hospital experience confirms this conclusion. If infection exists, it is preventible. If it exists, it is the result of carelessness, or of ignorance. "Contagion," as a doctrine on which distinct practical proceedings have been taken, appears to be of very modern invention, and it has been highly injurious to civilization and humanity, from the loss of life which has from time to time followed from the practices which it inculcates, and from the immense tax which it has entailed upon commerce.

Note C

"In 1788" (in the Hôtel-Dieu), "each bed was for two or for four sick."

"Much has been said about beds in two shelves, one over the other, in which up to eight and even twelve sick were said to have lain. Nothing in the archives justifies such an assertion. This tradition, derived from M de Pastoret,[8] doubtless originated in a passage of the Report of the Commissioners of the Académie des Sciences (1786, p 19), where it is said that in 1752 the sick were four and six in the same bed, and that some were lying on the testers of the beds, 'according to the testimony of a physician of the Hôtel-Dieu, who witnessed it.' This testimony is the more curious, because the 'Mémoire of the Physicians of the Hôtel-Dieu,' presented in 1756, makes no allusion to this circumstance, although the form of the beds takes up a very large share of the report."

"That, at times of extraordinary overcrowding, some of the sick should have been placed even on the wooden roof of the bed, as in 1752, when the Hôtel-Dieu had to receive more than 4000 sick, this fact would not be very surprising, but this was only a momentary expedient, and can only have taken place, if it did take place, from the period of the seventeenth century, for before that period the beds of the Hôtel-Dieu had no testers. It was then in beds that the sick lay, or rather were heaped up. In 1515, there were only 303 beds at the Hôtel-Dieu, 'in each of which, from want of space, are generally seen eight, ten and twelve poor in one bed, so crowded that it is a great pity to see them' " (Letters Patent of Francis I, 1515; *Archives of the Assistance Publique).*

"100 beds were placed in the new ward built by Cardinal Duprat in 1530. The following is an extract of the bargain made for the construction of these beds."

---

7 For citations see p 52 above.

8 Claude-Emmanuel de Pastoret (1755-1840), marquis.

"Jehan Morel, carpenter, living at Paris, has bargained with the governors to make proper beds to furnish the new ward which the legate is building to adjoin l'Hôtel-Dieu, i.e., up to the number of 100 beds, made as follows: each bed 6 feet long by 4 feet wide, the back 4 feet high, the division (or partition) the same height, all in plain panel, and all framed and open below; in the front of which beds two horizontal panels x x, on the pillow of which beds there shall be a board 6 inches in breadth, or thereabouts, for the service of the poor, under each of which beds there shall be a little form (bench) of the length of said beds, to be taken out to rest the said poor."

(Extract from the Registers, 1533.) The sick, being too many to lie all together in the same bed, necessarily relieved each other. And this little bench was no doubt intended to serve as a seat for those who were waiting their turn to lie down.

"In the seventeenth century, the beds of the Hôtel-Dieu were covered with a tester standing upon four massive feet, with curtains which, when drawn, completely shut in the bed."

"In 1781, Louis XVI[9] forbade more than two sick being placed in the same bed, and these were to be separated by a compartment or division. This did not satisfy the physicians of the Hôtel-Dieu, and it was decided:

1. That all the beds, single and double, should be 6½ feet high.
2. That all beds, single and double, should be 6 feet long overall.
3. That all single beds should be uniformly 3 feet wide overall.
4. That all double beds should be alike 5 feet 2 inches wide overall.
5. That the testers of all the said beds should have a strong crossbeam, for a cord to be solidly fastened, by which the sick can raise themselves" (*Deliberations, etc.*, 1781)."

"In 1791, the number of beds was still far from enough, as states a report of the Commission of Hospitals: 'In April 1791, there were only 1650 to 1700 beds, of which 580 to 590 were large beds; counting these for two, as well as those with divisions, the 1700 beds gave about room for 2300 sick, the sick who had a bed apiece being only 1700; 100 others lay two, three and even more in the large beds' (Report of the measures taken to accommodate at the Hôtel-Dieu, during the winter of 1792, 2500 sick, of whom 2000 in little beds, one in each bed, and 500 in large beds, *only two* together"; *Archives of the Assistance Publique.*)

2. Defects in Existing Hospital Plans and Construction

Considering, then, the conditions essential to the health of hospitals are principally these:

1. Fresh Air. 2. Light. 3. Ample Space. 4. Subdivision of Sick into Separate Buildings or Pavilions—let us examine the causes in the usual

9 Louis XVI (1754-93), king of France.

ward construction which prevent us from obtaining these and other necessary conditions. The principal causes are as follow, viz.:

1. Selection of Bad Sites and Bad Local Climates for Hospitals.

2. Construction of Hospitals on such a plan as to prevent Free Circulation of External Air.

3. Defects in Ward Construction injurious to Ventilation, including: Defective Height of Wards; excessive Width of Wards between the Opposite Windows; arranging the Beds along the Dead Walls; having more than two Rows of Beds between the opposite Windows; having Windows only on one Side; or having a closed Corridor connecting the Wards.

4. Defective Means of Natural Ventilation and Warming.

5. Defects of Drainage, Water Closets, Sinks, etc.

6. Using Absorbent Materials for Walls and Ceilings, and Washing Floors of Hospitals.

7. Defective Hospital Kitchens.

8. Defective Hospital Laundries.

9. Defective Accommodation for Nursing and Discipline.

10. Defective Ward Furniture.

1. *Selection of Bad Sites and Bad Local Climates for Hospitals.* As the object to be attained in hospital construction is to have pure dry air for the sick, it will be evident that this condition cannot be fulfilled if a damp climate be selected. It is a well-known fact, e.g., that in the more damp localities of the south of England, certain classes of sick and of invalids linger, and do not recover their health. Again, retentive clay subsoils keep the air over entire districts of the country always more or less damp. And soils of this character should not be selected as sites for hospitals. Self-draining, gravelly or sandy subsoils are best. River banks, estuary shores, valleys, marshy or muddy ground ought to be avoided. It may seem superfluous to state that a hospital should not be built over an old graveyard, or on other ground charged with organic matter, and yet this has been recently done. Although hospitals are intended for the recovery of health, people are very apt to forget this, and to be guided in the selection of sites by other considerations—such as cheapness, convenience and the like, whereas the professed object in view being to secure the recovery of the sick in the shortest time, and to obtain the smallest mortality, that object should be distinctly kept in view as one which must take precedence of all others.

Similar remarks are applicable to the erection of hospitals in large cities and towns. If the recovery of the sick *simply* is to be the object of hospitals, they will not be built among dense unhealthy populations. If medical schools are the object, surely it is more instructive for students to watch the recovery from, rather than the lingering in, sickness. Twice the number of cases would be brought under their notice in a hospital in which the sick recovered in half the time necessary in another.

According to all analogy, the duration of cases, the chances against complete recovery and, as has been shown, the rate of mortality, must be greater in town than in country hospitals.

Land in towns is too expensive for hospitals to be so built as to secure the conditions of ventilation and of light, and of spreading the inmates over a large surface area—conditions now known to be essential to speedy recovery—instead of piling them up three or four storeys high, in regions contaminated with coal smoke and nuisances.

In country towns, and even in the larger manufacturing and commercial towns, there is no great difficulty in building hospitals in the purer atmosphere of the open country or suburbs. The distance from any part of the town likely to send its sick or maimed can never be very great, and gratuitous medical and surgical service can be rendered without much inconvenience by the officers of the hospital. The distance, also, to be traversed by friends on visiting days is not so great as to cause undue loss of time. No legitimate excuse can therefore be urged for constructing hospitals amid the smoke, foul air and bustle of the densely peopled seats of commerce and manufactures. It is otherwise with such a place as London. Here the distances are so great, and the outward spread of the population so rapid, that the question of hospital position assumes quite another aspect to what it does in provincial towns.

The problem has been, besides, complicated by the nature of the hospital foundations which have been created at different periods of time, and under very different conditions of population. The various metropolitan hospitals have been erected, and their positions determined, on no general system of medical or surgical relief for the metropolis, and without any foresight, had it even been possible to exercise such, as to what would finally be the position of each hospital with reference to the population whose sick it was intended to receive.

The practical result has been that several of the largest and most important hospital establishments are concentrated within a comparatively narrow area of the metropolitan district. They receive their sick from a certain radius in every direction, extending often into and even beyond the district which would be allotted to other hospitals under a general system of hospital relief. And they receive their patients from distances of two, three, five or more miles, or even from the country round.

To illustrate this question as regards our metropolitan hospitals, I give a sketch plan of London, on which are shown the distances of all the larger hospitals in direct lines from one central point, St Paul's. Four hospitals only out of twenty-one are nearer than a mile. All the others are at distances varying from a mile to nearly five miles. The map shows that there are large areas of the metropolis which have to send their sick even greater distances than the average required by the French system, presently to be noticed, and that, practically, the question of distance has been little understood in controversies which have arisen on this subject.

One result which follows from this arrangement of the London hospitals is that a considerable proportion of the sick has been concentrated towards the heart of the metropolis, not unfrequently among dense masses of population and in unhealthy localities. It may be safely stated that, if all the existing general hospitals had been originally distributed at suitable distances from the middle of the metropolis, they would all have been placed as conveniently for the sick as they now are, and in much purer air. The question of moving existing hospitals has been mooted at different times, and has recently assumed a practical shape as regards one of them, St Thomas'.[10] A long and warm controversy has arisen on the subject, in which nearly every element incident to such questions has been discussed, with the ultimate probability that the future site of the hospital will be determined by no element incident to the question, but by circumstances only. It is worthwhile to consider briefly the main points which have been mooted in this important controversy.

The elements which ought to determine the position of a hospital are the following:

First, and before all others, purity of the atmosphere.

Second, the possibility of conveying the sick and maimed to it.

Third, accessibility for medical officers, and for the friends of the sick.

Fourth, convenient position for a medical school, if there be one.

---

10 For correspondence on this see p 775 below.

All of these elements are of importance, every one in its place. It is obviously of no use to build a hospital in the best air in the world if neither patients nor medical officers can get to it. It is only in applying common sense to such a question, and by always giving a preponderance to the condition of highest importance, namely, pure air, when the other conditions can be at the same time reasonably obtained, that the best will be done for the sick.

There is no doubt that suburban sites, nearest to the population likely to apply for relief, afford the best solution the case admits of with the ordinary means of conveyance. This is to a certain extent the system in Paris. Several of its best hospitals are in or close to the suburbs, and the sick are admitted under a rule which requires all applicants to appear before the medical officers at a central bureau, whence they are sent to the hospitals where there are vacant beds. Accidents and other cases of urgency may, however, be admitted at once into any hospital on certificate of one of the hospital physicians or surgeons. It will be seen that, under this system, the patient has to leave his home and present himself at the bureau, and from the bureau he has to go to the hospital. Some of the establishments are at a considerable distance from the bureau.

To illustrate the working of this system, I give a sketch plan of Paris showing the position of the Bureau of Admission, close to the Hôtel-Dieu, the distance in yards (in a direct line) from this bureau to each of the civil hospitals, and the number of beds they contain. It will be seen that four hospitals only are within a mile of the bureau, and that the remaining twelve are at distances of from a mile and half to two miles and a half in straight lines, to which probably a fourth should be added for bendings of streets, and from a third to a half for the average distance between the houses of the patients and the bureau. There appears to be no practical difficulty attending this, so far at least as the distance is concerned, but as already stated, urgent cases are admitted at any hospital at once on the certificate of a medical officer.

Of course the distances are all much less in Paris than they would be in London with a similar organization, and yet there are several special hospitals in London, e.g., those for consumption, smallpox and fever, which are at a far greater distance from some of the districts yielding them cases than are the distances in Paris.

All are agreed that fresh country air is better for the sick than impure town air, and hence the whole question narrows itself within the compass of one of the conditions enumerated above, namely, accessibility. Any site which can be obtained with pure air and sufficiently convenient means of access will fulfill the required conditions. It has been proposed to extend the distance by using railway conveyance. To this there can be no possible objection, if it is necessary. A few years ago no one could have predicated that a considerable portion of the metropolitan dead would be conveyed long distances by railway for interment, without inconvenience to friends or injury to their feelings, and yet it has been done. The truth is, however, that in regard to hospital sites, no precise general rule can be laid down.

If a new hospital is wanted, the true way to deal with the question is to determine whereabouts it must be; next, to seek out all the sites which there is a possibility of obtaining; then to have each examined by competent persons with reference to the elements already laid down, and to select the best.

This has been done in selecting recent hospital sites, and it has answered well enough in practice. The evil arising out of a contrary procedure is that parties are apt to be formed, especially among persons who are not sufficiently acquainted with the subject, one party advocating one site, another party another, and so the cause which all have at heart is injured.

If we could suppose such a thing as all the metropolitan hospitals being removed to the furthest accessible healthy points from their present positions, there cannot be a doubt that the sick would gain immensely by the change, except accidents or cases of severe and sudden illness. For these cases special wards would have to be provided at the points where they would be most required. There is no reason why all such cases should not be treated in this way, and sent to the suburban hospitals as soon as they were able to bear the journey. The hospital receiving rooms and dispensaries for out-patients might be attached to these accident wards.

Patients from the country would, of all others, benefit most by such a change, for they would be spared the additional risk of coming from the fresh air of their homes into the foul air of the metropolis—a change attended with more or less additional risk to them.

Even medical education would benefit by such a change. The quiet and studious habits of a college would be substituted for the desultory lecture hunting and hospital walking of London. Education might thus take the place of simple instruction.

2. *Construction of Hospitals on such a Plan as to prevent Free Circulation of External Air.* To build a hospital with one closed court with high

walls, or, what is worse, with two closed courts, is to stagnate the air even before it reaches the wards. This defect is one of the most serious that can be committed in hospital architecture, and it exists, nevertheless, in some form or other in nearly all the older hospitals, and in many even of recent construction.

The air outside the hospital cannot be maintained in a state sufficiently pure to be used for internal ventilation, unless there be entire freedom of movement. Anything which interferes with this is injurious. Neighbouring high walls, smoking chimneys, trees, high ground, are all more or less hurtful, but worse than all is bad construction of the hospital itself.

Examples of bad plan and construction are common enough. One of these (Fig. 1) is a block plan of the Hospital Necker at Paris.

In this case, it is true, the size of the inner court is so considerable that, to a certain extent, it obviates the objection. But where this principle of construction is applied in smaller buildings, the evil of it becomes obvious. Fig. 2 represents another form of the same defective plan. None of these arrangements should ever be used for hospitals.

All closed corners stagnate the air more or less, even where the building forms but three sides of a square, as in Fig. 3, unless the wings are so short that they can hardly be called wings.

The only safe plan with this form of construction is to leave the corners entirely open, as in Vincennes plan, where they are connected only by an arcade on the ground floor. (Plan No. 5).

Even in the true separate pavilion structure, unless the distance between the pavilions be double the height of the walls, the ventilation and light are seriously interfered with. For this, among other reasons, two storeys are better than three, and one is preferable to two, provided it be erected upon an arched basement.

To build a hospital in the midst of a crowded neighbourhood of narrow streets and high houses is to ensure a stagnation of the air without, which no ventilation within, no cubic space however ample, will be able to remedy. I shall return to this subject in discussing the question of what should be the relative position of different parts of a hospital.

3. *Defects in Ward Construction injurious to Ventilation.* One of the most common causes of unhealthiness in hospitals is defective construction and arrangement of the ward space, of such a nature as to lead to difficulty of ventilation, or want of light. The expression, "a good ward," comprehends something quite different from mere appearance. No

Figure 1
Block Plan of Hôpital Necker, Paris

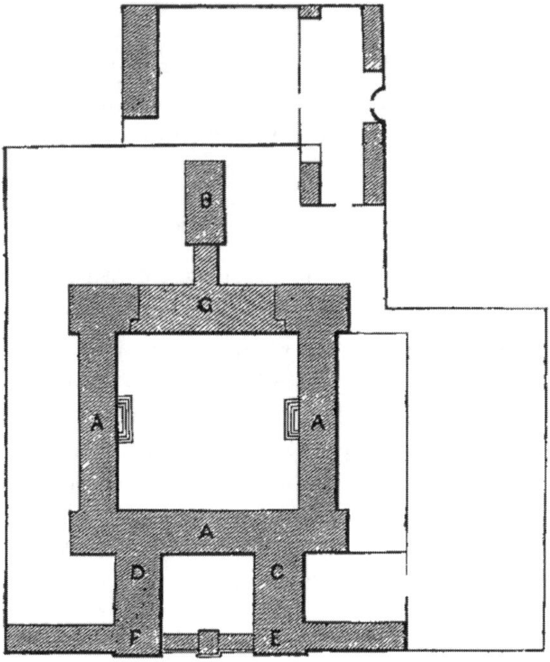

A. Wards.
B. Chapel.
C. Kitchen.
D. Pharmacy.
E. Offices and "Sisters."
F. Dwellings.
G. Gallery.

ward is in any sense a good ward in which the sick are not at all times supplied with pure air, light and a due temperature. These are the results to be obtained from hospital architecture, and not external design or appearance. Again, no one of these elements need be sacrificed in seeking to obtain another. Anyone who feels himself in a difficulty in realizing all three may rest satisfied that hospital architecture is not his vocation. A few of the more common errors may be here introduced as illustrative of this part of the subject.

Defective Height of Wards. It is not possible to ventilate sufficiently a large ward of ten or twelve feet high. And, again, it is not possible to ventilate a ward where there is a great height above the windows. A

Figure 2
Block Plan of the Royal Free Hospital, London

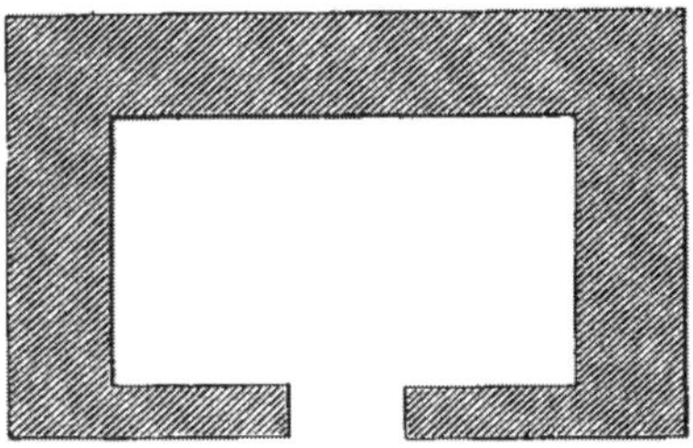

Figure 3
Block Plan of the London Hospital, London

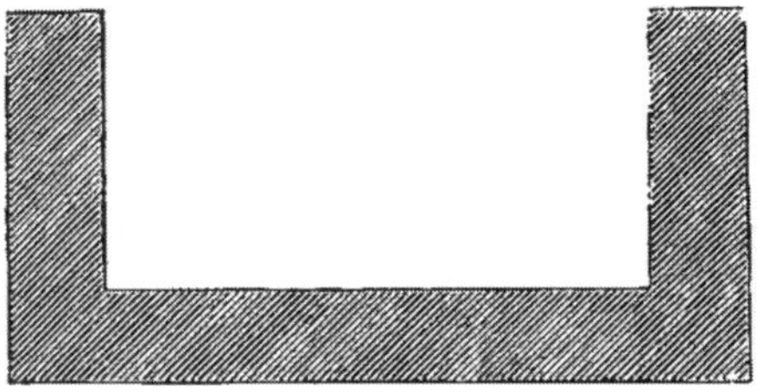

ward of thirty beds can be well ventilated with a height of about fifteen or sixteen feet, provided the windows reach to within one foot of the ceiling. Otherwise, the top of the ward becomes a reservoir for foul air. But a ward may be too high to be ventilated with sufficient ease. Good ventilation consists in emptying the hospital of foul air as speedily as possible. Why have a greater height of ward than will allow the windows and ventilating arrangements to be easily managed? It is more than probable that the decrease of facility for opening windows would lead to negligence, and so to the fine lofty ward becoming a reservoir of foul air.

Too Great Width of Wards between the Opposite Windows. It does not appear as if the air could be thoroughly changed if a distance of more than thirty feet intervenes between the opposite windows, if, in other words, the ward is more than thirty feet wide. This is the true starting point from which to determine the size of your ward and the number of beds you will have in it. If you make your length too great in proportion to this width, your ward becomes a tunnel—a form fatal to good ventilation. This was the case with the great corridor wards at Scutari.

If, on the other hand, you make your wards too short in proportion to this width, you multiply corners in a greater ratio than you multiply sick. And direct experiment has shown that the movement of the air in the centre of a ward is three or four times as great as it is at the corners. The movement of the air in a hospital ward should always be slightly perceptible over the face and hands, and yet there should be no draughts.

Arranging the Beds along the Dead Walls. This deprives the patient of the amount of light and air necessary to his recovery, and has, besides, the disadvantage that, when the windows are opened, the effluvia must blow over all the intervening beds before escaping. This arrangement is to be seen at Portsmouth Military Hospital (Fig. 4), Chatham Garrison Hospital, in the new part of the Edinburgh Infirmary, and at Netley Hospital (Plan 2).

Plan No. 2
Royal Victoria Hospital, Netley

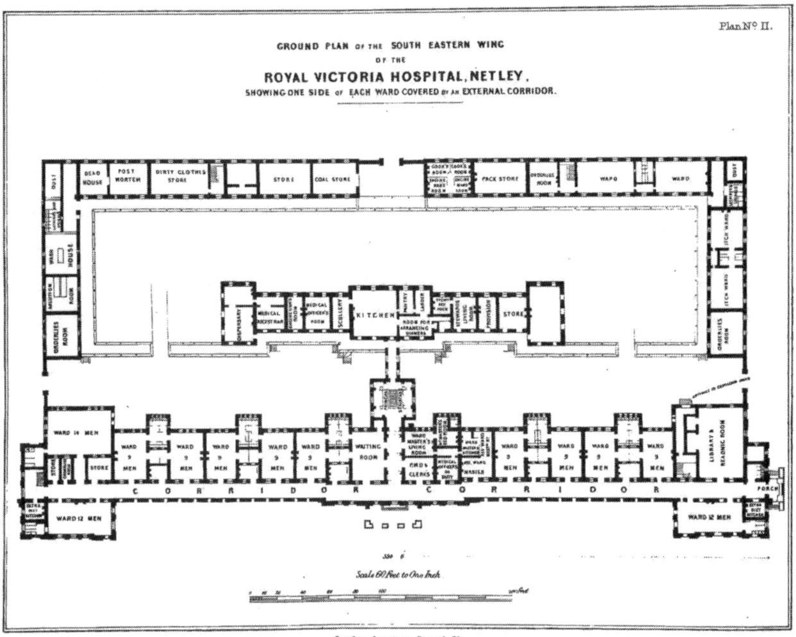

London Longman Green & C°

Another striking example of the same defect is given in Fig. 5, which formerly existed in the Accouchement Hospital at Paris.

Unfortunately, we have not to go abroad for existing examples of this construction. The following plan (Fig. 6), which represents the arrangement of a floor of Manchester Royal Infirmary, will tell its own tale.

Figure 4
Ward Construction—Portsmouth Military Hospital

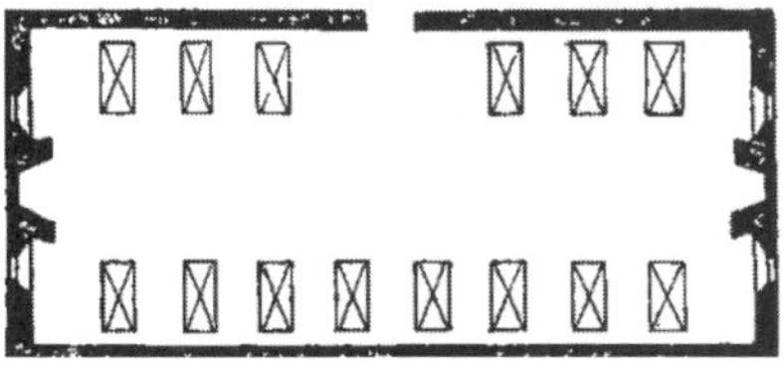

Figure 5
Hôpital de la Clinique, Paris

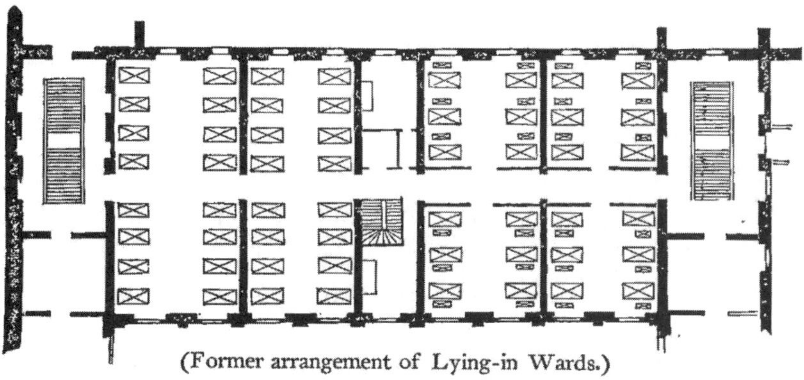

(Former arrangement of Lying-in Wards.)

It will be seen that, in all these examples, free renewal of the air is impossible, except for the beds close to the windows. It is needless to point out that plans of this kind should be abandoned in future. Another form of this arrangement is shown in Fig. 7, part of the old Marine Hospital at Woolwich. In this example there is no provision for ventilation worthy of the name, and the wards are so arranged that the sick must of necessity be supplied with common foul air.

Having more than Two Rows of Beds between the Windows. In the double wards, or wards back to back, of the new part of Guy's, of King's College and of the Fever Hospital, this arrangement is seen. It is objectionable on every account. These double wards are from twelve to nearly twenty feet wider than they ought to be between the opposite windows for thorough ventilation. The partition down the middle with apertures makes matters rather worse; complaint has been made that it beats down the draught on the heads of the inner rows of patients. It also prevents the head nurse from having that view of her whole ward at once which she ought to have for proper care of it. The following illustration, Fig. 8, from King's College Hospital, will show how these defects are produced.

Figure 6
Manchester Royal Infirmary

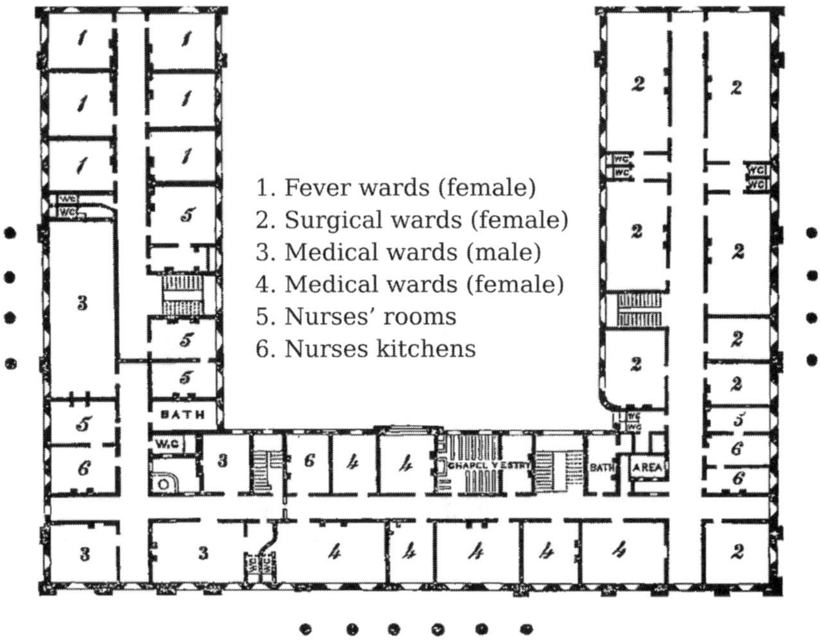

Figure 7
Wards of old Marine Hospital, Woolwich

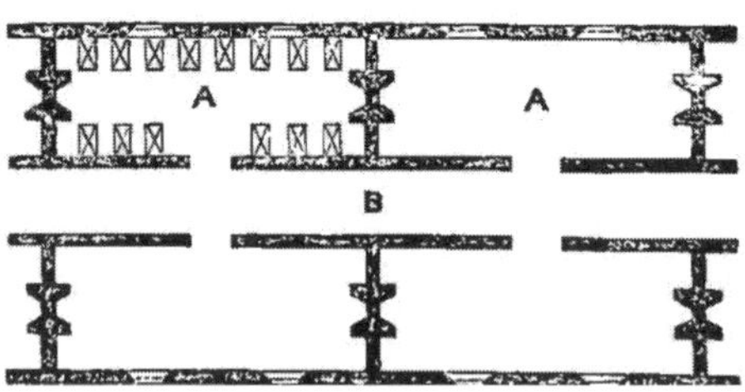

A A: wards; B: inner passage

FIGURE 8
Ward plan of Kings College Hospital, London

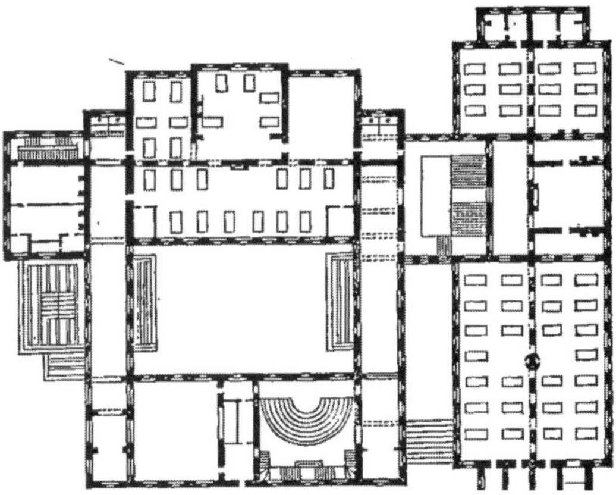

Having Windows only on one Side, or having a close Corridor connecting the Wards. As it is a necessity of hospital construction that every ward must have direct communication with the external air, by means of a sufficient number of windows on its opposite sides, and that every ward must have its own ventilation distinct and separate from that of every other ward, it follows that to have a dead wall on one side, or to cover one of the sides by a corridor, is directly to interfere with the natural ventilation of the ward. To join all the ward doors and windows on one side by means of a corridor is much more objectionable than even to have a dead wall, because the foul air of all the wards must necessarily pass into the corridor, and from the corridor into the wards indiscriminately. The whole hospital becomes in this way a complicated ward, and hence, without extraordinary precautions, such as are not usually nor likely to be bestowed on such matters, these corridors are the certain means of engendering a hospital atmosphere. A similar objection exists against any form of hospital construction in which a door connects any two wards. If anyone had wished to see the corridor plan in all its horrors, Scutari would have shown them to him on a colossal scale. But the evils connected with corridors may be seen on a smaller scale in some part of almost every hospital in London. Netley also has its corridor (*vide* [see] Plan No. 2).

I give another illustration, Fig. 9, from the Hôpital St Antoine, at Paris, in which it will be seen that the corridor, as well as the wards, is occupied by sick. This building was not, however, constructed for a hospital. The arrangement is obviously a bad one.

Figure 9
Hôpital St Antoine, Paris

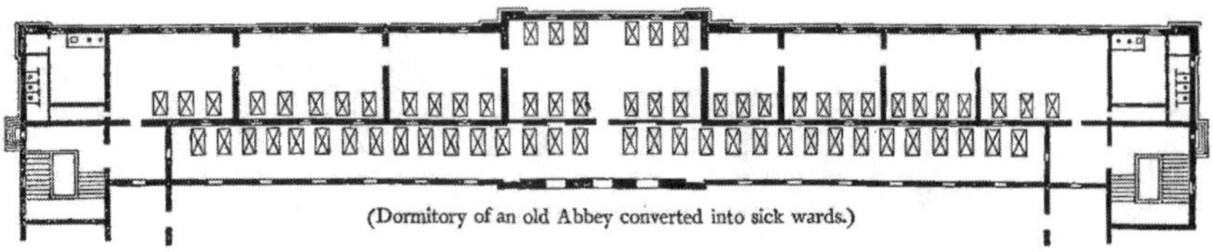

(Dormitory of an old Abbey converted into sick wards.)

Here is, too, another quite recent illustration, Fig. 10, of a grave structural defect in the new part of Glasgow Infirmary.[11] The intention in this instance was evidently to adopt sound principles of construction, but it will be observed that at one end of the ward there are three beds, and at the other four beds between the opposite windows. The small wards intended for the most serious cases are placed in the vicinity of the sinks, baths and water closet, and have a direct communication with the ventilation of the larger wards. These arrangements are to be regretted, on account of the example.

Figure 10
New part of Glasgow Royal Infirmary

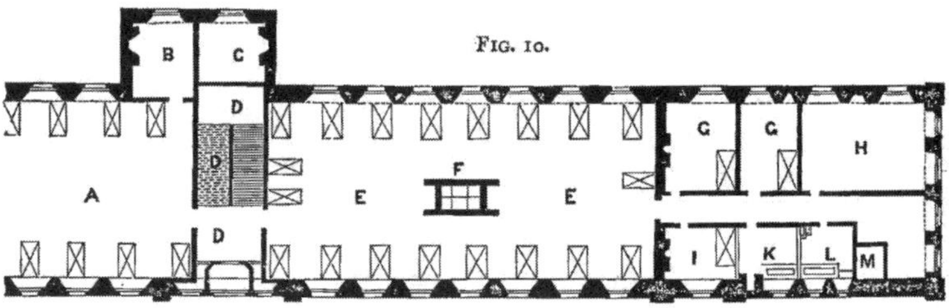

(Small wards, &c., entering from large wards.)

A. E. Wards. | D. Stair. | H. Day-room.
B. I. Nurses' rooms. | F. Chimney and ventilating shaft. | K, L. Baths, lavatories, water-closet.
C. Pupil. | G. Small wards. | M. Lift.

All of these defects in plan and construction of wards have a very serious influence on the question of defective ventilation and warming, which we will now discuss.

4. *Defective Means of Ventilation and Warming.* When the question of ventilation first assumed a practical shape in this country, it was supposed that 600 cubic feet of air per hour were sufficient for a healthy adult in a room

11 Presumably the Surgical Block, 1861, for correspondence on which see p 532 below.

where a number of people are congregated together. Subsequent experience, however, has shown that this is by no means enough. As much as 1000 cubic feet have been found insufficient to keep the air free from closeness and smell, and it is highly probable that the actual quantity required will ultimately be found to be at least 1500 cubic feet per hour per man.

In sick wards we have more positive experience as to the quantity of air required to keep them sweet and healthy. It was found in a certain Parisian hospital, in which the ventilating arrangements were deficient, that pyemia and hospital gangrene had appeared among the patients. These diseases are said to have disappeared on the introduction of ventilating arrangements whereby 2500 cubic feet of air per bed per hour were supplied to the wards. Notwithstanding this large quantity, however, the ward atmosphere was found not to be sufficiently pure. In other wards, the quantity of air was increased to as much as 4000 or 5000 cubic feet per bed per hour. But again we say, do not trust to artificial means: without natural ventilation the air will never be *fresh*.

I have, in a preceding page, stated generally the importance of the method of ventilation and warming employed to the state of the ward atmosphere. I will only repeat here that, if our object be to obtain a wholesome state of the air round the sick, we must have no air except what comes direct by windows or ventilating openings from the outer atmosphere, and we must have no other warming apparatus than the open fireplace. It is the safest warmer and ventilator. Air cooked by metal surfaces is especially to be avoided. It seems likely that we shall soon be enabled to have open fireplaces in the middle of wards, the draught being carried under the floor. It is obvious that fireplaces in the side walls are in the wrong place. There is great loss and unequal distribution of heat in consequence. But in order to obtain the benefit of a central fireplace, it is certainly not necessary to carry the chimney stalks up in the wards as has been done at Glasgow and in one Guards' hospital in London, making it look more like an Egyptian temple than a hospital.

5. *Defects in Drainage, Water Closets, Sinks, etc.* Hospital sewers may become cesspools of the most dangerous description, if improperly made and placed. In one hospital I knew [Scutari Barrack Hospital], if the wind changed so as to blow up the open mouths of the sewers, such change was frequently marked by outbreaks of fever among the patients, and by relapses among the convalescents from fever. Where there are no means for externally ventilating the sewers, no traps, no

sufficient water supply, no means for cleansing or flushing them, and where the bottoms are rough and uneven, such occurrences cannot fail to take place. The emanations from the deposits in the sewers are in such cases blown back through the pipe drains into the water closets and sinks, and thence into the wards. Where sewers pass close to or under occupied rooms, the walls or covers being defective, exhalations will infallibly escape into those rooms. There are hospitals where such things exist at the present time.

There can be no safety for the sick if any but water closets of the best construction are used, as also if they are not built *externally* to the main building, and cut off by a lobby, separately lighted and ventilated by cross windows from the ward. The same thing may be said of sinks. I have known outbreaks of fever even among the healthy from an ill-constructed and ill-placed sink in this country.

The smell of latrines which are not water closets, as used in French hospitals, is quite perceptible at the end of the ward nearest to them, and becomes, indeed, a very serious taint to the atmosphere, which might, with proper water closets, be secured so fresh by their admirable plan of building in pavilions. The whole drainage should be carefully studied and provided for, otherwise one may build a magnificent hospital, with abundant ventilation, and yet be distilling foul air from sewers into every ward of it.

Not very long ago five fatal cases of fever occurred in rapid succession among the nurses in one of our civil hospitals, which were traced to a defective drain.

6. *Using Absorbent Materials for Floors, Walls and Ceilings of Hospitals, and Washing Floors.* The amount of organic matter given off by respiration and in other ways from the sick is such that the floors, walls and ceilings of hospital wards—if not of impervious materials—become dangerous absorbents.

The boards are in time saturated with organic matter from this cause, as well as from accidental filth and want of due attention to cleansing, and only require moisture to give off noxious effluvia. When the floors are being washed, the smell of something quite other than soap and water is perfectly perceptible, and there cannot be a doubt that washing dirty floors is one cause of erysipelas, etc., in some hospitals.

Common plaster is the material most usually employed for ward walls and ceiling. The objection to it is its being porous, and its faculty of absorbing emanations from the sick. When the surface is recently finished, plaster thus tends to purify the air of a sick ward. But, after a time, it becomes saturated with impurity. Occasionally a minute vegetation appears upon it, which can be scraped off and examined by the microscope, and also chemically. When ward walls and ceilings become fouled in this way, hospital diseases are very apt to invade the wards. It has happened that workmen employed in scraping and cleansing such wards have themselves suffered from severe illness. The usual remedy is frequent limewashing with periodical scraping. Caustic lime decomposes the organic matter or covers it with a thin film for the time. The process is objectionable, because to be of use it requires to be frequently repeated, and the wards to be evacuated during the cleansing and drying. The latter part of the process requires to be very complete before the ward is reoccupied, to prevent accidents to the sick.

Plastered walls, when not cleansed sufficiently, have led to increased impurity of the ward air, and to hospital diseases.

7. *Defective Hospital Kitchens.* Two facts every careful observer can establish from experience:

1. The necessity for variety in food, as an essential element of health, owing to the number of materials required to restore and preserve the human frame. In sickness it is still more important because, the frame being in a morbid state, it is scarcely possible to prescribe beforehand with certainty what it will be able to digest and assimilate. The so-called "fancies" of disease are in many cases valuable indications.

2. The importance of cooking so as to secure the greatest digestibility and the greatest economy in nutritive value of food. Feeling the importance of this element in recovery, I have often been surprised by the primitive kitchens of some of our civil hospitals, with which little variety of cooking is possible. It shows how little diet and cooking are yet thought of as sanitary and curative agents. There still exists a confusion of ideas about "spoiling" the sick, about "too much indulgence" of the patients, and even yet comparatively little is practically known as to what is, and what is not, essential for restoration to health.

A hospital cook, instead of being the best obtainable cook, is sometimes put to the work because she is fit for little or nothing else, and her utensils are often as faulty as her performances. I have often seen the sick unable to eat the messes prepared for them in the name of diets, not so much because they were bad in quality, as because the cook had no clear idea of the class of stomachs for which he or she had to provide. It is singular that, while so much care is taken to provide good medicine properly made up, so little care is bestowed on the cooking of that which is of more importance than most medicines. The nurse or doctor only finds out, perhaps next day, that the patient has lost appetite, or been sick, or has had a relapse, and nobody suspects that the men or women in the kitchen had occasioned it.

Steps have been taken to educate hospital cooks for the army, so that in this department of the public service there will be less chance of the sick suffering, as I have seen them suffer, than there was formerly.

But the generality of civil hospital kitchens have little to boast of, and defective hospital kitchens and bad cooking may be classed as among the causes of hospital unhealthiness. Besides this, the kitchen is not unfrequently situated in objectionable proximity to the wards, at the foot of a staircase leading to them, if not under them. This should not be. In all except the smallest class of hospitals, for a few beds only, the kitchen should be detached, to keep the damp and fumes of cooking away from the sick.

8. *Defective Hospital Laundries.* Not very long ago there was scarcely an army hospital which had such a thing as a laundry. The bedding was washed by contract. And the body linen in the smaller hospitals was generally washed, if such a term ought to be used, in a small washhouse, or lean-to shed, with or without a boiler, and without any means for drying, getting up or airing linen. The linen was taken out of the damp washhouse, possibly into the damp air, and there hung up for a longer or a shorter time, and if the "orderly" were careful of his patients, he would complete the process by drying the linen, before it was put on, in front of the ward fire. In provincial hospitals, even of our largest cities, there is sometimes a too infrequent change of bed linen, and fresh patients have been put into the last patients' sheets.

The Barrack and Hospital Improvement Commission has led to great changes, still in progress, in this important part of hospital administration, and some of the best laundries in existence are now to be found attached to army hospitals of the larger class. The importance of a good laundry to a hospital is by no means sufficiently appreciated. Neither are its dangers, if improperly placed. It would not be difficult to point to hospitals in which all the linen is washed within the hospital boundary, close under the ward windows, or in the basement of the hospital itself. I have even seen recent hospital plans in which it was proposed to place the laundry in this position, or even under the sick wards. A moment's consideration of what is likely to be the result to the atmosphere, and consequently to the sick of a hospital, by impregnating it with the steam of linen fouled by the excretions of a number of sick people, would surely be sufficient to put a stop to such errors in construction! May not some of the anomalous outbreaks of disease in hospitals be traced to this, among other causes?

A great deal has been said about the communication of "infectious" disease, both in civil and military hospitals, from patients' linen to washerwomen. The usual conclusion arrived at on such occasions is that such and such a disease is "very infectious"; e.g., I was lately told in a civil hospital that the washerwomen became infected with fever from the patients' linen. Have those who put forward this doctrine of inevitable "infection" among washerwomen ever examined the process of washing, the appliances by which it is done and the place where the women wash? If they will do so, they will very generally find a small, dark, wet, unventilated and overcrowded little room or shed, in which there is hardly space to turn about—so full of steam loaded with organic matter that it is hardly possible to see across the room. Is it surprising that the linen is badly washed, that it is imperfectly dried and that the washerwomen are poisoned by inhaling organic matter and foul air? An ordinary hospital washhouse is a very likely place indeed to contract disease in, but it supplies equal reason for demurring in toto to the doctrine that the occurrence is inevitable, or that the disease is to blame.

Ignorance and mismanagement lie at the root of all such presumed cases of "infection." And it would better serve the cause of humanity if, instead of citing such facts—if they be facts—as illustrations that such and such a disease is infectious, people would reform these washing establishments and convert them into proper laundries, from which properly cleansed and prepared linen could be supplied to the sick, and in which the health of the servants could be preserved from injury.

Let hospital laundries be constructed in proper situations, with sufficient area and cubic space for each washer, with abundance of water, with proper means of drainage, and of ventilation for removing the vapour, and with properly constructed drying and ironing rooms; it will be all the better for the sick, and we shall cease to hear of washerwomen "catching" fever.

9. *Defective Accommodation for Nursing and Discipline.* Want of simplicity of construction in not a few hospitals is destructive to discipline. Effectual and easy supervision is essential to proper care and nursing. And as everybody knows, a patient may often be saved by careful nurs-

ing when everything else will fail. It is at this point that the hospital architect may either facilitate or prevent recovery to the extent to which his plan renders nursing easy, or the reverse.

Every unneeded closet, scullery, sink, lobby and staircase represents both a place which must be cleaned, which must take hands and time to clean, and a hiding or skulking place for patients or servants disposed to do wrong. And of such no hospital will ever be free. Every five minutes wasted upon cleaning what had better not have been there to be cleaned is something taken from and lost by the sick.

But, on the other hand, there must be conveniences. From one of our most recently constructed hospitals, complaints have been made that there were no sufficient nursing conveniences, that nothing was at hand, that everything had to be sought. Where this is the case, the hospital administration must necessarily be both inefficient and costly.

There are four essential points of construction as regards nursing and discipline in which hospitals are generally deficient, from want of due consideration on the part of hospital architects. They are those points required to ensure: (1) economy of attendance, (2) ease of supervision, (3) convenience as to number of sick in the same ward and on the same floor, so as to save extra attendants and unnecessary waste of time and strength on the stairs [and] (4) sufficient accommodation for nurses so as to overlook their wards.

First. *Economy as to Attendance.* I would rather not enumerate the instances where, often from the most various causes, one result arises, viz., that more time and care are given to passages, stairs, etc., than to the sick. Extreme simplicity of construction and of detail is essential to obviate this. A convenient arrangement of lifts, and the laying of hot and cold water all over the building, economize attendance—certainly as much as one attendant to every thirty sick.

Secondly. *Ease of Supervision.* The system of scouts, watch, alarm, is well understood in many wards where patients would be puzzled to give the things names. Some patients will know both things and names. Attendants require inspection as well as patients. Whatever system of hospital construction is adopted should provide for easy supervision at unexpected times. The Vincennes plan (No. 5) is better adapted for this than the Lariboisière plan (No. 4), inasmuch as there is a greater number of patients on the same level, and stairs are spared.

Third and Fourth. *Distribution of Sick in Convenient Numbers for Attendance, and Position of Nurses' Rooms.* Four wards of ten patients each, taking the average of patients as in London, cannot be efficiently overlooked by one head nurse. Were it allowable to have forty patients in one ward, this number could be fully overlooked by one head nurse. She ought to have her room so placed that she can command her whole ward, day and night, from a window looking into the ward. This cannot be the case if she has four wards. If she has two, they ought to be built end to end, with her room placed between and looking into both wards.

Four wards of ten patients each cannot be attended by one night nurse, taking the average of London cases. Forty patients in one ward can be fully attended by one night nurse. Small wards are indeed objectionable in working a hospital.

If we are to be guided, however, by the results of recent experience in hospital building, we shall probably come to the conclusion that, taking sanitary and administrative reasons together, thirty-two patients is a good ward unit.

Let us see what we have done in our older military hospitals at home. The first thing that will strike anyone in most of our old regimental hospitals is the extraordinary number of wards and of holes and corners, in comparison with the number of sick. In a hospital for a battalion 500 or 600 strong, you find eight or ten little bedrooms, miscalled wards, a little kitchen—everything, in fact, on a little scale, like a collapsed hospital. How much more sensible would it be to have one, or at most two, large wards from twenty-eight or thirty-two sick each, with a small "casualty" ward! How much less the expense of erection and administration, how much easier the discipline and oversight, how much better the ventilation! In the recently erected military hospitals these errors have been avoided.

To return to large civil general hospitals. The "casualty" wards, as they are called, for noisy or offensive cases, are much better placed apart, with a completely appointed staff of their own, than attached one small ward to each larger one. Patients requiring much attention, whose condition fits them the most for small wards, cannot be put there, because either they are more or less neglected, or they unduly monopolize the service of the ward attendants. If convalescent patients are put into them, they are comparatively removed from inspection, and often play tricks there. If separate "casualty" wards are provided, as they ought to be, the small ward (often seen in French hospitals), at the end of the larger ward, is only an incubus [devil].

10. *Defective Ward Furniture.* Hospital bedsteads should always be of iron, the rest of the furniture of oak. Hair is the only material yet dis-

covered fit for hospital mattresses. It is not hard nor cold. It is easily washed. It does not retain miasma. Straw has the advantage of being easily renewed, but it is not desirable. It is too hard and too cold not to render necessary the use of a blanket *under* the patient, which use is likely to encourage bedsores. I speak from actual experience of the fatal effect of using the paillasse with patients much reduced. It may lower their vital energy beyond repair. Patients also say the straw feels to them "like sticks," and "put their hands under them to move it."

Among defective ward appurtenances very liable to be undervalued in the results may be enumerated: eating, drinking, washing vessels, of tin or any other metal, on account of their greater difficulty in being kept clean. It requires some care to ensure that any dark-coloured vessel is clean, and any means by which extra care of this kind can be avoided in a hospital are cheap and safe. Notwithstanding the greater amount of breakage and of expense, glass or earthenware is therefore best. Some kinds of tin vessels cannot by any amount of cleaning be freed from an unclean smell.

The more common and avoidable causes of hospital unhealthiness having been here enumerated, we will now discuss the principles on which hospitals should be constructed.

Note. On the Proportion of Attendants to Sick in Different Classes of Hospitals

It is singular how little, even in civil hospitals, attention has been directed to the comparative cost of nursing in larger and smaller wards. In two civil hospitals in London, I found the annual cost of nursing each bed about one third *more* in the one than in the other. It is true that the average number of constantly occupied beds was about one third less in the former than in the latter hospital. But the difference of cost seems mainly attributable to the difference of the number of beds in each ward. And the efficiency of the nursing was certainly not less in the latter than in the former hospital.

In civil hospitals the proportion is one to every seven, generally of attendants to patients, but is mainly determined by the size of the ward.

In one of the hospitals alluded to, where there are quadruple wards of forty-four or forty-eight patients, eleven or twelve in each compartment, the number of attendants is seven to each quadruple ward. In exceptional cases, extra night nurses, sometimes extra day nurses, serve particular patients. The labour, both of cleaning and of night nursing, is much increased by the compartments being four, and separated by a large lobby.

In the other hospital the proportion of attendants to sick in the different wards was as follows:

PATIENTS		ATTENDANTS
22 24	there were to each ward	1 Sister 2 Nurses
30	"	1 Sister 2 Nurses 1 Scrubber
34	"	1 Sister 3 Nurses
40	"	1 Sister 3 Nurses 1 Helper

In the Lariboisière Hospital at Paris, where the wards hold thirty-two beds, one sister, one nurse and two orderlies on the men's side, one sister, two nurses and one orderly on the female side, serve the ward efficiently. In this hospital there are no lifts.

In all naval hospitals, the regulation number of attendants is one to every seven patients, or two attendants for each ward containing more than seven patients and up to fourteen.

In military hospitals, the regulation number of orderlies is one to every ten patients, irrespective of the size of the wards.

The largest sized wards in the older class of military hospitals hold no more than twenty patients. But a ward of twenty patients cannot be efficiently served by two orderlies, nor (if the orderlies be men) with less than

½ head nurse, female
3 orderlies.

And the other ward of this head nurse ought to be on the same floor.

The same number would quite as efficiently serve a ward of thirty-two patients, provided there be lifts and a supply of hot and cold water all over the building.

The army system of one orderly to ten patients, with a number not exceeding ten patients to a ward, is upset as immediately by one bad case among the ten, as by nine to the ten.

Lifts and a supply of hot and cold water laid on all over the hospital make, on an average, the difference of one attendant to every ward of thirty-two patients. And, other things being equal, it is certain that a ward with the appliances and without the extra attendant will be better served than a ward without the appliances and with the extra attendant.

Another thing is certain. A nurse must not be a scrubber. And a scrubber cannot be a nurse.

Also, every night nurse and every ward attendant, scrubber included, must sleep and live and be entirely attached to the hospital which she serves. Otherwise it is obvious she will not serve it; she will serve someone else—probably her family at home. Also, every nurse on night duty must have regular night refreshment supplied her by the hospital.

One orderly should be trained to be *frotteur* to each military ward. He should also be the porter to fetch and carry everything to and from the ward.

The following is an illustration of the cost of nursing in two military hospitals, one with large, the other with small wards:

A ward of nine sick would require one day and one night orderly, and a third of a nurse (that is, a nurse could superintend three such wards).

A ward of thirty-two sick would require two day and one night orderlies and one nurse = four persons in all. Or if two such wards were on one floor, one nurse could serve both.

We cannot count the cost of orderlies and nurses, including lodging, rations, wages, at less than £50 a year, which, when capitalized at 3 percent (thirty-three years' purchase), would amount to £1650 for each.

A ward of nine sick would cost in nursing £1650 × 2⅓ = £3850, or £427.15s.6d. per bed.

A ward of thirty-two sick would cost for nursing, in perpetuity, £1650 × 4 = £6600 = £220 per bed. (One nurse to each ward is here allowed.)

The cost of the two plans relatively for a hospital of 1000 sick would stand thus:

Wards with 9 beds	= £427,775
Wards with 30 beds	= 220,000
Capitalized difference of cost in favour of large wards	= £207,775

Suppose there be twenty-five sick to a ward, the cost would stand thus:

For each ward 25 sick, 3 orderlies, at £1650	= £4950
If two such are built in line close to each other, with the nurse's room between them, one nurse could superintend both wards, or half a nurse to a ward. The cost would be for the ward	= 825
[total]	= £5775

Or cost for each bed 5775/25 = £231.

The comparative cost of wards with nine beds and twenty-five beds would stand thus for 1000 sick:

Wards with 9 beds	= £427,775
Wards with 25 beds	= 231,000
Saving	= £196,775

3. Principles of Hospital Construction

The first principle of hospital construction is to divide the sick among separate pavilions. By a hospital is meant a detached block of building capable of containing the largest number of beds that can be placed safely in it, together with suitable nurses' rooms, ward sculleries, lavatories, baths, water closets, all complete, proportioned to the number of sick, and quite unconnected with any other pavilions of which the hospital may consist, or with the general administrative offices, except by light airy passages or corridors. A pavilion is indeed a separate detached hospital, which has, or ought to have, as little connection in its ventilation with any other part of the hospital as if it were really a separate establishment miles away. The essential feature of the pavilion construction is that of breaking up hospitals of any size into a number of separate detached parts, having a common administration, but nothing else in common. And the object sought is that the atmosphere of no one pavilion or ward should diffuse itself to any other pavilion or ward, but should escape into the open air as speedily as possible, while its place is supplied by the purest obtainable air from the outside.

The question of a general hospital plan resolves itself, first of all, into obtaining the most healthy structure of the pavilion, and, second, into arranging all the pavilions in the way best suited to obtain free, external ventilation, plenty of light on all sides, and convenient means of communication. To realize these advantages, pavilions may be placed side by side, or in line.

The arrangement of pavilions side by side should be adopted for hospitals of above 120 beds; the arrangement in line is most suitable for small hospitals with fewer than 120 beds. In the larger class of hospitals, the arrangement of pavilions side by side diminishes the distance to be traversed from block to block, and thus materially facilitates the administration. Besides this, it allows covered communications to be kept up between all parts of the hospital, without interfering with the lighting or ventilation of the wards.

The distance between the blocks should not be less than double the height of the blocks. This rule is specially applicable to English climates, in which it is necessary to preserve as much space as possible for sunshine. A greater distance would be better, but this would involve a greater cost for land, and a greater distance to be traversed by the hospital staff. Generally the distance between the pavilions should be greater than twice their height in low confined localities, where there is not a free external movement of the air. If the wards are raised on basements, the rule as to distance should apply only to the height of the pavilion from the floor of the ground-floor ward. In very close positions it is difficult to say what distance will be found sufficient for free ventilation. Such localities are precisely those where no hospitals should be built.

The first thing, however, is to determine the best construction for a pavilion, and in doing this the following principles require to be kept in view:

1. Number of Floors in a Pavilion

There should not be more than two floors of wards to the block.

The most healthy hospitals have been those on one floor only, and this because they require less scientific knowledge and practical care in ventilation. If another floor is added, a community of ventilation exists between the ward below and the ward above by the common staircase, and by filtration of air upwards through the floor. The risk from this can be diminished by constant care in the use of doors and windows, and by introducing impervious floors. But, unfortunately, systematic care in these matters is not to be looked for, especially that constant supervision necessary to keep the ventilation of three or more floors of wards quite independent of each other. (Whoever sees this, even in a private house, where there is an invalid?) And hence there is a strong conviction in the minds of careful hospital physicians, surgeons and nurses that patients do not recover so well on upper floors. And there are instances in which the mortality of patients on upper floors has been higher than that of the floors below. Moreover, a *sick population* requires more surface for health than a healthy population. And it is clear that, if patients are placed on three floors instead of on two, overcrowding is increased by one third, unless the distance between the pavilions is increased in a corresponding ratio. But the general administration of lofty hospitals is also far more difficult and fatiguing than of those of moderate height; any increase of distance between the pavilions will add to the difficulty, and both difficulty and fatigue are very important considerations for efficiency and economy in this branch.

To sum up. Hospitals on one floor require least care; hospitals on two floors can be kept healthy with moderate average care and intelligence. Beyond this, care, intelligence and fatigue, such as are rarely likely to be bestowed, are essential to maintain a moderate average amount of health, among either wards or nurses. Nobody but those who have had to do with running up and down lofty hospitals can have any idea of the waste of time and strength it entails. The objection usually urged is that hospitals in two floors cost more than in three or more floors. But I submit that this is not the question before us, which is how to construct a hospital with the requisite facilities for ventilation, administration, nursing and health.

The mode of construction in hospitals is, it is presumed, to be determined by that which is best for the recovery of the sick. If any other consideration is taken, such or such a percentage of mortality is to be sacrificed to that other consideration.

But it so happens that the safest for the sick is in reality the most economical mode of construction.

2. Number of Wards to a Floor

If the pavilions are single, i.e., if each staircase gives access to the end of the pavilion, as in the Lariboisière and Lisbon plans, Nos. 4 and 11, there should be only one ward on each floor. The pavilion should never be divided so that a second ward or wards is placed beyond the first, to be reached by passing through the first. The reason is that the floor, however divided by cross walls, can never be other than a single ward. The cross walls only obstruct the ventilation. If the doors are accidentally left open, the foul air in one ward passes into the next, and the greatest improvement in ventilation would be to pull down all the partitions and throw the pavilion open from end to end, so as to have only one ward on the floor.

To illustrate the meaning of this, here is a plan (Fig. 11) of one wing of the Hôpital Necker at Paris, in which it will be seen that an excellently constructed ward, with windows on all sides, is cut up by partitions into four wards. If the partitions were removed, one cannot fail to see that the ventilation would be better, but in this case the ward would be too large.

Figure 11
Plan of a wing of the Hôpital Necker, Paris

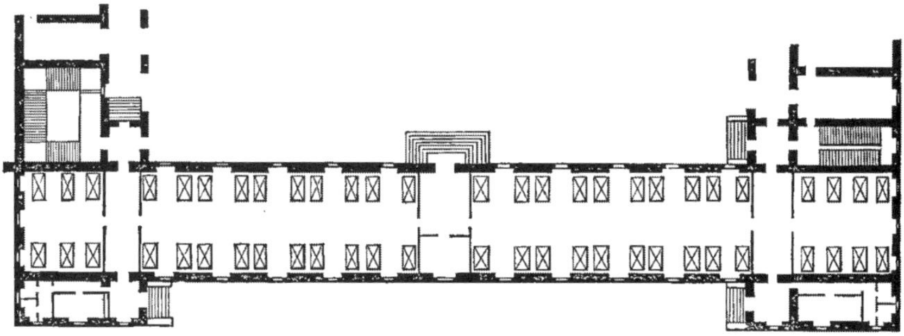

If the pavilions are double, i.e., if each staircase gives access to a ward right and left off the staircase, as in the Herbert Hospital, No. 6, and in the regimental hospital plans, Figs. 20 [and] 21, provided the staircase be of spacious size, and thoroughly ventilated sides and top, two wards may be placed on each floor with safety, and with this great advantage, that administration, nursing and discipline are all facilitated, while expense in construction is saved. One staircase does the work of two for the same number of sick, or rather one staircase answers for double the number of sick.

3. Size of Wards, Pavilion and Hospitals

The question, what is the best number of beds in a ward? has been but little considered in England in regard either to health, economy or efficiency of service. The more beds in one ward, the fewer the attendants necessary in proportion, and, within a certain limit, the greater the facility of supervision. But the sanitary necessities of cubic space per bed, etc., impose the limit. After we have attained a certain number of beds per ward, the height of the ward becomes too little for its other dimensions. The ventilation becomes impeded, a circumstance which can only be guarded against by making the ward higher than necessary. Additional cubic space has thus to be given, and the construction ceases to be economical. Without the most perfect ventilation, there is always more danger of effluvia being driven by a draught till it accumulates in one part of a very large ward, as was the case in the long corridors of Scutari. Besides which, you may make your ward too large for the chief attendant to overlook the whole at a glance, which he and still more *she* ought to be able to do. And you would have to double your supervision. (See Note to Section 2 on the relation which the size and arrangement of wards bears to the question of nursing and supervision.)

Wards of a small size are decidedly objectionable, because unfavourable to discipline, inasmuch as a small number, when placed together in the same ward, more readily associate together for any breach of discipline than a larger number.

It has been proved by experience that the presence of head nurses, whether male or female, one to each ward, is essential to discipline, and a sufficient number of such nurses cannot be allotted in smaller wards. One head nurse can easily overlook all the patients in one large ward. In four small ones it is almost impossible.

The best size of wards for ensuring the two conditions of health and facility of administration and discipline is from twenty to thirty-two sick. Wards smaller than of twenty beds multiply both the attendance unnecessarily, and the corners, unfavourably for ventilation, in proportion to the number of patients. Wards larger than of thirty-two beds are undesirable, because they require a greater height of ceiling, and are hence more costly in construction and difficult to ventilate.

In the event of a death taking place in the ward, the survivors, when they are few in number, are far more likely to be affected by it than a larger number.

Wards, again, much smaller than of twenty beds are more difficult to ventilate by natural means alone. A certain amount of space is requisite for diffusion in order to secure perfect natural ventilation. Wards of a moderate size, like those indicated, are better for the purposes of ventilation than wards half the size, and are less subject to a hospital atmosphere than wards of double the size.

Where clinical instruction is intended, to admit even a class of six students into a ward of twelve sick is increasing the population in the cubic space by one half. There is more than twice the room proportionally for students in a ward of double the size. On the other hand, if the number of students be very large, a ward of twenty patients, it must be at once admitted, is too small. The size of the ward must be increased, and with it its height and its cubic space, for, be it remembered, the whole of the proportions of the ward, not only its length, must increase with its number of beds, for if the ward be very long in proportion to its height and breadth, it becomes not a ward but a corridor, and all corridors are objectionable for sick, because it is impossible to ventilate them safely, because, as already stated, in admitting air, the effluvia may be driven from one end and be accumulated at the opposite end faster than they can be taken out. The right proportion is a fixed one.

As to the size of the pavilion, if the pavilion be single and in two floors, it will of course contain under one roof no more than the sick of the two wards, i.e., of thirty-two beds each, or sixty-four in all. With double pavilions and intervening staircases, the number would be double, i.e., 128 beds. Where small wards for special cases are required, they can always, as a point of construction in small hospitals, be attached to the pavilion, which would add a few more beds to the number which can be accommodated under a single roof. In good existing examples small wards have been thrown out separately from the staircase.

Guided by these considerations, a hospital consisting of two end-to-end pavilions, such as would be required for a county establishment receiving a small number of sick, would contain, say, sixty-eight beds under one roof, i.e., thirty-two beds in each of the large wards, and two beds in each of the small wards. A double pavilion hospital would contain double that number. It would thus be safe, so far as plan is concerned, to construct a large hospital of any administrable size of separate double pavilions, each containing, say, 136 beds. But in large hospitals the smaller class of special wards should always be grouped together, and completely separated from the other wards, because they are intended to contain either the most dangerous and important cases, or noisy cases, or cases with offensive discharges, which it is always safest to remove from the general wards; besides, small wards require, if possible, purer air than larger wards, and therefore more care in construction; and in order to insure those cases which really require most nursing from neglect, they should always be placed under a completely appointed staff of their own, and *not* attached, one to each large ward, which renders proper attendance extremely difficult.

The next point is to determine what ought to be the size of a hospital, in other words, how many beds it can contain with safety. But from what has been said, it will be observed that this question resolves itself into the previous one, viz., what should be the size of each hospital pavilion? Because, if a pavilion of healthy construction is obtained, it is evident that the only limit to the size of the hospital will be an administrative one. A hospital may be constructed for any number of sick until a point is arrived at when some portion of the administrative arrangements, material or personal, has to be provided in duplicate. Any further extension beyond this ceases to be economical.

Considering each pavilion as a separate unit in the hospital construction, any number of single or double pavilions could be put together up to accommodation for, say, 1000 beds, beyond which it would be difficult, if not impracticable, to have good administration with one set of officers. It is to be hoped, however, that few hospitals will ever be built for such a number nowadays. The fewer hospitals required, and the smaller their number of sick, the better will it be for civilization. All I submit is that the pavilion construction may, not should, be safely used up to this extent.

4. Space and Area to the Bed

Having determined the number of beds per ward, the next point is to ascertain what amount of cubic space should be given to each patient. There is scarcely a point of hospital construction in which there has been so much error as in this. The chief element in the question, and that one which has been very generally overlooked, is the superficial area per bed. If it be—as it is—an essential condition to the healthy state of a hospital that there should be ample facility for the air moving around and in the immediate vicinity of the sick, it is quite clear that, if the beds are placed as close as they can stand, it matters very little whether you give your patient 1000 cubic feet or 20,000 cubic feet. To show the importance of this, it may be sufficient to state that, if a large building, say, a church, be selected for a war hospital, on account of its spacious, light, cheerful aspect, if it be measured to ascertain its cubic contents, its height being no more than 60 feet, in such a building the very liberal war hospital allowance of 1200 cubic feet per bed would render it necessary to place the beds on the floor so close together that not even a pathway would be left between them. Has not this, in times past, been one cause of the frightful mortality in these hospitals? In some splendid new hospitals in India, where they give above 1000 cubic feet per bed, the superficial area for each patient is only 24 square feet. But then the architect has made such a spacious ward no less than 42 feet high (!), that it is supposed to make amends.

Let us inquire what is the smallest amount of superficial area we can do with. Hospital beds are generally from 3 feet to 3 feet 6 inches wide, and 6 feet 3 inches long, the bed space being increased to 7 feet by the bed being a little removed from the wall. The mere surface required to hold the bed is hence from 21 square feet to 24½ square feet. It is quite clear that, whatever surface area is required for ventilation, administration or for clinical instruction, must be in excess of this amount. There should be space sufficient between the sides of adjacent beds to avoid stagnation of air altogether. There should also be room for free movement of three or four persons, for the use of a night chair, without annoying the next patient, and also for a portable bath when required. The distance from foot to foot of opposite beds should be sufficient to afford space for a moveable dresser or table, benches on either side, and easy passageway. In a well-constructed civil hospital in England, occupying a healthy airy position, it cannot be said that 80 square feet, *besides* the bed space, are too much. In round numbers, the superficial area per bed should be not less than 100 square feet.

Wards for the numbers of beds already given need not be higher than 15 feet, which would allow 1500 cubic feet per bed. This ought to be quite sufficient in a well-constructed hospital in a healthy position, and for the average class of cases received into civil hospitals. For small wards, however, neither this superficial area nor cubic space would be sufficient. In these wards the space per bed should be, as near as may be, 2500 cubic feet, and this partly from the more severe nature of the cases, partly from the greater difficulty of ventilating this class of wards.

If, however, a hospital is built in the centre of a large city, where pure air is not to be had, or in a locality where the circulation of air outside is deficient, it is hard to say what amount of space would make the building healthy. We know of hospitals where 2000 cubic feet per patient are not sufficient to make the wards safe. But these hospitals should not be there at all.

A good proportion for a ward of twenty patients would be 80 feet long, 25 (or 26) feet wide and 16 (or 15) feet high. This would give 1600 (or 1560) cubic feet to each bed. It would give 11 (or 12) feet between foot and foot, which is not too much where there is a clinical school. It would give an average of 16 feet to each two beds in width. Half the sick are supposed to be on each side the ward.

5. Number of Beds to a Window

One window at least should be allotted for every two beds, the window to be not less than 4 feet 8 inches wide, the sill within 2 or 3 feet of the floor, so that the patient can see out, and up to within a foot of the ceiling.

The pair of beds should have the width of the window between them on one side, and in the wall space between the windows the beds should be not less than 3 feet apart. With a very bad fever case, I would leave one bed empty, for the sake of isolating the patient. Miasma may be said, roughly speaking, to diminish as the square of the distance. With good ventilation, it is not found to extend much beyond 3 feet from the patient, although miasma from the excretions may extend a considerably greater distance.

Windows are to be placed opposite each other, and to be either double or filled with plate glass; the former would be preferable as affording the opportunity of indirect ventilation in all weather. But attendants find them too difficult to manage and to clean so as to be cheerful.

Windows opening as at Middlesex and Guy's Hospitals, in three or more parts, with an iron casting outside, to prevent a delirious patient from throwing himself out, are the best form of plate-glass window.

No part of the ward ought to be dark. This is of the utmost importance in many cases. The light can always be modified for individual patients. But even for such patients to have light in the ward is not the less important.

There are three reasons for this multiplicity of windows:

1. Light.
2. Ventilation.
3. To enable patients to read in bed.

The necessity of light for health is established by scientific inquiry and experience. The proportion of window space to cubic space in a room, but especially in a ward, is a point of the first importance. It has been lost sight of in English architecture, owing to the unfortunate window tax, which has left its legacy in giving us a far smaller proportion of light than in French houses. In huts the proportion of window space to cubic space is far greater than in buildings. One main cause of the unhealthiness of large numbers of men congregated in one large building, even with sufficient cubic space, is the disproportionately small window space.

For the same purpose of ensuring a sufficiency of light, the walls should always be light coloured, excepting perhaps for some few cases of ophthalmia.

6. Material for Walls and Ceilings of Wards

One of the most difficult points in ward construction is to find a good material for walls and ceilings.

An impervious material capable of receiving a polish on a white or tinted surface would make the best lining for a hospital ward. What is wanted is such a surface as can be washed frequently with soap and water, without its being absorbed into the substance, and dried with towels so as not to interfere with the current use of the ward. Parian cement[12] is the nearest approach to a good material for this purpose hitherto discovered. But the polish is rather costly. And what is of more consequence, the manufacture has not yet reached such a point of perfection as to afford a surface of one uniform colour. Even the best becomes blotchy after a short time, and is liable to crack, especially when applied to ceilings. If manufacturers wish to bring this substance into general use for hospitals, they must improve the material until the cement can be applied over any required extent of wall, and retain a uniform texture, colour and polish. Various silicated surfaces have recently been introduced for walls. Some of these are worthy of trial—always bearing in mind that a good colour, and not a dull dirty one, is necessary in all sick wards. It is possible that a sufficiently good surface might be obtained by applying some of the better class of light-coloured paints in repeated coats over unpolished Parian, and then varnishing and polishing the surface.

All the woodwork should be painted and varnished in such a way as to admit of ready washing and drying. But the best material is pol-

12 Named from the fine white marble of the island of Paros.

ished or varnished wainscot oak. It is the cleanest, most durable and most satisfactory in use.

7. Ward Floors

The materials used for floors may be oak wood, pine wood or tiles. Oak wood, well seasoned, is the best. No sawdust or other organic matter capable of rotting should be placed underneath the floor. Concrete, or some similar indestructible substance, would be the best for the purpose. The floors at the new Herbert Hospital, Woolwich, are formed of concrete, supported by wrought-iron joists, over which the wood is laid. They are consequently fireproof, as all hospitals floors ought to be.

The reason for using oak wood is that it is capable of absorbing but a very small quantity of water. And it is very desirable to diminish even that capability by saturating it with beeswax and turpentine. Beeswax is an inalterable substance. This floor should be cleaned like the French *parquet*, by *frottage*.

A hospital floor should never be scoured. A very good hospital floor is that used at Berlin, which is oiled, lacquered and polished so as to resemble French polish. It is wet-rubbed and dry-rubbed every morning, which removes the dust. Its only objection is want of durability.

Both processes render the floor non-absorbent—both processes do away with the necessity of scouring altogether. The French floor *stands* the most wear and tear, but must be cleaned by a *frotteur*, which cleaning is more laborious than scrubbing, and does not remove the dust. The Prussian floor requires repreparing every three years. But the wet- and dry-rubbing, or process of cleaning, is far less laborious than either *frottage* or scrubbing, and completely removes the dust and freshens the ward in the morning. By either process the sick would gain much in England. The Berlin flooring is by no means perfect, on account of this deficient durability of surface, and might be improved. Practically, with care, a well-laid oak floor, with a good beeswaxed surface, can always be kept clean by rubbing, but the means of producing a really good impervious polished surface, with little labour, have yet to be discovered.

The joints of the flooring must be fitted well together, and cemented with any impervious substance. The object is, of course, to prevent any water from entering the floor.

Impervious, non-absorbent cement or composition would make a capital floor, used as it is in Italian houses. But, on account of its great conducting power, it would be necessary to furnish each patient with a pair of list shoes,[13] and a small bedside carpet. Flooring of this kind, or of tiles, is better suited for a warm than for a cold climate.

The stairs and landings should be of stone. The corridors should be floored with diamond-shaped flags or tiles, which stand better than those laid in the usual manner. The terraces over the corridors might be either covered with asphalt or glazed tile, to admit of convalescents walking on them, and of patients in bed being wheeled out on them.

8. Sisters' Rooms and Sculleries

There should be a "sister's" room on one side of the ward door. This room must have superficial area enough to be the nurse's bedroom and living room, being, as she is, the head nurse or "sister" of her ward, and therefore in immediate command of it, night and day. A scullery should be attached to each ward, on the side of the passage opposite the nurse's room. The scullery must be supplied with complete, efficient, simple apparatus for its various purposes, places for washing up and cleaning and for *ward* cookery, so that the "sister" can warm the drinks, prepare fomentations, etc., without jostling the nurses or orderlies who are washing up. The best sink for a scullery is the new white porcelain sink recently introduced, with hot and cold water laid on. Care must be taken that the waste pipe has no direct communication with a closed drain, otherwise foul air is certain to find its way into the hospital. The scullery should be large enough for the assistant nurses to sit in to have their meals comfortably.

9. Bathrooms and Lavatories

Every hospital of any large size should have a separate bathing establishment at a convenient distance from the pavilions, but connected by the corridors. The walls of the bathhouse should be of white tiles, or cement, the floors of wood. The apartments should be suitably ventilated and warmed. They should contain hot and cold water baths, sulphurous water, hot air, medicated and vapour baths, shower baths and douche.

There should also be a small bathroom with one fixed bath of white glazed terra cotta, supplied with hot and cold water, adjoining each large ward. Terra cotta has the advantage of retaining the heat longer than almost any other material, and of being always cleanly.

---

13 Shoes made of fabric, or slippers.

A lavatory table with a row of sunk white porcelain basins, with outlet tubes and plugs, each basin supplied with hot and cold water, should be placed in the same compartment as the bath, but separated from it by a partition and door. It is a common mistake to place these lavatory basins too near each other to be used conveniently by men patients standing abreast.

There should also be room for a portable bath to each ward, with a hot and cold water supply at hand, and means of running off the bath water after it has been used.

10. Water Closets and Sinks

The water closets should be placed at the end of the ward opposite the entrance, and separated by a lighted and ventilated lobby. They should never be against the inner wall, but always against the outer wall of the compartment in which they are placed. They should be of the best construction. A syphon water closet of a hemispherical shape, *never of a conical shape*, and abundantly supplied with water to flush it out with a large forcible stream, is by far the best contrivance of the kind for a hospital. The cost of water is a bagatelle in comparison with the advantages. The sink for ward slops, bedpans, expectoration cups, etc., which should have a compartment of its own adjoining the water closet, should be a high, large, deep, round, pierced basin of earthenware, above a *large* hole, with a cock extending far enough over the sink for the stream of water to fall directly into the vessel to be cleansed. This is far preferable to the usual oblong sink. The scullery sink is, of course, to be entirely separate, and for entirely different purposes from this. The only way to ensure dryness and cleanliness in the compartments where the water closets and lavatory accommodation are placed is to cover the walls with white glazed tile, enameled slate or cement.

It is, perhaps, hardly necessary to say that there must be private water closets for the hospital officers, for the nurses, who should not be compelled to use those of the patients (and, of course, *never* those in the men's wards), also water closets for the patients when not in their wards; patients should not be allowed to use the ward ones, except when confined to their wards. All these water closets fall under the same rules of health as those laid down.

As the arrangement of this part of a hospital, viz., lavatories, water closets, etc., is one of primary importance, a measured plan of the most improved arrangement of ward offices, such as has been introduced into recent military hospitals (Fig. 12), is given next page.

FIGURE 12
Plan of Lavatory, Baths, and Water Closets for Hospital Wards

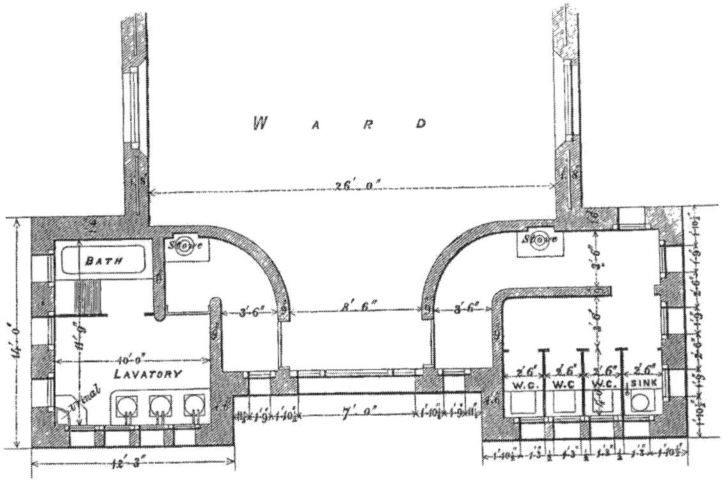

11. VENTILATION OF WARDS

The doors, windows and fireplaces should be the chief means of ventilation for properly constructed wards. If a hospital must be ventilated artificially, it betrays a defect of original construction which no artificial ventilation can compensate; it is an expensive and inefficient means of doing that which can be done cheaply and efficiently by constructing your building so as to admit the open air around.

In countries where fuel is dear and cold severe, the problem complicates itself, because it is supposed to require a smaller consumption of fuel to warm the fresh air as you admit it.

Artificial ventilation means the use of some machine or method whereby air is drawn from without—sometimes, it is to be feared, without due care whence it comes—bringing the air into forcible contact with heated surfaces, generally of hot-water vessels, and then introducing it into the ward for the use of the sick. The foul air is either expelled or drawn out of the ward by some mechanical means, and the fresh (if it is ever fresh) warmed air takes its place. In certain Parisian hospitals where this system is applied, the fresh warmed air enters the ward by pedestals down the centre, and the foul air is extracted by openings close to the floor between the beds—the presumption being that the foul air is in this way taken off before mingling with the general air of the ward.

It is a fact that one hospital at least in which this system is in full operation yields, notwithstanding its otherwise excellent construction, a very high death rate among its inmates. English physicians and surgeons who have examined this hospital concur in stating that the ward atmosphere is by no means so pure as it is in a London hospital. These facts have led to considerable discussion, which it is necessary to notice. Here we have one of the best constructed hospitals in existence, professing to afford to each of its beds from 2500 to 5000 cubic feet of "fresh warmed air" per hour introduced, and the foul air removed, in accordance with strictly correct scientific principle—and yet here is the result.

It strikes one on examining this process that it is not in accordance with Nature's method of providing fresh air. She affords air, both to sick and healthy, of varying temperature at different hours of the day, night and season—always apportioning the quantity of moisture to the temperature, providing continuous free movement everywhere, and warming not by warm water in iron pipes, but by radiant heat. We all know how necessary the variations of weather, temperature, season are for maintaining health in healthy people.

Have we any right to assume that the natural law is different in sickness? In looking solely at combined warming and ventilation, to ensure to the sick a certain amount of air at 60 degrees, paid for by contract, are we acting in accordance with physiological law? Is it a likely way to enable the constitution to rally under serious disease or injury, to undercook all the patients, day and night, during all the time they are in hospital, at one fixed temperature? I believe not. On the contrary, I am strongly of opinion, I would go farther and say, I am certain that the atmospheric hygiene of the sick room ought not to be very different from the atmospheric hygiene of a healthy house. Continuous change of the atmosphere of a sick ward to a far greater extent than would pay a contractor to maintain, together with the usual variations of temperature and moisture given by nature in the external atmosphere, are elements as essential as any other elements to the rapid recovery of the sick in most cases.

The best way to cure these beautiful but unhealthy buildings would be to remove the warming and ventilating apparatus, to put in chimneys, with good radiating open fireplaces, and to trust to their magnificent supply of windows for fresh air. (Why do not all learn the lesson taught by the experience of the invasions of France in 1814-15? At that date the hospital administration of Paris, not knowing where to receive the sick and wounded, fitted up three of the unfinished "*abattoirs*" slaughter houses] for 6000 patients—several of the buildings fortunately had neither doors nor windows, and had the wind blowing through them. The mortality was one half among the patients in the "abattoirs" of what it was in the ordinary hospital establishments. Husson, *Étude*, p 39.) (This is done in Russia, where it is far colder than at Paris.)

The administration would complain of the additional cost of fuel. But I would reply, you must consider how much you prolong the stay of sick in your hospital, and what percentage of recoveries you prevent or delay by this combined warming and ventilation. It does not matter what the present saving may appear to be; the object of your magnificent charities, perhaps the finest in the world, is to recover the largest number of sick in the shortest possible time. It is to be feared the statistics show that this end is not obtained.

Natural ventilation and open radiating fireplaces are the only suitable means of renewing and warming the air in hospitals. Whenever the weather permits of it, the windows of every sick ward should be more or less open. During cold, boisterous weather, and at night, a sufficient renewal of the air can always be obtained, even if the windows cannot be opened, by the method recently introduced into English military hospitals of carrying up a few air shafts from the ceilings of the wards to above the roof, and allowing fresh air to enter by means of Sherringham's ventilators at the top of the ward walls, close to the ceilings. No other system is required but this, and it costs little or nothing, besides which it takes advantage of the natural laws of varying temperature and moisture.

Fig. 13 shows the ventilating arrangements for a ward in plan. A foul air shaft is carried up in each alternate wall space between the windows, and a Sherringham's ventilating inlet is placed close to the ceiling in each alternate wall space opposite the shaft.

Fig. 14 gives a section of the shafts and inlets. The shafts are louvred at the lower ends to prevent chance down draughts falling on the beds. Fig. 15 is Sherringham's ventilator used as an inlet. It can be opened or shut by a weighted cord to regulate the amount of fresh air.

If with these simple means, including windows, attendants cannot be trained to keep the rooms ventilated without draughts, there is a defect of intelligence, and attendance on the sick is not their calling.

There should be one or more open fireplaces, according to the size of the ward, but lofty, so that the throat of the chimney shall be above the patient's head and bed.

FIGURE 13
Plan of Ward Ventilation, showing the position of Shafts and Inlets

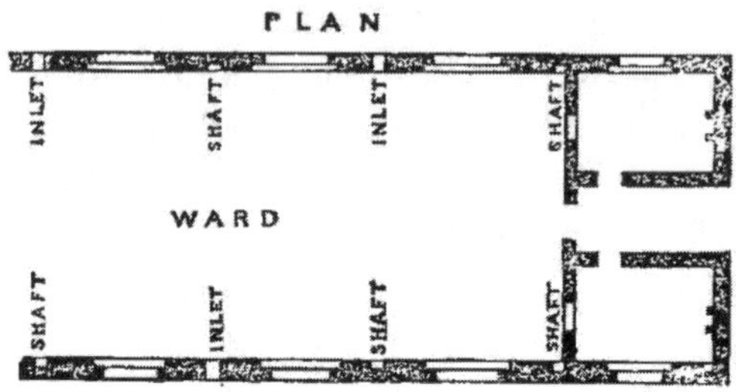

FIGURE 14
Section of Ward Ventilation

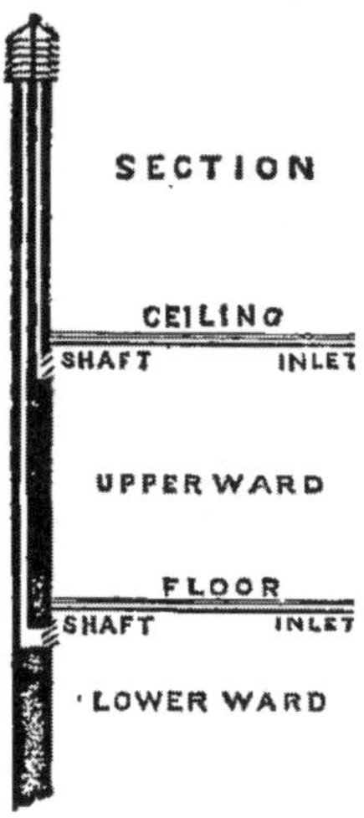

FIGURE 15
Sherringham's Ventilating Inlet

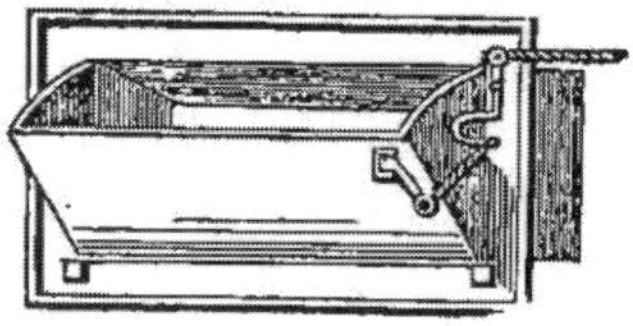

The chimney is indispensable as a ventilating shaft; the fire sets it acting; it takes the air from the ward so successfully that, as has been proved by direct experiment, a single chimney will, in certain states of the wind, remove 60,000 cubic feet of air in an hour, or as much as the French contract system allows for twenty-four patients.

12. WARD FURNITURE

White window curtains are used in some French hospitals, not to exclude the light, but to look cheerful. In most French hospitals, and in some in this country, the beds have curtains. They are not necessary. They interrupt ventilation and entail additional cost in washing. Where seclusion of a patient is required, a low movable screen, not higher than the patient's head when he is sitting up in bed, is far preferable.

Oak furniture should be supplied for wards. There should be a light chair for each bed, two or three spare armchairs for patients who get up for the first time to sit at the ward fire; there should be a small open bed table for each bed; two or more tables or moveable dressers down the centre of the ward, according to its dimensions; one or two forms with backs would be found very useful. In some hospitals the allowance of furniture is more liberal, but the less ward furniture, speaking generally, the better. The use of glass or earthenware for all eating, drinking and washing vessels is recommended from its great superiority in cleanliness, and in saving time and labour in cleaning. Tin vessels of certain kinds cannot, by any amount of cleaning, be freed from smell.

13. Bedding

No bedding but the hair mattress has yet been discovered that is fit for hospitals. Hair is indestructible. It does not readily retain miasma. And, if it does, heat easily disinfects it. It may be washed. It is not hard to the patient. It saves the objectionable use of a blanket under the patient. There have been repeated objections to the use of horsehair on account of the current expense. But this, under careful administration, is much less than is generally supposed. From special inquiries, I find that, allowing 5 percent for deterioration, the cost would stand as follows:

	Per Bed per Annum
Cleaning and remaking	2¼d to 2½d
Loss of hair	1½d to 2d
Interest at 5 percent	2s
Total	2s 3¾d to 2s 4½d

Straw paillasses, as already stated, are inadmissible. They are cold, and in some cases the abstraction of heat from the spine lowers the patient's vital energy to a degree which does not leave him a chance of recovery. I am of opinion that the loss of life must have been great during the war from laying our patients on paillasses, which were either placed on wooden divans, on the flagged corridors, with only a mat between.

All bedsteads for hospital use should be of wrought iron, frequently painted of a light cheerful colour. This costs little, and yet it has a far greater influence on the general appearance and comfort of a hospital ward than most people are aware of. Just in proportion to the discrepancy between the spacious, cheerful ward and its shabby, dirty-looking furnishing, is the air of general discomfort which it presents. A head shelf to the bed is useful. The French military hospital bedsteads have one at the feet too.

Sacking bottoms are preferable to iron bottoms, which are stated to harbour vermin between the interlacings, and it is said that the edges of the iron bands cut the bed ticks. The Rheocline open iron springs, like snakes sitting on their bottom ring, make the easiest, best ventilated, freshest bed I know; save your bed ticks by sewing a sacking under them. Some cases, like compound fractures, require a firm bottom to the bed for the splints and apparatus to rest upon. A wooden frame or such like may be made to fit the bedstead for such cases.

Every hospital should have dropsy and surgical bedsteads for raising a patient when he cannot be moved, for inclining him at a certain angle, etc., also water and air beds. For many purposes different forms of new spring bedsteads will be found very useful.

14. Water Supply

One of the most essential sanitary provisions for a hospital is an abundant supply of pure, soft water. The obtaining of such a supply presupposes a careful examination of the sources, and a chemical analysis, both quantitative and qualitative. It has frequently happened, especially in warm climates, that waters of a most impure character, containing poisonous amounts of dissolved organic matter, have been used for sick, without suspicion that the diarrhea or dysentery of which they were dying was nothing more than a *water disease.* Absence of colour, taste and smell is no criterion of sufficient purity, for some of the most impure waters are often the most agreeable, as, e.g., the water drawn from wells supplied by filtration through old graveyards is often clear, bright and sparkling, from being charged with carbonic acid derived from human remains in the soil, and, during an epidemic, poisonous.

Hard water containing sulphates or carbonates is unfit for most hospital purposes—especially so for dressing wounds. Filtered rainwater is generally the best for this purpose. In small hospitals, either spring or well water should be selected after analysis, and, if found to be hard, the roof water should be stored for surgical purposes. In large hospitals where no other than a *hard* water supply can be obtained, it will be possible to soften the water by the lime process. But in large hospitals where engine power is used, there is often much waste steam, which can be usefully condensed for soft water. Of course, for all pharmaceutical purposes, the softer the water the better, and the same rule holds for the cooking, especially of vegetables.

Having obtained the best available water source, all the water required for ordinary ward purposes should be laid on at pressure, hot and cold, all over the building, for sinks, ablution basins and baths, but never from a cistern within the hospital. This would be to expose the water to impurity, and the hospital to damp.

The consumption of water for an English hospital, including, besides patients, all its officers and servants (who may be roughly estimated as 150 for 500 patients), is on an average of 25 gallons for each person per day. This includes baths, brewing, washing the pavements, but *not* laundry work, farther than the necessary wringing out of soiled sheets, etc., before sending to the laundry. Of this amount two thirds at least should be soft water for personal use—one third being for domestic purposes may be hard. In the laboratory of a hospital of this size, the steam boiler will supply 500 gallons of condensed water per day, to be used for all mixtures, decoctions, infusions, etc., and collected in iron or slate cisterns for the purpose. One gallon of soft water per patient per day is thus on an average required for the pharmacy. I may just allude to the difficulty, if you have one tap of soft water and one of hard, of making sure that the attendants never use the hard for soft-water purposes.

There should be convenient means in or close to the wards for obtaining pure filtered drinking water for the sick.

15. Drainage and Sewerage

No drain should ever pass under a hospital; all sinks, water closets, lavatories and baths should be so placed that the drainage should be conveyed directly away, without passing under any part of the hospital. And for this purpose all drain pipes from them should be placed in the outer walls, but never against any inner wall of the building.

All drains or pipes for the purpose of conveying away water from any part of the hospital should be carefully trapped between the outer wall of the building and the sewer, and all drains should be ventilated. An excellent arrangement has been adopted at the Herbert Hospital, by which all the ward drainage is discharged into vertical drain pipes in the outer walls, which drain pipes are carried from a trap in the main drain below, straight up above the roof of the building, where they are left open to the air. This ensures thorough ventilation of the pipe, and prevents the possibility of the regurgitation of foul air into the building. A perforated box of charcoal is placed over the upper opening of the drain pipe to destroy any noxious gas that might otherwise escape into the air above the building.

16. Kitchen

The kitchen should be placed away from the wards. Its walls and ceiling should be of light-coloured cement, for plaster has a tendency to fall off from the vapour and effluvia of the kitchen.

Hospital cooking apparatus should be capable of doing two sets of cooking: (1) all the ordinary "diets," [and] (2) casual diets and "extras" for emergencies.

It has been said that a good cook can cook with anything, but cooking in a hospital is a very important part of the general administration, and requires to be done with the utmost regularity, efficiency and economy. In providing apparatus, it is necessary to consider how many "diets" of the same kind will be required, also what the nature of the cooking should be. Usually this consists of soups, farinaceous preparations, including puddings, stewed vegetables, roast joints, baked meat or meat roasted in a roasting oven, broiled beefsteak or mutton chop (there should be no frying in a hospital, except for fish, and even fish cooked after the French plan, in oil, is better; if a patient can digest a fried steak, it is the best proof that he is fit to be discharged from hospital), tea and coffee. The "extra" articles usually required are beef-tea or warmed beef juice, sago, etc. There should always be plenty of boiling water.

The dimensions, as well as the number of parts of which any hospital cooking apparatus should consist, will depend, of course, on the size of the hospital. The cheapest fuel for boiling liquids on a large scale is common coal. Where stewing has to be done on a large scale, steam is the best agent. For stewing on a small scale, and preparing extra articles at irregular times, gas is by far the most convenient fuel. But its use requires to be carefully restricted to such purposes, otherwise it will be found too costly. Roasting is now very well and economically done in ovens constructed for the purpose, with ordinary fuel. Gas ovens are sometimes convenient, but they are more expensive. Lately, many improved forms of hospital cooking apparatus capable of performing these various processes, have been introduced. For small hospitals, all the parts are generally combined in one small apparatus placed in an ordinary kitchen fireplace. For large hospitals, the different parts are better separated. Of course, the same cooking apparatus and kitchen which answer for the patients are sufficient also for officers, nurses and servants, although tea and breakfast will probably be made in the respective quarters of each.

The cooking apparatus, boilers, ovens, etc., if placed in the centre of the kitchen, after the French plan, instead of against the walls, will afford twice the amount of fire space.

17. Washhouse

How to Dispose of the Foul Linen. Of course it should never be treasured up in any ward, scullery or closet in the hospital. The sooner it is sent away and in the washtub the better. In hospitals of a few beds it should be thrown into a basket and carried straight away immediately, but in large hospitals, where changes are constantly going on, it is necessary to have ready means of conveying it out of the building, and for this purpose nothing answers so well as foul-linen chutes. These should be built in the wall. The best material for them is glazed earthenware piping, 15 to 18 inches in diameter. They should have an open mouth, also of earthenware, with a door, opening not near a ward, but from a staircase or well-ventilated passage. And they should end below in a small closet, out of and removed at once to the washhouse. To be quite safe, the pipe should be carried up to the roof of the building, though of a smaller diameter, to secure that the shaft is well ventilated.

Hospital washing should never be done in or close to a hospital. In a small hospital, the kitchen may be put in the basement, provided it is not under a ward, and it is very well ventilated, but the washhouse *never*. It at least should be always detached, and if within the hospital grounds at all, at the farthest attainable point in them, and to leeward. The reason, of course, is that pure air in a hospital is the sine qua non [without which nothing], while the surest method of obtaining foul air is to combine the excretions of the patients with the steam of hot water, and give access for this combined result to the sick by staircases or open windows.

The excellent new washing, drying and wringing machines lately invented are so numerous that it would take too long to enumerate them. On the whole, the laundry at the Wellington Barracks, which also washes for all the Guards' hospitals and barracks, and the new laundry at Haslar Naval Hospital, are the best I have seen. But every day brings in fresh inventions, and a reformer is always adopting the good ones. Admirable ones are attached to the new Herbert Hospital at Woolwich, and to Netley Hospital. The former is intended to wash for all the troops in garrison, as well as for the sick. I do not think that any reliable comparison has yet been made between the French system adopted at the Salpêtrière and Lariboisière hospitals and the English system. The French consists in filtering hot ley[14] through the clothes, which are placed for that purpose in large tubs, with a compartment at the bottom, from which the ley is pumped up by machinery, and allowed to flow over the top of the linen, through which it filters into the compartment, to be again raised by the machine.

This plan is stated to be the most economical which has been tried in Paris.

The essential characteristic of the Haslar one is boiling by steam, the linen being afterwards placed in a rotating washing machine. The method in use in the Wellington Barracks consists in passing the linen through slowly rotating washing tubs, in which it undergoes a process of *waulking* by wooden rods. This latter plan is both economical and effectual.

To ascertain which is the most really economical of the French and English plans, it would be necessary to inquire, not only into the relative cost of washing, but into the relative wear and tear. The hardness or softness of the water must also be taken into account. The softer water is the cheaper, both in the consumption of soap and the wear and tear. Now the Paris water is in hardness to that of London as 20 to 16, and as 20 to 2 to that of Glasgow. Probably the Paris method is the only economical one with the Paris water. All the water used at the new Herbert Hospital, including that for the laundry, has a hardness of 13 degrees, which will be reduced to 5½ degrees by Dr Clarke's softening process. This will effect a large economy in soap and linen, in addition to the advantage of having softer water for general hospital use.

Clean Linen Room. After passing through the laundry, the linen is returned to the hospital for use, and anyone who wishes to see perfect arrangements for storing and issuing clean linen must go to the Paris hospitals. Each hospital there is provided with one or more large well-lighted rooms containing every arrangement for the mending, classification and issuing of ward linen. The linen is *stacked* in open framework so as to admit currents of air through the piles—a thing of great importance.

---

14 Ley, an alkaline solution for disinfection.

This is a point of administrative detail in which all English hospitals are woefully behindhand. Even in the most recent plans I have seen, there has either been no provision of the kind, or it has been a mere half-dark closet. The mending room ought to be a separate room from the clean linen store, and adjoining. There should be, besides, on each ward a lock-up movable press, best placed under the sill of the large end window, with a table leaf on hinges for folding, for such articles as may be stored in the ward.

18. Operating Theatres

I need not say that surgical cases should never be placed higher than the first floor. It is important that an operating theatre should not only be on a level, but central between men's and women's surgical wards. An operating theatre in a third storey is very objectionable, particularly if patients have to be carried up a narrow flight of stairs and back after the operation has been performed. The proper place for an operating theatre is to be built out at the back of the centre, and the board room may be under it. It is not uncommon, in small country hospitals, to have a recess or small room leading from the operating theatre, in which the patients remain until they have recovered, or at least recovered the immediate effects of the operation. But it is more and more becoming the practice of the best London hospitals to carry such patients back to their own ward, where it is believed (a belief in which I entirely concur) they have, if the ward is what it should be, better advantages, better chances, better care, nursing and supervision. Of course there are exceptional cases, as in ovariotomy, trephining, etc., which may require to be by themselves. But this is for the surgeon to decide upon.

Operating theatres are best lighted by a good large skylight and a steady northern light from one large window, quite up to the ceiling. There must be no conflicting lights from different windows, and no southern aspect. Now, as the operating theatre is the only room in the hospital which ought to have one sole north light, this is very convenient, because it may occupy a situation which would not do for a ward.

We will next consider the application of these principles to the improvement of hospital plans.

4. Improved Hospital Plans

Within the last few years very considerable advances have been made in hospital architecture in this country. A number of hospitals have been improved and added to on correct principles. Several new hospitals embodying these principles have been built, and the plans of many more are at present under discussion. The subject has also awakened renewed attention abroad, and quite recently two works of great importance have appeared on the subject in Paris. One of these is the *Étude sur les hôpitaux*, by M Armand Husson, director of the General Administration of the *Assistance Publique*, the other the *Rapport sur les hôpitaux civils de la ville de Londres*, by Mm Blondel and Ser,[15] of the same bureau. These works afford information of great interest on the whole question of hospital administration, and I am indebted to them for several illustrations introduced into these pages. I have had the opportunity also of examining a number of new hospital plans for buildings which it is proposed to construct in different parts of the country. They have all borne marks of careful study of the subject, but there are one or two points in which all of them present certain defects in common. I shall merely allude to these as points of experience, before proceeding to the general subject of this section.

One of the most common mistakes in hospital plans, even in some of the most recent of those I have seen, is mixing up together, in the same block, sick wards and administrative offices of all kinds. It need hardly be pointed out that such an attempt must necessarily lead to a very complicated structure, containing large wards and an indefinite number of rooms of different sizes, all connected by passages and stairs more or less dark, badly ventilated and diffusing a common atmosphere throughout the building. By this arrangement of parts, all the old complications of badly constructed hospitals are reproduced in another form. The usual excuse is that it is cheaper than to separate the sick from the administration, which is extremely doubtful. One thing is not at all doubtful, that such an arrangement exposes both sick and administrators to very unnecessary risks, and is one of the causes of fever among the latter, already mentioned, a danger which should never be incurred on any plea of economy.

It is possible, no doubt, to ventilate more or less effectually a complicated building of this sort, but practically it will never be done.

---

15 Louis Ser, *Rapport sur les hôpitaux civils de la ville de Londres au point de vue de la comparaison de ces établissements avec les hôpitaux de la ville de Paris.*

Wherever any form of hospital construction requires much thought to be applied to its ventilation and other sanitary arrangements, it may be considered quite certain that the hospital is not a safe one for sick. Practically it is impossible to escape from this, viz., that safe hospital construction must, at whatever (apparent) cost, contain a maximum of facility and a minimum of difficulty for keeping every part of the building healthy.

It is a fundamental principle that the pavilions, whether single or double, should contain nothing but the sick and the offices immediately required for the ward. Everything else, board rooms, chapels, quarters for officers and servants, except for the head nurse or nurses of each ward, stores, kitchens, laundries, should be placed in a separate building or buildings. It would be better even that convalescent rooms, where it is determined that there should be such rooms, should be out of the main building, but accessible under cover, for the obvious reason that convalescents require change of air which cannot be obtained under any circumstances in a hospital. The matron should always have her rooms as near to the nursing staff as possible. And as it is highly desirable that the day and night nurses of each ward should be kept as a separate staff, lodged as near to the head nurse as possible; if room can be found for these near their own pavilion, it is better.

Simplicity of construction, involving, as it should always do, a provision of abundant light and ventilation through every part of the hospital in which sick are placed, can only be secured in hospitals of any size by separating the administrative part from the sick part. The smallest country hospital should consist of at least two blocks of building.

The utmost simplicity of plan is an essential of good hospital construction. Complication of plan interferes with light, ventilation, discipline, facility of supervision. Every hole and corner, every passage, every small ward which need not have been there interferes with these four vital conditions of a good hospital. Every skulking place which can be spared must be avoided. As an invariable hospital rule, rather more than elsewhere in military hospitals, publicity may be considered as the best police and the best protection. It is far better that thirty patients should see the nurses's door than one or none. It is quite necessary that the chief ward attendant should be able to see the whole of her or his patients at once.

When the architect has arrived at a clear idea of what a hospital pavilion means—what it should contain and what it should not contain—the next important matter is to determine how the pavilions are to be arranged so as to form a hospital. From what has been said, it will be obvious that the arrangement of parts will depend on the number of beds for which the hospital is to be built. The following principles will enable a good block plan to be made.

Plan No. 3
Bucks Infirmary

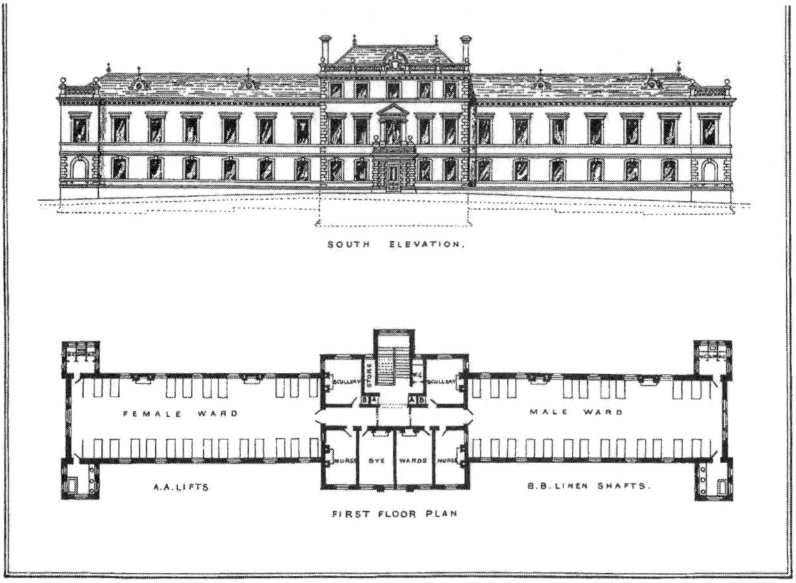

1. Small Hospitals

For hospitals intended to consist of two pavilions in line, the arrangement shown in Fig. 16 might be followed. It consists of two wings, containing one ward on each floor of the wing, and a centre block for the administration.

Figure 16
Two Pavilions in line

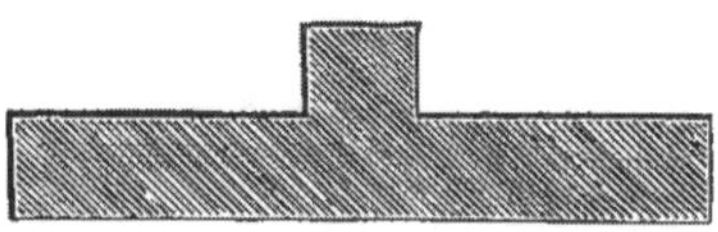

A block plan of this kind, if erected in an airy position, would possess every requisite for health. The size of the administrative part of the building will depend upon the nature of the hospital management, and upon whether or not out-patients are to be received within the hospital.

When the administration is of very limited extent, the arrangement in Fig. 16 would be unobjectionable. But, as a general rule, and especially where out-patients have to be received, as much of the administrative part of the building as possible should be detached behind the main line of the hospital, in the manner shown in the regimental hospital plans, Figs. 20 [and] 21.

The plan and elevation of the New Bucks Infirmary (No. 3), intended for fifty-two beds, with the offices on the ground floor, and wards 16 feet on the first floor, built by Mr Brandon,[16] is the most recently completed civil hospital on the new plan, and has been found to answer very well.

When the number of beds for which the hospital is intended exceeds what can be accommodated in a double pavilion of this form, the plan shown in Fig. 17 may be adopted. This figure shows a building consisting of two double pavilions and a centre. Wherever this form is adopted, the pavilions should be entirely cut off from the centre by spacious staircases carried up where the centre joins the pavilions. In a hospital of this form, the centre should be one floor in height; the pavilions would be in two floors.

FIGURE 17
Hospital of Two Double Pavilions and Centre

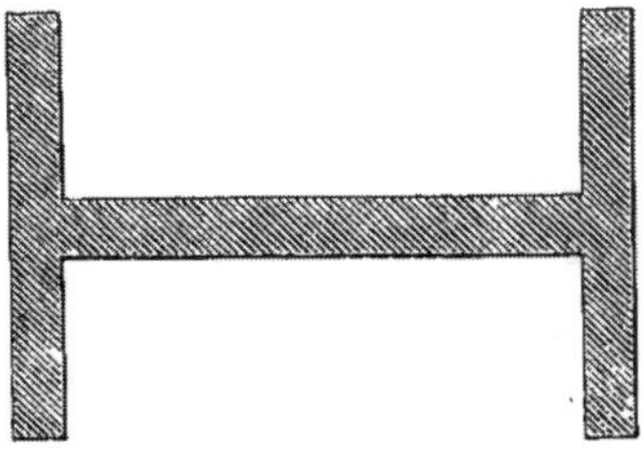

A similar arrangement of parts is shown in Fig. 18. In this case the administration is a separate block, two or three floors in height, connected with the pavilions, two floors in height, by a centre one floor in height.

16 David Brandon (1813-97), architect of the Bucks Infirmary.

Figure 18
Hospital of Double Pavilion Wings with central administration

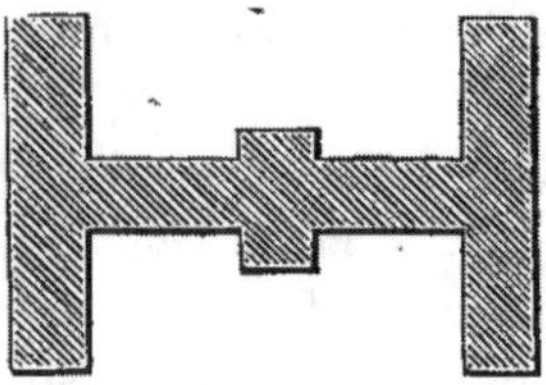

Fig. 19 is one half of Fig. 17 and consists of three pavilions radiating from a common centre. If this plan is adopted, there should be a large central staircase at the point of junction.

Figure 19
Double Pavilion Hospital with projecting Centre

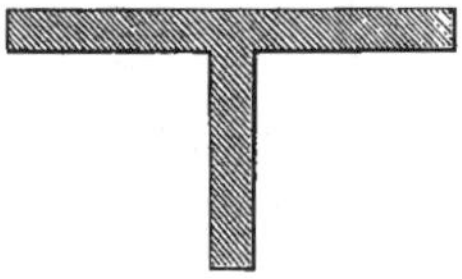

Another application of the pavilion principle is shown in Figs. 20 and 21, and is adapted for regimental hospitals, either for cavalry or infantry. For a full cavalry regiment, one floor is sufficient. For an infantry regiment, double the accommodation is required, and the building is then erected in two floors. This is simply one of the double pavilions of the Herbert Hospital, with so much of the administration as is absolutely necessary arranged between the wards, the remainder being in a block behind.

Figure 20
Ground Plan of a Regimental Hospital for 120 Beds

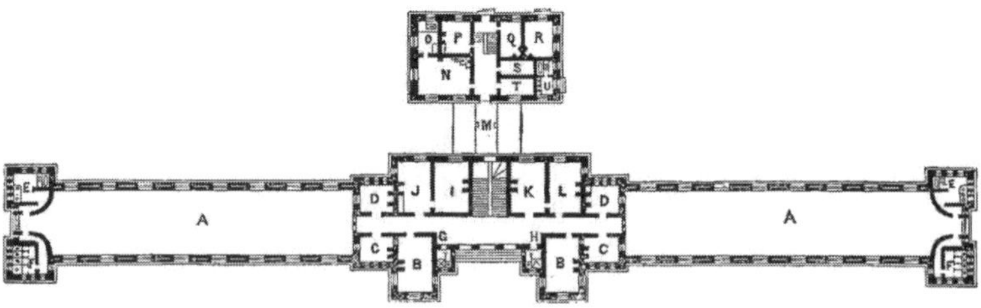

Figure 21
First Floor Plan

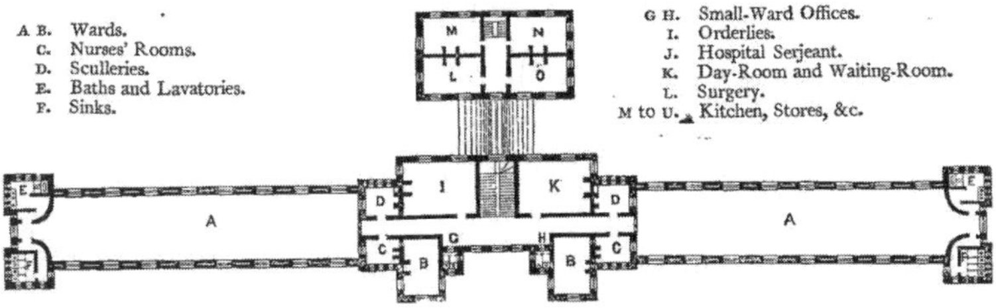

Several cavalry hospitals on this plan have been constructed, and they are found to answer admirably. A pavilion hospital on the same plan is proposed for Malta, to receive the sick from barracks on the Cotonera side of the great harbour.

These examples of block plans are taken from existing hospitals. The object, in buildings of this class, is to bring all parts of the hospital under one roof, more with a view to facility of communication throughout than to securing the sanitary state of the hospital. Such plans can only be used within certain limits. As a rule it is safer to consider every pavilion containing the largest number of sick a pavilion ought to contain as a separate hospital, and to connect all the pavilions together in such a way as to insure a separate ventilation for each block.

2. Large Hospitals

I next ask, what should be the arrangement of parts in the larger class of hospitals?

Fortunately we have a number of examples in different parts of Europe of excellent arrangement of parts in block plans. No doubt all the older hospitals of this class admit of considerable improvements in detail. But the block plan can be studied by itself with great advantage. I shall choose a few examples illustrative of existing hospitals—of hospitals in the progress of construction, and of plans completed but not yet carried into execution.

Fig. 22 is the block plan of St Bartholomew's Hospital, showing four pavilions arranged at right angles to each other, with the corners open to admit of the circulation of air. In such a hospital each block might be a double pavilion, each in two floors, and each pavilion might contain two wards with their offices on each floor. The advantages of this plan are compactness of structure and a corresponding facility in administration, together with open angles to allow of circulation of air in the court. The disadvantages are that the means of communication must either be in the open air in all weathers, or under a verandah or corridor carried along one side of the lower floor wards, partially obstructing the light and ventilation. All the sides of the hospital could not be thoroughly exposed to the sun's rays, summer and winter, although this ground of the objection would be diminished by placing two of the open opposite angles north and south.

Figure 22
Block Plan of St Bartholomew's Hospital

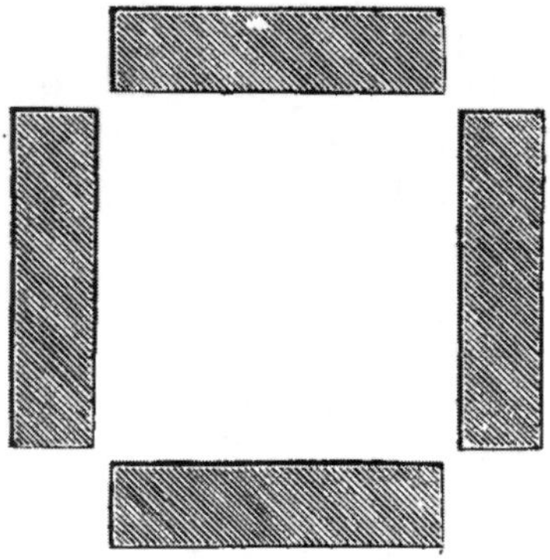

Fig. 23 is an illustration of the same block as it exists at Yarmouth Naval Hospital. This is a very good building, one of the best, indeed, of the older hospitals in Great Britain. The pavilions are on two floors only; they are wide enough apart at the corners to admit the sea breeze into the court, and every part of the building is connected by an arched corridor along the ground floor. This corridor of course partially obstructs the light of the wards. The ward details, as shown in the plan, are not altogether in accordance with modern requirements, but they could easily be made so in any future applications of the same principle. And the lower floor wards should be raised on basements to such a height as to admit of the connecting corridor, being carried round the building below the level of the ward windows.

An exceedingly simple arrangement of pavilions is shown in Fig. 24, which gives a ground plan of the "Fondation Brezin," at Garches. All the administrative parts of the building are in separate blocks. The pavilions and chapel are also separate, and all are connected by a simple corridor carried past the end of the blocks.

FIGURE 23
Ground Plan of Naval Hospital, Yarmouth

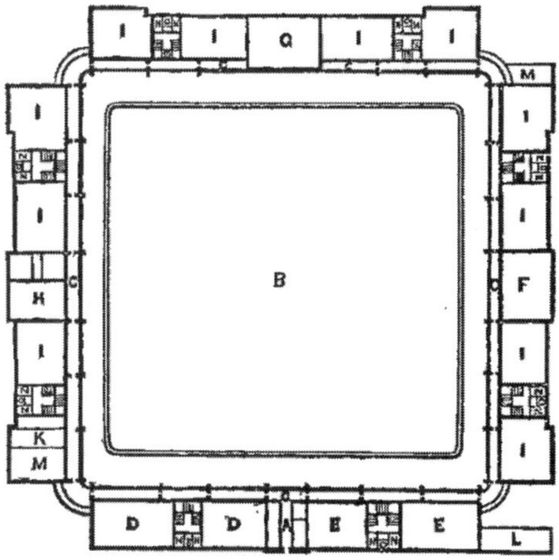

A Entrance Archway.
B Garden.
C Open-arched Corridor, one story high, surrounding the garden.
D Rooms for sick officers.
E Steward's stores.
F Chapel.
G First Floor, Operating Theatre: Ground Floor, Billiard Room.
H Committee Room, Surgery, &c.
I I I Wards, 14 beds each.
K Padded Room.
L Bath Rooms, Wash-house, &c.
M M Sculleries.
N N Nurses' Rooms.
O O Water Closets.

I do not propose this as a *hospital* plan. It will be seen at once that it is deficient in proper hospital details. But it contains the pavilion arrangement reduced to its utmost simplicity for purposes of health and facility of administration. (This building is in fact planned for infirm, and not for sick.) It contains the germ of the hospital construction adopted for Lariboisière, of which here is a plan (No. 4).

The famous Lariboisière Hospital consists of six detached single pavilions for sick, two pavilions in the front for administration, two behind for the sisters and nurses and for the washing establishment, with chapel, operation room, baths, etc., in detached buildings at the end furthest from the entrance. Between the pavilions is a range of one-storey rooms used for dining rooms, etc. The pavilions contain three floors of wards, one large ward for thirty-two beds, and one small ward for two beds at the far end of it, on each floor. Each floor has a sister's room and scullery, and a spacious staircase gives access to

Figure 24
Fondation Brezin (Hospice de la Reconnaissance) at Garches

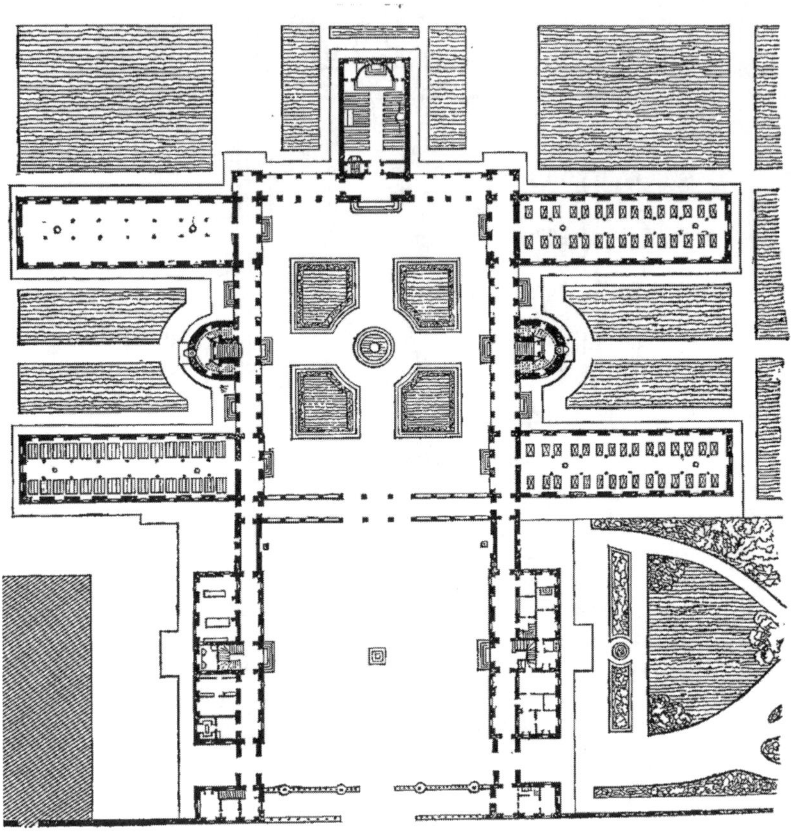

the wards. All the pavilions are connected by an arched glazed corridor, one floor in height, over which is an open terrace, used by convalescents, and also as a means of access between the first floors, when the weather permits. The hospital contains 612 beds, divided amongst six separate pavilions, which are just as much distinct hospitals as if they were miles from each other. The block plan of this hospital is excellent, but the pavilions are too close together for their height, or rather there should have been only two floors of wards instead of three. The small wards are badly placed, away from the sister, and close to the *open privies* of the ward. This hospital is warmed and ventilated, unfortunately, by artificial means, and has presented the anomaly, easily resolved by those acquainted with the sanitary requirements for sick, of one of the best hospitals in existence, so far as the block plan is concerned, yielding one of the highest rates of mortality.

PLAN NO. 4
Paris Hôpital de Lariboisière

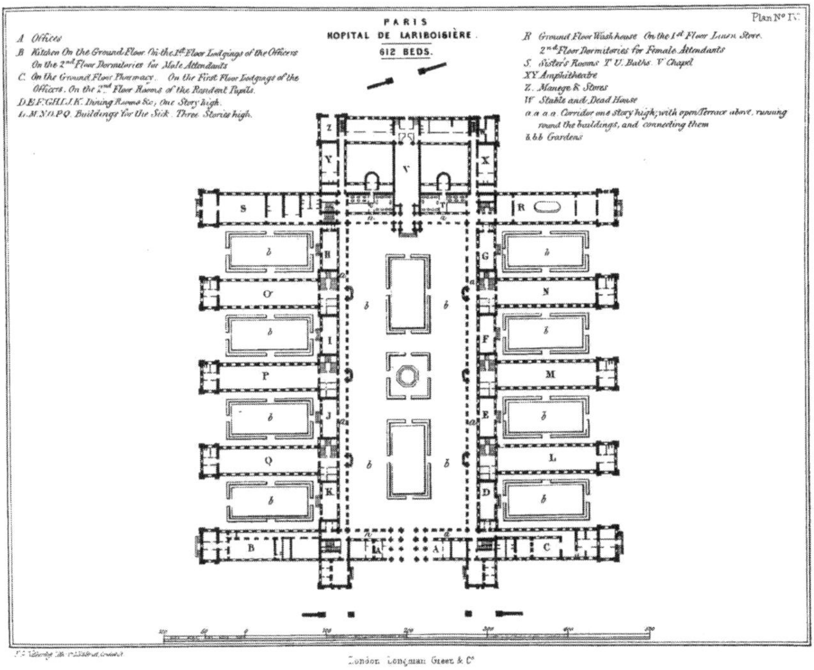

There is another hospital, the St Jean, at Brussels, built upon a similar plan, and also a hospital at Bordeaux.

The Vincennes Military Hospital, for 637 beds, of which I give a ground plan (No. 5), shows another arrangement of pavilions. In this example, the pavilions for sick are double, with wards for non-commissioned officers, and rooms for sisters at the two extreme ends, but cut off by separate staircases. These pavilions form two sides of a square; the third side is formed by a block containing the chapel and the administrative offices and quarters. The fourth side of the square is open to the country. Each pavilion consists of three floors and an attic, and is connected with the administration by a glazed corridor as far as the central staircases. It consists, in fact, of two hospitals, one for 308, the other for 332 sick, connected with one administration common to both. The disadvantages of the plan are that, if the whole building were used, there would be three floors and an attic occupied by sick, instead of two floors only. The ward details are also objectionable in some important points.

Plan No. 5
Vincennes Military Hospital

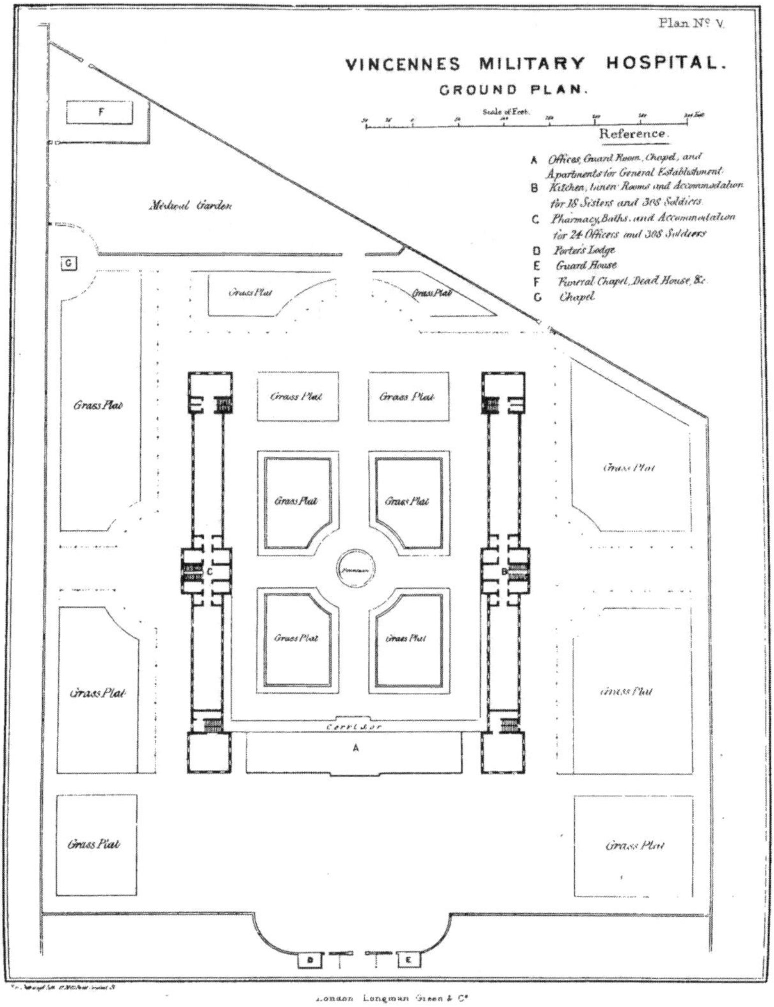

One advantage of the double pavilion adopted in this plan must be mentioned, and that is the facility with which a large number of sick can be superintended and nursed on the same floor, instead of entailing on the attendants the amount of running up and down stairs required in the Lariboisière plan. The Vincennes wards, however, are built for rather too many beds. But, on the other hand, the building is in an open, elevated situation in the country, and each pavilion is divided from top to bottom by an unusually spacious staircase up to the roof. It is ventilated and warmed by the draught of a chimney and hot water vessels.

All the advantages of the Vincennes and Lariboisière plans, without any of their disadvantages, and with greatly improved sanitary arrangements, will be realized in the new Herbert Hospital now under construction at Woolwich (Plan No. 6).

Plan No. 6
Herbert Hospital

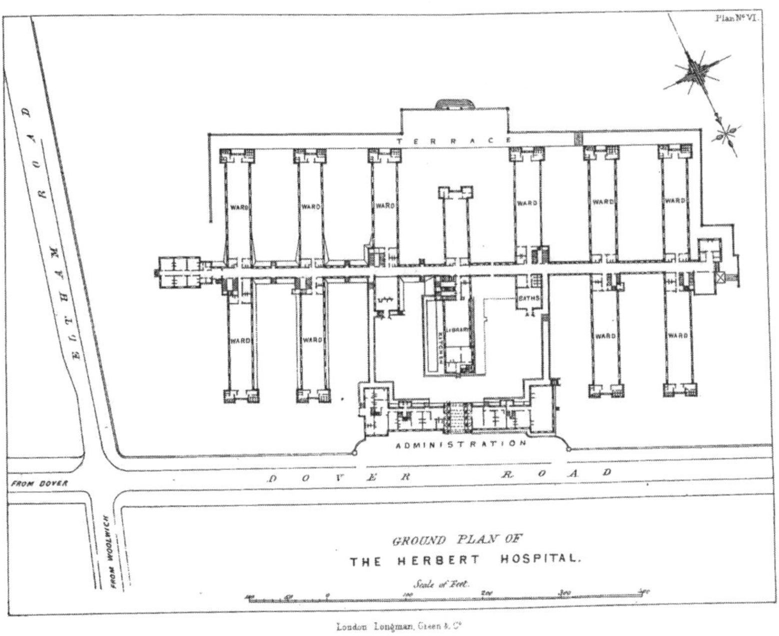

This, when completed, will be by far the finest hospital establishment in the united kingdom, or indeed in Europe. It consists of four double and three single pavilions, with the ends in the free air. All the wards are raised on basements, those at the lower end of the ground are so lofty as to afford excellent accommodation for the museum, library, medical officers' rooms, boardrooms and stores. There are only two floors of wards to each pavilion, and the distance between the pavilions is double the height of the pavilion, measured from the floor to the lowest ward. Every ward has a large end window, commanding beautiful views, and the ablution and bath accommodation, together with water closets, is placed in the free atmosphere at the end of the wards. Each large ward contains from twenty-eight to thirty-two beds, with windows along the opposite sides, one for every two beds, and each ward has a nurse's room and scullery.

Unfortunately the army regulation number of cubic feet per bed has limited the height of the wards to 14 feet. There is a convalescents' day room in the central pavilion. The kitchen is in a basement, also in the centre; over it there is a library, and over the library the chapel. All the administrative offices and quarters are in a separate block in front. The axis of the wards is a little to the east of the north, and each side will receive the sun's rays during some part of the day. At one end of the hospital there are separate lunatic wards with separate offices. At the other end is the operation theatre, with a few small wards for special cases. The total accommodation is for 650 beds, in seven detached buildings, all connected together through the centre by a corridor one floor in height, with a basement corridor beneath, through which the whole of the service of the hospital, so far as regards the conveyance of diets, medicines, coals and the removal of dust and foul linen, will be carried out. This is effected by a system of lifts and chutes. And the result will be that the usual bustle observed in hospital passages will be altogether avoided.

This hospital embodies the great administrative principle of an entire separation between what is immediately necessary for the sick and what is not so, and yet without interfering with the efficiency of the administration. Over the corridor there is an open terrace, to which convalescents in the first-floor wards will have easy access in fine weather. And the covered corridor below will be available for exercise in wet weather. Each ward is 26½ feet wide and 14 feet high, and each bed has 93 to 97 superficial feet and 1200 to 1400 cubic feet. The walls will have a polished light-coloured surface. It is intended to warm the wards by two open fireplaces along the centre of the wards, the flues being carried under the floor, and used for warming the air admitted to the wards. The floors are of iron beams, filled in with concrete, and covered with oak boarding. The whole will be fireproof, and the sick in the lower wards will not suffer from noise in the wards overhead. Hot and cold water will be laid over the entire building, and the supply, which is taken from chalk, and hard, will be softened by the lime process before being transmitted to the hospital.

In Malta it is proposed to erect a general military hospital on the pavilion principle for 300 beds, with the pavilions differently arranged from any existing example. A ground plan of this proposed hospital is given in Plan No. 7. The site, chosen as the most healthy in the garrison, is limited, and the arrangement of parts has to be conformed to the shape of the ground. But so flexible is the pavilion construction that it suits itself readily to this requirement. There will be six pavilions arranged side by side, each containing two floors of wards, and the whole connected by open arcades sufficient to afford shelter for sun and rain, but to leave ventilation perfectly free. The entire administration is detached and placed in front of the hospital, but all parts of it are connected by convenient staircases with the corridors. The walls on the sides towards the sun and the roof will be double to ensure coolness. The hospital will overlook the sea at a height of 170 feet above its level.

Plan No. 7
Proposed General Military Hospital, Valetta

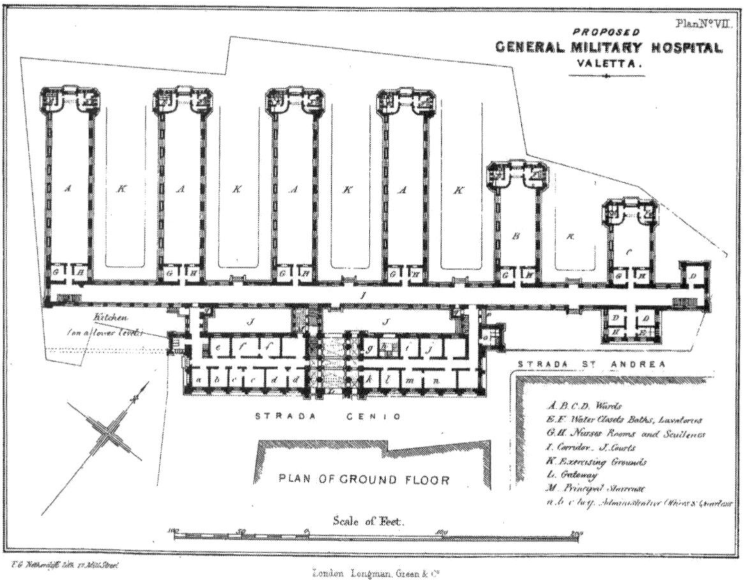

Other two establishments are proposed to be erected by the enlightened local government of Malta. One of these is an asylum for 1000

aged and infirm persons, 500 of each sex. A ground plan of this proposed establishment is given, Plan No. 8. It consists of eight pavilions, each two floors in height, arranged in two squares, containing in all twenty-nine wards for beds, with dining rooms on the ground floor. To each square there is a day room placed in the centre. The whole establishment is connected by open arcades, with terraces over. Every block throughout the entire establishment is detached from every other. And the latrines, lavatories and baths, which will be on the most improved English construction, are in detached square blocks in the angles, and accessible from the wards under open arcades. The administrative portion of the building is very complete, and the whole exemplifies an arrangement which, with some alterations in detail, might be adopted for a hospital of the same number of sick, if it ever were considered necessary to bring so many together.

Plan No. 8
Asylum for the Aged and Infirm, Malta

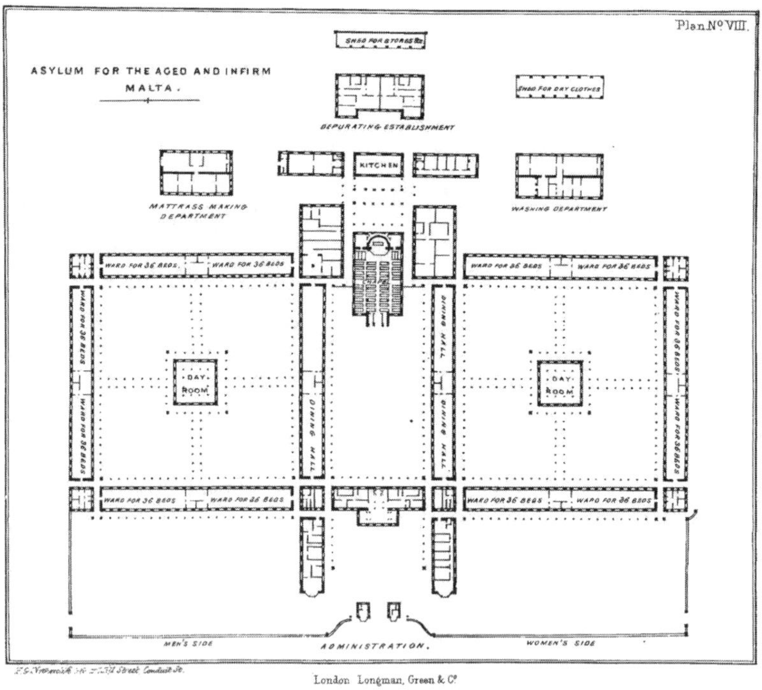

Connected with this establishment, it is proposed to build a hospital for 300 beds, on a plan shown in No. 9. This consists of two long pavilions similar in construction to those of the Herbert Hospital, and two smaller detached blocks for the treatment of special or offensive cases. It will be observed that each of the larger blocks has a dining room and day room—a matter of necessity in this building, for a considerable proportion of its inmates will be incurable, not acute cases.

PLAN NO. 9
Hospital for Incurables, Malta

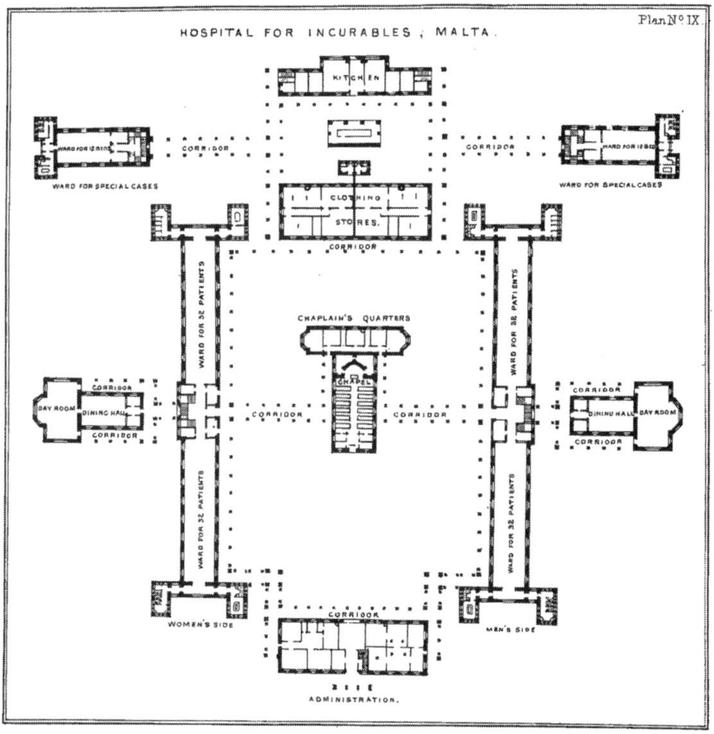

The sanitary details of both plans contain everything required for ensuring a healthy state of the buildings. They were prepared at the instance of the government of Malta, by Mr T.H. Wyatt,[17] and when completed they will place this small island in the foremost rank as regards its charitable institutions.

---

17 Thomas Henry Wyatt (1807-80), hospital architect.

These illustrations of hospital construction, when compared with what has been the past practice in this country, will show at once what ought to be done, and what ought not to be done, in planning buildings to be occupied by sick or maimed.

Some recent plans, however, have, alas! reproduced all the old errors in a novel form. Sometimes the wards have been improved in proportions, in light and facilities for ventilation, while the arrangements for baths, lavatories and water closets have been most objectionable. In other instances, kitchens and other offices have been placed under the sick wards, while the wards themselves were good. Again, as already mentioned, the administrative parts of the building have been so mixed up with the portions allotted for sick as to introduce all the old objectionable dark corners and useless passages which constitute so large a proportion of the worst class of hospital buildings. Mistakes such as these can only be avoided by a very careful study and application of the principles laid down. It should never be forgotten that the first thing to be considered is what is best for the sick, not what may appear to be cheapest—for the cheapness is only apparent—not what will make a good architectural elevation, for this is a point quite beside the question.

The very first condition to be sought in planning a building is that it shall be fit for its purpose. And the first architectural law is that fitness is the foundation of beauty. The hospital architect may feel assured that, only when he has planned a building which will afford the best chance of speedy recovery to sick and maimed people, will his architecture and the economy which he seeks be realized.

5. Convalescent Hospitals

It is a rule without any exception that no patient ought ever to stay a day longer in hospital than is absolutely essential for medical or surgical treatment. What, then, is to be done with those who are not yet fit for workaday life? Every hospital should have its convalescent branch, and every county its convalescent home.

The first necessity of a convalescent hospital is that it should not be like a hospital at all, and the very best kind of convalescent hospital would be a string of cottages. The reason for this is fourfold:

1. To get rid of the idea of being in hospital altogether from the minds of the inmates, and to substitute for it that of home. As long as they are hospital inmates, they feel as hospital inmates, they think as hospital inmates, they act as hospital inmates, not as people recovering.

2. To secure a more free and bracing atmosphere than can ever be secured in any building containing a large number of inmates.

3. Because cottages may be more slightly built, and therefore are less expensive than large, complicated, solid buildings.

4. Because in the point of view of moral discipline it is yet more important to separate men from women among convalescents than among the sick. And of course this can be done much more easily and efficiently, and with far less trouble to the administration, in separate houses than in separate parts of the same house.

It is almost needless to repeat the A B C of all sanitary lessons—that the best building intended to hold a large number of inmates can never be made so healthy as a cottage for a small number, if well constructed.

All rules against curtains, against washing in the dormitory, etc., which *must* be maintained in hospitals, may be relaxed, at all events on the female side, in a properly built convalescent home. It should be a home. Each bed should be separated by a rod and iron staple, and curtain, about 6 or 7 feet high (to be pulled far back in the daytime) from the next bed, and a wash-hand stand should be permitted within this compartment.

The number of beds for which each ward, whether for men or women, is constructed, should not exceed six, or be less than three: almost every hospital condition, in fact, is reversed.

The indispensable hospital rule, that no patient should be sent to or admitted into the kitchen or ward scullery, is also reversed in a convalescent home, where the more the patients are occupied the better. The men who are able for it should be employed in the garden, which is better for them than their indoor trades. The women who are able for it should do nearly all the household work, at least on their own side, and a little sick cookery may well be taught them in the kitchen, but on a hot plate, as convalescents should not be called upon to stand long at a hot kitchen fire.

That all this must be done with discretion, and in subordination to the necessity of giving the convalescents constant fresh air, and as much as possible of it out of doors, it is almost needless to say.

Some convalescents will want entire rest, and this, with fresh air and good food, will be the main element of their recovery. This will be the case with those forms of uterine disease now sadly common among young female servants, from the use of stiff stays and form of petticoats hanging from the waist. Others will be able to walk and yet not able to use their arms to do household work. With all, much care will be needed to prevent them damping their feet or clothes.

The medical officer and head sisters will have to exercise constant vigilance in this matter of occupation.

There are as yet few convalescent establishments. And as it is most probable that this class of accommodation will be extended, it is important to observe correct principles in future plans. Here are two or three illustrations of different kinds of buildings.

Fig. 25 is a plan of the first floor of the convalescent institution at Walton-on-Thames. On the left are four women's wards, opening from a common inner passage. There is a corresponding number of men's wards on the right-hand side of the plan. There is one ward for nine beds, two wards for eleven beds each, one ward for twelve, one for thirteen, two for fourteen and one for fifteen. The projecting ward behind, called the Ellesmere Ward, is for eighteen beds. The cubic feet per bed vary from 459 to 874, the average being about 628 cubic feet per bed. There are 117 beds on a floor, all of which, except eighteen (in the Ellesmere Ward) are in rooms opening from inner passages, and having windows on one side only. The Ellesmere Ward has windows on three sides. In general construction the building can only be considered as an inferior model of a provincial hospital. It is a praiseworthy attempt to meet a great want, but its details should certainly not be followed in future institutions.

Figure 25
First Floor Plan of the Convalescent Institution, Walton-on-Thames

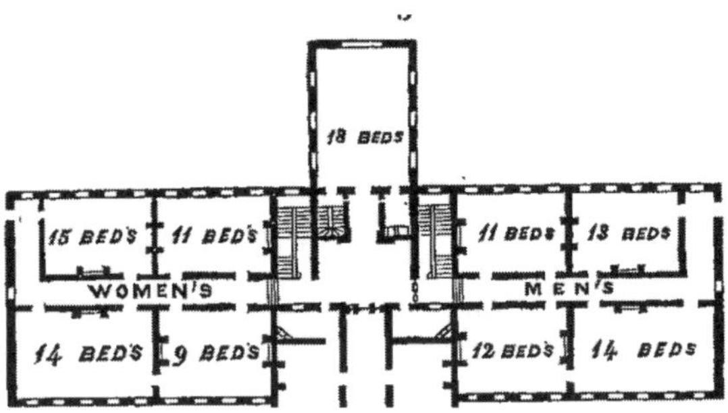

Fig. 26 is a sketch plan of the male convalescent institution founded by the emperor at Vincennes.[18] It is constructed on a totally different

18 The military hospital at Vincennes, which opened in June 1858, was commissioned by Napoléon III during the Crimean War.

FIGURE 26
Sketch Plan of Male Convalescent Institution, Vincennes

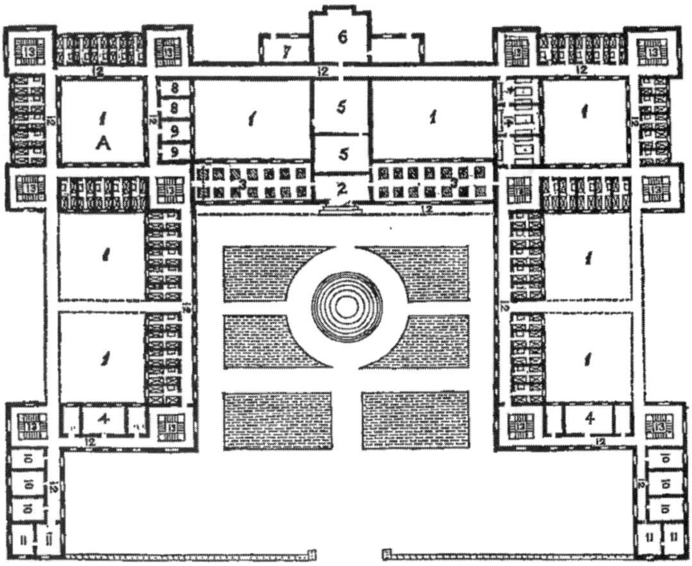

1	Courts.	8	Pharmacy.
2	Chapel.	9	Stores.
3	Refectory.	10	Bureaux.
4	Parlour.	11	Directeur.
5	Kitchen.	12	Connecting Corridors.
6	Laundry.	13	Staircase.
7	Baths.	14	Lingerie.

2ND FLOOR.

Centre Pavilion over the Chapel, the Bibliothèque.
Over the Refectories, the 'Salle de Chant' and the 'Salle de Jeu.'
Attics of main Building contain Workshops.
Infirmary Ward is in Court A.

principle from the English one. It consists of a long series of three-bedded rooms, bent on itself at right angles, so as to form partial courts, the whole being connected by a corridor for communication. The arrangement of parts is simple and ingenious, while it enables a large number of rooms to obtain the benefit of direct light and air through the outer wall. For an interesting account of this establishment, vide [see] Note, p 116, and the following sketch plan (for it is only a sketch to show the general arrangement), I am indebted to

Colonel Clark-Kennedy, who was kind enough to go over the establishment for the purpose.

It will be seen at once wherein this building differs in design from the preceding. In the first place, it has no internal corridor. It has a corridor along one end of all the rooms, but the arch of the corridor, the door of the room, and the window at the opposite end of the room, are all in one line, so that a thorough ventilation is easily effected. Again, the rooms are intended each for three beds only—a number of which diminishes materially the objections to corridors as a means of communication, provided they be ventilated with ordinary care. The whole suite of rooms on one side of a court of this building would hardly contain more beds than a single ward in a hospital. All the rooms are ventilated and warmed artificially on the usual Paris hospital method.

The plan consists simply of a number of separate rooms connected by a corridor, in which the convalescents sleep at night, while during the day they are out in the air or following some occupation. The corridor construction, if properly ventilated, or, what is much better, if wholly or partially open, is not objectionable as a means of communication in a building of this kind intended for convalescents, who spend most of their time "out and about." For a hospital whose inmates are always confined to their wards the structure would be objectionable.

This building, together with its economy, is worthy of careful examination by those engaged in planning convalescent establishments. It is, I believe, the largest building of the kind hitherto specially erected for the purpose. Of course, were it possible, it would be better to have more than one window for a bedroom to be occupied by three persons. And it would be highly advantageous if windows could be placed on two sides of the room.

The best arrangement of buildings for convalescents is, however, doubtless that of a series of cottages, and here is a sketch of such a building (Plan No. 10) made at the request of the committee for the Herbert memorial of the county of Wilts. It consists of four detached cottages, intended for twenty men and women. Two of the cottages are intended, one for men and one for women. The centre cottage contains the sister's room, etc., together with two small wards for sick, or relapses, one for men and one for women. The fourth contains the kitchen and the men's and women's dining and day rooms. It is intended to make the establishment as like a home and as unlike a hospital as possible, and to provide, at the same time, for strict discipline over the inmates.

PLAN NO. 10
A Design for Convalescent Hospital Arranged as Cottages

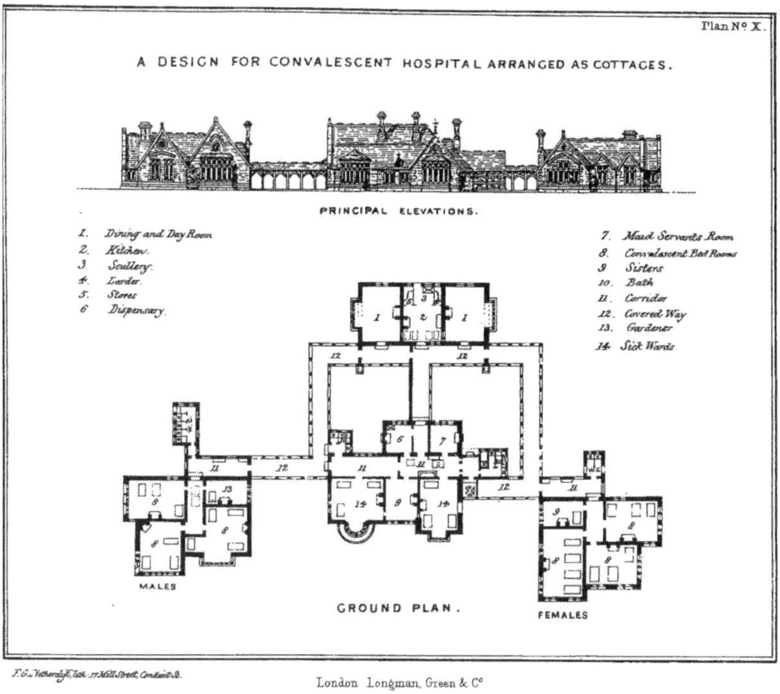

A plan such as this, while possessing all the advantages of a home, would admit of extension, merely by the addition of similar parts. The working plans were made by Mr Thomas, of the War Office.

It is scarcely necessary to say that convalescent establishments should be placed in healthy, cheerful positions, varying in local climate according to the class of cases for which they are intended. The best climates can easily be determined by the usual practice adopted by physicians with private convalescents. Certain irritable chest cases do best in the moist relaxing seaside climates of the S.W. of England. Diseases requiring a medium character of climate are usually sent to the southern districts and to the Isle of Wight. If bracing seaside climates are required, the S.E., E. and N.E. coasts and part of the N.W. coast are generally chosen. A large class of convalescents suffering from general constitutional debility are benefited by certain inland climates, such as Malvern, Clifton, Derbyshire, etc. I merely allude to this subject of climates because it should not be overlooked in providing for the relief of convalescents. There are many places round London on dry, comparatively elevated, gravelly soils, which would afford excellent sites for convalescent institutions.

If convalescent homes are necessary for adults, they are doubly necessary for children; the rule never to keep a patient a day longer in hospital than is absolutely essential applies rather more to children than to any others.

It is necessary to say a few words on another proposal for convalescents, namely, providing convalescent wards and day rooms in hospitals. In dealing with this proposal, it is right to repeat:

1. That no patient should be kept in hospital a day longer than is absolutely essential, i.e., for medical or surgical treatment.

2. That many, nay, most patients are quite unfit to return to a workaday life, even when they would be much better out of hospital. Where, then, should they go?

3. Every county and every hospital should have its convalescent branch, as unlike a hospital and as like a home as possible—the best a string of cottages—where such can be received.

Do day rooms in hospital answer this want? No. It is found practically impossible to keep such supervision over day rooms as will prevent patients in them from playing tricks and from doing themselves more harm than good. Recovery has been found to be actually retarded by days in the day rooms.

It has been suggested that a day room should be attached to each ward, in order that patients in the day room might be under the supervision of their own nurse. But the advantages of this supervision are more imaginary than real: practically a nurse can really supervise only as many persons as she can see from one point. Even in two wards in one line, and where everybody is in bed, an experienced nurse knows perfectly well how much really escapes her supervision. It would be doubly impossible for her to know what is going on in a day room at the same time as in her ward, especially as it is quite out of the question that a day room and ward should open out of one another. There might be one men's and one women's day room for the whole hospital, with a head nurse over each. But it is very undesirable to mix the patients of the several wards when they have to return to them. They meet only for gossip; they prefer this gossip to out-of-door exercise. And even if a head nurse be spared—which she will not be—to manage them, she will succeed but with difficulty.

Practice differs widely from theory in these things. Practically it will be found that all patients, as long as they need to remain in hospital at all, had better be in their own wards, under their own nurse, provided those who *can* go out have as much out-of-door exercise as possible.

It has been objected that *no* ventilation can keep a sick ward fresh enough for semi-convalescents. Then how can it be fresh enough for sick?

It has been objected that semi-convalescents disturb the ward for serious cases. The serious cases, generally, think the ward very "dull" without them, and call a large, full ward "so cheerful."

In military hospitals it is totally different. For (1) a soldier must either be in hospital or in barracks; (2) in a general hospital, a non-commissioned officer can always be placed over the day room.

Do convalescent wards in hospital answer the want of a convalescent "home"? Certainly better than day rooms, because convalescent wards are, or ought to be, always under a regular nursing staff, the same as sick wards are. But they would answer it much better still if they were totally out of and away from hospital, in an institution of their own.

Convalescent wards are absolutely essential to a military hospital, especially in India, because you cannot send the semi-convalescent back to barracks, much less keep him in the fever and dysentery wards. Day and dining rooms are also absolutely necessary for military convalescents, especially in India, if it were only for the plague of flies..

But day and dining rooms are objectionable in a civil hospital. Taking the general run of cases, when patients can go into day and dining rooms, they had better go out of hospital, not home, but into a convalescent institution. And even if there be none such to go to, their recovery and discharge from hospital is rather retarded than otherwise by day and dining rooms.[19]

6. Children's Hospitals

The first thing to decide is whether you will have a children's hospital at all. On the one hand, none but the hospital experienced can possibly guess how important public opinion is to keep a hospital in any way straight. Ay, even with the best religious order for nurses. Now, among children, there can be no public opinion. They cannot make their complaints, and even if they do, it is always unwise for doctors or

19 At this point Nightingale incorporated an article by John Clark-Kennedy, "Note on the Male Convalescent Hospital at Vincennes," April 1861.

visitors to take part with the children against the nurses, who are always with them, and ought to be in authority over them. And the nurses will take their revenge (and cannot help doing so) upon the children. For certainly the children are not in authority over *them.* Also, each sick child may almost be said to require a nurse to itself. Where adults are mixed with them, the woman in the next bed, if the patients are judiciously distributed, often becomes the child's best protector and nurse. And it does her as much good as it does the child.

It is a matter of universal hospital experience that this intermingling of ages is essential. Let the age of admission be, at all events, raised so as to include fifteen years, especially on the female side, if you decide on a children's hospital. To have the best religious order as nurses does not all guarantee the child patient from, at least, indifference, since there is a tacit idea among some "religious" that it is better for the children to die than to live. Indeed, more tenderness has been shown to them sometimes among the commonest hospital nurses. It is not enough to be merely conscientious and patient with sick children.

There must be a real genuine vocation and love for the work, a feeling as if your own happiness were bound up in each particular child's recovery. Nothing else will carry you through the perpetual wear and tear to the spirits, of the fretfulness, the unreasonableness of sick children—not that I think it is greater than that of many sick adults—but it is more wearing, because the strain is never off you for a minute. This hearty love of and companionship with sick children, such as the Wilderspins[20] felt for their *well* pupils, is essential for a nurse in a children's hospital. It is to be found just as often and just as seldom among mothers as among nuns. The true *maternal* feeling may be in the girl and the old maid. But wherever it is, there only must the good nurse for children be looked for. Duty and conscience must come in too, of course, because no natural feeling will stand the fatigue and anxiety always.

These are the peculiarities of children's hospitals, to be weighed before such are decided upon. Shall you find nurses sufficient of this kind?

The only idea of many (doctors and others) about a child's hospital is that it is a place where children are to be admitted and to be recovered, or dead and buried as soon as possible. Such is not our idea. But, whatever you do, do not have children's wards in a general hospi-

---

20 Samuel Wilderspin (1792-1866), infant educator and pioneer of playgrounds for children.

tal. There at least mix up the children with the adults. For a children's ward in a general hospital combines all the disadvantages with none of the advantages of a children's hospital.

(There are, besides, certain children's habits, which I can do no more than allude to here, perfectly well known to all who have had much to do with children's wards, which render the strictest supervision necessary, and this is much more likely to be obtained in a special children's hospital, all under the same responsible management, and with every special means of treatment and exercise and occupation, than in any children's wards in a general hospital, where sick children are only received and dealt with as a portion of the hospital inmates, yet without the protection and amusement of being with the "big" inmates.)

On the other hand, the advantages of a children's hospital are that there they do not see the things which they had much better not see, and which it is impossible to prevent their seeing in an adult hospital, and that children's hospitals require and obtain far larger recreation and exercise grounds and more appliances than hospitals for adults.

Paris exhibits and London does not what is justly thought necessary in this respect. Physical exercises in and out-of-doors are a part of the treatment, in all but acute cases. So is teaching, secular as well as religious. So is bathing.

It must never be forgotten that children can never be left alone for a moment—and that a separate staff must be provided for every room—I had almost said a nurse for every child.

The bathing establishment forms a most important branch of a children's hospital. In all children's hospitals abroad, the classification is

1. Medical
2. Surgical
3. Cutaneous [skin diseases]

And in all continental hospitals the proportion of the cutaneous is large. I speak of the Continent, because England, indeed, affords no large experience as to children's hospitals.

The bathing establishment must, therefore, consist of four separate bathing places:

1. For boys
2. " cutaneous
3. For girls
4. " cutaneous

And neither sex should ever come on the side appropriated to the other.

Each bathing place must be under the charge of a separate competent "sister," with one or more attendants under her; otherwise the lists of accidents, by drownings and scaldings alone, will be fearful.

Each bathing place must have a number of small baths, separable by a curtain or slight partition, with one or more large baths in which several children may be bathed at once. The girls must bathe alone, the infants together, unless the disease is something special. The medical officers must decide when the age comes when boys should bathe alone.

Girls should always be bathed in frocks, unless the special disease prevents it.

Outdoor patients are always (to their own great advantage and to the in-patients' great disadvantage) admitted to baths and gymnastics in these institutions. This must be taken into account.

In regard to the water closets, as a general rule, there should be no possibility for a child to fasten itself in, or to communicate with another child when in. They should be self-acting, and well lighted day and night.

It is almost needless to say that the lavatories for children must not be lavatories for adults, as to height, handiness or anything else, and that the children who will have to be washed in ward are much more numerous than adults in hospital, consequently there must be a much greater provision of portable basins, etc. On this point foreign hospitals are woefully deficient. To prevent a child's skin from becoming chafed (in certain diseases) it has to be partially sponged many times a day.

The bathroom at the end of each large ward should contain two small baths for acute cases or infants. There should also be a portable bath.

A large garden ground, laid out in sward and grass hillocks, and such ways as children like (*not too pretty* for the children to be scolded for spoiling it) must be provided—or rather four such grounds for:

1. Boys
2. " cutaneous
3. Girls
4. " cutaneous

These must be combined with gymnastic grounds and halls *in* and *out-of*-doors. A professor (a man) must be attached to superintend these exercises; otherwise the children, especially the girls, will injure themselves.

I have already said that out-patients are always admitted to these, which form a very important part of the treatment. Singing in chorus should accompany some exercises. A "sister" must superintend each of the playgrounds, besides the professor for all. The gymnastic covered place may also be used as a playroom and day room, and as a schoolroom.

In foreign children's hospitals two schoolrooms—one for boys and one for girls—are generally attached. And these again are each under the charge of a "sister," who teaches *besides* the teaching in the wards and the teaching by the chaplain.

The chapel should be contrived so that secular as well as religious teaching may be conducted there by the chaplain. Boys and girls may sit on opposite sides of the chapel. This is the only place where they should meet.

Special care should be taken to occupy the children enough, and only enough, to conduce to their recovery. Prizes and suchlike incentives may be given.

All experienced children's doctors lay immense stress upon this, viz., that *every* child's hospital ought to have a *convalescent* branch at a distance, in the most healthy spot that can be found—probably by the sea, or at a watering place. And this, however munificently the hospital itself may be furnished with air and exercise.

In all hospitals (in a child's hospital much more than in others) the patient must not stay a day longer than is absolutely necessary.

Finally, I must remark that the perfection of all these arrangements abroad, and the obstinate mortality of the children, are equally remarkable. Sometimes an epidemic disease will sweep a whole ward. One child out of five has actually died (from 1804 to 1861 inclusive) at the "Enfans Malades" at Paris, the greatest and oldest child's hospital in the world.

The only plan of a children's hospital which realizes all the various conditions laid down is that to be erected at Lisbon, of which here is a sketch (No. 11). This plan possesses peculiar interest on account of its being the embodiment of a desire of the late king of Portugal, to commemorate his lost queen.[21]

Our own beloved Albert,[22] who is always present in the longing and grateful recollection of her majesty's faithful subjects, had every stage of the plan brought to him, and made constant suggestions—it being his anxious wish to introduce into Portugal in a model building all the recent improvements in hospital construction made in this country. The architect was Mr Humbert,[23] to whom the design was entrusted by the prince consort.

---

21 King Pedro V of Portugal (1837-61); Queen Estefania, née Princess Stephanie of Hohenzollern-Sigmaringen (1837-59).

22 Prince Albert (1819-61), consort of Queen Victoria (1819-1901).

23 Albert Jenkins Humbert (1822-77). For correspondence on the planning of the hospital see p 526 below.

PLAN NO. 11
Plan of Children's Hospital, Lisbon

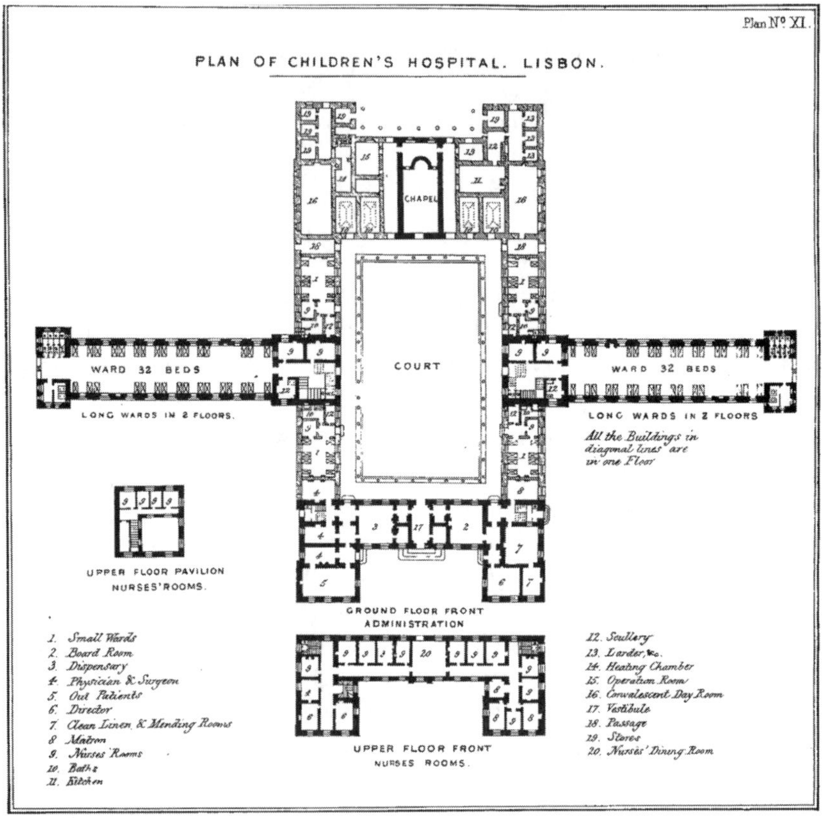

The building is arranged along a parallelogram, 135 feet long by 75 feet wide, surrounded by an open corridor and terrace. It consists of two pavilions, similar in construction to those of the Lariboisière. These pavilions are two floors in height, and the upper wards are reached by wide open staircases. One peculiarity of the pavilion is that the nursing staff is all accommodated in the staircase end of it. This is effected simply by putting an additional floor at the top of the staircase. Each ward contains thirty-two beds. The water closets, bath and lavatory, are at the farther end of the long wards. They are specially planned for children's use. Each closet is ventilated separately, and is also cut off from the body of the compartment in which it is placed, so that all of them are surrounded by a considerable mass of constantly moving air passing through the compartment by windows on three sides, *in addition to* a window for each separate closet. If any foul air were by chance to escape from the closet, notwithstanding its ventilation, into the compartment, the foul air would at once be mingled with a large body of moving air, and carried outside the building. Escape of foul air into the ward is thus rendered impossible.

Each large ward is provided with two small baths, children's size, having hot and cold water laid on. Each ward is 128 feet long by 30 feet wide and 18 feet high, and gives 2160 cubic feet per bed. They will be the most magnificent wards in Europe. There are nine windows and one fireplace on each side. Besides the wards in the pavilions, there are four small wards of eight beds each, placed on the sides of the court. They are provided with nurses' rooms, scullery, water closet, etc. The front of the hospital contains the administrative offices and quarters for the director, medical officer, matron and sisters not attached to the beds. This part is two floors in height. The chapel is placed as in the Lariboisière plan, and on each side of it are the general baths of the establishment. In this same part of the hospital are two day rooms, also kitchen, stores and other offices.

It will be observed that the only buildings which exceed one floor in height are the administration, the two pavilions and the chapel. And although there is a closed court, the sides of the court consist essentially of one-floor buildings. The general bathing arrangements, day rooms and exercising grounds are all made in conformity with the principles already stated. Taken as a whole, the building has been well considered in its details, and will, no doubt, prove a healthy structure.

If children's hospitals are to be built at all, this is the kind of plan that should be adopted. But every variation from it will require as much careful consideration as was bestowed on the original plan.

Note on the Attendance Required in Children's Hospitals

If the nurses' quarters ought to be separate in a military hospital, certainly the men's ought to be separate in a child's hospital. Not one woman more than is absolutely essential ought to be in a military hospital. Not one man more than is absolutely necessary ought to be in a children's hospital. The only men who ought to sleep in a child's hospital are: (1) resident medical officer (supposed to be a man of weight and experience); [and] (2) porter (who should be as far off the wards as possible). The director (or whatever he may be called) and the chaplain (if this is conformable with the usage of the clergy) are the only other men who may sleep in the building. The cook and her assistant should be women.

Women must be in undisputed charge of a child's hospital, saving, of course, as above-said, the direction and the medical service. On the Continent, where men do far more of household work than with us, the necessity of having as few men as possible in children's hospitals is fully recognized.

All cleaning which *must* be done by men should be done by men not attached to the hospital. No male attendants must ever be attached to children's wards. A children's hospital requires far more attendants than an adult hospital. All must be women, and all ought to sleep near their respective wards.

The two schoolmistresses are the only women who need not live in the hospital.

Reverent decency in the deadhouse, so much neglected in England, is peculiarly desirable in children's hospitals. It should be a separate building in a quiet corner, beyond the possibility of being overlooked, with two separate entrances, one into the *post-mortem* room, the other opening from the outer wall, for the relations to come in.

7. Indian Military Hospitals

The Report, Evidence and Stational Reports issued by the Royal Commission on the Sanitary State of the Indian Army contain a large amount of exceedingly interesting information as to the condition of military and female hospitals in that part of the empire, the results of which I purpose to give, with the view of deducing from the inquiry principles which might be applied in future hospital buildings for Indian climates.

The Indian hospitals, though planned on simple principles, admitting of admirable details, are, as a rule, exceedingly bad as regards points considered essential to health and administration even in this country. What would be, e.g., thought in this country of a hospital without a water closet, or bath or means of personal cleanliness? Such a hospital would be considered as a mere makeshift till accommodation fitter for recovery could be provided.

The "means of ablution" in Indian hospitals are often "a tin pot, with which the sick pour the water over themselves." Or, as at Bombay [Mumbai], they "take water to bathe themselves from a trough." Elsewhere, they have "one tub, one basin, to 100 men." The means of washing, as at Ramandroog, a convalescent station, are "two shallow earthenware pie dishes," "on a form in a room" ("very chilly in damp" weather) "adjoining where the night stools are." At Rangoon the "bathing accommodation" is "hitherto nothing but a tub of water, without basin, soap or towel." There may be a bathroom. But "all apparatus is entirely wanting." The sick "can always, if they please, get a skinful of water thrown over them by the water carriers," as at Hazareebaugh.

One may safely say that when the sick are able to bathe in India, it is a sufficient test of their being able to leave hospital, as has indeed been discovered to be the case at some home stations.

At Nynee Tal the sick bathe in the lake. Darjeeling says, "in fact, the inducements to remain dirty are, especially in the case of sickly men, greater than those to be clean."

There does not appear to be a single well-placed orderlies' or nurses' room in any of the hospitals, from which the sick can be seen at all times, and where the nurses themselves can be inspected. The surgeon's and "nurses' " quarters are sometimes three quarters of a mile or a mile off, so that they (the medical and nursing attendants) are represented as spending their whole day in going backwards and forwards on the road.

The hospital is generally surrounded by a "high prisonlike wall." At Ghazeepore [Ghazipur] it is said, "of course all the buildings generally are most unsuitable for hospital purposes." Proper ventilation is represented, as at Baroda, as "next to impossible." At Kolapore [Kolhapur] the rain beats in through the cowls, and "makes the wards so damp that charcoal has to be used to dry them." The water for drinking may be brought, as at Bangalore, from a tank which receives the whole sewage of the cantonment, and which "just now is not very clean," from which "hundreds of bullock loads of impure matter are removed year after year when the tank is low and smell from it most offensive." Or the water may be brought (cholera also being brought with it) from wells into which the said tank drains. The drainage may be by an open ditch into the tank, whence the hospital derives its water. Or the water supply may, perhaps, have to be carried from half a mile off, or even from two miles off, as at Madras [Chennai]. But "no improvement is required in this respect." (!) The privies are everywhere either "highly offensive" or "not more offensive than the best of such places usually are in this country." Or the privies are "without seats," and are "kept pure by burning salt in them." "Arrangements admit of improvement."

Scarcely ever is there any provision of separate wards for convalescents, although in a country whose scourge is dysentery, to leave men convalescing from dysentery in the same place and under the same circumstances as those suffering from dysentery, is just to ensure as far as possible their *not* convalescing. The same may be said of fever and of bowel diseases generally. Convalescents pass their whole twenty-four hours in bed, except during their time of exercise (*where* they have means of exercise) on elephants, in sick carts or doolies. They have not even a room to take their meals in, but eat their food upon their knees, sitting on their beds, "possibly with dying men around," or they are sent to barracks and put on barrack rations, and "marched out under a non-commissioned officer morning and evening for exercise."

Where there is no guardhouse, the "men on guard occupy a corner of the hospital verandah, where they eat, drink and smoke at their discretion." No hospitals have dining rooms, although all ought to have them because of the pest of flies in India. Not one has a day room for men who can leave their beds.

The "sanitary state" is generally represented as "good," although at the same time we are told, as in certain cases, that the hospital is "unfit for accommodation of European patients," or that "epidemic disease has appeared in it," that "sores become erysipelatous," that, as at Bangalore, "one of the flags" in the floor being removed, "the smell from the opening was so offensive that" the surgeon was "obliged to run," that "gangrene and phagedena[24] have appeared when the hospital was crowded," that the "privy is a nuisance to one ward," that the "cesspools are always more or less offensive," or that the "outhouses are in a very dirty and unwashed condition." At Muttra the contents of the latrines are "carted away every morning for combustion in one of the many brick kilns which surround the station, and help to poison the air." At Madras the "sanitary state" is called "good," and the commander-in-chief himself adds, "if the vile, stinking river Kooum were not under the very noses of the patients." Both cholera and gangrene have appeared at times in the hospital. The latrines are placed to windward; "unfortunately," "tubs only are used." The privy is washed daily and charcoal "burned in it." It is called "not offensive," the commander-in-chief again adding, "a year ago it was odiously offensive."

No wonder it is stated, as at Bangalore, that "sick men are reluctant to come into hospital from barracks," and that the medical officer does not want "convalescent wards," because he finds it better to send his convalescents to barracks, where they recover faster.

From some hospitals the "impurities" are removed by hand carriage to 30 yards from the hospital. In another, the privy is said to be a "disgrace to the nineteenth century." One wonders to what century it would be a credit.

At most hospitals the bedsteads are of wood instead of iron, and the men break them to pieces in their "efforts to expel vermin." As at Ramandroog, where men are sent for their health, "the building swarms with bugs." And so of every barrack and hospital where these

24 A spreading ulcer.

wooden bedsteads are used. One surgeon complains of the serious injury to his sick occasioned by want of sleep from vermin. The bedding is of hemp or straw, instead of hair. Hair it ought always to be in hospitals, and hair is now the regulation in all queen's hospitals. It appears from several reports that sheets are not provided except for dysentery and fever, and certainly in no hospital deserving the name should the inspector general feel himself called on to recommend that "a good mattress, a blanket, *sheets* and pillowcases should be provided for every bed," as does the excellent inspector general of the Madras presidency.

FIGURE 27
Plan and Elevation of Horse Artillery Hospital, Bangalore

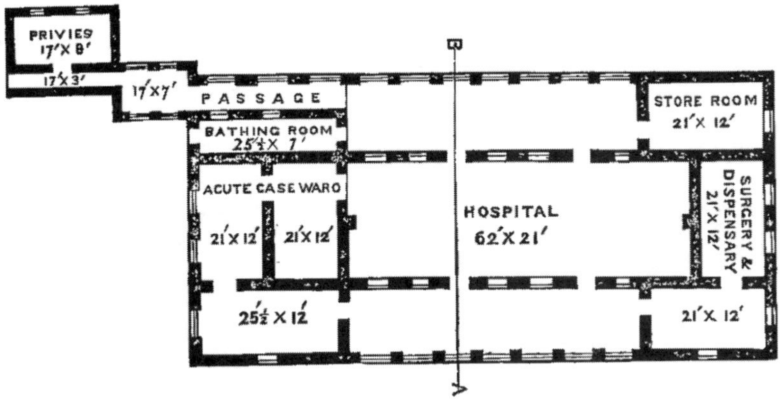

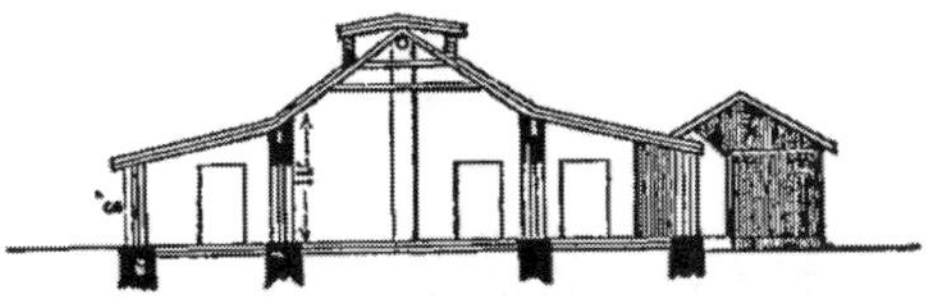

Section on A B.

Horse Artillery Hospital, Bangalore

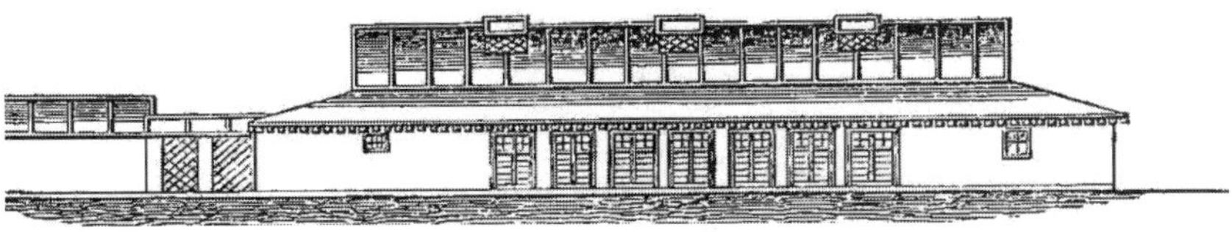

Figure 28
Plan and Elevation of Artillery Hospital, Belgaum

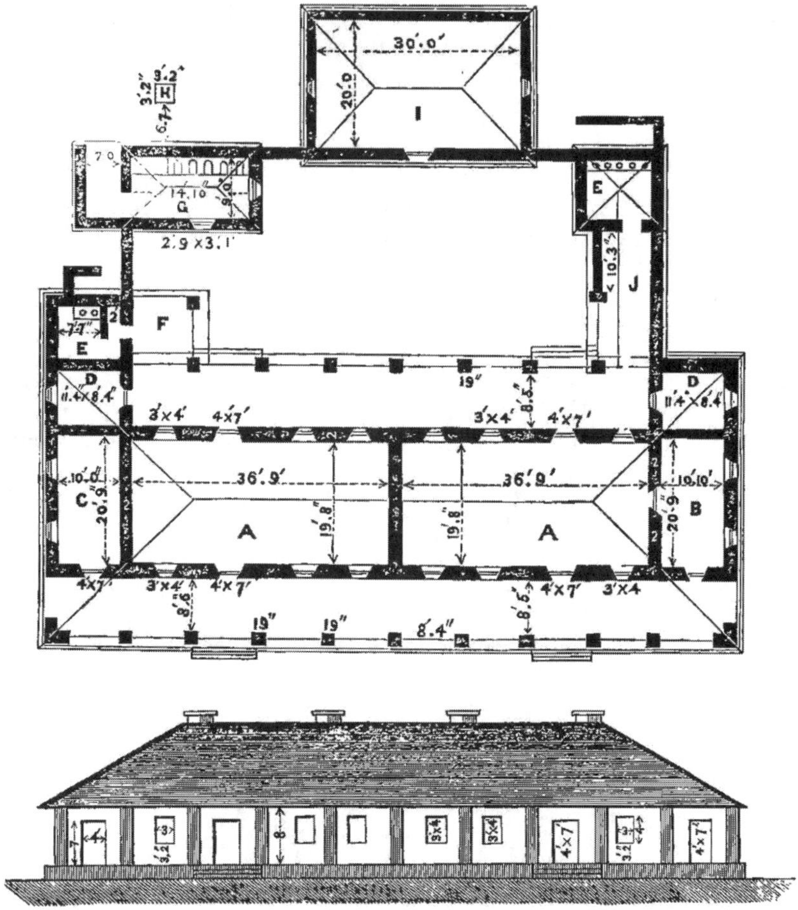

Figs. 27 [and] 28, are illustrations of the smaller class of regimental (British) hospitals. Fig. 27 shows the simpler form of construction, a single large ward, partially enclosed by other rooms for sick, all communicating and having a common ventilation, the arrangement good and simple up to a certain point, and then marred in the details. There are privies in place of water closets, with covered passages, to conduct foul air to the sick in certain states of the wind. Bangalore gives a reason for "the covered way to the latrines," which we never should have thought of. It is a "covered place for exercise." It will be seen that the hospital is entirely destitute of proper ward offices.

Fig. 28 shows a somewhat better construction of hospital, but there is the same defect in detail. Either plan might answer for temporary camp purposes in default of better, but that is all.

Indian hospitals generally, so far as all conveniences and comforts are concerned, appear to be simply camp hospitals, good, because the best possible for field service, but by no means good or the best possible for permanent stations.

There is no instance, except at Wellington, where the hospital, if on one floor, as is usual, is raised from the ground with any current of air beneath. These hospitals are stated, as at Bangalore, to be "always damp in wet weather." And often the floor is merely the ground bricked over. Rangoon and Tonghoo live like the beavers, and raise their barracks and hospitals on piles, with free passage for air underneath. The [Fig. 28] consequence is, that in those jungly swamps, they are more healthy than at most other Indian stations where the men sleep close to the ground.

As at Allahabad, Barrackpore, Dinapore, Meerut, Kurachee [Kurachi] and Secunderabad, vast wards of from 100 to 150 beds, and even up to more than 200 beds, exactly the same as the barrack rooms, are in use.

Here is a plan and section of one ward at Dinapore, which is nothing but a passage 633 feet long with 150 beds in it.

FIGURE 29
Plan and Section of Hospital, Dinapore

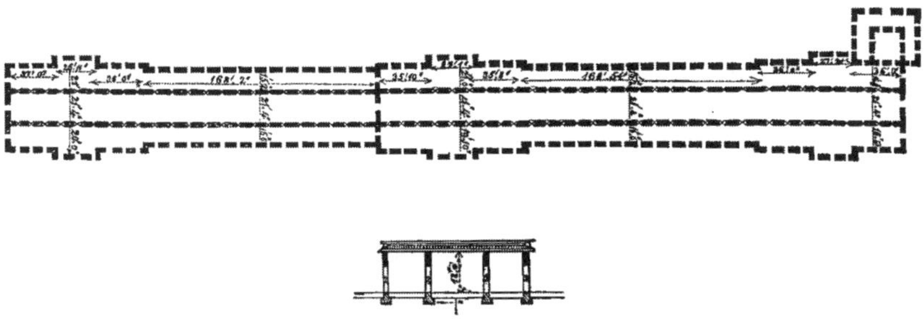

The wards can never be said to be light or airy: "as a general rule, hospitals are badly lighted and gloomy"; doors are more common than windows. And these doors, when closed, leave the ward, if not absolutely dark, yet absolutely dismal and close. Indeed a dark ward must always be a close ward. Or "light enters from a couple of panes in the doors near the top, and when closed darkness is almost complete." There is in

Indian hospitals hardly a room light enough to perform a surgical operation. And operations, it is stated, have to be performed in verandahs.

The inner verandahs are generally used for sick wherever more room is wanted, the outer ones sometimes cut up for lavatories, destroying what ventilation there is.

The superficial area per bed is almost invariably too small, and the wards almost as invariably too high, the result to the sick being that, with an apparently sufficient cubic space, the surface overcrowding is excessive. One of the worst examples of this is the recently constructed hospital at Trimulgherry (Secunderabad), which consists of three wards, two of which contain no fewer than 228 beds each; the wards are 42 feet high and afford 1001 cubic feet per bed, but the surface area per bed is only 24 square feet. This surface overcrowding is greater than I have ever seen it in the smallest or the largest temporary war hospitals. Such facts strike one very forcibly in connection with the high mortality among sick entering these and similar hospitals.

Figure 30

Plan of Hospital Ward, Trimulgherry (Secunderabad), 228 Beds

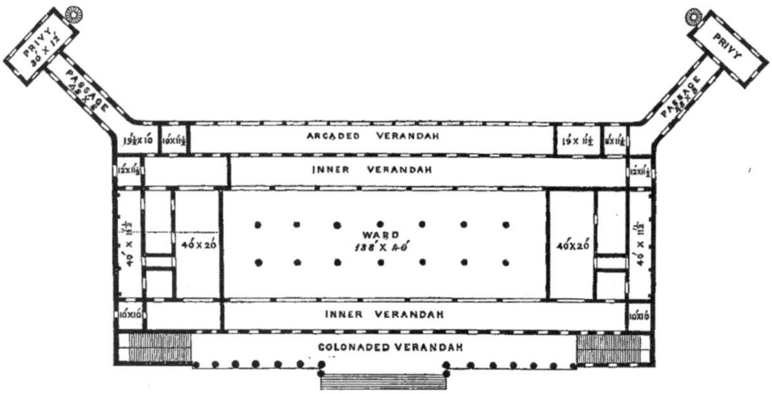

This Trimulgherry hospital is an immense hall supported on pillars and arches, and the surface crowded with beds. The distance from outer air to outer air, free of the building, is about 80 feet.

The general hospital at Madras is constructed on a different principle from any others, but on as bad a one. It consists of a centre and two wings, and appears to be intended for four rows of beds between the opposite doors and windows.

All the sanitary defects of barracks reappear and with worse consequences in the hospitals, viz., bad water supply, bad ventilation, no drainage; (Ferozepore [Firozpur] says, "drainage not necessary"), offensive latrines, so offensive indeed that the patients have sometimes to leave a particular ward, no means of bathing and hardly any of cleanliness.

FIGURE 31
Plan and Section of General Hospital, Fort St George, Madras

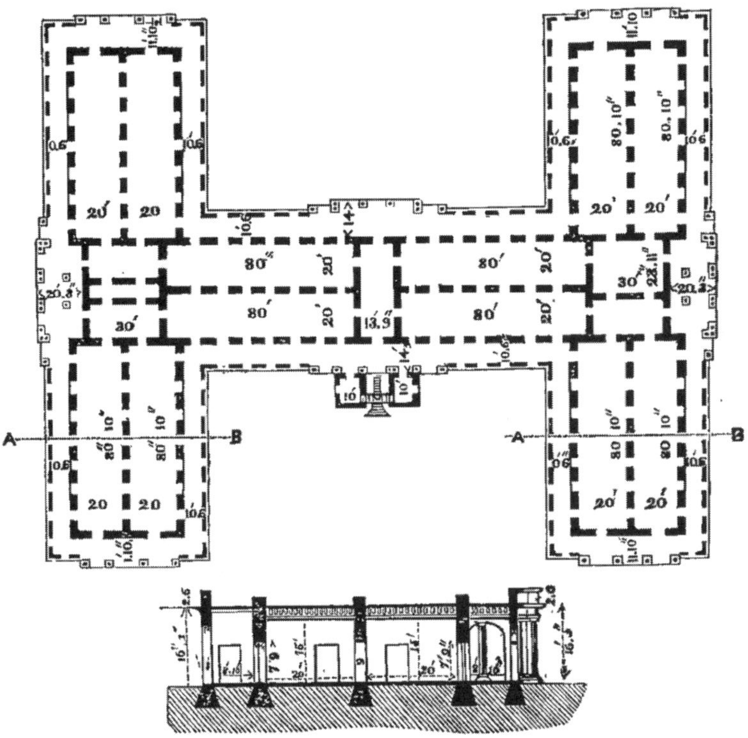

Section on A B

There are besides, however, two grave defects not felt in barracks, but peculiar and fatal to hospitals. These are the cooking and the attendance. It is in several reports complained that under the present system the cooks (natives or Portuguese), are nothing but "miserable pretenders," because the pay is so small, that the kitchens are no better than, but just the same as, the barrack kitchens. They are often small open sheds without chimneys, the smoke finding its way out as it can, and with but few utensils; sometimes the food is prepared on the ground. "But we are accustomed to this in India." It is added, that though common food is tolerably well prepared, there is nothing whatever that can be called sick cookery, nothing whatever to tempt the appetite or spare the digestion of the sick man, whom the hospital is for.

In hospitals at home, trained cooks of the Army Hospital Corps are now in charge of the cooking, under the direction of the purveyor, who is responsible that the diets are properly cooked. In India the chief quality in native cooks appears to be the "pursuit of cooking under difficulties"; their ingenuity in bringing about an *apparently* good result, in a rude and often bad way, is frequently admired by the reporters, as if the end of cooking were "to make a pair of old boots look like a beefsteak."

In England where the grass-fed meat is so much better than in India, it is found necessary to put the purveying of meat for hospitals under the charge of the purveyor, for the sake of always obtaining the best quality. There does not appear to be any provision of this kind in India, where all is under the Commissariat.

As to the attendants, they are just the same as would be supplied to idle healthy men. Quantity, it would seem, is supposed to supply quality. In serious cases a "waiting man" is supplied "from the battalion, who is relieved daily." That is, he goes on guard for twenty-four hours, as in the guard room, so in the sickroom. It appears that mounting guard in the sickroom is disliked, and the guard sometimes neglects his patient.

As to supposing that any nursing is required, the thing is totally out of the question. There are neither trained orderlies nor female nurses. A matron is sometimes "sanctioned," but "only for a complete battalion." If there are fewer sick they must do without. Every severe case, as has been stated, is allowed to have its comrade to itself in from the ranks, i.e., the case which requires the best nursing is to have the worst nurse. Something more is needed to make a nurse, as well as a surgeon, than mere kindness. Wherever the above comrade practice is found, we know beforehand that there can be no nursing, no discipline in that hospital, and any amount of drink.

There is generally one hospital sergeant and a "plentiful supply of ward coolies." The hospital sergeant is for discipline, and under him are seventy-nine coolies and bheesties [water carriers] in cold weather, 240 in hot weather. This for an European corps. The general impression, as regards the native attendants, is that they are in some sense kind, but "as a rule, very inattentive," and when there is any pressure of sick they are "lazy" and "apathetic," and the sick, it need hardly be said, neglected, and "averse to be waited on by them."

(And here comes in again the difficulty of difference in language. Our men dislike and despise the natives, and are regarded by them in return more as wild beasts than fellow creatures. The native, however, makes much more effort to learn the Briton's language than does the Briton to learn the native's. It is difficult to give an idea of the evil effects of the gross ignorance of all that relates to the country in the ranks of our army in India. The commonest attempt at conversation gives rise to feelings of impatience and irritation, too often followed by personal ill-treatment. Where the Briton is sick, it is of course worse.)

When at a hill station, as Landour, the hospital sergeant is taken at random from the sick men themselves sent up for convalescence; it is needless to point out the consequences. This grievance has been repeatedly represented, but in vain. Nynee Tal has one hospital sergeant, one barber, one orderly, for its attendance.

Lady Canning[25] introduced female nurses at Allahabad, who are mentioned (in the stational return of Allahabad) as being a great comfort to the sick. Wherever there are general hospitals there should be female nurses, but only under the organization laid down by the Medical Regulations of October 1859. It is a great mistake to put down a few women among a parcel of men (orderlies and patients) without exactly defining the women's duties and place.

Lastly, there appears nowhere in India to be provided any means of drying hospital linen, even during the rains. It is often complained that the washing is very bad and that the native washermen tear the linen, and at one cavalry hospital this keeps two tailors constantly employed in repairing the rents and injuries, for native washing is done by beating the linen against large flat stones or wooden boards. If the British military hospitals are such, what must be said of those for our native troops? Here the patients "diet *themselves*."

Native Hospitals. As regards construction, where native hospitals have been specially built, they resemble the smaller class of British hospital. One of the most complete of these is shown in Fig. 32. There are wards within wards, completely enclosed by other rooms, of which, although there are plenty, not one is suited for ward offices.

But it must not be supposed that native hospitals are all as good as this. They are generally nothing but a shed, perhaps a "gun shed" or a "cattle shed," as at Kolapore [Kolhapur], converted into a hospital,

---

25 Charlotte Canning, late vicereine of India and a colleague on nursing issues from the Harley St. establishment.

FIGURE 32
Plans, Sections, and Elevation of Native Hospital, Kurnool Fort

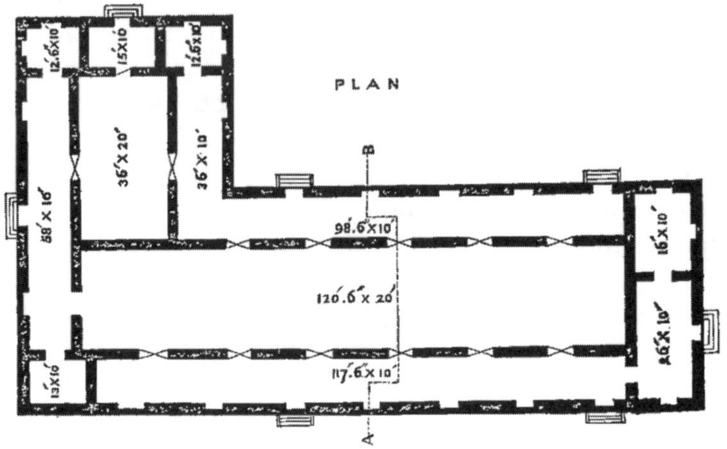

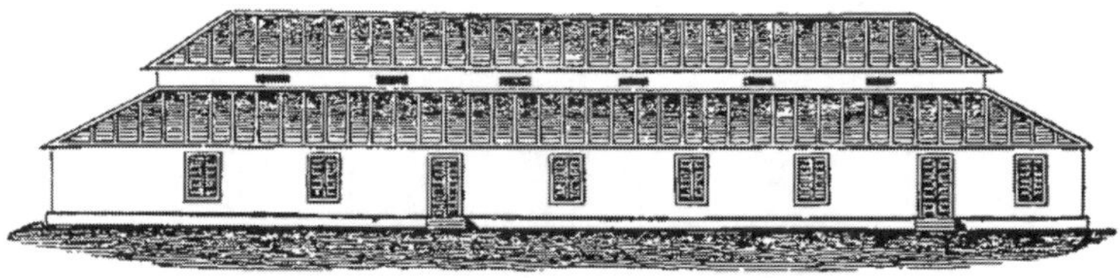

Kurnool Fort Hospital.

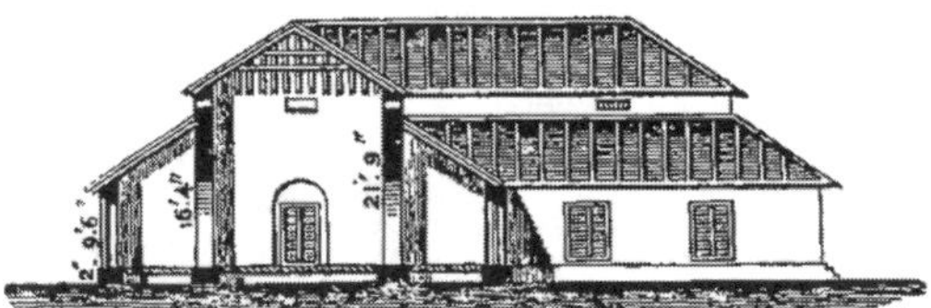

Section on A B.

PRIVY

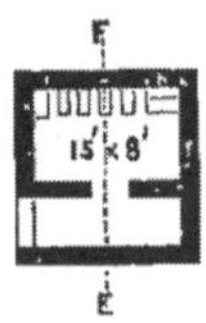

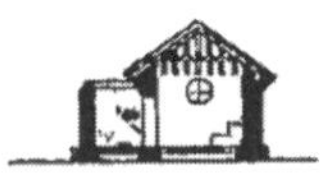

Section of Privy.

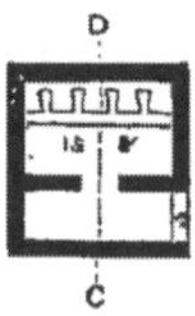

COOKROOM

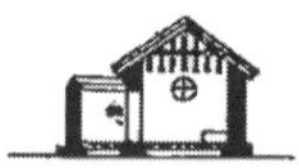

Section of Cook-room.

where the sick receive nothing but medicine. The patients cook their own diets, eating and drinking what they please. Or when too ill to cook for themselves, an orderly friend is detailed for the purpose. There are no conveniences; sometimes the sick go home to wash, or bathe themselves in a tank. Such are the "ward offices usually provided for these establishments." In one native infantry hospital at Secunderabad it is stated that hospital gangrene frequently occurs from overcrowding, from the cachectic[26] state of the patients, *owing to the unhealthy character of their lines*, and from a cesspool in the hospital enclosure, which last is, however, being remedied.

At Rangoon, it is stated that the privies for native regiments are built of matting, "which is most objectionable, as allowing the escape of noxious effluvia." Is it then desired to keep the "noxious effluvia" *in*?

It is supposed that "caste" prejudices are such as to prevent native hospitals being properly built and supplied with requisites for sick. But this has to be proved by giving natives a properly constructed and provided hospital. There are plenty of "caste prejudices" in this country against good hospital construction, but good hospital construction advances nevertheless.

At Loodiana, one native doctor, one cooley, one water carrier, one sweeper are the attendants "sufficient for the ordinary wants of the sick." The present arrangements for the female hospital are said to be "sufficient" (which means *none*). (Loodiana is now a native station.)

These native hospitals, again, combine all the disadvantages of civilization without any of its advantages. In one place the hospital was so overcrowded that for two years "gangrenous and spreading sores" were "frequent." In another it was so much out of repair that "it would before long be a ruin" (the best thing that could happen to it). If there is a privy, it is a "small room with no place in which the excrement can go to be cleared away." If there is a small lavatory or bath, it is "two tubs out of repair" (does that mean that they cannot hold water?). If there is a kitchen, as at Mercara, it is under the same shed as a privy, and cannot be used for the stench. Indeed the medical officer proposes that it should be turned into a privy. The sick generally cook under the nearest tree, and, if unable to do so, a comrade cooks for them under the tree. Linen is washed and dried by caste comrades, or by the patients when not too ill. Each patient brings in his own bed-

26 A depraved condition from malnutrition.

ding, generally his own bedstead. "Each patient defers bathing, according to custom, till he is cured, when he retires to the nearest well, draws water and undergoes the bath of cure," i.e., when he no longer wants it. Every report begs for a bathroom.

These are the facts with regard to the constructive arrangements for sick and for administrative purposes in the various classes of Indian hospitals. Some of the recent military hospitals are superior to those described. They are erected on what is called the standard plan, supposed to contain every necessary requirement, and issued for the guidance of local authorities.

FIGURE 33
Standard Plan and Section of Hospital, Hazareebaugh

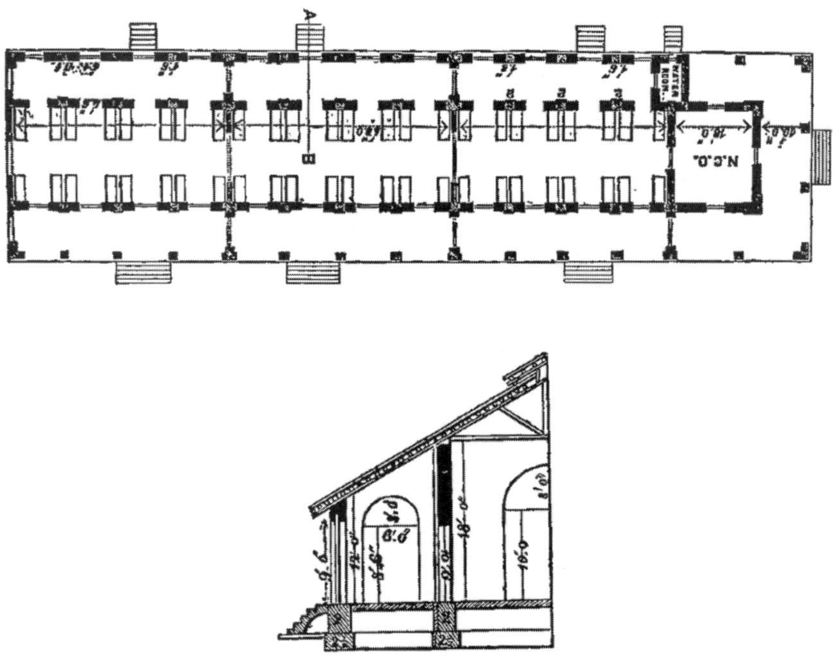

Fig. 33 shows half of this plan. It consists of a large hut with sloping roof, supported by longitudinal and transverse arches, the latter of which divide it into six divisions, called wards, each of which is 48 feet long, 20 feet wide and 18 feet high to the top of the wall. The building from end to end is intended for 96 beds, virtually in one long ward, at 1080 cubic feet and 60 superficial feet per bed. The floor is raised 4 feet above the level of the ground, but there is no circulation of air beneath the floor.

There are six open fireplaces in the closed verandah, which runs along one side of the hospital. The verandah on the other side is open. There is roof ventilation along the entire length. There is a non-commissioned officer's room at each end, with a door opening into the ward.

There are several favourable points in this construction, but it cannot by any means be taken as representing good hospital construction for a warm climate. There is no circulation of air beneath the floor; the hut forms, in reality, one long ward with 96 beds in it—just four times too many, and as it is the ventilation is obstructed by the transverse arches. The closed verandah along one side is inadmissible if closed by anything else but jalousies [blinds], except, indeed, in very exposed situations, subject to high winds. But even in such positions it is better to place the end of the building to the wind, and to leave the sides without closed verandahs, than it is to turn the side to the wind with closed verandahs.

The wall space per bed is smaller than I ever remember to have seen in any European hospital; pairs of beds appear to have only about 7 feet allotted to them. It is true there is a door or window between every two pairs of beds, but these, if used for ventilation, will necessarily expose the sick in the beds directly to draughts of air, which cannot fail to be injurious in not a few distances.

This plan exhibits no improvement in hospital lighting, for, although the ward is 18 feet high, exclusive of the open roof, the openings in the verandahs and the arches in the longitudinal walls are only 9 feet high. There are no ward offices, and the building can only be considered as an improved camp hospital.

It is very important to inquire on what general principles hospitals for Indian climates should hereafter be constructed. The defects in the present plans, taken in connection with the local conditions described in the reports appear to indicate what these principles should be—e.g., malaria is a constant product of the Indian soil. It rarely rises more than a few feet above the surface of the ground, but all who sleep within its sphere suffer more or less.

1. Out of this fact comes one great general principle, viz., that sick men in India should always sleep as high above the ground as the circumstances of the case admit of; the height will vary with locality. In high, well-drained positions, 4 or 5 feet will be enough, but in low, malarial districts, the sick should always be placed on upper floors. In every instance there should be a free current of air between the ward floor and the ground.

2. In a warm climate it cannot be safe to agglomerate a large number of sick in one ward. It is unsafe in Europe. It cannot be less unsafe

in India. What is wanted in a warm climate is a very free movement of the air around the sick, without exposing them to blasts or great variations of temperature. And all emanations from the sick should be discharged at once into the open air. To realize these advantages, the best method obviously is to subdivide the sick in separate detached buildings, containing, say, twenty-four beds each or thereabouts, so arranged as to obtain the full benefit of prevailing healthy winds.

3. In all hospitals, but especially in hospitals in warm climates, the question as regards space is not simply one of cubic feet per bed, but it is mainly one of superficial area. What is wanted is a large body of comparatively pure air around each bed. The extent of area and space will of course differ according to the healthiness of the position. In high, airy districts the surface area might approach to that of a cooler latitude, viz., 100 square feet, with 1500 cubic feet, which is now the regulation in her majesty's service for warm-climate hospitals. In low, hot, moist, malarial localities, it would be better to have no hospitals. But as there must be sick, the space and area per bed should be increased in a corresponding degree, from 100 up to, say, 120 or 130 square feet, with from 1500 up to, say, 2000 cubic feet.

4. In a sick ward, simplicity of construction is essential to good ventilation. There should be no transverse arches or thick pillars, no double verandahs, nor corridors. The ward should be perfectly open from end to end, and from side to side. The window space and door space should be sufficient for light and ventilation. Dark hospitals are unfit for sick. It is not necessary for light and heat to go together.

The doors and windows should be on opposite sides. Verandahs are required for shelter from the sun. They should always be single and open, and of sufficient width to afford the requisite shade. Verandahs should never be constructed or used to supplement the sick accommodation, or for dining rooms, or for convalescent day rooms. All such accommodation should be provided at the end of the block and not along its sides.

5. In permanent hospitals the wards should be ceiled. They are more comfortable, cooler and they look cleaner. The space between the ceiling and the roof should be freely ventilated to allow the hot air to escape. Double walls, where practicable, having a ventilating space between the outer and the inner wall, with openings above and below to allow a current of air to pass up, will always be cooler than any other construction, except the walls be very thick.

6. The question of wall space for beds is of great importance in hot climates. It is inadmissible to place a bed close beside an open door.

Any arrangement of doors and windows which allows the wind to blow directly upon the sick should be avoided in future. There should be a space of at least three and a half feet between every two adjoining beds, if the beds are arranged in pairs. But it would be much better to construct wards which would allow the beds to stand at equal distances from each other. If each bed is allowed, as a minimum, 100 square feet of surface, and 1500 cubic feet, the bed might have from 8 to 10 linear feet of wall space. With wards 15 feet high, which is quite enough, an 8 feet wall space would enable the ward to be about 25 feet wide. A 10 feet wall space would reduce the width to 20 feet, which is rather narrow for comfort.

When the larger amounts of cubic space and superficial area are given, the wall space per bed need not exceed 10 feet, and the additional surface should be thrown into the width of the ward, the height (15 feet) being retained.

As, in hot climates, all convalescents *must* be removed to convalescent wards, and as thus only serious cases, generally of fever or dysentery, will remain, the conclusion is, how doubly important a sufficient space and area!

7. Each ward should have its own ward offices. Or if two wards are placed in line end-to-end certain of the ward offices might be placed in the space between them outside the verandahs. These might be the ablution and bathrooms and scullery. The hospital sergeant's room must always be attached to and overlook one ward, if not both, and if not both, the orderly's room must overlook the other. Each ward should have a separate water closet accessible from the verandah, but so arranged as to prevent the patient going out or holding communication with persons outside, and yet with a perfectly free cross-ventilation between the closet and the ward.

8. Each ward, in such a climate as India, should have a bath with hot and cold water laid on. There should be a basin stand with sunk basins and water laid on.

9. Were it not that there is not a hospital in India which is drained, it might appear quite superfluous to have to state that no building is fit for sick that is not thoroughly drained to an outlet.

10. Every hospital should have an abundant supply of pure water *laid on*, for all purposes. The present supply by water carriers and bullocks is perfectly absurd.

11. Ventilation should always be ensured by a sufficient number of louvred ventilating turrets carried straight from the ceiling of the

ward through the roof. They should be so louvred as to prevent rain beating in, and they should be protected at the ceiling in such way as to prevent casual blasts of air in high winds from blowing upon the sick. Fresh air should always be admitted abundantly at the eaves. The fresh air ventilator should be carried all the way round the hospital; there should be louvres to throw air currents up towards the ceiling; the ventilation should be sufficient at ordinary times without doors or windows, but the doors and windows should be jalousied to be used for increasing the ventilation in still weather. The windows should always be glazed, which they are not at all invariably in India.

12. Each hospital kitchen should be supplied with improved cooking apparatus.

13. All the administrative offices should be in one block by themselves; the wards should only be for sick. If the hospital were on an upper floor, the administrative offices and stores might occupy the ground floor.

14. The medical and nursing attendants should never have to pass all their day upon the road in going backwards and forwards, as is not at all unfrequently the case in India. Convenient quarters should be provided, and the regimental orderlies' rooms should be attached to their respective wards.

15. Each hospital should be provided with a covered ambulatory for convalescents.

16. Convalescent wards, and especially convalescent day and dining rooms, are a necessity of all hot-climate military hospitals, more particularly during epidemics, because a soldier must be in hospital or in barracks. To leave him, when recovering from fever or dysentery, among the fever and dysentery cases, or to make him return from a day room to sleep among them, is to consign him to an almost certain relapse. He should sleep in a convalescent ward, and eat and live in a convalescent day room. But these convalescent wards must have a completely appointed nursing staff of their own, the same as sick wards have. Otherwise the convalescents will play tricks, and make themselves worse instead of better. And the day room must be included in the supervision.

Convalescent accommodation will enable the hospital to be cleared much sooner than if convalescents are left to sleep, eat and pass their time among men in all stages of the same epidemic malady from which they themselves may be recovering.

8. Hospitals for Soldiers' Wives and Children

Of late years a small number of hospitals for sick wives and children of soldiers have been erected in this country, on account of the very defective accommodation in married soldiers' quarters, rendering due care of the sick, especially of cases of confinements, all but impossible. These new hospitals are constructed on the same plan as that adopted for regimental hospitals, Figs. 21, 22. One half of the building is set apart for general cases, and the other for confinements. A small delivery ward is provided at one end of the long ward, instead of the bathroom, which is not required, but in every other respect the plans are similar. Each hospital has a matron and such additional attendants as she may require. Wherever these hospitals have been provided, they have been of the greatest use.

There are female hospitals also in India, but they are constructed on a totally different plan. Some of them, as at Kurrachee [Kurachi] and Deesa, Lucknow, Raneegunge and Ferozepore [Firozpur], appear to be very complete, with female attendants. In the Madras presidency, they are too often, as at Bangalore, Trichinopoly and Kamptee, merely men's wards appropriated to women, and justly stated to be "objectionable in every way." Elsewhere they are rather bare. Indeed, as at Baroda, Kirkee, Poona [Pune], Darjeeling, the sick women and children "have to be attended at their own quarters," either because "there is no matron," or because the "ward is too small," or etc. Curiously enough, it is generally stated that the "present arrangement is conducive to comfort." What arrangement? of having no matron? while it is added that a lying-in ward and a matron are "much wanted." At Darjeeling, the women and children are treated in their own quarters, which "would be satisfactory enough if the married quarters were not so dark and damp as they are." Sometimes it is said that "the arrangements are quite equal to those for the men."

The construction of these hospitals appears to be the same as that of small regimental hospitals. The following plan and section of a female hospital at Meean Meer [Mian Mir] (one of the most recently built in India) shows that they require quite as much structural improvement. It is a nest of rooms within rooms, and the same may be said of it that one of our engineers said of the pasha's new fort on the Dardanelles, that "he would be much safer outside of it."

Figure 34
Plan and Section of Female Hospital, Meean Meer

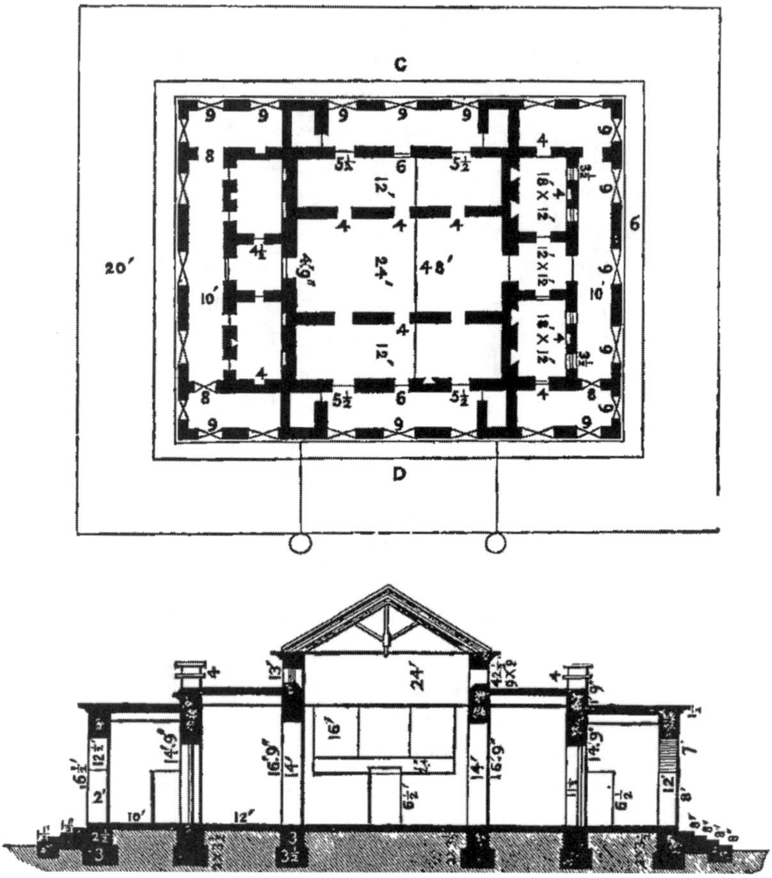

Section on C D

9. Hospital Statistics

In the first edition of my *Notes on Hospitals,* the defects of existing systems of hospital statistics were pointed out, and it was proposed to collect and tabulate certain elements for each hospital on one uniform plan. This plan was laid before the London meeting of the International Statistical Congress,[27] and was adopted by the congress with a few additions. The special question of statistics of surgical operations

27 Related in *Society and Politics* (5:83-85), and further discussed (see p 48 above).

had subsequently to be considered. In the present section will be given the substance of my former communications, as well as the new proposal for tabulating all operations on one uniform plan.

These methods, if generally used, would enable us to ascertain the mortality in different hospitals, as well as from different diseases and injuries, at the same and at different ages, the relative frequency of different diseases and injuries among the classes which enter hospitals in different countries, and in different districts of the same country. They would enable us to ascertain how much of each year of life is wasted by illness, what diseases and ages press most heavily on the resources of particular hospitals. For example, it was found that a very large proportion of the limited finances of one hospital was swallowed up by one preventible disease, rheumatism, to the exclusion of many important cases or other diseases from the benefits of the hospital treatment.

The relation of the duration of cases to the general utility of a hospital requires also to be shown, because it must be obvious that, if by any sanitary means or improved treatment, the duration of cases could be reduced to one half, the utility of the hospital would be doubled, so far as its funds are concerned.

This section is divided into two heads, the first referring to the general method laid before the congress, the second to an additional proposal for a uniform method of recording the results of surgical operations.

A. General Statistics of Hospitals

In the appended table for registering hospital statistics, the nomenclature agreed to at the Paris meeting of the Statistical Congress has been adopted, with two or three slight modifications, referring chiefly to rare diseases, and the proposed classification is essentially the same as that used by the Registrars-General of the United Kingdom.

The form itself has been in use for many years in the Registrar-General's office, for the registration of deaths, and has hence the advantage of having been fully tried by experience. Each table is divided vertically into columns containing the ages in monthly and yearly periods from under one year to five. Above five the ages are given quinquennially.

The disease list is divided into two sections, one printed on the left hand, the other on the right of the sheet. The left-hand division contains the diseases more frequently admitted into hospital, the right hand the rarer forms of disease. This arrangement is necessary for the purpose of limiting the size of the tables. In allotting the diseases between these two columns, advantage has been taken of the experience gained in filling up the forms by different hospitals.

Hospital General Statistical Form

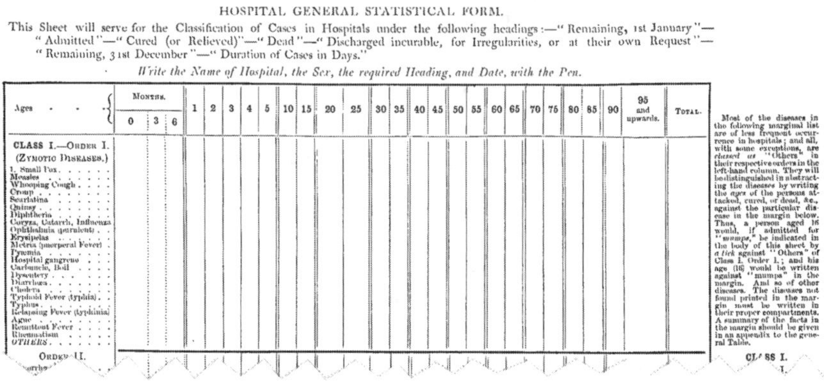

HOSPITAL GENERAL STATISTICAL FORM.

This Sheet will serve for the Classification of Cases in Hospitals under the following headings:—"Remaining, 1st January"—"Admitted"—"Cured (or Relieved)"—"Dead"—"Discharged incurable, for Irregularities, or at their own Request"—"Remaining, 31st December"—"Duration of Cases in Days."

Write the Name of Hospital, the Sex, the required Heading, and Date, with the Pen.

Ages	Months 0	3	6	1	2	3	4	5	10	15	20	25	30	35	40	45	50	55	60	65	70	75	80	85	90	95 and upwards	Total
CLASS I.—ORDER I. (ZYMOTIC DISEASES.)																											
1. Small Pox																											
Measles																											
Whooping Cough																											
Croup																											
Scarlatina																											
Quinsy																											
Diphtheria																											
Coryza, Catarrh, Influenza																											
Ophthalmia (purulent)																											
Erysipelas																											
Metria (puerperal Fever)																											
Pyæmia																											
Hospital gangrene																											
Carbuncle, Boil																											
Dysentery																											
Diarrhœa																											
Cholera																											
Typhoid Fever (typhia)																											
Typhus																											
Relapsing Fever (typhinia)																											
Ague																											
Remittent Fever																											
Rheumatism																											
OTHERS																											
ORDER II.																											

Most of the diseases in the following marginal list are of less frequent occurrence in hospitals; and all, with some exceptions, are *classed as* "Others" in their respective orders in the left-hand column. They will be distinguished in abstracting the diseases by writing the *ages* of the persons attacked, cured, or dead, &c., against the particular disease in the margin below. Thus, a person aged 16 would, if admitted for "*mumps*," be indicated in the body of this sheet by *a tick* against "Others" of Class I. Order I.; and his age (16) would be written against "mumps" in the margin. And so of other diseases. The diseases not found printed in the margin must be written in their proper compartments. A summary of the facts in the margin should be given in an appendix to the general Table.

CLASS I.

The facts in regard to the diseases in the left-hand column, being those of most frequent occurrence in hospitals, are to be entered directly in the columns of the table. The name of any disease not found in the left-hand column is to be looked for in the right-hand one, and the ages of the persons affected are to be placed after the name. The *class* and *order* in which the case stands is then to be sought for in the left-hand column, and a mark or marks, as the case may be, are to be placed in the "age" column in the line "others." Should any very rare case present itself not included in the right-hand column, it should be written in under its proper class and order, and entered in the left-hand column under the head "others" as before.

[Text of the form follows.]

This Sheet will serve for the Classification of Cases in Hospitals under the following headings:—"Remaining, 1st January"—"Admitted"—"Cured (or Relieved)"—"Dead"—"Discharged incurable, for Irregularities, or at their own Request"—"Remaining, 31st December"—"Duration of Cases in Days."

Write the Name of Hospital, the Sex, the required Heading, and Date, with the Pen.

Class I

ORDER I

(ZYMOTIC DISEASES.)

1. Small Pox
Measles
Whooping Cough
Croup
Scarlatina
Quinsy
Diptheria
Coryza, Catarrh, Influenza
Ophthalmia (purulent)
Erysipelas
Metria (puerpural Fever)
Pyemia
Hospital gangrene
Carbuncle, Boil
Dysentery
Diarrhea
Cholera
Typhoid Fever (typhia)
Typhus
Relapsing Fever (typhinia)
Ague
Remittent Fever
Rheumatism
OTHERS

ORDER II

Gonorrhoea
Primary Syphilis
Secondary Syphilis
Tertiary Syphilis
OTHERS

ORDER III

Scurvy
Purpura
Alcohol:
a. Delirium tremens
b. Intemperance
OTHERS

ORDER IV

Thrush
Porrigo
Scabies
Worms
OTHERS

Class II

ORDER I

(CONSTITUTIONAL DISEASES)

Gout
Dropsy
Cancer
Canker (noma)
Mortification
OTHERS

ORDER II

Scrofula
Tuberculosis Mesenterica
Phthisis
Haemoptysis
Pneumothorax
Hydrocephalus (with tubercular deposit)
OTHERS

Class III

ORDER I.

(LOCAL DISEASES.)

A. Brain, spinal marrow and nerves
Meningitis
Cephalitis (including acute hydrocephalus)
Paralysis
Chorea
Mania
Epilepsy
Hysteria
Tetanus (idiopathic)
Convulsions
OTHERS

B. Sense organs
Ophthalmitis (not purulent)
Cataract
Amaurosis
Glaucoma and other diseases of the eye
Otorrhoea
Otitis
Deafness and other diseases of the ear
OTHERS

ORDER II

Carditis
Pericarditis
Endocarditis
Disease of Heart Valves
Heart Hypertrophy
Heart Atrophy
Heart Fatty degeneration
Aneurism of heart
Aneurism of aorta, etc.
Angina Pectoris
Fainting
Phlebitis
Varix
OTHERS

ORDER III

Epistaxis
Laryngitis (Edema of the glottis
Bronchitis
Pleurisy
Pneumonia
Asthma
OTHERS

ORDER IV

Gastritis
Enteritis
Peritonitis
Constipation
Colic
Ileus (Obstruction of bowels)

Intussusception
Hernia
Stricture of aesophagus
Stricture of intestinal tube
Ulceration of intestinal tube
Dyspepsia
Pyrosis
Gastralgia
Haematemesis
Apoplexy
Melena
Haemorrhoids
Fistula
Pancreatic disease
Spleen disease
Hepatitis
Jaundice
Gall Stones
Cirrhosis
Ascites
OTHERS

Order V

Nephritis
Ischuria
Nephria (Bright's diaease, Albuminuria)
Diabetes
Stone (uric Acid, etc.)
Gravel (uric Acid, etc.
Haematuria
Cystitis
Disease of Prostate Gland
OTHERS

Order VI

Varicocele
Hydrocele
Ovarian Dropsy
OTHERS

Order VII

Synovitis
Ostitis (including Periostitis and endostitis)
Exostosis
Curvature of Spine
Caries
Necrosis
Muscular Atrophy
OTHERS

Order VIII

Phlegmon
Whitlow
Abscess (external)
Ulcer (external)
OTHER SKIN diseases

Class IV

Order I.

(Developmental Diseases.)
Spina bifida
OTHER malformations
Teething
OTHERS

Order II

Chlorosis
Childbirth (Miscarriage, Abortion, etc.
Paramenia (including Amenorrhoea, Leucorrhoea, Turn of Life, Climacteria)

Class V

Violent Deaths or Diseases

Order I

(Accident)
Burn
Scald
Fracture
Contusion
Concussion
Gunshot wound
Cut, stab
Poisoning
OTHERS

Order III

(Homicide)

Order IV

(Suicide)
Gunshot wound
Cut, stab
Poisoning
OTHERS

Sudden deaths (cause not ascertained)
Causes not specified or ill-defined

Total

Most of the diseases in the following marginal list are of less frequent occurrence in hospitals; and all, with some exceptions, are *classed as* "Others" in their respective orders in the left-hand column. They will be distinguished in abstracting the diseases by writing the *ages* of the persons attacked, cured or dead, etc., against the particular disease in the margin below. Thus, a person aged 16 would, if admitted for "*mumps*," be indicated in the body of this sheet by *a tick* against "Others" of Class I, Order I; and his age (16) would be written against "mumps" in the margin. And so of other diseases. The diseases not found printed in the margin must be written in their proper compartments. A summary of the facts in the margin should be given in an appendix to the general Table.

Class I

Order I

varioloid
varicella
miliaria
mumps
erythema
dysentery with abscess of liver (placed to *dysentery*)
yellow fever

Order II

leprosy (Greek elephantiasis
yaws
glanders
hydrophobia
malignant pustule
necusia*

* *Infection by puncture in dissection or by handling the parts of dead animals*

Order III

rickets
bronchocele
cretinism
ergotism

Order IV

Phthiriasis-Hydatids, tape worm, and other entozoa should be distinguished here. In the capital table they will be added to the head "Worms."

Class II

Order I.

anaemia
lupus
dry gangrene
bed sore
melanosis

The several forms of cancer comprised in the capital table under the head "Cancer" should be distinguished as under; the ages and parts affected should also be specified:

Soft
Colloid
Osteoid
Scirrhus
Epithelial

Order II

psoas abscess
scrofulous abscess of joints (placed to *scrofula*)
tubercular peritonitis

Class III

Order I

myelitis
shaking palsy (placed to *paralysis*)

The parts affected, in all cases referred to "paralysis" in the capital table, should be distinguished here, and the ages states.

monomania (placed to *mania*)
dementia (placed to *mania*)
laryngismus stridulus

The different parts of the eye attacked by inflammation should be distinguished here.

neuralgia (tic douloureux)
neuroma

Order II

arteritis
atheroma (of arteries)

Order III

hydrothorax
empyema
pleuripneumonia (placed to *pneumonia*)
congestion of lungs (placed to *pneumonia*)
emphysema (of lungs)
spurious melanosis

Order IV

glossitis
stomatitis
pharyngitis
aesophagitis

Distinguish here the following varieties of hernia, all of which are classed in the capital table under hernia:

congenital
femoral or *crural*
inguinal

scrotal
umbilical
ventral

Order V

diuresis
stricture of urethra
(not a consequence of gonorrhoea)

In cases of stone and *gravel, the composition of substances should be specified here.*

Order VI

orchitis
hysteritis
ovarian tumour
uterine tumour
polypus of uterus

Order VII

fragilitas ossium
mollities ossium

Order VIII

roseola
urticaria
eczema
herpes
pemphigus
ecthyma
impetigo
acne
mentagra
lichen
prurigo
psoriasis
pityriasis
ichthyosis

In abscess and ulcer the parts affected should be distinguished here.

Class IV

malformations
anus imperforatus
cyanosia
decay of old age
atrophy and debility

Class V

Order I

explosion of powder, gas, etc. (placed to *burn*)
chilblains
frost-bite
lightning (where struck and how?)
sun-stroke (state circumstances)

The circumstances attending deaths by violence should be shown in detail; as, for example, how many persons, at their several ages, were burnt by their clothes taking fire, how many died by falling from scaffolds or heights, how many were poisoned by arsenic, opium, quack medicine, overdose, etc. Gunshot wounds should be distinguished as regards the species of weapon—rifle, pistol, cannon, etc.; other wounds, as whether inflicted by knife, dagger, etc. When cases of privation, drowning, hanging, suffocation, fall within observation, they should be placed to "Others" in the general Table, and the particulars should be stated here. All violent deaths should fall under one or other of the three orders: Accident—Homicide—Suicide.

These exceptional cases will only afford statistical results of value after periods of years, and they should be extracted separately.

It is proposed that one and the same form should be used for each statistical element. Seven elements are required to enable us to tabulate the results of hospital experience; they are as follow:

1. Remaining in hospital on the first day of the year.
2. Admitted during the year.
3. Recovered or relieved during the year.
4. Discharged incurable, unrelieved, for irregularities, or at their own request.

5. Died during the year.
6. Remaining in hospital on the last day of the year.
7. Mean duration of cases in days and fractions of a day.

These seven elements, printed as separate headings and attached to copies of the same form, or written in, would furnish us with the means of tabulating every fact we require. Provision can be made for different sexes in one of two ways: the column for each age may be subdivided for males and females, or it might be more convenient to have two sets of forms, one for each sex.

Again, surgical cases and injuries may be included in the same form with medical cases, or in large hospitals a separate set of forms might be devoted to surgical cases.

For small hospitals, one set of seven forms might easily be made to contain the annual statistics of ages, sexes and diseases (medical and surgical), but for very large hospitals possibly four sets might be required.

The primary object of these tables is to obtain a uniform record of facts from which to deduce statistical results, among which the following may be mentioned:

1. The total *sick population*, i.e., the number of beds constantly occupied during the year by each disease for each age and sex.
2. The *number of cases* of each age, sex and disease submitted to (medical or surgical) treatment during the year.
3. The *average duration* in days and parts of a day of each disease for each sex and age.
4. The *mortality* from each disease for each sex and age.
5. The annual proportion of *recoveries* to beds occupied and to cases treated for each age, sex and disease.

In reducing the data to give the annual results, either percentages or per thousands may be used.

The number of beds constantly occupied may be obtained by taking the mean of the numbers remaining at the beginning and end of the year, if the hospital has been fully occupied, or the mean of the numbers remaining at the beginning and end of each quarter, or oftener, if the hospital be irregularly occupied or the total number of days spent in the hospital by all the cases during the year might be obtained, and by dividing the sum by 365, the mean daily sick would be arrived at. (The total daily "*diets*" issued during the year divided by 365 would give the same result.)

The "*sick treated*" during the year may be obtained by taking the mean of the admissions, and of the discharges from all causes, including deaths.

With fixed data, arrived at on these principles, we can readily obtain the proportionate mortality, not only of the whole hospital, but of every ward of it, and also the proportionate mortality and duration of cases for each age, sex and disease. It need hardly be pointed out of what great practical value these and similar results would become, if obtained over a large number of hospitals.

The laws which regulate diseased action would become better known; the results of particular methods of treatment, as well as of special operations, would be better ascertained than they are at present. As regards their sanitary condition, hospitals might be compared with hospitals and wards with wards. The whole question of hospital economics, as influenced by diets, medicines, comforts, could be brought under examination and discussion.

The liability of particular ages, sexes, occupations and classes of the community to particular forms of disease might be ascertained; other data, such as "married" or "single," previous attacks of illness of the same or of different kinds, birthplace, etc., might be added for comparison, and hospital experience might thus be made to subserve sanitary improvement. The data for these latter comparisons would have to be kept separately, as indeed they generally are in all well-regulated hospitals.

The present proposal for improved hospital statistics is confined to those points bearing directly on the welfare of sick admitted to the wards.

The work has been materially assisted by the kindness of the authorities of St Thomas', University College and St Mary's Hospitals, who have been at great pains in having the experimental sheets (sent to them) accurately filled up, and to whom grateful acknowledgments are here expressed. These forms are now in use in St Bartholomew's Hospital and in London Hospital, and the recommendations of the Statistical Congress have led to a greater uniformity in keeping the records of several other large hospitals.

The forms are intended solely for the tabulation of cases, whether of in-patients or out-patients, but the congress considered it to be advisable that certain other data should be recorded, and it made the following recommendations, in which I cordially agree:

1. The publication in the annual report of a TABULAR STATEMENT, not only of the total number of patients, but also of the total number of *cases of disease*, under the various heads, distinguishing the diseases which have supervened in the hospital.

2. That, in the *registration of cases*, not only the disease for which the patient is admitted, but also those by which he is subsequently affected, be separately recorded.

3. That not only the date of admission into hospital, but the date of attack be recorded.

4. That the date of admission be noted, so as to be compared with the disease, occupation and age of the patients.

5. That in transferring patients from medical to surgical wards, or vice versa, a uniform method of record be adopted.

6. That the exact locality in which the disease originated should, as far as possible, be recorded.

7. That a system of registration of *out*-patients at hospitals and dispensaries be adopted on a similar classification (as far as practicable) to that of the in-patients.

8. That in hospital statistics the average proportion of empty beds be noted, both for the whole year, and also for the different seasons.

9. That the average cost of each *in*- and *out*-patient be noted under the different heads of (*a*) food, etc., (*b*) officers and nurses, (*c*) drugs, etc., (*d*) sundries.

10. That in all hospitals supported by private subscriptions, both the number of *in*- and *out*-patients be noted, and also the number of letters of recommendation be given.

11. That previous diseases of patients, and diseases and habits of parents, be (as far as possible) noted.

12. That in hospitals there be tabulated:

the number of beds,
the number of storeys,
the number of wards,
the length, breadth and height of wards,
the number of beds per ward,
the cubic feet per bed,
the superficial area per bed,
number of windows, with their dimensions,
means of ventilation,
drainage,
water closets or latrines,
water supply.

The following heads for a Hospital Admission and Discharge Book will afford a ready means of collecting the data required for filling up the annual forms proposed in this section. They also include those particulars in regard to cases of disease contained in the additional propositions adopted by the Congress.

Hospital Admission and Discharge Book.

No. of Case	Date of Admission	Name	Age	Sex, M. or F.	Residence, and Place where taken ill, or Injured	Trade or Occupation	Disease or Accident	Date					Duration of Case in Hospital in Days and Quarters	Remarks — (Previous Diseases of Patients and of Parents)
								Of Attack	Of Recovery	Of Death	Of Discharge (Relieved), or (unrelieved), or otherwise	Of Transfer to other Division of Hospital		

Note. If a patient admitted for one disease (such as ulcer) is attacked by another disease (such as erysipelas), unconnected with the former, the patient *should not be "discharged."* The new disease should simply be entered as *another case*, and the date of recovery from the first disease (ulcer) should not be filled up until the ulcer is healed. At the same time as the entry of the new disease (erysipelas) is made, a note should be written in the discharge column of the admission for ulcer, simply referring to the new number under which the case is entered, thus (See No.   ). The date of recovery, death, etc., from the second disease, erysipelas, must be entered in the proper column opposite that disease.

The following Annual Tabular Abstracts for the Yearly Report of the Hospital embody the other recommendations of the Congress.

1. IN-PATIENTS

Periods	No. of letters of recom-mendation*		Admissions		Total cases of disease treated†		Deaths		Recoveries		Otherwise discharged		No. of beds occupied					
													Maximum		Minimum		Average	
	M	F	M	F	M	F	M	F	M	F	M	F	M	F	M	F	M	F
1st Quarter																		
2nd Quarter																		
3rd Quarter																		
4th Quarter																		
Total for the year																		

* These columns are only required for hospitals for which Letters of Recommendation are necessary.
† This column includes cases of disease occurring in patients *after* admission to hospital.

2. Out-patients

Periods	No. of Letters of Recommendation*		No. of patients	
	Males	Females	Males	Females
1st Quarter 2nd Quarter 3rd Quarter 4th Quarter				
Total for the year				

*These columns are only required for hospitals for which Letters of Recommendation are necessary.

3. Cost of Each Patient

	Food, etc., wine, spirits, malt liquor	Officers and nurses	Drugs, etc., instruments	Other expenses			Total
				Washing	Firing and lighting	Sundries	
In-patients Out-patients							

4. Sanitary Statistics of Wards

Number of wards	No. of beds per ward	Dimensions of wards			Cubic feet per bed	Super-ficial feet per bed	Windows			No. of fire places	Ventila-tion if by (windows) or (ventila-tors), and its suf-ficiency by day and night	Number of		
		Length	Breadth	Height			Number	Height	Width			Water closets	Baths	Ablu-tion basins
Ground Floor														
No. 1														
No. 2, etc.														
First Floor														
No. 1														
No. 2, etc.														
Second Floor														
No. 1														
No. 2, etc.														

State of Drainage {
- Good
- Indifferent
- Bad
- Cesspits, etc.

State of Water-Supply {
- Quality { Good / Indifferent / Bad
- Quanity { Sufficient / Insufficient

B. Proposal for Improved Statistics of Surgical Operations

Some time ago the attention of the medical profession was occupied with an important discussion on the mortality from surgical operations, resulting in certain conclusions as to the causes of this mortality in different hospitals and in different countries.

Having been engaged some time previously in endeavouring to further a more uniform system of hospital statistics generally than had previously existed, I was naturally interested in the discussions alluded to, and a very cursory examination of the statistical data adduced was sufficient to satisfy anyone that the real mortality due to operations had not as yet been ascertained with sufficient accuracy to enable a just comparison to be made. The data employed may be described as follows:

So many operations of such and such a nature, without reference to age, sex or cause of the operation, followed by so many deaths, without reference to age, sex or complications. Given these elements, divide the one by the other, and you get the mortality.

A statistical proceeding such as this can at best lead to very loose approximations. It can convey but a very imperfect idea of the real state of the case. And one thing is quite certain, that it can lead to no practical result whatever, either as regards the true causes of the mortality, or how these may be mitigated.

The first step in the way of improvement is to obtain a terse and accurate registration of the elements of the problem. Every well-kept hospital record ought to contain these. But for the sake of uniformity, I enumerate them as follows:

1. Age.
2. Sex.
3. Occupation.
4. Accident or disease leading to operation.
5. Date of accident and of operation, or date of operation if from disease.
6. Nature of operation.
7. Constitution of patient.
8. Complications occurring after operation.
9. Date of recovery or of death.
10. Fatal complication (*a*) resulting directly from the accident, (*b*) occurring after the operation.

These elements are of so much importance that it would be well to enter them in a separate operation book. Having obtained them, the next step is to tabulate them for use, and, to do this properly, two forms are required:

1. Including all the operations, with their results.
2. For registering fatal cases.

Copies of these forms are appended.

Table 1 is for tabulating the surgical operations performed. In this table, the ordinary English nomenclature of operations is adopted (with its numerous Anglicized Latin and Greek words) as the one most generally in use. The great operations are classed under two separate heads: those resulting from injury, those rendered necessary by disease. By so doing, we are able to eliminate the effect of shock, and also of the state of health of the patient, the former consequent on the accident, the latter as influencing the result of the operation.

After several trials, the sexes and the ages have been given for quinquennial periods up to twenty years, thence to sixty by decennial periods, and from sixty onwards again, by quinquennial periods. This enables the influence of each (sex and age) on the result of operations to be ascertained. For the purposes of abstracting, the disease or injury requiring operations should in every instance be tabulated in a word or two. A column has therefore been provided for this purpose.

The most important perhaps of all the elements are the complications occurring after operation. It is these which mainly determine the result of the case, while they at the same time afford the most insight into preventible causes of mortality. As it is a matter of primary importance to adopt a common nomenclature of complications, one has been prepared, which is printed on each form for reference.

In filling up the column of complications, this nomenclature should be as far as possible adopted. It has been tried on an experience of upwards of 800 operations, in 141 of which there were distinct complications. The first result of the tabulation was to show that sixty-six of these complications were referable to pyemia, cellular inflammation, erysipelas, sloughing, suppuration, gangrene, diarrhea and bedsore, diseases notoriously connected with defective sanitary conditions in wards, or with constitutions in patients so bad as to render doubtful the propriety of operating at all.

Table 2[28] is intended to tabulate the fatal complications and causes of death. It is constructed to correspond with Table 1, in order that,

28 Table 2 is to report fatal complications and causes of death, using the same headings as in Table 1.

Name of Hospital

Period included in this Table: from   to

(*The Period should he the same as in Table 2.*)

Table 1: Surgical Operations Performed

Operations	Age and sex																										Results				Diseases or Injuries Requiring Operation	Complications Occurring after Operation [After each complication, give the age of the patient.]	Average Duration in Days from Operation to Result†	Remarks on Constitution of Patient, etc.
	Under 5 Years		5–		10–		15–		20–		30–		40–		50–		60–		65–		70–		75 & above		Total		Re-covered		Died					
	Male	Female	Male	Female	Male	Female	Male	Female	Male	Female	Male	Female	Male	Female	Male	Female	Male	Female	Male	Female	Male	Female	Male	Female	Male	Female	Male	Female	Male	Female				
Amputations* (for injury) *Primary*:																																		
Hip Joint																																		
Thigh																																		
Leg																																		
Foot																																		
Toes																																		
Shoulder Joint																																		
Arm																																		
Forearm,																																		
etc., etc., etc.																																		

* Under amputations through any part of the limb should be included amputations through the joint next above, e.g., under amputations of the leg those through knee-joint, unless where the amputation at the joint is expressly named.

† As a general rule, the result should be considered as attained at the date of the healing of the operation wound.

by simple arithmetical processes, the mortality from each operation for each sex and age, and also for each complication, may be readily ascertained. The same nomenclature, both of operations and of complications, is adopted in this as in the other table, and two columns are added in which to enter the average duration of the cases (in days) from the date of the operation to that of the death.

The causes of death in 482 fatal operations have been compared in this way, and one result has been to discover that 190 deaths (or nearly 40 percent of the total mortality) were occasioned by pyemia, phlebitis, cellular inflammation, erysipelas, sloughing, suppuration, gangrene, diphtheria, pneumonia and fevers, typhoid and hectic. No less than fifty deaths occurred from these two last diseases. Another result has been to ascertain the great difference in relative frequency of complications in different hospitals.

Thus out of three large hospitals, one returns 25 percent of its mortality after operations as being due to the fevers mentioned above, while the other two hospitals return not a single death from fever. In one of the hospitals, 27 percent of the deaths are returned as due to shock, in another 2½ percent, in another less than 1 percent are attributed to this cause. In one hospital, 33 percent of the deaths are attributed to peritonitis, in another 3½ percent, and in the third 22 percent. The deaths from pyemia are returned from one hospital as amounting to 12 percent of the total mortality, from another at 4½ percent, and from a third at 14 percent. Cellular inflammation, erysipelas, sloughing, suppuration and gangrene together yield in one hospital a proportion of 2 percent, in another 6 percent, in another 15 percent of the total mortality.

The comparative frequency of complications not attended by fatal results varies in an equal degree. The facts already ascertained, imperfect as they are, point to the following consequences. First, that the sanitary condition of the hospitals has a much greater effect on the result of operations than could have been anticipated. Second, that in describing the complications, the same name is not always used to signify the same thing. The data at my disposal are too limited to allow of the comparative effect of age and sex on mortality being discovered, but, incomplete as they are, they all go to prove the necessity for adopting a uniform nomenclature of complications and a uniform method of tabulation. The one drawn up will, I believe, be found suitable for every purpose; it has been tried on a somewhat large scale and has been found to answer.

Every annual hospital report should contain a digest of the previous and past years' statistics, including those of its operations, on a uniform plan. For the general registration of cases, the forms and method given above, which were submitted to the Statistical Congress, and laid before the meeting of the Social Science Association at Dublin, will be found to answer the purpose, and the forms for registering operations I now submit complete the work I took in hand.

It will not, of course, be necessary to print the entire forms in each annual report. In most hospitals, not above a dozen or fifteen lines will be required every year. In the trials I have made, I find that the complications following on 811 operations can all be included in thirty-four lines, and this is a much larger number of operations than is ever likely to be registered in any one year in any hospital. In the smaller class of country hospitals, the annual table would rarely exceed half-a-dozen lines, so that no one need be alarmed at the apparent magnitude of the tables.

I am fain to sum up with an urgent appeal for adopting this or some *uniform* system of publishing the statistical records of hospitals. There is a growing conviction that, in all hospitals, even in those which are best conducted, there is a great and unnecessary waste of life, and that, as a general rule, the poor would recover better in their own miserable dwellings, if they had proper medical and surgical aid and efficient nursing, than they do under more refined treatment in hospitals. But few have had so sad or so large an experience as I have had to lead them to this conviction. It is imperative that this impression should be either dissipated or confirmed.

In attempting to arrive at the truth, I have applied everywhere for information, but in scarcely an instance have I been able to obtain hospital records fit for any purposes of comparison. If they could be obtained, they would enable us to decide many other questions besides the one alluded to. They would show subscribers how their money was being spent, what amount of good was really being done with it, or whether the money was not doing mischief rather than good; they would tell us the exact sanitary state of every hospital and of every ward in it, where to seek for causes of insalubrity and their nature, and, if wisely used, these improved statistics would tell us more of the relative value of particular operations and modes of treatment than we have any means of ascertaining at present. They would enable us, besides, to ascertain the influence of the hospital with its numerous diseased inmates, its overcrowded and possibly ill-ventilated wards, its bad site, bad drainage, impure water and want of cleanliness—or the reverse of all these—upon the general course of operations and diseases passing through its wards, and the truth thus ascertained would enable us to save life and suffering, and to improve the treatment and management of the sick and maimed poor.

NOMENCLATURE OF OPERATIONS INTENDED TO BE USED IN FILLING UP TABLES 1 AND 2

(The operations should, for the sake of uniformity, be inserted in the table in the order in which they stand in this list.)

AMPUTATIONS (FOR INJURY)
- *Primary*
  - Hip joint
  - Thigh
  - Leg
  - Foot
  - Toes
  - Shoulder joint
  - Arm
  - Forearm
  - Hand
  - Fingers
- *Secondary*
  - Hip joint
  - Thigh
  - Leg
  - Foot
  - Toes
  - Shoulder joint
  - Arm
  - Forearm
  - Hand
  - Fingers

AMPUTATIONS (FOR DISEASE)
- Hip joint
- Thigh
- Leg
- Ankle joint
- Foot
- Toes
- Shoulder joint
- Arm
- Forearm
- Hand
- Fingers

HERNIA
- *Inguinal*—Radical Cure
  - Herniotomy—Opening Sac
    - Without opening
- *Femoral*—Radical Cure
  - Herniotomy—Opening Sac
    - Without opening
- *Umbilical Hernia*—Opening Sac
    - Without opening
  - LITHOTOMY
  - LITHOTRITY
- *Urethrotomy*—For Calculus
  - For Stricture

EXCISION AND REMOVAL OF TUMOURS
- Cancer of Breast
- Other Tumours of Breast
  - (State nature)
- Cancer of Lip
- Encysted of Scalp
- Glandular
  - (State nature)
- Exostosis
- *Other Tumours*, Cancerous or Recurrent
  - (State nature)
- Not Cancerous
  - (State nature)
- *Polypi*—Nasal
  - Uterine
  - Others
    - (State nature)

EXCISION (including TREPHINING) OF BONES AND JOINTS

For Disease
Humerus
Ditto, Head of
Clavicle
Scapula
Elbow joint
Ulna
Radius
Carpus
Metacarpus
Fingers
Hip joint
Pelvis
Femur
Knee joint
Tibia
Fibula
Ankle joint
Tarsus
Metatarsus
Toes
Cranium
Jaw, upper
Ditto, lower
Vertebra
For Injury
Humerus
Ditto, Head of
Clavicle
Scapula
Elbow joint
Ulna
Radius
Carpus
Metacarpus
Fingers
Hip joint
Pelvis
Femur
Knee joint
Tibia
Fibula
Ankle joint
Tarsus
Metatarsus
Toes
Cranium
Jaw, upper
Ditto, lower
Vertebra
Removal of Sequestra—From Head
From Trunk
From Upper Extremities
From Lower Extremities
Tracheotomy
Laryngotomy
Oesophagotomy
Abdominal Section—Ovariotomy
Gastrotomy
Opening of Colon
Caesarean Section
Reparatory Operations
Cicatrices and Contractions (from Burns and Other Injuries)
Deformities from Disease
Deformities from Injuries
Deformities Congenital—Harelip
Others
Cleft or Defective Palate
Paracentesis
Abdominal
Hydrocele
Ovarian
Thoracic
Vesical
Cephalic
Spinal
Evacuation of Cysts and Tumours
Sections of Soft Parts
Perineal Section
Fistula
Anal and Rectal Ulcers
Hemorrhoids
Partial Excision of Organs
Extraction of Loose Cartilages
Extraction of Balls and Other Foreign Bodies
Internal Division of Stricture
Urethra
Of Rectum
Others
Tenotomy
Myotomy
Removal of Parts by Ligature
Naevi

Hemorrhoids
Tongue
Others
REMOVAL OF PARTS BY ECRASEUR
LIGATURE OF ARTERIES
For Aneuryism
(State nature)
For Hemorrhage
For Other Diseases and Injuries
(State nature)
OBLITERATION OF VEINS
OPHTHALMIC OPERATIONS
Extraction
Dislocation
Keratonyxis
Artificial Pupil
Strabismus
Excision of Eye

NOMENCLATURE OF COMPLICATIONS OCCURRING AFTER OPERATIONS

The same nomenclature is to be used in filling up the column of FATAL *complications in Table 2.*

(In filling up the column of complications in Tables 1 and 2, it is proposed, for the sake of uniformity, that the following nomenclature of the more common complications be adopted.)

Shock
Accidents from chloroform or other anaesthetics
Exhaustion, from accident
Exhaustion, from operation
Delirium tremens
Delirium traumatic
Tetanus
Coma
Hemorrhage, continuous
Hemorrhage, recurring
Hemorrhage, secondary (state in a note the times of its recurrence)
Acute inflammation, in or near the seat of operation, such as:
Peritonitis
Peritonitis, hernial
Pleuritis
Pyelitis
Cystitis
Pneumonia
Of Brain or Membranes
(Distinguishing such as are the direct result of the wound in operation by adding the word "traumatic")
Necrosis
Fistula
Pyemia, acute
Pyemia, chronic (Including:
Purulent infection
Purulent diathesis
Putrid infection
Pyemial pneumonia)
Gangrene:
Primary
Secondary
Hospital
Diphtheria of wounds
Phagedena
Sloughing
Sloughing of intestine (hernial)
Erysipelas, simple
Erysipelas, phlegmonous
Cellular inflammation (including purulent edema, sloughing, and suppuration of cellular tissue)
Extravasation of urine
Phlebitis
Inflamed lymphatics
Fevers, typhus
Fevers, typhus hospital
Fevers, typhoid
Fevers, hectic
Fevers, scarlet
Measles
Diarrhea

Tuberculosis, phthisis, etc.
Scurvy
Diphtheria
Bedsore
Vomiting
Cancerous cachexia
Continuance of disease
Recurrence of disease
Croup
Croup (after tracheotomy)
Internal strangulation (hernial)
Secondary diseases of liver
Secondary diseases of heart
Secondary diseases of kidney, etc.

(Any other complication, not included in this list, may be inserted under its usual name.)

Appendix

On Different Systems of Hospital Nursing

In the important question of accommodation for nurses, so much depends upon the method of nursing chosen, that an appendix is devoted to this.

The methods of nursing the sick adopted in the public hospitals of Europe may be distinguished under five classes.

1. Where the nurses belong to a religious order, and are under their own spiritual head, the hospital being administered by a separate and secular governing body. *Examples:* the hospitals of Paris, of King's College Hospital, London, the Protestant institutions of Bethanien at Berlin, Kaiserswerth on the Rhine, many Roman Catholic institutions at Rome and all over Europe, also Anglican sisterhoods at home.

2. Where the nurses are secular under their own head, the hospital having its own separate and secular governing body. *Examples:* the Protestant institutions of Bethanien at Berlin, Kaiserswerth on the Rhine, many Roman Catholic institutions at Rome and all over Europe, also Anglican sisterhoods at home.

3. Where the nurses are secular under their own head, the hospital having its own separate and secular government. *Example:* the hospitals of London.

4. Where the nurses are secular, and under the same secular authority as that by which the hospital where they nurse is governed. *Examples:* the great general hospital at Vienna, the Charité at Berlin.[29]

5. Where the nurses are all men and seculars, and under the same secular male authority as the hospital. *Example:* the military hospitals of Germany, and till a recent period of England, France and Russia.

(With regard to English army hospitals, this odious system of autocracy is done away with in a twofold sense, both in regimental hospitals, where female nursing is not—and cannot be—introduced, and in general hospitals, where it is. Thus, in regimental hospitals, the hospital buildings, furniture, diets and all supplies required for the sick, except medicines, together with the washing, are in the hands of the purveyor, who is responsible to the War Office. The regi-

29 Nightingale's visits to these different institutions are related in *European Travels*, volume 7.

ment stands in the relation of temporary tenant of the hospital. It brings with it its specially trained hospital sergeant and its specially trained orderlies, who, as long as they are competent, are attached solely to the service of the sick, and cannot be called on for any regimental duty. The nursing must be done to the satisfaction of the medical officer, who again is responsible to his commanding officer and to the director general of the Army Medical Department. For everything, then, connected with the building, lodging and dieting of the sick, the purveyor is directly responsible—he being responsible, as above-said, not to the commanding or medical officer, but to the secretary of state for war, through the purveyor-in-chief. The purveyor supplies everything according to a fixed scale to prevent disputes, which scale, fixed after much consideration, is most liberal. And the regiment is responsible for the loss or breakage of all articles thus issued by the purveyor for its use.

In general hospitals, the governor, who is specially commissioned by the War Office, is responsible for everything, except for female nursing and medical treatment. All officers of the hospital are his officers, and are under him not only as regards military discipline, but as regards the due performance of their special duties. The governor has, by regulation, power to provide all manner of supplies and furniture through the proper officer, who is his purveyor or steward. He has jurisdiction over all orderlies through the captain of orderlies, and is responsible for their discipline and their care in nursing the sick. He can suspend medical officers or female nurses. But the medical officer is responsible for the performance of his duties solely to the director general, as are the nurses to the superintendent general of nurses. No extraneous military authority has any jurisdiction within the walls of the hospital.)

Of these systems of nursing:

No. 1, where the nurses belong to a religious order, and are under their own spiritual head—the hospital being administered by a separate and secular governing body—is, on the whole, best calculated to secure good nursing for the sick, and the general well-being of both patients and nurses.

Of the great hospitals of Paris, four, Hôtel-Dieu, St Louis, Lariboisière and La Charité, are nursed by the Augustinians; four, La Pitié, Beaujon, St Antoine and Cochin, by the Soeurs de Ste Marthe, one, Necker, by the Soeurs de St-Vincent-de-Paul; two for children are nursed, one, Les Enfans, by the Soeurs de St-Thomas-de-Villeneuve, one, Ste Eugénie, by the Soeurs de St-Vincent-de-Paul. The administration of all these, it is needless to say, is in the hands of secular men, the Assistance Publique.

Great have been the "scrimmages" from time to time between the administration and the orders, and great have been the benefits accruing to the sick from such "scrimmages." A testimony which will probably be considered fairer than mine, and which certainly would err on the side of the orders, if at all, has spoken out so much more strongly than I could venture to do, that I cannot forbear quoting him. La Rochefoucauld-Liancourt[30] says, in his Seventh Report, p 3,

---

30 François Alexandre Frédéric, duc de la Rochefoucauld-Liancourt (1747-1827), ed., *Journal de Paris.*

"We cannot but believe that it is principally to the power exercised by the nuns in the Hôtel-Dieu, and to their resistance to all authority, that the perpetuity of many abuses must be attributed, and of very great evils, of which we do not hesitate to denounce here the grievous effects." This was in 1790. Now the balance is most happily established. The administration complains of the sisters, and the doctors wish the sisters "were completely under them." The sisters complain of the administration, and wish that the order "had it completely under itself." And all are the best possible friends, and the collision and competition does the greatest possible good. And all work much better for it, and none know how much evil it prevents, how much good it secures.

But in giving this unqualified opinion in favour of nursing by sisterhoods, *provided* the administration be secular, I must add a caution against two mistakes, whether committed in France or in England, in Roman Catholic or in Protestant institutions, viz., (1) the female head of the sisters *must* reside in the institution nursed by them, and neither in a "nurses' home" or "maison mère" [mother house] *not* the hospital, nor in a "home" where other works of charity, not hospital ones, are carried on. If she has other works of charity which appear to her more important, then she had better not undertake hospital ones.

Hospital nursing is jealous, and demands her whole heart. It will not have a divided allegiance. It will not be too much of her whole life to gather experience and learn to govern such institutions. If she has several hospitals, as the Augustinians of Paris, the female head must live where the novices, or probationers, or whatever they are called, are trained. She must be at once matron of the hospital, which means of the nursing in it, and superintendent of the nurses. It will not do for her to head the nurses or probationers in their "home," and to leave the heading of them in the hospital to a matron or other superior.

(2) The sisters must not be the heads of wards merely in order to use "moral influence," as the inexperienced sometimes fancy will be sufficient. If a lady has, in addition, the same knowledge and experience as an old-fashioned hospital head nurse, which indeed many nuns, but only in secularly governed hospitals, have, good; she is fit to be sister or head nurse; if not, not.

No. 3, where the nurses are secular under their own secular female head, the hospital having its own separate and secular government, is, unquestionably, the system which secures the best nursing, after No. 1.

Out of the other systems of nursing, Nos. 2, 4 and 5, in each of which there is but one sole authority, although in No. 2 a religious one, in Nos. 4 and 5 a secular one, over both nurses and administration, are equally to be deprecated.

Nos. 4 and 5, because the nurses, whether male or female, are under the sole command of the male hospital authorities; in this case the arrangements as to hours, proprieties and sanitary rules generally would strike anyone as all but crazy. Such are the rules which give nurses twenty-four hours "on duty" in a ward—or which put them to sleep with the sick, of which the extreme case is where a female nurse is made to sleep in a man's ward, etc.

In No. 2, on the contrary, the nursing staff, whether Protestant or Roman Catholic, whether its heads be male or female, or both, is in entire and sole command of the hospital; in this case the arrangements are generally nearly as crazy as in the former, although the objects and results are widely different. Such are the letting a patient die of a bedsore, because the nurse may spread the dressing for it, but must not look at it, the leaving the wards at night, or at times when the "community" assembles, in sole charge of subordinates, etc.

In Case No. 4 the nurses are destroyed bodily and morally, but the patients are generally, not always, better nursed. In case No. 2, the patients are not always but generally worse nursed, the sick are less cared for, while the spiritual good of the nurses is consulted. But the care of the sick is the object of hospitals.

The collision, often disagreeable but generally salutary for the care of the sick, between the secular administration and the nursing staff (whether this consist of nuns, brothers, deaconesses or nurses), as is the case in the hospitals of London and Paris, keeps each belligerent party to his duty, and reacts beneficially on the interests of the sick. Even the mutual impertinence, just as often to be heard between nuns and doctors, as between doctors and nurses, is far better for the management of a hospital, and any neglect of the sick is far less likely to pass unnoticed, than where the authority is solely invested in one of the two ways above-mentioned, i.e., either vested in the secular male authorities of the hospital, as is the case in the great general hospitals of Germany, or in the spiritual head of the nursing establishment, as is the case in German hospitals, nursed by either Protestant or Roman Catholic orders. Take the nuns, brothers, deaconesses out of the parent institution, and set them to work in a great secular hospital, in daily contact with the (often vexatious) exigencies of doctors and governors, and they will work admirably.

Take Case 2. Theory differs widely from practice in these things. If we were perfect, no doubt an absolute hierarchy would be the best kind of government for all institutions. But, in our imperfect state of conscience and enlightenment, publicity, and the collision resulting from publicity, are the best guardians of the interests of the sick. A patient is much better cared for in an institution where there is the perpetual rub between doctors and nurses or nuns, between students, matrons, governors, treasurers and casual visitors, between secular and spiritual authorities (for this applies quite as much to Roman Catholic as to Protestant institutions) than in a hospital under the best governed order in existence, where the chief of that order, be it male or female, is also sole chief of the hospital.

Taking the imperfect general run of human things, for we are considering men, and not angels, public opinion is a higher average standard than individual opinion. For many years I have been trying to find out how this could be, since public opinion is made up of individual opinions. I think it is because A will be much more rigid in making B mind B's business than in minding his own. Public opinion is good for this. The remark is not a high-minded one, but it is true.

Orders, whether Roman Catholic or Protestant, unless held in check by the rude curb of public opinion, or by the perpetual rub and collision with the secular authority of the hospital, are inclined to make into a special object the spiritual (often fancied) good of their members, and not the general and real good of the inmates of the hospital (for whom, nevertheless, the hospital was intended, and not for working out the salvation of the order).

It is bad for the activity of anyone to have always his own way. And if it were only for this, viz., that no great sanitary or administrative improvements have ever come out of orders, or out of seculars, whose authority is undivided, it would be enough to condemn them.

Nos. 2 and 4, where the nurses, religious or secular, are governed by the same authority, religious or secular, which governs the hospital, the destruction of health of the members, both of orders and secular institutions, often takes place in a period of about five years. This consumption of human beings is the worst policy in every sense. Its operative causes are underfeeding, want of proper sleep, want of the most ordinary sanitary precautions—the result of austerity in orders, of an ignorant economy in secular institutions. In the latter, want of the most ordinary means for propriety and morality is often a fourth cause.

No. 2. In some institutions nursed by brotherhoods, abroad, a good Augustinian nun, or good hospital nurse from London, would turn everything out of window (though the former could not do all she would wish), and be as disgusted as we are with their pestilential filth. But, alas! this has been seen even in those nursing *sisterhoods* where the salutary check of the secular administration was not.

No. 2. Where institution and sisterhood alike are under the same authority. The following remark applies exclusively to orders, and to orders where no secular authority is in play, but much more to Protestant than to Roman Catholic orders, which latter have better sense. There is a constant change of occupation of each member of the order, for the sake of detaching said member from earthly things. Today he or she is in the kitchen, tomorrow in a surgical ward, next week in a medical ward, the week after in the laundry. The perplexed medical attendant, when giving his directions about the patients, sees a new face at least every fortnight to give his directions to.

In the best Roman Catholic orders, especially where, as in 1, the secular authority comes into action, there is far less latitude given to individual character and scope to individual capacity than we are at all aware of. Each member is much more independent in his or her own occupation than is the case under arrangement No. 2.

Nos. 2, 4 and 5, where there is but one authority over both hospital and nurses, whether that authority be religious or secular. The following remark applies alike to some institutions, both religious and secular, to all military and to some civil, to Protestant and Roman Catholic establishments.

The want of one definite head in permanent charge of each ward, or set of wards, invariably acts disastrously for the patients. There should always be some one person in acknowledged responsibility for the nursing, with servants—call them lay sisters or brothers, or assistant nurses, or what you will—under the head.

Religious motives, in some orders, a want of any practical system of nursing, in many military and some civil hospitals, reproduce the above defect, in the most varied forms, in institutions of the most opposite character.

No. 4, where nurses and institutions are under the same secular authority. The following remark applies solely to institutions secularly nursed.

The practice of having man and wife in joint charge of a ward or wards has in it more evil than good for the patients. It is true that a woman had better flirt with her husband than with a student or patient; it is true that the common phrase "settling" (which means marrying in some classes) has signification here—for some women never are "settled" till they are married. But it is no less true that the interest of the husband henceforth comes before that of the patients, in honest as in dishonest ways. The woman is no longer attached to her ward, but to her husband, and the patients are, more or less, neglected. This is still more eminently the case in regimental hospitals, where it is a common practice to choose married hospital sergeants as being more "respectable," and to have the wife to live in the hospital. As well might the hospital head nurse have her husband to live with her in the room off her ward.

Nos. 1, where the sisters are of a religious order, but the nurses are secular, 3 and 4, where all the nurses are secular, whether governed by a separate head from that which governs the hospital, or by the same head. The cardinal sin of paid nurses, of all classes, of all nations, is taking petty bribes and making petty advantages (of many different sorts and sizes) out of the patients. From this sin all orders, whether Roman Catholic or Protestant, are exempt, but from it their servants are by no means exempt.

The rules of hospital head nurses in London, were they really religious women, who would neither take any present themselves, nor be guilty of any kind of impropriety, would enable them to exercise a far more efficient surveillance over assistant nurses, as to both these things, than can be exercised by Roman Catholic or Protestant orders living in community. All kinds of things between nurses and patients may and do go on in the sisters' wards when the sisters are out of the way. A hospital head nurse is (or ought to be) always in command of her ward. *To sum up.* Case 1. There is a higher average care of the sick and a higher universal sense of morality among hospital sisters, Protestant and Roman Catholic, provided the hospital authority be a secular one. Case 2. There is a lower average care of the sick, although an equally high morality, among hospital nuns, Protestant and Roman Catholic, if the hospital authority be not a secular one. Case 3. There is a far greater average care of the sick, although a lower morality, among nurses under a secular female head, the authority of the hospital being a secular and separate one, than in Case 2, and there is a somewhat higher average care of the sick in Case 4 than in Case 2, and no morality at all, but an awful destruction of both life and soul, among nurses, where both nurses and hospital are under the same secular (male) authority. Case 5. There is no care of the sick and no morality, nor even discipline, in hospitals where the nurses are men, and where both nurses and hospital are under the same secular (male) authority. This is the worst state of things of all. Case 2 is perhaps the second worst. For, take it which way you will, the idea of the "religious order" is always, more or less, to prepare the sick for death, of the secular, to restore them for life. And their nursing will be accordingly. There will be instances of physical neglect (though generally unintentional) on the part of the former, of moral neglect on that of the latter. Unite the two, and there will be fewer of either.

Of course to all this there are exceptions. This appendix is dealing only with systems of nursing *as systems.*

Note. Two excessively foolish books by the same woman, calling herself an "English Sister of Mercy,"[31] on this question of sisterhoods, in which the diffi-

---

31 Margaret Goodman, *Experiences of an English Sister of Mercy*, 1862, and *Sisterhoods in the Church of England*, 1863.

culty is not to find what is false, but to find what is true, and which I should never have thought of referring to, but that she has been quoted by grave divines in consistory, give every reason for the comparative usefulness or uselessness of sisterhoods but the right one, viz., that if a sisterhood cordially and frankly co-operates with and works in a secular institution, it is useful, if not, not.

Distribution, Reviews and Response to *Notes on Hospitals*

Editor: The book was still being printed when Sir John Lawrence was leaving for India and Nightingale wanted him to take a copy with him. She had the press "put up this one copy for your start," she explained to his secretary and special sanitary commissioner for Calcutta, Dr Charles Hathaway, suggesting that Lawrence might "have some time to glance at it on the voyage."[32] She also had a small number of quarto-sized copies printed, as a note to her family indicates:

> *Notes on Hospitals* by Florence Nightingale, third edition, enlarged etc., *Longmans* is out—a small quarto. As it has been entirely rewritten and printed in a large type, on purpose that my family may know as much of what I have been doing as other people, please order your copies. I am sorry to say it is to be 18/. But it is full of pictures and a standard book. And as my family has been very tempestuous on account of my former small print, they ought not to complain of price. This is a good library book.[33]

The book was out by 14 December 1863, the anniversary of the death of Prince Albert, as a letter to Colonel Clark-Kennedy, who had assisted her with information on convalescent institutions, explains:

> Would you allow me to send you a copy of my 3rd edition of *Notes on Hospitals*, which unlucky book has only just seen the light. And, if so, where may I send it? I shall always remember that you, a great man, went out of your way to assist little men in tiresome details, which you mastered, although somewhat out of your province, for the sake of your fellow creatures.
>
> I have always looked upon this power and willingness of mastering detail as the true mark of a great man. At least, it was that of two with whom I have had the privilege to work, poor Sidney Herbert and Albert, second anniversary of translation to a yet higher path of usefulness we this day sadly celebrate. My book is too technical to

32 Letter 9 December 1863, Florence Nightingale Museum 1085.2.
33 Note, Wellcome (Claydon copy) Ms 9000/157.

be fit for any but hospital physicians, builders and matrons like me. And therefore I make an apology for offering it.[34]

On the day of publication Nightingale sent inscribed copies to James L. Thomas at the War Office, dedicated "from a fellow-worker F.N.," and to civil architect T.H. Wyatt.[35] William Farr got an early copy, for he thanked her for the "3fold gift, black cock, wild duck and the *Notes on Hospitals*!!![36] She arranged for a copy to got to a German doctor, Varrentrapp, who had attended the International Statistical Congress of 1860 (see p 582 below). Another copy went to India, for Sir Charles Trevelyan, then the finance member at Calcutta: "If it will amuse you to cut it open on the voyage, pray do. But (except the recommendations at the end of the section on Indian hospitals) its principles of construction are adapted only for temperate climates."[37]

The anonymous review of Nightingale's *Notes on Hospitals* in the *Medical Times and Gazette* was largely negative,[38] and in places sarcastic. The reviewer particularly objected to Nightingale's choice of indicator for London hospital death rates, which has the effect of making the rates look high. It uses the number of deaths for the year, divided by the average number of patients per day. Thus 90.84 percent, the figure for London hospitals, does not mean that 90.84 percent of patients died, but that over the 365 days of the year there were 90.84 deaths per 100 beds. This the reviewer called "legerdemain" and then cited the fictional "Lord Dundreary" to poke fun at her. As well as the remark that hospital death rates were "almost wholly independent of sanitary condition" (129), there were sarcastic references to "forward schoolboys—what is the quotient of a hundred apples divided by fifteen red herrings?" Nightingale was an "authoress" and "lady," and her views on children's hospitals were "what a woman only could frame" and thus of "most sterling worth." On the other hand, he also wished that Nightingale's views on moving St Thomas' Hospital might "carry due weight" (130).

William Farr promptly wrote a letter to the editor defending Nightingale's analysis and choice of indicator, which was of course also his.[39]

---

34 Wellcome RAMC 801/9/20.

35 Add Mss 46123A f7 and Florence Nightingale Museum 0442.

36 Farr letter 22 December 1863, Add Mss 43399 f162.

37 Letter to J. Pattison Walker 11 January 1864, in *Wars and the War Office* (15:397).

38 *Medical Times and Gazette* 30 January 1864:129-30.

39 William Farr, "Miss Nightingale's 'Notes on Hospitals,'" *Medical Times and Gazette* 13 February 1864:186-87, and, as a further reply, "Hospital Mortality" 27 February 1864:242.

He justified the use of what he called an annual death rate for a hospital, asylum or workhouse infirmary as a better alternative to a rate over admitted cases. Nightingale had allowed that either method could be used, and given a fair comparison between the two. Farr was especially offended by the sexism (my word) of the reviewer's remarks, and defended her stoutly:

> What a refreshing contrast does the woman's book afford to the man's review! She has not walked through—she has lived in hospitals during many of the fairest years of her life. She understands the whole economy of these institutions; she has watched thousands of patients enter their portals and leave their wards after long illnesses, which she has softened by science and by kindness.

He went on to praise Nightingale's powers of observation and her knowledge of medical statistics.

> She probes all the defects which make hospitals ways of death to their inmates. She collects plans; she consults engineers, and she brings the whole of the facts together in a clear, practical form, and holds out hopes that general hospitals may yet benefit mankind directly, and not merely as pathological observatories and medical schools.

Her third edition of *Notes on Hospitals* was "the most judicious, complete and masterly treatise that has recently appeared on any subject" (187). A St Thomas' doctor, J.S. Bristowe, however, attacked Farr for sharing Nightingale's negative assessment of hospitals.[40]

The editor of the *Medical Times and Gazette* followed up Farr's letter with his own analysis. He endorsed Farr's commendation of Nightingale, acknowledging that she was reforming what their own profession had "not yet been able fully to carry out" (187). The editor thought Nightingale was wrong on the issue of contagion and about her opposition to isolation wards for infectious cases, and challenged Farr to advise hospital committees to follow her dictum not to isolate infectious cases. In the end, however, he thought her book was of "immense value," though she was wrong "about one or two incidental matters."

The editor's critical remarks on Nightingale's views of contagion and infection were, in my view, fair. In his review he referred variously to "special poison," "vegetable spores or germs," "minute animal atoms,

40 Letter, *Medical Times and Gazette* 20 February 1864:211, discussed in correspondence (see p 657 below).

pus globules" and "organic particles in a state of chemical change," using the terminology of the time to describe infection and contagion. The spread of all diseases might be hindered "by free ventilation and cleanliness," he wrote, yet all precautions could fail, so that without decrying the powers of ventilation and the virtues of air, sensible people practised "quarantine" in their homes as well, separating an infectious person. To his mind, Nightingale was guilty of "ignoring one truth in order to exalt another" (188).

One assumes that Nightingale and Farr must have discussed her opinion that infectious patients could be mixed in with others without harm, but there is no surviving correspondence on the point. Farr's endorsement of her views on quarantine, as "not too strong," pointedly omitted mention of her dismissal of the need for isolation wards. This omission might be taken as a tacit rejection of that particular view. Nightingale soon stopped giving that advice, and indeed over time became ever more stringent in calling for isolation measures. The terms "isolation ward" begin to appear with favour in her work, although more often the term she used was "separation ward." She was not so fast or thorough in abandoning her dislike of the term "contagion," however, retaining her narrow, etymological definition based on the word's Latin roots, to do with touch.

There is not space here to discuss other reviews of *Notes on Hospitals*. *The Lancet* gave it detailed attention, objecting to her treatment of contagion and infection, among other things, while *The Builder* gave it a long and thoroughly positive review.[41]

Nightingale's *Notes on Hospitals* was influential and for many decades, as will be seen in the correspondence to come. During the American Civil War, which took place soon after the book's publication, *Notes on Hospitals* was used in the planning of war hospitals by both sides.[42] In 1871, the Nightingale Fund Council offered to supply a copy to any hospital board proposing to erect a new building. This prompted many requests for copies across the country, from institutions such as North Lonsdale, Croydon General Hospital, Huddersfield Infirmary, West Kent General Hospital and the Queen's Hospital, Birmingham. By the late nineteenth century, airy "Nightingale wards" became common in hospital construction in North America as well as in Britain and Europe. Not until the major reconstruction that took place after

41 "*Notes on Hospitals*," *The Builder* 22,1094 (1864):53-54.
42 See *Wars and the War Office* (15:592-602).

World War II were they replaced by high-rise hospitals, with rooms of one, two or four beds.

Nightingale was still receiving royalties for the book in 1877, as a payment of £5.8.5 is listed in her diary for that year.[43] In 1879, she sent a spare copy of the book to the Edinburgh Royal Infirmary matron, A.L. Pringle.[44] However, by the following year Nightingale had no more spares when asked by a correspondent and the book was out of print, so she sent this correspondent her own copy.[45] It seems that the book was never translated, unlike *Notes on Nursing*, which appeared in many languages. It is now available online.

A facsimile reprint of *Notes on Hospitals* appeared in 1989, with a scant and inadequate introduction written by Charles E. Rosenberg, an enthusiastic endorser of F.B. Smith's negative opinions of Nightingale.[46] More could not have been expected, for he had already convicted Nightingale of being a "liar, a careerist, a bully, a callous manipulator of friends" and a "power-hungry psychopath" in his review of Smith's book.[47] In the (unpaged) introduction to the reprint, Rosenberg charged Nightingale with failing to distinguish between the moral and the material in hospitals, individuals and the community. "Her certainty was strident and uncompromising," he wrote, and furthermore she had an "obsession with cleanliness and ventilation," a point apparently to be disparaged. Rosenberg completely failed to take into account the science of the time Nightingale wrote *Notes on Hospitals*, 1858-63, which predates the ground-breaking work of Louis Pasteur and Joseph Lister. He nowhere acknowledged that Nightingale's views of germ theory and disease etiology changed over time as medical science developed. "In her explicit rejection of the germ theory," Rosenberg stated, "Nightingale was to draw gradually further apart from the consensus of medical opinion during the last third of the nineteenth century."[48] But it is clear that Nightingale's views did change, and not

43 Entry end December, ADD MSS 45847 f101.

44 Extract, University of Edinburgh 7 May 1879 58.

45 Letter to Mrs Harrison Blair 22 July 1880, Florence Nightingale Museum (LMA) H1/ST/NC/SU170.

46 Charles E. Rosenberg, ed., *Florence Nightingale on Hospital Reform.*

47 Charles Rosenberg review of F.B. Smith, *Florence Nightingale: Reputation and Power, Medical History* 27 (1983):93.

48 Rosenberg, ed., *Florence Nightingale on Hospital Reform*, preface.

long after medical doctors themselves gradually moved to the new theory. The great bacteriologist W.M. Haffkine wanted to meet Nightingale in 1895, evidently seeing no conflict between their positions.[49]

Rosenberg was wrong also in another paper about Nightingale, where he called her "resolutely hostile to the idea of specific contagion," and "sceptical of the existence of specific disease entities."[50] Here he saw Nightingale as failing to distinguish between the social or moral and biophysical spheres. A social scientist would say that she saw the causal influences going both ways.

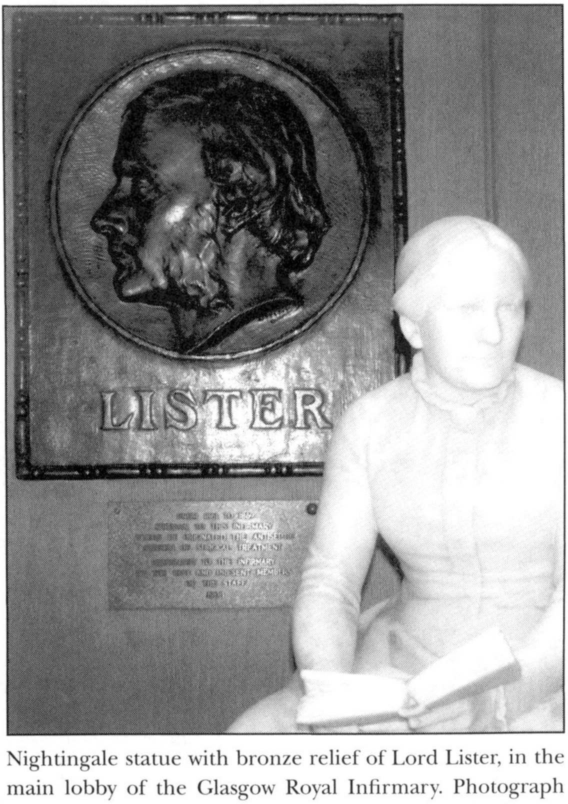

Nightingale statue with bronze relief of Lord Lister, in the main lobby of the Glasgow Royal Infirmary. Photograph courtesy of the NHS Greater Glasgow and Clyde Archives.

49 See *Nightingale School* (12:18).

50 C.E. Rosenberg, "Florence Nightingale on Contagion: The Hospital as Moral Universe," in C.E. Rosenberg, ed., *Healing and History: Essays for George Rosen* 126-27.

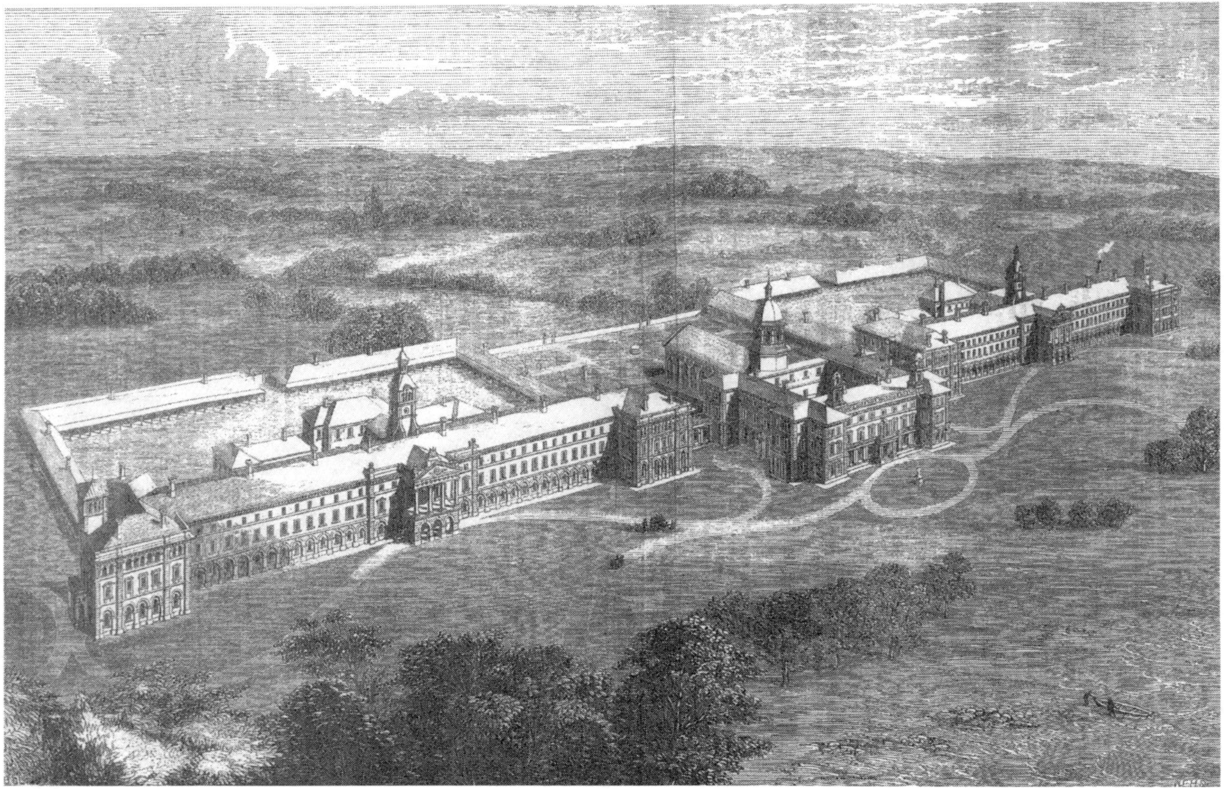

Royal Victoria Hospital, Netley, the massive army hospital on Southampton Water, with a magnificent facade, but long corridors with double wards on each side, and no cross-ventilation. See the contrast with the pavilion army hospital on p 232. From *The Builder* 23 August 1856, 459.

Military Hospitals: Letters, Notes, Articles and Reports

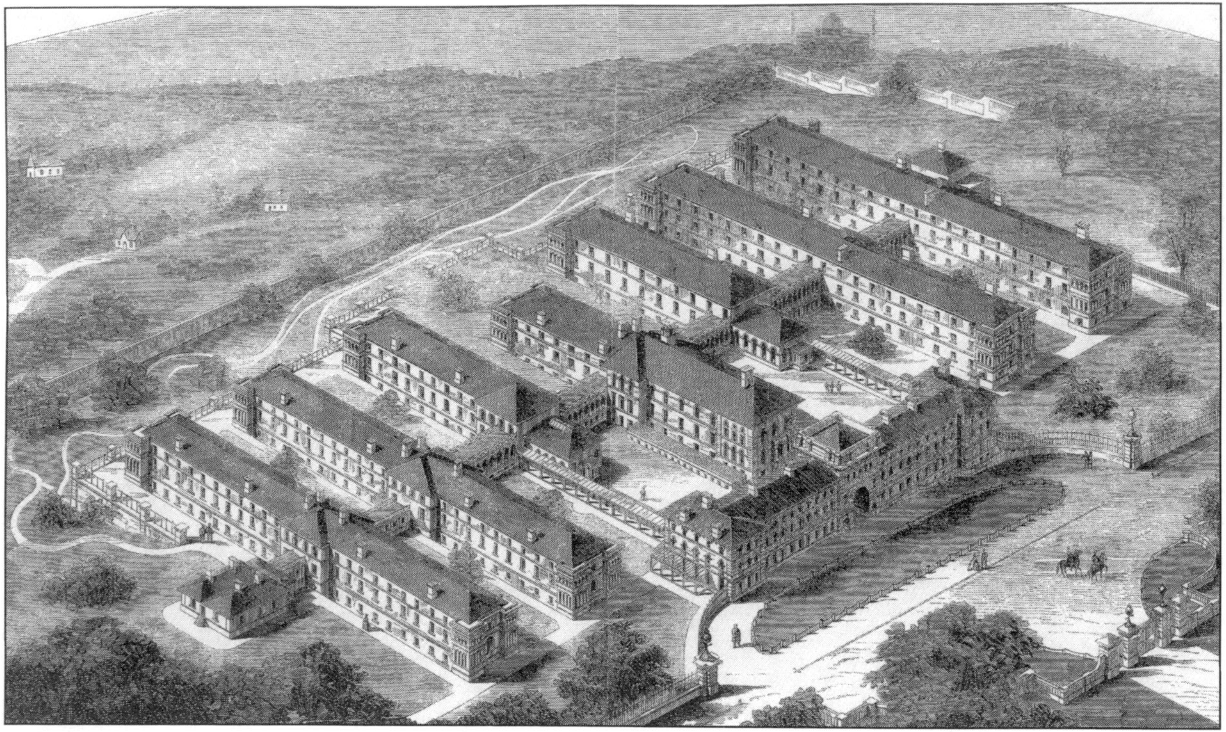

Herbert Hospital, Woolwich, the model army pavilion hospital designed by Douglas Galton, with much input from Nightingale; the narrow "spokes" were wards, with a row of beds on each side, windows facing each other for cross-ventilation, now private residences, the "Royal Herbert Pavilions" (see picture p 493). From *The Builder* 14 April 1866, 269.

Military Hospitals: Letters, Notes, Articles and Reports

The great impetus for Nightingale's work on hospital reform came from her own experience of the horrendous defects in British Army hospitals during the Crimean War. The analysis she did to ascertain what went wrong in them led to her first papers on hospital reform, and in time to her comprehensive 1863 *Notes on Hospitals*. The similarities between civil and military hospitals are obvious from that early writing, and they appear again in the correspondence on civil hospitals later in this volume. However, a sufficient number of differences between the two remain to make a separate section on military hospitals useful. This section is also the place to report related health concerns in barracks and stations, and such issues as nutrition and healthier lifestyles for soldiers. As with civil hospitals, Nightingale considered better statistics to be crucial for planning reforms and tracking their implementation and results.

The dominant concern in the period immediately following the Crimean War was the building of a new and massive hospital at Netley. Nightingale's opposition to the project is clear right in her confidential report, *Notes on the Health of the British Army*. Correspondence here shows that she, with her team, initially tried to get the project cancelled, and then to have it modified substantially when it could not be stopped. Nightingale proposed making Netley into an invalid hospital or even a barrack instead of a full general hospital (see p 258 below), ideas which were again rejected. Correspondence here will show, however, that the team was successful in getting significant alterations made to the design. By 1 July 1857, Nightingale could describe the revised plans as having "very great improvements," listing five crucial points (see p 253 below). In January 1858, she went so far as to declare the hospital to be "not now" unhealthy, although not what "a great military hospital of the British Empire should be" (see p 258 below). The assessment of Nightingale's Netley work as being one of her "recorded failures" seems to have missed the point, given how much change was achieved.[1]

The impetus for building Netley on such a grand scale came from the director general of the Army Medical Department, Andrew Smith, who also strongly defended the estuary site.[2] In March 1855, while the Crimean War was still producing large numbers of sick and invalids, the war secretary, Lord Panmure (1801-74), instructed Sir John Burgoyne (1782-1871), inspector general of fortifications, to appoint an officer to assist in the selection of a site for a new military hospital to accommodate 1000 patients. Appointed was Captain Robert Michael Laffan (c1821-82), R.E., who, with Dr Henry Mapleton (1815-79), head of the Medical Board at the War Office, looked at potential sites in the Portsmouth area.

Sir James Clark (1788-1870), a Nightingale ally, objected to the first site selected as being too close to the Naval Hospital at Haslar. Clark marked a map for Laffan at what ultimately became the settled-on location, the ruins of an old abbey at Netley, on the south coast near Southampton. Laffan inspected and approved the proposed location, and a committee was established in January 1856 to prepare a plan. Panmure told it that the new hospital should be in a form like French pavilion hospitals such as Bordeaux. Andrew Smith, however, who opposed the pavilion model, succeeded in getting a quite different plan made of one vast building, 1400 ft. in length, with a central block and two long wings of 554 ft. each. The only ventilated wards were at the extreme ends of the two wings. The long corridors would facilitate the transmission of disease from ill-ventilated ward to ill-ventilated ward. Moreover, the wards were small, to accommodate twelve to sixteen patients each, a size Andrew Smith favoured, but one, from Nightingale's perspective, that made them impossible to nurse. Separate kitchens, dining rooms and other offices were planned for each wing, adding to the expense.

The design made for a magnificent impression, with a facade a quarter mile long facing the sea. Nightingale, of course, had known another hospital with a magnificent facade facing the sea: the Barrack Hospital at Scutari, one with a high death rate.

---

1 Keith J. Williams, "Reappraising Florence Nightingale," *British Medical Journal* 337 (2008):a2889.

2 Andrew Smith (1797-1872); see the biographical sketch in *Wars and the War Office* (15:1039).

Panmure made his decision in favour of Smith's plan on 15 May 1856 and the queen laid the cornerstone on 19 May of what would bear her name, the Royal Victoria Hospital, Netley. He and Nightingale did not meet each other until after she returned from the war in late September, when both were guests of the queen at Balmoral Castle. After that meeting, Panmure sent the plans to her as a courtesy and she, jointly with Dr Sutherland, prepared a response (her covering letter and the report are the second and third items below).

The assessment by Sutherland and Nightingale was highly negative, for reasons that will appear repeatedly in the correspondence. To begin, the ward windows did not open into outdoor air on at least two sides; windows on the corridor took in effluvia from other wards; and the few windows which opened onto fresh air faced the cold northeast. Lord Palmerston (1784-1865) joined in the fray, accusing Lord Panmure of sacrificing the comfort and recovery of patients to the vanity of the architect, whose sole object, it seemed, was to make a building "to cut a dash" at Southampton River. "Any sacrifice of money" to correct the errors would be better than persevering with bad arrangements."[3]

George Godwin, editor of *The Builder*, began to campaign against Netley in 1856. An editorial on many aspects of hospital design referred to "serious mistakes" in the ground plan, citing especially the placement of baths and toilets. Should the proposed arrangements be carried out, more disease would be generated than cured, he said.[4] Godwin published two further critical articles on Netley in 1857, by persons other than Nightingale. He also published articles favourable to the royal commission on the Crimean War and other reforms.[5] Nightingale's articles of 1858 built on these.

In February 1857, a committee was appointed to consider the objections raised about the Netley design and report to the secretary for war, along with advice from doctors at the Middlesex, Guy's, St Thomas' and other civil hospitals. The committee reported in May

---

3 George Douglas and George Dalhousie Ramsay, eds., *Panmure Papers* 2:233-34.

4 Editorial, The *Builder* 14,711 (20 September 1856):509-11.

5 "The Victoria Military Hospital, Netley," The *Builder* 15,749 (13 June 1857):340-41; "Netley Hospital and Aldershot" 15,753 (11 July 1857):396; "The Sanitary Commission in the East" 15,739 (4 April 1857):188; and "Sanitary Arrangements for Barracks and Hospitals" 15,770 (7 November 1857):647.

1857, but only minor changes were made as the work was so far along. Alterations to corridors were possible. A building was removed.

Early in 1858, Lord Panmure appointed Sidney Herbert to inspect the works at Netley and to examine its plans with Dr Sutherland, Dr W.H. Burrell (c1795-1866) and Douglas Galton. They reported on 12 March 1858 with a scathing indictment, which was, of course, in line with the objections Nightingale had been raising all along.

The succinct report Nightingale and Sutherland wrote for Lord Panmure strongly defended the pavilion principle, and credited the French for advances in hospital architecture that they believed the British should follow (see p 241 below). To her brother-in-law Nightingale described the French as "the only hospital builders of the present day," and the British had to "copy them if we desire hospitals to be places of recovery." After the plans for Netley were altered, it was "very greatly improved," but she thought that they should adopt what was known to be "best," rather than to "improve what is known to be bad" (see p 255 below). The improved Netley was "better than any London hospital," but still "behind the day": hardly a compliment, but far from failure. She also saw Netley as faulty for its expensive administration. On the other hand, it could be approved as an invalid hospital, and it would make a "model" barrack (see p 258 below).

When the able and conscientious Thomas Alexander was made director general of the Army Medical Department, early in 1859, Nightingale could see some positives for the hospital and even the site. Alexander would see to it that the hospital was used effectively for pulmonary cases, for which the river situation would be beneficial (see p 310 below).

Construction at Netley was completed early in 1863 at a cost of £350,000. It received its first patient on 11 March 1863. Queen Victoria made the first of her many visits to the hospital on 8 May 1863. It was her first public appearance after Prince Albert's death in 1861.

Netley soon began to receive the sick and wounded from India and other colonies where British troops were based, and it was used for the sick and wounded from the Egyptian campaigns of 1882 and 1885. However, the hospital was not fully occupied until the Boer War, and then not again until World War I. It was the home of the Army Medical School from its opening until 1902. Netley was largely demolished in 1966 and effectively closed in 1978. The central section was made into an information centre for visitors.

The errors of Netley comprise a major theme running through all the correspondence on military hospitals: the long corridors, lack of cross-ventilation and the bad building site. Contrast was often made between Netley and the new military hospital at Woolwich, whose superiority derived from the lessons learned from the Crimean War.

The royal commission on the Crimean War made numerous recommendations for building renovation and replacement, which later budget cutbacks made impossible to implement. Debate on the estimates in the House of Commons was fraught with trouble, as MPs sought economies and did not understand the importance of the expenditures planned. In Nightingale's "human capital" approach, "the life of the soldier is the most costly article," so that measures to preserve it were good expenditures (see p 399 below). While many planned buildings were dropped in the cost-cutting, Sidney Herbert managed to hold on to the new hospital at Woolwich.

Plans were well under way for Woolwich Hospital when Sidney Herbert died on 2 August 1861. Nightingale pressed for, and succeeded, in having it named after him. She told her sister, quoting from Virgil's last ode, "at my request, the new magnificent Woolwich Hospital is to be called after him: Exegi monumentum aere perennius [I have raised a monument more durable than bronze]."[6] It had all of the advantages of Vincennes and Lariboisière, both exemplary hospitals, with none of their disadvantages.

What Nightingale and her allies did not succeed in getting for Netley they worked mightily to obtain for Woolwich. Douglas Galton was the architect and the two worked closely together on the plans. Nightingale gave much advice on the materials to be used in the hospital, and was insistent that details about the walls, flooring, fittings and other materials be included in the plans.

Nightingale's active involvement in the design is clear both in Galton's letters to her, many of which survive, and those reproduced here by her to him. For example, while at Malvern she wrote Sidney Herbert, "We have the plans sketched out, but cannot go on with them till we all meet in London." Galton's draftsman had sent "the first draught to me here," she noted (see p 313 below).

Next, Nightingale had to fight to keep the War Office from cancelling the new hospital for reasons of cost, as Sidney Herbert had earlier (see p 399 below). It was opened on 1 November 1865, without ceremony. The first British hospital deliberately built on the pavilion

6 Letter 7 August 1861, *Life and Family* (1:328).

principle for reasons of health, it became a model both for civilian and military hospitals. The Herbert Hospital acquired the "Royal" title after Queen Victoria visited Boer War soldiers there in 1900. It was closed, as superfluous to military needs, only in 1977. Left vacant but not demolished, it was bought in 1990 and renovated into luxury apartments. Its new name proclaims its proud past: the Royal Herbert Pavilions.

Almost all of the material on military hospitals concerns army hospitals, general and regimental. There are several places where the Royal Navy, and the Navy Medical Department, are at issue. Nightingale even joked to Sidney Herbert that she was talking to the navy partly "to shame" the army into taking more action, but "I cannot forget my first love, nor marry another department again so soon" (see p 245 below). The visits she made to navy hospitals in 1857, however, at least enabled her to draw useful comparisons with those of the army (see pp 245 and 246 below).

Only a month after her return from the Crimean War, Nightingale had a two-hour interview on naval hospitals with Sir John Richardson, a retired inspector general of hospitals for the Royal Navy, for which a Crimean War colleague, Colonel Lefroy, seems to have been the intermediary.[7] Richardson recorded the discussion in a letter to his wife the day after:

> Yesterday I went by appointment to the Burlington Hotel at five o'clock to wait on Miss Nightingale, and talked with her till seven, during all that time answering questions, and occasionally making some remarks on the present state of the public departments and hospitals. I was glad to find that our opinions were precisely alike. She wished to know the mode of conducting the naval hospitals, and how the medical officers obtained alterations, amendments and supplies. After I had detailed my experience, she remarked that it was nearly as bad as in the army, and believed that both were branches of the Circumlocution Office. The only advantage which I could point out was that the Admiralty are much more liberal in their supplies. There is the same difficulty in introducing the improvements of modern science, from the number of channels through which every suggestion must pass, until the head of the office is

---

7 Richardson (1787-1865) was also a famous Arctic explorer and naturalist; John Henry Lefroy (1817-90), scientific adviser to the secretary for war; letter to Lefroy 2 December 1856, in *Crimean War* (14:471).

> called upon to decide regarding a matter of which he knows nothing, all the reasons for the change having filtered away in the progress upwards of the proposal. "The weary Treasury," she says, "is at the root of all the evil."[8]

He further described Nightingale as "an earnest reformer of the right sort." She did not have much faith "in public men," and believed "that the grievous failures of the past will not produce much future amendment." She was "very like the print of her at Lancrigg," their home in Scotland, he told his wife. He would have "known her at once," but she had "much more intellect of the countenance."

> She has a most brilliant and intelligent smile, a very pleasant and not patronizing address, but always perfectly self-possessed, quick in comprehending a subject, and distinct in her questions, which were calculated to bring out a correct view of the subject [571].

The correspondence begins with Nightingale's visit to the Registrar-General in quest of comparative hospital data to be used for her several reports, and then moves on to Netley.

Source: Notes from a visit to the Registrar-General, ADD MSS 43402 ff164-65

24 November 1856

Through kindness of Registrar-General,[9] went over, with him, all his books. Sir C. Campbell[10] declared his shame when he compared Sardinian troops with ours. Had our G.O.s [general officers] but information enough to feel the shame they ought, when comparing civil registration with theirs. All needed to determine causes of disease and means of removing them to be found in former. All needed to leave H.M.'s ministries in ignorance as to state of H.M.'s troops, to be found in latter.

When one businesslike head set to accomplish one object, if that object to make beer, we see the result in, say, the Burton Breweries. When one mathematical head set to accomplish one object, that of classifying and registering the great statistics and discovering the causes

8 Excerpt of letter 4 December 1856, in John McIlraith, *The Life of Sir John Richardson* 250-51.

9 Major George Graham (1801-88), Registrar-General 1842-79, William Farr's superior.

10 Sir Colin Campbell (1792-1863), later Lord Clyde, commander of the Highland Brigade, commander-in-chief in India.

of the various events in a population, we see the results in the magnificent organization—magnificent because of its simplicity economy and efficiency—in the Registrar-General's Office.

When we see the good of a great army bested in various departments with *different* objects and under different authorities, we see the results in delay, inefficiency and death. A weekly published return, such as Registrar-General's Office of disease, might have saved our army. It did the Sardinian. The Commissariat [illeg] hardly, in face of such, have gone on supplying as with salt meat and biscuits. But, to effect this, and secure us the benefits of publicity, essential that those who make the returns should not be those whose interest it is to conceal them. Registrar-General showed me a correspondence between himself and War Department on February 1855, in which he had urged civil registration of soldiers' deaths and been refused. They already have it in France where nearly useless, because [the] French do on purpose what we do from stupidity. In January 1855, losing at the rate of 576 per 1000, corresponding week of January 1856 rate of 17 per 1000.

The more I think of these things, [the] more I feel both absolute necessity of ripping up our army system and impossibility (almost) of your gaining evidence to do so. Hall now preparing with Smith army statistics.[11]

Source: From a draft letter or copy to Lord Panmure, Wellcome (Claydon copy) Ms 8997/12

4 December 1856

Private. I have completed the report which you directed me to make, with the assistance of Dr Sutherland, upon the new "Victoria Hospital" at Southampton. But, as I know that you will not read it, I would come and *say* it to you at any place (except in the newspapers) that you might be pleased to direct. I beg to remain, dear Lord Panmure,

your faithful servant

Florence Nightingale

It appears that there is no time to be lost, if your lordship intends making any alteration in the said plans.

---

11 The last tables and charts in Andrew Smith's official report were by John Hall, on meteorological observations and diseases. See Andrew Smith, *Medical and Surgical History of the British Army which Served in Turkey and the Crimea* vol. 2.

Source: John Sutherland and Florence Nightingale, Confidential Report on the Plans of the Royal Victoria Hospital, Southampton, Add Mss 45825 ff132-35.

[ca. December 1856]

The site selected for the hospital possesses certain advantages for the treatment of chest affections, but it may fairly be doubted whether the relaxing local climate and the large extent of muddy beach exposed at low water close to the site be advantageous as regards other classes of disease.

The hospital is intended to consist of three flats of wards, one over the other. It would have been much better adapted for the successful treatment of the sick had these been two flats only.

As far as can be judged from the plans, the wards themselves are deficient in some important sanitary requirements. The larger wards, generally speaking, are deficient in window space and it does not appear that the direct sunlight will be admitted as plentifully as experience has shown to be necessary in hospitals.

One of the smaller wards appears to have one window only communicating with the external air, and there are others which appear to have no direct window light, but are lighted from the corridor.

The arrangement of the wards and corridors seems to be based on that of the General Hospital at Scutari, namely, two windows on one side of each of the larger wards, opening to the external air, and two windows and a door on the opposite side, opening into the corridor. Though the General Hospital at Scutari has been followed to this extent, there are some important particulars in which its arrangements are better than those of the Victoria Hospital, while the hospitals at Scutari cannot be considered as equal in their ward arrangements to other existing hospitals.

The introduction of the corridor is a decided improvement, if it be properly done. The fault of those in the Scutari hospitals is that they lead to the intermingling of the foul air of different parts of the building with the air of the wards, because, from the position of the latter, the only means of obtaining a thorough cross-ventilation is by admitting the air from the corridors into the wards.

To obtain the advantage of the corridor, without its disadvantages, each ward should have a row of windows on two opposite sides, independently of the side next the corridor, as is the case with the great hospital at Bordeaux and at the Hôpital de Lariboisière at Paris, which represent the latest improvements in hospital construction. It is a fact well known that medical and surgical treatment are by no means so successful when the sick are massed together under one roof, and it was to obviate this that the great improvement of breaking of large hospital buildings into smaller connected pavilions, as shown by these hospitals, was introduced.

The improvement is effected by projecting the ward straight out behind the corridor, so that each block of two wards, when the hospital consists of two flats, constitutes in reality a separate hospital, with a row of windows on each side, and independent ventilating arrangements. As each block of wards stands by itself, with a space intervening between it and the adjoining block, the corridor serves the purpose of connecting the blocks together. The corridor should not be a long passage with windows, but should consist of arched "loggie"[12] open from top to bottom, and the whole space should be filled with glass, the framework of which should be so constructed that it can be thrown open entirely in fine weather. Each corridor should have ventilating arrangements quite distinct and separate from those of the wards.

In one particular, the position of the water closets, as shown on the plans of the Victoria Hospital, is not so good as in the hospitals at Scutari. In the great Barrack Hospital, there the latrines are placed not only away from the wards, but outside the building altogether, while the plans of the Victoria Hospital represent them as being situated between the wards. There cannot be a moment's doubt as to the risk to health from the arrangement.

If each block of wards were built detached as in the Hôpital de Lariboisière, the proper position for the water closets and urinals would be in the free air at the end of the wards, opposite the entrance from the corridor. They should have a ventilation of their own, quite independent of that of the wards, and should be cut off by double doors, and by a ventilating lobby or passage, from the body of the ward.

No arrangement can be considered safe for the sick in which there is a possibility of any effluvia from them entering the wards. It is hardly necessary to state that water closets of the best construction should alone be permitted beneath the roof of a hospital.

The whole drainage of the hospital should be conveyed away in impervious glazed earthen pipes, well cemented, and if possible without passing under any part of the building used for the sick. The drains should be all trapped, and should be provided with the means of flushing. The outlet sewer should be carried sufficiently far into the

12 Loggie or loggia, a gallery or arcade with at least one side open to the air.

estuary to open under low water, and the main sewers should have free ventilating, opening at a distance from the hospital, to prevent the rise of the tide from forcing the sewer gases into the buildings. The baths and lavatories for each ward should be entirely separate from the water closets.

Whatever plan may have been adopted for ventilating the wards, it should be sufficient to keep the wards free of odour by day and by night. It might be useful to examine and inquire into the merits of two systems of ventilation which have been in use and on trial, one against the other, for a considerable time in the Hôpital de Lariboisière. Some useful hints could be obtained from the ventilation of this hospital.

The true principle of ventilating a hospital is to introduce a sufficient amount of fresh air at as many points as possible, and to withdraw foul air at as many points as possible. One or two openings in the floor with corresponding openings above in the ceiling will only allow air to pass, but without renewing the body of the air within the ward.

It would be found useful to place the steam engine in such a position that the steam might be used for washing and for heating the drying closet and the engine power would be of service for mangling and wringing.

The washhouses appear made for the size of the building.

The laundry and the dirty and clean linen stores should be placed near each other. All the buildings used for washing and laundry purposes should be very finely ventilated at the roof. It would be advisable to have clean linen stores on each flat of the hospital.

There should be a kitchen for extra diets on each flat, or even in each division of sick.

Accommodation for female attendants should be provided distinct and separate from that of the male attendants.

Source: Notes, Add Mss 45751 f15

[c1857]

This present report leaves altogether untouched the question of site [Netley]. We made certain objections regarding deficiency of light and means of ventilation, which appear to have been obviated as far as [the] nature of [the] plan previously adopted permitted. Great improvement to abolish smaller wards with borrowed light. Arrangement in end wards seems simplified, so that they have now better means of light and ventilation. In regard to corridor, its open space towards the external air has been very considerably increased, and no doubt advantageously. And the danger of the atmosphere of the different wards intermingling will be correspondingly diminished. But everything will depend on air in corridor being at all times in a state of purity equal to that of external air.

Although corridors improved to this important extent, I still retain opinion that a corridor should not extend along any side of [a] ward from which it obtains light and ventilation, and that if [a] corridor is to be introduced into hospital construction at all, it should be solely with view of connecting detached blocks of wards with a comparatively small number of sick in each, and not made to cover the whole surface of one side of a hospital block intended for from 400-500 sick.

Editor: Naval nursing became an issue again in 1857 when Nightingale was actively courted for her advice on naval hospitals by the director general of the Navy Medical Department, Sir John Liddell (1794-1868). It is not known if her earlier discussions with Sir John Richardson, a senior but retired naval official, who was never director general, played any role in this next development (see p 238 above). A mutual family friend with Liddell, H. Seymour Tremenheere (1804-93), wrote Nightingale on Liddell's behalf.[13] The letter is marked answered. The first item below simply reports the planned meeting. Nightingale next wrote to Sidney Herbert that Liddell was to take her down to Haslar "almost immediately."[14] There were complications about timing as she was also visiting other hospitals.

What precise proposal was made to Nightingale to advise on navy hospitals is not clear. Liddell evidently asked her to review the navy's Blue Books on hospital statistics. She subsequently told Sidney Herbert that the mortality was lower than she had expected, but that the data were almost as bad as the army's. That said, the navy took better care of its sailors than the army of its soldiers. In addition to its early pavilion hospitals, it was known to provide more nutritious food than the army. Notably, the navy figured out how to prevent scurvy long before the army did—scurvy appears frequently in the first year of the Crimean War.

---

13 Tremenheere letter 6 January 1857, Add Mss 45796 f127.

14 Letter 16 January 1857, Wiltshire County Record Office, Pembroke Collection 2057/F4/66.

Source: From a letter to Parthenope Nightingale, Wellcome (Claydon copy) Ms 8997/30

13 January 1857

I dine at Tremenheere's on Thursday to meet Sir John Liddell, who wishes to talk with me on introducing female nursing in the naval hospitals.

This is done by Sir John Liddell's own desire, who wishes of course to see me as quietly as possible, and I have not mentioned it even to Uncle Sam.[15] It may lead to much.

Source: From a letter to Sidney Herbert, Wiltshire County Record Office, Pembroke Collection 2057/F4/66

16 January 1857

Private. I think, as my professional foster mother (a curious position, by the way, for you to stand in towards me), it is my duty to inform you that the director general of the *Navy* Medical Department is making serious proposals to me, viz., to occupy the position of fulfilling the same duties in the *naval* hospitals at home which you assigned me in the war hospitals. Sir John Liddell is to take me down to Haslar almost immediately. I will confess to you that, if I accept, it will be mainly because I think it will shame the *army* hospitals into doing what they require so much more. I cannot forget my first love, nor marry another department again so soon.

I was shocked and scandalized by the Woolwich Artillery Hospital when I visited it with General Williams,[16] and longed to be "at it." Lord Palmerston even spoke of giving me (when I saw him) a permanent commission to visit and inspect the Woolwich and Aldershot hospitals. But I have heard nothing of it since.

I should consider it by no means breaking but entering into the spirit of the kind of engagement I am under to your Fund,[17] to include the naval and military female nursing in my work. But I will not enter into any engagement without consulting you. I will only ask you to mention this *to no one*, for two reasons: Sir J. Liddell is, for obvious causes, anxious to keep it all quiet till all is settled.

15 Samuel Smith (1794-1880), Nightingale's maternal uncle.

16 William Fenwick Williams (1800-83), later 1st baronet, commander at the siege of Kars, during the Crimean War.

17 The Nightingale Fund, for which Sidney Herbert had been a major advocate; he chaired the first meeting of its council, held at the War Office.

2. Mr Bracebridge and I are almost as wide apart in our courses as Sir J. McNeill and Colonel Tulloch.[18] He wishes me to liberate my soul, as he calls it, say as many disagreeable things, i.e., as I can, and then have nothing to do ever with government again. I, on the other hand, mean to stick to the army hospitals as long as I live, and do not see at all how I liberate my soul with regard to them by "speaking my mind" so that it would eject myself, even if that mind were a true one.

Please to be so good as to return me those notes of mine I troubled you with, as I have no copy. It does not signify about your reading them, as I could tell it you all in half an hour if you have "your commission."

Source: From a letter to Sir John Liddell, Harvard University, Countway Medical Library

17 January 1857

I find that the only days I have at liberty next week are Tuesday *or* Wednesday, on either of which days I could remain the night at any hotel near Haslar, returning to London the next day.

As I can hardly expect that, with your multifarious occupations, you should happen to have the same days at your command, I will ask you to give me one line of reply, when, in case of its being in the negative, we will try to make an appointment for the ensuing week.

Editor: Liddell took Nightingale on the Haslar inspection soon after the above letter. He made some kind of proposal to her, which is missing, on which Sidney Herbert commented in a subsequent letter.[19] In planning a second trip, for 25 March, this time to Chatham, Liddell sent Nightingale a charming letter about the arrangements:

> If nothing has occurred to prevent you undertaking the journey to Chatham tomorrow, I shall wait upon you at a quarter past nine, by which time I trust you will have made a more substantial breakfast than the dry biscuit and cold coffee which constituted that scanty

18 Charles Holte Bracebridge (1799-1872), family friend who, with his wife, accompanied Nightingale to the Crimean War; Sir John McNeill (1795-1883), head of the supply commission in the Crimean War and a major ally of Nightingale's; Alexander Murray Tulloch (1803-64), later Sir, member of the supply commission. Bracebridge and McNeill were members of the original Nightingale Fund Council.

19 Herbert letter 25 January 1857, Add Mss 43394 ff13-18.

> repast the last time I saw you at your frugal meal. It is surely not necessary, in this land of plenty, to limit yourself to the starved system that prevailed in the Crimea and to which you have been so long accustomed. . . . I would beg to remind you that you have a long and hard day's work before you tomorrow.[20]

An undated note, probably a little later, shows Nightingale examining navy statistics, the next item below.

A later letter of Nightingale's recalls that she made inquiries about the nursing at Haslar on her visit, to find out that the character of the nurses there was "notorious" (see p 408 below).

Source: From an undated note for Sidney Herbert, Wiltshire County Record Office, Pembroke Collection 2057/F4/67

[1857-58]

I applied to Sir J. Liddell to give me data for the period *after* 1843. He cannot, but will send approximate data, if he can. The result of my examination of his Blue Books up to 1843 is astounding. The mortality is even lower than we thought. For (*excluding* the unhealthy stations) while the highest mortality at a foreign station is 11 per 1000, that at the home station is under 7. Now a ship is more difficult to ventilate than a barrack. What can make the mortality of our Guards in home barracks nearly three times as much?

These are quite authentic and fair to use. At the same time, while abusing Tulloch for his unfairness in getting at his results, it would hardly be right not to say that these are almost as bad. Upon looking in Tulloch's Blue Book for what you pointed out to me, it is obvious that his way of calculation may tell anyway. For, unless the proportion is constant between the mean force of each period of two different populations, you may bring out a perfectly identical result (by adding the deaths and dividing by the number of periods) from data which tell exactly the other way, and vice versa.

Source: From a draft letter to Lord Panmure, Add Mss 43397 f11

8 April 1857

When last you were kind enough to afford me the opportunity of some conversation with you about army medical matters, you may perhaps remember that you allowed me the privilege of reporting to you

20 Liddell letter 24 March [1857], Claydon House bundle 295.

personally anything connected with existing military hospitals which I might see desirable to bring before your notice. You kindly said, apply to me whenever you like. I have seen the Chatham hospitals and, if you still continued to wish it, shall be ready to report some easy and possible improvements to you.

Editor: Panmure replied promptly that he would call on her on "Tuesday" the 14th, if it suited;[21] however, no correspondence from their meeting is available. The following rough note, undated, may have come from that meeting:

1. Southton [Southampton] Hospital: four requisites by laws of God refer back to us. John Bull and national gall.
2. Précis—official Instructions.
3. Woolwich Artillery. Medical School. Aldershot plans. Nurses' clothing. Portsmouth sanitary state.
4. Admiralty people at me.
5. Aldershot: three reading rooms (two South Camp, one North) for coffee and games.
6. Finnerty about to be referred to him.
7. Commission.

Lord Panmure always just.[22]

Source: From a letter to Sidney Herbert, Wiltshire County Record Office, Pembroke Collection 2057/F4/66

Good Friday [10 April 1857]

I have had your letter of the 31st [missing], and you have had by this time Sutherland's of the 1st, asking your orders about serving on the *new* Netley commission.

I think what you think is probably the best, viz., to let them have their wicked way and to fight the thing in the House of Commons and before the public. I have seen Galton, who allows (a wonderful admission for a R.E.), that Laffan knows nothing about sanitary construction.

---

21 Panmure letter 11 April 1857, Add Mss 43397 f12.
22 Note, Add Mss 45825 f141.

Source: From a letter to an unnamed recipient,[23] Add Mss 45796 ff177-78

Granton House
Edinburgh
10 April 1857

Sir John McNeill has persuaded me to stay in order not to hurry my business here. And he thinks you can do very well without me there. So do I, if you will but make a good stand-up fight? But in that I conceive I am the better soldier of the two, am not I? I think we were perfectly agreed as to the ventilation, corridors, window space, water closets.

N.B. There is an ingenious little steward at St Mary's, Paddington, who has fitted up the ventilation of his sinks and water closets there with great success. When we get so far as fittings, I should take his advice.

With regard to the female nursing, Lord Panmure distinctly said, at Balmoral, that there were to be female nurses, and directed me to see that there was accommodation for them. If Andrew Smith has persuaded him otherwise, I have received no intimation of it. I, therefore, propose that there shall be accommodation for twenty-four nurses and one female superintendent (twenty-five total), i.e., one woman to forty patients, supposing the patients to be 1000, all the nurses to be of the class of head nurses in the civil hospitals, since the assistant nurses will be *men* (of the Medical Staff Corps) in a military hospital.

For the performance of their duties, I propose that each nurse should have a little day room (with a fireplace) *adjoining* every cluster of forty patients, a clean linen store and small extra-diet kitchen to each flat in each wing. The sleeping accommodation for these twenty-five women may be on the upper storey, or on the other side the court. All should be together and away from the patients. About the fitting up of the sleeping rooms (if in stalls, *there must be a window to each*), there is perhaps no immediate necessity to decide. There should be a common room for the nurses and an office for the matron, the first *adjoining the sleeping rooms*, the second conveniently near the patients. (N.B. Lock-up cupboards in each of the nurses' day rooms. But you are not come to that yet.)

As I do not know how you have modified the corridor and what you call the "odd corners," I cannot say how these things are to be done, without seeing the plans. But I hope you will stand up to these principles—and you will work out the details better than I.

---

23 Sue M. Goldie, comp., in her *Calendar of the Letters of Florence Nightingale*, lists William Aitken as the recipient, but the content suggests Douglas Galton; neither was given the appointment referred to in the letter.

I should very much urge working the "lift" by hydraulic press rather than by engine, if the water lends itself to the plan without too much expense. The advantages of the former over the latter are so numerous.

I take for granted that the lavatory to *each* ward will not be neglected in the alterations, and that all the new improvements of steam power for laundry and washhouse (carried out at Haslar [Naval Hospital]) will be seen here. (There was no laundry on the plan.) N.B. Pray remember that the *shaft* ventilation at Guy's is a failure.

Are you aware that the medical officers of Middlesex Hospital sent in a remonstrance to Lord Panmure after ours, almost, I believe, of the same tenor?[24] Lord Panmure, with his usual candour, did not tell me of this which, I have no doubt, considerably strengthened our hands.

I suppose you know that Dr Alexander is arrived.[25] I saw him last week in London. I have reason to think that Lord Palmerston and Lord Panmure are preparing the House of Commons for your appointment as sanitary adjunct to Andrew Smith. But probably you know more than I do. . . .

I suppose Captain Laffan is on your committee. Who else?

Source: From a letter to Douglas Galton, Add Mss 45759 ff1-2

20 April 1857

I want to see one reform in the Chelsea Hospital[26] (which won't require a bill in Parliament and which I know that Mr Robert Lowe both could and would, and that no one else would carry out). I have waited till Mr Lowe's head was mended, which it was a disgrace to us to have broken at Kidderminster.[27] And I would ask you, as I am not

24 Memorial to Lord Panmure respecting the Royal Victoria Hospital at Netley, *Reports from Commissioners* (Session 3 December 1857-2 August 1858, Vol. XIX), 45-47; signed by Francis Hawkins and ten others.

25 Nightingale succeeded in getting Thomas Alexander (1812-60) returned from his posting in Canada, to be a member of the royal commission on the Crimean War. See the biographical sketch in *Wars and the War Office* (15:1039).

26 The Royal Hospital, Chelsea, for aged soldiers, known as the "Chelsea Pensioners," opened in 1692.

27 Robert Lowe (1811-92) was attacked by a mob at an election meeting, his skull fractured and his life saved only thanks to bystanders pulling him away unconscious and bleeding; *Times* 30 March 1857:12 and 31 March 1857:9. He was narrowly elected, but the result was subsequently declared to be void.

acquainted with him, to put me kindly into personal communication with him, either by letter, or if he would let me see him for one half hour, I could tell my whole story in that time.

It is by no means a terrific matter, but the governor and commandant of Chelsea Hospital are not men to move in it. If, however, you should see any objection to what I ask, pray do not hesitate to tell me so—for I can arrive at Mr Lowe in another way.

Source: From a copy of a letter to Sir John McNeill, Wellcome (Claydon copy) Ms 8997/42

11 May 1857

I have carefully looked over the plans which you did me the honour to show me—and the suggestions which I would beg to offer merely is as follow:

pivot the wards round, pillar the corridors, fill up the space with glass.

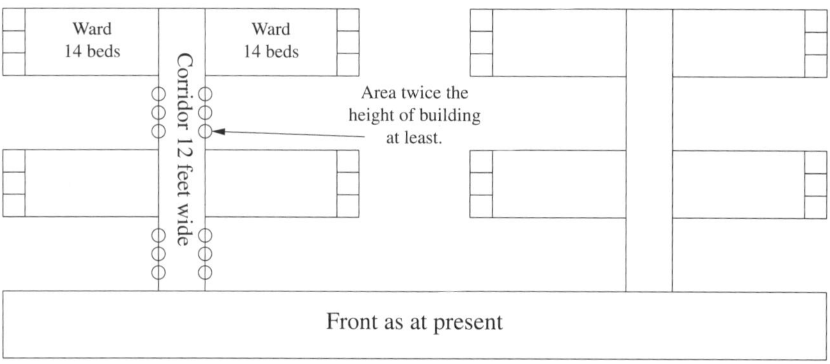

What is the exposure?

I have damaged my own cause by not drawing it to a scale which would give a greater distance between the wards.

As you were kind enough to consult me, I ought to explain what I said about Scutari, which is an historical instance of sufficient importance to furnish us with much absolute knowledge, no longer within the domain of hypothesis. It is true that the sanitary arrangements adopted brought the mortality down to 1.8 percent in the latter year of the war. But on what condition? That of not allowing above 1000 patients in a building, 700 ft square, 3 flats in height. Had this building been differently distributed as to its construction, it might easily have accommodated 3000 patients with good recovering conditions. It is ruinous to build after this fashion. The question is to find a construction which will accommodate the greatest number of patients upon a given area with the greatest facilities for recovery.

I do not hesitate to say that the causes of the great catastrophe of Scutari were want of ventilation, [want of] draining, cleanliness (too disgusting to detail farther), [want of] hospital comforts, frightful overcrowding.

However good the construction and ventilation of the corridors, if you fill them up with patients, it is the same as building two hospitals back to back. In all our experience, whether of healthy, or of sick men, such a construction generates disease. And our knowledge is now somewhat absolute on these points.

If it is objected that the condition of the men sent down from the Crimea and during the first winter was such that they could not have recovered under *any* circumstances, I answer that the Land Transport Corp sent us down men in exactly the same condition the second winter, and that under different circumstances they did recover, witness our ratio of mortality—1.8 percent. But again, it was at the expense of limiting a building upwards of 700 ft. square to an extravagantly small number of patients.

Our mortality from "diseases of stomach and bowels" was *at Scutari* 23.6 percent, *in Crimea* 18.3. Why this fatal increase? The condition of the building at Scutari is a sufficient answer. You will observe that we lost at Scutari nearly 25 percent more than we did in the Crimea from this cause alone. And the disease was chiefly generated within the building itself.

I would furnish the amplist details on this all-important subject to anyone interested in it officially as I have already done to H.M.

Source: From a copy of a letter to R.G. Whitfield,[28] Boston University 2/1/3

12 June 1857

I am truly obliged for your most kind offer to help us, which I am going to snatch.

Neither civil physicians nor surgeons, still less military ones, are, generally speaking, at all conversant with sanitary things, and I assure you that you yourself, with two or three other men whom I could name, who have had large sanitary experience in London, are the only per-

28 Richard Gullett Whitfield (d. 1877), resident medical officer at St Thomas', 1858-72.

sons who have at all apprehended the real cause of our disaster in the East. Of course I say this in private, as I have never animadverted on my masters, whatever may have been said as to my doing so.

I will tell you exactly what has been done about the Netley Hospital. And I should extremely like to hear some portion of the large experience which you have been accumulating. If you could come to me on Wednesday evening at 8 o'clock and have a cup of tea, or if you do not like to leave your charge at that hour, if you could come to me on Thursday at 4, or on Friday at 1, I shall feel myself very much indebted to you.

Both you and I are so driven with business that I will ask you to write one line to say "when."

Source: From a letter to Lord Panmure, National Archives of Scotland GD45/8/337/9

1 July 1857

Private. I have seen the revised plans for Netley Hospital, which have undergone very great improvements, viz., the throwing open the corridor, (2) the giving more window space in the wards, (3) the abolition of borrowed lights and odd corners, (4) the ventilation and separation of the appurtenances, (5) the abandoning of the idea of artificial ventilation and trusting to air shafts, doors and windows, and giving the fire air to itself.

Captain Laffan has done the very best that could be done with the impossible problem given him to solve. Now the best plans I have ever seen for a field hospital were those made by Mr Brunel[29] for the *Renkioi* Hospital, sent out by you to the East, in huts. The principle applies equally to permanent hospitals. Should Lord Panmure wish for another opinion before he finally decides on the revised plans for Netley Hospital, Mr Brunel's opinion would be the very best, probably, to be had—his hospital having been tried and succeeded. I would only suggest, should the above idea be at all taken into consideration, that before a consultation be held over the patient (viz., the hospital) Mr Brunel should see the revised plans first, without any other engineer—consultations are always fatal.

Editor: Panmure's cordial reply to the above letter is dated 6 July 1857.[30]

---

29 Isambard Kingdom Brunel (1806-59), designer of the prefabricated hut hospital at Renkioi, in the Crimean War.

30 National Archives of Scotland GD45/9/337.

Source: From a letter to an unnamed recipient, Columbia University, Presbyterian Hospital School of Nursing C36

Bury House [Malvern]
3 September 1857

I have not yet been allowed to leave my room, from illness. At the same time, I am so deeply interested in the fate of Netley Hospital that, should you be about to stay some few days longer, I should be glad, if you could propose the latest day you can, to see you on this subject as you suggest. I believe that we shall find that our opinions entirely agree in this matter, although mine are only practical and yours are scientific.

I enclose a copy of some evidence lately given by me before a commission, and have placed a paper where it touches the point of *hospital construction.* I should be glad, if you have time, that you should glance over it, and will ask you to return it to me, and to consider it "confidential" till the Blue Book comes out.

Source: From a letter to Sidney Herbert, Wellcome Ms 5482/22

9 November 1857

Herewith comes the first draft of Regulations for type, including

1. General Duties of Medical Officers;
2. Regulations as to General and Regimental Hospitals.

We shall require several proofs of this before we are satisfied with it ourselves. For it is an affair of memory and comparison. And therefore I would not, if I were you, trouble myself more than to glance over it, and certainly make no further use of it before we have looked over it several times. For it is a matter of no little time to put consistency, logical arrangement and so on into these Regulations. (The Amended Health Act took two years' preparation.)

The General Hospital Regulations, herein specified, are at present only transcripts of my little report, and will require much careful sifting on our parts. The sooner I can have a proof of all this the better for me. . . . You shall have the rest tomorrow.

Source: From two letters to Harry Verney, Wellcome (Claydon copy) Ms 8997/49 and 51

26 November 1857

I return the letter from Lord Palmerston, which was sent by my people to me, with, as I understood, your desire for any suggestion. I can only make the same as I sent down, viva voce [out loud] by my aunt the day you were good enough to call here.

The principal objection stated by Lord Palmerston against the plan of the Lariboisière Hospital is the distance between the blocks. But this is a mere matter of *detail*. The difference in *principle* between the Lariboisière and Netley is a final one. The former represents the sanitary science of the present age—the latter the sanitary neglects of a century back.

Netley, as amended, is very greatly improved. But could we not adopt what is known to be best, rather than improve what is known to be bad?

The French are the only hospital builders of the present day. We must copy them if we desire hospitals to be places of recovery. As a British hospital, Netley is not bad. As a French hospital, it would be detestable. And, anyhow, it is no fit monument of the Crimean War of the queen's reign, or of Lord Palmerston himself, who deserves more of us than either.

Dr Sutherland re-echoes every word of this.

2 December 1857

With regard to Netley Hospital and Mr Tite,[31] the latter sent me his letter to Lord Palmerston, before it was sent. The chief point of it was to urge a reference of Netley to London architects. And in proof of the desirableness of this, Mr Tite sent me a plan of the new part of King's College Hospital by his friend, a London architect,[32] which is twice as undesirable as Netley. Netley, as improved, is better than *any* London hospital. And, if they will not give us the Lariboisière principle, they had much better let it alone. The defect in the Lariboisière details, which Lord Palmerston mentions, we deplore the most. The principle we stick to.

I do not apologize for writing in this dogmatic manner, because these sanitary principles are neither my discovery nor my invention. They are recognized by all the advanced sanitary reformers of Europe, of whom Mr Tite is not one, nor any London architect that I know of. If we put sick in Netley corridors, it would then be as bad as the King's College Hospital, which he, I believe, advocates. . . .

Dr Sutherland quite leads the forlorn hope of the sanitary reformers and is a safe counsel in everything of this kind, which I have only learnt from a dreadful experience.

---

31 William Tite (1798-1873), later Sir, a leading London architect, MP and later a governor at St Thomas'.

32 Thomas Bellamy (1798-1876); for Nightingale's objections to his plans see p 112 above.

Editor: After the Crimean War, Nightingale strongly encouraged her most able matron, Jane Shaw Stewart (c1821-1905),[33] to gain the needed experience to become an effective hospital matron. In 1858, she organized introductions for Shaw Stewart to European hospitals, both civil and military. For this she sought the help of her old friend, Henry Manning (1808-92), a Catholic convert and later cardinal, to gain access to the hospitals nursed by Roman Catholic orders.[34] She wrote the (last) commander of the French Army in the Crimean War, Marshal Pélissier (1794-1864), for help with entry to military hospitals. Both came through and Shaw Stewart spent months in those hospitals. Later, when Nightingale sent Marshal Pélissier copies of her confidential report on the Crimean War, she described Shaw Stewart as having had four months in "his" hospitals, receiving instruction and information, and thanked him for his "intervention."[35] Shaw Stewart sent Nightingale letters with her observations from the various hospitals.[36] Serious problems with Shaw Stewart's management at Netley, however, soon emerged, which are related largely in *Wars and the War Office.*

Source: From a letter to T. Graham Balfour,[37] Add Mss 50134 ff33-34

Gt. Malvern
14 January 1858

Thank you very much for your letter of this morning. Could you send me the dietary of your boys? I have the one (but in London) you were once good enough to give me. But I was asked yesterday to recommend one. And, thinking yours the best, I promised to ask you for it at once. If it will take you any time to look it up, pray put it off till you are less busy. . . .

I mean the dietary of your *well* boys, as well as of your sick ones. I am going to write to Greenwich for theirs. But I think it was inferior

33 See the biographical sketch in *Wars and the War Office* (15:1037-38). Shaw Stewart had had no hospital experience pre-Crimea.

34 Letter to Manning, in *Theology* (3:269).

35 Draft letter in French ca. July-August 1859, Add Mss 45797 f56.

36 See Shaw Stewart to Nightingale 6 January 1858, Florence Nightingale Museum (LMA) H1/ST/NC2/V1/58.

37 Thomas Graham Balfour (1813-91), surgeon general, secretary of the Royal Commission on the Sanitary State of the Army, and head of the statistical branch of the Army Medical Department.

to yours. If you recommend the one at the Caledonian Asylum,[38] could you let me have it at your leisure?

Source: From four letters to Sidney Herbert, Wiltshire County Record Office, Pembroke Collection 2057/F4/67, and draft/copy, Add Mss 43394 ff260-61, the first three from Great Malvern

20 January 1858

I sent you this morning, "as directed," a rough estimate of the comparative cost of attendance on wards of thirty, twenty-five and nine patients respectively. But, for fear it should be made use of "to our disadvantage," I pray you to listen to what I now want to say (*not* "as directed") upon the different alterations of Netley in your letter.

Any alterations you may see fit to advise with regard to the wards at Netley must, in the first place, provide for the *direct* lighting and ventilation of *every part* of every ward. This is not the case. No throwing of wards together, no causing parts of wards to project behind, will compensate for the evil produced by ill-lighted and ill-ventilated *other parts* left in doing so.

The chief ward improvement made by the first commission, on the old plan, consisted in clearing out all corners. And in attempting to improve the new plan, the old defects must not be restored. Again, the back buildings are much too close to admit of any projecting wards or parts of wards being thrown out behind. You would have two wells or "culs de sacs," with stagnant atmosphere, on each side the corridor leading to the back buildings.

If you throw out wards behind, you would require to pull down all the kitchen and dining room buildings and remove them to a greater distance. If left, they would hinder ventilation and light. Also, in such a plan, every ward projected out behind would interfere materially with the lighting and ventilation of the whole building.

The projections in the old original plan of the chapel and dining rooms across the line of lighting were bad, and every ward projected would make it worse—unless indeed the distance between each projection were at least 101 feet, as at Aldershot, which is impossible at Netley.

If, Plan 2, the adjoining wards are thrown together so as to produce long wards, with beds along the back and front, then the ward windows into the corridors would have to be altered from the present

38 The Royal Caledonian Asylum School for Educating and Maintaining Children of Scotch Parentage.

plan (in which these windows are in reality glass doors) so as to leave a sufficient wall space between each two windows for two beds.

The plan of joining two wards by *excavating* a dark passage through the orderlies' room would not do. These seem to me the principles to be kept in view in making the alterations. To some of them I should say directly, if I were you, *I won't have it.* Of others, I should like to see the plans, as you have kindly proposed, VERY much.

The cost of attendance must also be considered. I see no alteration of plan which will not involve sacrifice of bed space, and the hospital will not accommodate the number its vast size ought to do—this will be another source of outlay.

23 January 1858

1. The glass in Netley corridors is intended *to open* double—not to be removed at all. (It would be impossible to remove it.) Such, at least, was the last plan I saw sanctioned by the committee upon it.

2. It is better that there should *not* be an architectural correspondence between the arches of the corridors and the doors of the wards, for sanitary purposes. The piers are so thin that neither light not ventilation are impeded.

3. The hospital would not now be *unhealthy*. At least, it would be more healthy than any London hospital. But it is quite behind the day. It is most expensive for administration. It is not at all what the great military hospital of the British Empire should be. It would make a model barrack for 2000 men.

4. To propose a GOOD hospital plan will be the keynote to your report—giving *plans, details, estimates.* This would, in itself, condemn Netley and prove your case. Otherwise, the government would find fifty architects to swear that Netley is the best hospital they ever saw, which is true now.

5. The site cannot be other than unhealthy.

6. In regard to the principles to be kept in view in alterations, you cannot afford to sacrifice any of those which we have laid down together. I send you a plan for the illumination of your commission, provided they will not sacrifice the site:

(1) Propose to provide for 800 sick. You will never have more. (2) Keep your foundations. (3) Have your corridor one storey, with open terrace above. (4) Throw out four pavilions, 100 feet apart, behind the corridor on each side, the pavilions to contain three wards in tiers 101 ft. long, 25 ft. wide, 16½ ft. high. (5) Remove the kitchens altogether from the centres of the square and place them behind. The dining rooms will be on the ground floor between the pavilions (or

they may be made room for in the front of each pavilion *middle* floor). Part of the foundations will come in for this. The rest must be laid.

31 January 1858

I do not see that you could say less—or more—than what you propose about Netley—for it is the exact truth.

I cannot help hoping that they will adopt your barrack suggestion for it. Sir Harry Verney's fear of large hospital wards, because the French have small prison wards, reminds me of the argument used by the first Netley projectors against light (in hospitals), *because* Colonel Jebb[39] found small windows good for solitary prisoners!!

I had heard that Panmure is very mad about Netley. It does not much signify, I suppose. If God *would* make sanitary laws, we are not responsible for them. We are not the inventors or even the discoverers of them.

But I really have nothing to trouble you with, except that I am very sorry you still have neuralgia, and glad you are going to Paris, and not by night.

9 February 1858

I really trust you *are* better, as I saw your name in the House last night. That is the first thing.

I dare say you have seen all your Paris commissioners.[40] They seem to have come back strengthened in the "*pavilion*" view of the hospital question, thinking that no further alteration can be made in Netley, and that all that can be done is to recommend it as a barrack.

I am come back, as you see. I did not write to you because I was afraid you would say, "Don't, we don't want you," when it would have been sheer impertinence in me to have come.

I think it is curious, in the *Times* article of this morning, to see A. Smith coming out in the character of a *complainant* and a reformer about the barrack and hospital question. And I wish it would not attack Prince Albert and the duke of Cambridge,[41] which sets them

39 Jebb's Pentonville Prison, where prisoners were held in solitary cells, had small windows to the outside.

40 Drs Sutherland and Burrell and engineer Douglas Galton were appointed to review the Netley plans; they visited French pavilion hospitals early in 1858.

41 George, duke of Cambridge (1819-1904), cousin of Queen Victoria, commander-in-chief of the British Army.

against us, men who both are certainly far more progressive than A. Smith. . . .

I hope your Netley report will give, once for all, all that is known of sanitary principle regarding hospital engineering. We are sadly behind the rest of the world.

Sir H. Verney came to Malvern to see me about it. He is ignorant but *agog.*

Source: From a letter to T. Graham Balfour, Add Mss 50134 ff35-36

Gt. Malvern
5 February 1858

I have not been able to thank you yet for your *great work,*[42] which I received on the 2nd. I admire him very much—I think he looks very handsome. And I cannot help congratulating you on the successful conclusion of this part of your labours.

I cannot find that the *Times* has noticed it yet. I rather think that there are so many things now to engage people's attention that the effect may be slower but not less sure than we wish.

The only misprint that I can find is at p xiii, Report: it says, "Appendix *P.*"[43] I was very much obliged for your kindness in sending me so early a copy. Lady Tulloch says I make my pillow of Blue Books. It certainly has been the case with this.

Also, many thanks for your dietaries. You shall have all the others back. Yours is much the best. I found it afterwards in your own evidence.

I shall be in town very soon, when I shall hope to see you. . . .

I was quite satisfied with Mr Herbert's answer to Dr Smith.

Source: Note on a letter of William Farr, Add Mss 43394 f296

[after 14 February 1858]

I should lay down broadly:

1. Diffusion necessary for good ventilation;

2. With opposite windows, ward twice the size has better ventilation than ward half the size, *within certain limits*;

3. With the Netley construction, wards half the size undoubtedly have a better *chance* than wards double the size. I would not put size of wards upon facility of administration. I don't mind having to fight it.

---

42 The "great work" was the royal commission report, for which Balfour was secretary.

43 The misprint refers to the royal commission report, where Farr's diagrams, in the Appendix, are given Roman numerals.

Source: From a letter to R.G. Whitfield, Florence Nightingale Museum (LMA) H1/ST/NC1/58/1

23 February 1858

Your kindness encourages me to ask you what offices you think a ward in a military hospital, after the pattern of Lariboisière, should have. I believe three superimposed wards of twenty-four sick each have been decided on for each pavilion. At the further end of the ward:

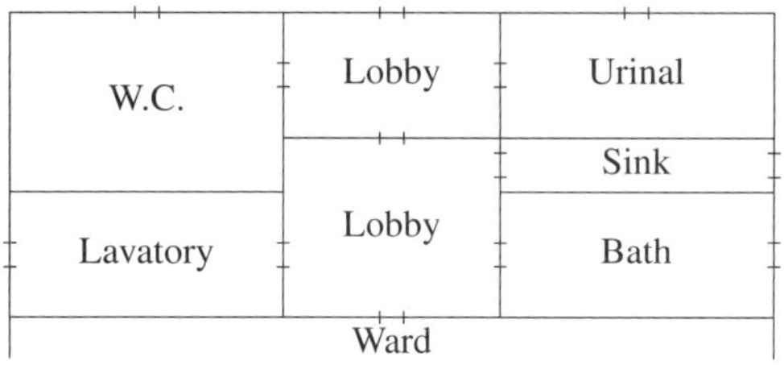

Do you think this a bad place for the sink in a man's ward, where the head nurse is the only woman?

At the near end of the ward.

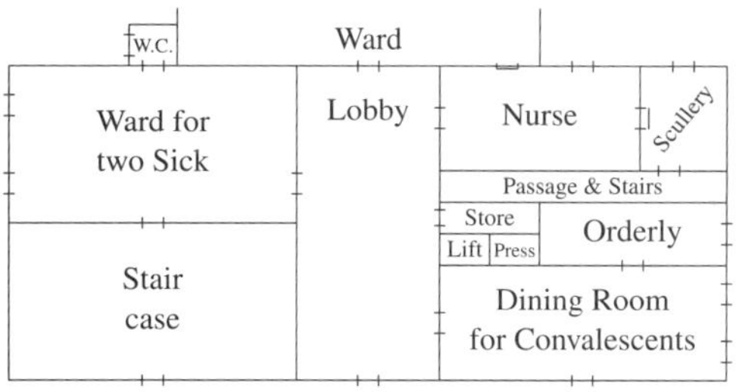

This is not drawn to a scale, and it is rather about the disposition than the size of the offices that I want to consult you. (I suppose all cooking, whether for sick, nurse or orderly, to be done *out of* the pavilion.)

1. The scullery is for warming food and for poultices, etc., for sick. Do you think it in an inconvenient place? Or do you consider it better that all these things should be done in the ward?

2. The store is merely for the pots and pans. I suppose it is better for all dressings, stimulants for the day, etc., to be kept in the ward.

3. Do you think it better to compel the orderly to be in the ward, or to let him have a day room? (Our allowance is one orderly to ten patients. But this is often exceeded.)

4. I suppose it is not desirable to have the scullery and storeroom *through* the nurse's room, as the orderlies must help her in these. (These trifling arrangements will make a very large item in the success or fail-

ure of a new plan. And, therefore, I make no apology for soliciting your kind assistance.)

5. On the ground floor, instead of the ward for two sick, will be the wardmaster's day room and the medical officer-on-duty's day room.

Since I wrote this, I have received your kind packet, and glanced over your notes, which will be very useful. I do not know how to thank you for your magnificent offer of visiting Vincennes for us. But it is one I feel too much scruple in accepting. We had just sent over a government commission, consisting of Dr Sutherland, Dr Burrell and Captain Galton, R.E., and though they have not brought back all the information I wanted, and if I were able to move I would go myself, yet I have no excuse to ask you.

Editor: Sidney Herbert wrote Nightingale on 20 March 1858 with "the final plans for Netley." She responded on the 29th that: "General Peel[44] has referred your Netley report back to the 'second Netley commission,' which means, I suppose, Laffan, Mapleton and Co. Perhaps this was unavoidable. Perhaps you knew it. Anyhow this requires no answer." A further letter he wrote her on 1 April 1858 again opposed the plans.[45]

Source: From a letter to Douglas Galton, Add Mss 45759 ff3-4

10 April 1858

Dr Sutherland desired I would further the kitchen plan for the Wellington Barracks, for which, it appears, you are waiting. So I sent up to Soyer, who is ill, for it, found it was done, sent it (with the necessary direction) to Smith and Phillips in Skinner St. and expect it back today at Soyer's. Soyer wishes it to be looked at *here* first, by you and Dr Sutherland and Captain Grant, and appoints Monday.

I do not know his reason for not going at once to the place where it is to be put up. But I think, if you could fix any hour between 1 and 4 on Monday to come here, it would be as well to do as he wishes. I see

44 Jonathan Peel (1799-1879), MP, twice secretary war; although he was a Conservative he supported inquiries into abuses and generally was supportive of Nightingale's concerns.

45 Herbert letters 20 March and 1 April 1858, Add Mss 43395 ff20 and 39; Nightingale letter 29 March 1858, Wiltshire County Record Office, Pembroke Collection 2057/F4/67.

no occasion to trouble Captain Grant[46] to come, to whom you will give the necessary information. But *you* will judge. Soyer gives up about the men dining in the kitchen and admits that it is undesirable.

Source: From a letter to Harry Verney, Wellcome (Claydon copy) Ms 8997/64

13 April 1858

I see your motion for tonight about the Netley report.

Perhaps you are not aware that Mr Herbert is not and will not be in town till Thursday, and that General Peel has referred the report in question back to an old and adverse commission. For both these reasons, I would ask you not to press your motion till Mr Herbert comes back, as I think the effect of it now might be that General Peel would make a statement in the House, which there would be no means of answering.[47]

Source: From a letter to Thomas Alexander, Columbia University, Presbyterian Hospital School of Nursing C38

23 April 1858

We enclose your proposed diet tables, with Dr Christison's letter,[48] which we shall be glad, if you will return, as soon as you have done with it.

We should be glad if you would kindly consider the whole subject over again, and write out the scheme of nine diets in full, stating in each case what the patient is to have for breakfast, dinner, tea or supper—in short, completing the scheme of diets and preparing it for the press. Also, adding at the end such general instructions as you may think requisite for the system of dieting in field hospitals.

If you think it impracticable to draw up a scheme of preserved provisions for the purpose, will you look at Soyer's diets for the Crimean hospitals and consider whether they would be generally applicable for field purposes, with or without alteration? And, if so, whether it would be advisable to introduce them by way of information or of regulation?

Will you be kind enough to return the whole manuscript here as soon as you can?

---

46 Captain John Grant, who re-organized cooking at Aldershot.

47 Verney presumably withdrew it, for it does not appear in Hansard, *Parliamentary Debates.*

48 Robert Christison (1797-1882), expert on nutrition; letter 20 April 1858, Add Mss 43395 f45.

Source: From a letter to Douglas Galton, Add Mss 45759 f5

30 April 1858

That Soyer came after you were gone, and will come again today at 2 for the chance of seeing you. We (i.e., Soyer and I) think, however, that a repetition of the proposed scheme for Wellington kitchen will do for Chatham, if the former succeeds, and that the drawing for a kitchen which you brought of --? will neither be economical nor efficient in its cookery.

Source: From a letter to T. Graham Balfour, Add Mss 50134 ff44-46

18 May 1858

I shall be delighted to see you at any hour tomorrow if you will kindly fix the time by a verbal message, through the bearer.

I do not think that Dr Farr has asked for anything in his report or in his forms but what you have yourselves recommended in your great report and what you and Colonel Storks have paved the way for in your admirable labours of the last twenty years. It is for the Army Medical Department now to carry out those labours systematically itself.

About the practical ways of doing this, you are, of course, a better judge than any of us. About the principles we shall, I am sure, not differ.

I am too unwell to discuss anything. But I shall be particularly anxious to hear from you all your objections and propositions.

With regard to the sentiment I do entirely agree with you that I wrote to Mr Herbert that it must *come out* particularly three pages near the end. And so it shall. And he agrees. . . .

What has Dr Smith done with his great Blue Book? He has been a long while writing it. He must be learning to write.

Source: From a letter to Harry Verney, Wellcome (Claydon copy) Ms 8997/70

9 July 1858

I send you a privately printed document, drawn up in anticipation and in answer of one (in favour of Netley) to be presented to the House of Commons tonight—in anticipation too of your kind assistance, whenever you leave home again. . . .

The enclosed is to be presented to General Peel, who will not be able to understand one word of it. Perhaps you will help him when you see him again.

Source: From a letter to Edwin Chadwick, Add Mss 45770 ff20-23

14 July 1858

We have just had one of those checks which people who are fifty years behind the age are so fond of inflicting upon the poor workers, who are fifty years before the age, viz., a verdict given in favour of Netley Hospital, of which you must have heard. The answer to it, a privately printed paper presented to General Peel, but not yet to the House of Commons, I venture to enclose and to ask you to read and to assist us to make known.[49]

We are going to try to do something in the House of Commons and in the newspapers about it still.

Source: From a letter to Lord Stanley,[50] Liverpool Record Office 920 Der 146/3

4 August 1858

The Netley inquiry, of which you may have heard, shows this. It is alarming—not because we have lost a good army model hospital by it—though that is a great loss—but because it shows what an amount of error in opinion and information is always at the command of government.

Nightingale's Articles on Netley

Editor: Nightingale biographer E.T. Cook described Nightingale as organizing "a vigorous press campaign" against Netley in July and August 1858, based on the large collection of newspaper clippings he found in her papers. He listed two items as clearly hers and four others as "probably hers," but some likely by friends.[51] My assessment is slightly different from his. I do not think the 24 July article in *The Builder* is her writing, and so omit it, but consider *The Lancet* articles of 31 July and 14 August to be hers. Each article refers to the other such that both or neither must be hers (the articles immediately below). The writing style is somewhat less lively than usual in the 14 August article, but the content is very much hers, including remarks on nursing that

49 Chadwick obliged by denouncing the Netley site in an article, for being on the "banks of a large tidal river, offensive mud at low water and mushy ground on both sides," in "Our Army in India," *North British Review* 29 (August-November 1858):242.

50 Edward Geoffrey Smith Stanley (1826-93), later 15th earl of Derby.

51 Edward T. Cook, *The Life of Florence Nightingale* 2:438.

architects did not normally make. The articles in the *Leeds Mercury* and the *Saturday Review*, of 21 and 28 August, respectively, are very obviously hers in style (following *The Lancet* articles). No article or letter in the *Times* could be found for this period, although Cook has one on his list and there are references to a *Times* letter in correspondence with her sister.

Her three articles in *The Builder*, in August and September 1858, follow, with further introductory remarks. Neither Cook nor I had any doubts about them, not the least for her own references to them in correspondence. A wry comment to her sister states:

> Two things I never expected to come to, to drink ether and write in the newspapers. I am come out upon Netley in *Examiner, Daily News, Lancet, Builder* and shall be in *Times* and *Saturday Review.* I shall then write an article upon the beautiful unanimity and *common* sense of the British press.[52]

Still, a recent commentator claimed that the three articles in *The Builder* "previously attributed" to Nightingale were, in fact, by Manchester doctor John Roberton.[53] The articles were published without attribution, the normal practice at that journal at the time. However, Nightingale not only called these articles her own in correspondence, but reprinted them with her name on them in the 1859 edition of *Notes on Hospitals*. Consequently, if this author were right about Roberton's authorship, she would be twice guilty of plagiarism. The 1859 edition, moreover, thanks the editor of *The Builder* for permission to reprint, which would make him complicit in a publishing fraud. That *Notes on Hospitals* was influenced by Roberton Nightingale herself acknowledged, and he in turn wrote favourably about her own work.

---

52 Letter to Parthenope Verney 14 August 1858, Wellcome (Claydon copy) Ms 8997/72.

53 A.D. King, "Hospital Planning: Revised Thoughts on the Origin of the Pavilion Principle in England," *Medical History* 10 (1966):361. Not only was King wrong on these three articles, but Nightingale published one further, short comment, "Preventible Disease," in November 1858 (see p 514 below), and three on the site for St Thomas'. For more on Nightingale's consultations on the articles see p 780 below.

Source: Two anonymous articles in *The Lancet* 31 July 1858:121-22 and 14 August 1858:175-77

On the 28th of December last, some time after the Report of the Royal Commission on the Sanitary State of the Army was sent in, the minister at war requested the "Barrack and Hospital Improvement Commission" to report upon the Royal Victoria Hospital. The commission had in their report pointed out the defects in the present system of construction, administration and attendance in army hospitals. It had shown the necessity for the public service of introducing into those institutions an efficient and economical method of administration and attendance upon the sick, and it had pointed out the defects of the present army hospitals, and the necessity for avoiding these in all future structures.

Assuming that the intention of the minister was to ascertain how far the plans, etc., of the Victoria Hospital, if carried out, would realize the objects aimed at in the report already sent in, the commission of course proceeded to deal with the whole question from such a point of view. Having done so, they arrived at the conclusion that, for such purposes, the hospital was generally unadapted from its construction, and that even if it were used, the cost of the administration would be so great that it would be cheaper to abandon it altogether, or rather to turn it into a barrack. The main circumstances leading the "commission" to this unfavourable judgment appear to us to be well substantiated as facts, and the reasoning founded upon them as fully warranting the adverse opinions expressed in the report.

The commission do not deny the apparent salubrity of the Netley district for healthy men pursuing ordinary avocations, but they maintain that it is not well adapted for the recovery of sick men confined to their beds—a distinction which, although it has been called in question, decidedly holds good. The commission assert that, as regards the district itself, there are ten square miles of mud exposed in the estuary twice in twenty-four hours, and that opposite the site of the new hospital there are seven eights of a mile of mud exposed at low water. In the next place the proposed hospital is to be built upon earth from which bricks are or were being made, a sufficient proof of the defective character of a sub-soil for such an institution. Farther, it is shown that, although on a clear bright day the country for miles around the site of the hospital is dry and self-draining, the *immediate site itself* is not so, and the inspection of the building had to be carried on by crossing upon planks over the mud and water lying upon the surface.

The commission place much stress upon the soft and relaxing, instead of dry and bracing, character of the local climate of Southampton. This they rightly affirm not to be the climate which should be desired, as it will retard or prevent the recovery of the particular class of invalids intended to occupy the Victoria Hospital. In fine, the following data being give to the commission, the rectitude of its judgment appears to us unimpeachable.

Site: Close to an estuary, with ten square miles of mud exposed at low water. Mud, containing vegetable matter and sulphurs, and saturated with mixed fresh and salt water.

Climate: Soft, mild, relaxing. Brick earth on the site of the hospital.

Conclusion: The shores of Southampton Water are not a desirable spot on which to erect a hospital for the majority of such cases as will be sent there for treatment.

In coming to a judgment upon this important matter, it is most essential to keep in mind the class of patients who would constantly inhabit Netley. They would, of course, be composed chiefly of invalids form the tropics, men suffering from chronic diseases of the digestive organs, the sequelae of fevers, etc., diseases, indeed, belonging to the same category as those described by good authority as common to the hospital locality itself. Mr Ranald Martin[54] has shown that all kinds of tropic invalids, whether suffering from fevers or from bowel complaints, thrive best in the *bracing* localities of the United Kingdom. They recover most rapidly in the highlands of Scotland during a summer and autumn residence, apparently from a union there of the ocean and mountain air—a union which appears to be especially advantageous to sick persons from the topics. However advantageous, then, the humid and warm climate of Southampton Water may be for certain pulmonary affections, for delicate persons and women and children who dread a little freshness and cold, we agree with the commission in viewing it as quite unsuitable for the recovery of persons suffering under the sequelae of tropical affections.

The unfavourable conclusions arrived at by the "commission" have been reviewed and answered in a "Report of the Committee of the Royal Victoria Hospital." In this antagonistic reply, however, it appears to us that the "committee" has not dealt with the report fairly. On the contrary, it has simply accumulated as large an amount as possible of

54 J. Ranald Martin (1793-1874), later Sir, member of the royal commission.

professional opinion against *certain only* of the points the commission raised, leaving the others untouched, and then considering the *whole report* as fully and satisfactorily answered.

We shall return to the consideration of this subject.

So far as relates to the expression of our opinion concerning the unfitness of the climate and locality of the Netley Hospital for invalids suffering under the *sequelae* of tropical diseases, we might rest satisfied with what we have already said. But there are two other important points in respect to the new hospital, and the counter statements of the committee which we cannot pass over, and are hence obliged to recur to this subject. In the first place, we must observe that there are certain opinions introduced into the report which tend to discredit the latest improvements in hospital architecture, and which, if they remain unanswered, might be productive of serious consequences in the future. What is called the "pavilion" or "block system" was rightly adopted as the best form of hospital by the royal commission, after ample inquiry into the matter. According to this system, the patients are separated into a number of detached groups, with the air freely circulating around them. Hence one of its chief advantages is its facility for subdividing the sick and for ventilating by *opposite windows.*

Even in the larger metropolitan hospitals (as in Guy's, e.g.), this latter advantage of the older wards can be at once compared with the difficulty of ventilating the new back-to-back wards, with windows on one side only, even with the aid of what is termed "artificial ventilation." The result of many years' experience is that the best observers have been gradually led to adopt the block principle as that which is most conducive to the recovery of the sick. The late and the present director general of the Army Medical Department (as members of the royal commission[55]) have both very wisely affirmed this principle in the Parliamentary Paper No. 361 (11 May 1858). The "block" form of construction for the new hospital at Aldershot, and the main sanitary reasons for employing it, are alluded to in the following terms:

> The board approved unanimously of the general principle to be adopted in the construction of the future building, which consisting of a series of detached structures (each a separate hospital, connected by an open corridor running along the ground storey), will

55 Andrew Smith and Thomas Alexander.

effectually prevent anything like an undue accumulation of the miasms unavoidably generated, more or less, in all hospitals, but more particularly where large numbers of sick are congregated under the same roof.[56]

The new hospital at Aldershot was then proposed to be built on this "pavilion plan," with even as few as 100 patients under one roof. The system, indeed, admits of much variety and accommodation, according to circumstances of extent and means of expenditure, as may be seen by comparing the Melville Hospital at Chatham, the Royal Marine Hospital at Woolwich, the plans of the proposed new civil hospital at Blackburn and the hospitals of Lariboisière and Vincennes at Paris. Thus not only the highest army and navy medical authorities and the "royal commission" agree as to the best constructive arrangements for a hospital, but the most eminent civil practitioners go hand in hand with them.

Now, the plan of the Netley Hospital, differing from the "block system," the "commission"[57] affirmed that such hospital was not the kind of structure best adapted for the speedy recovery of the sick and for facility and economy of administration. Its report demonstrates the great cost of the Netley construction from the duplicate arrangements of buildings and offices required for its future administration, i.e., regarding it as a general hospital for patients sufficiently ill to be confined to bed. To reply to this that Netley is a good arrangement for an *invalid* depot would not be to the purpose, for the "commission" did not and had not to regard it from this point of view. So far as the "commission" was concerned, the point at issue was "Is Netley the best form of structure for a *general hospital for the sick* in its sanitary, administrative and economic capabilities?"

In the next place we have to remark that if, in order to evade the question of administrative expense, we are to take for granted that the present system of nursing—peculiar, we believe, to the British army hospitals—is to be continued there, we can but deplore the continuance of a method not even permissible in an *invalid depot.* This system is to make those invalids able to walk about nurse those who cannot. The principle on which such practice is based has been condemned by the

56 Report of a Board of Medical Officers, 20 November 1856. Aldershot Hospital.

57 Chaired by Sidney Herbert, with Drs Sutherland and Burrell and Douglas Galton.

Poor Law Regulations even in workhouses, and its continuance in any army hospital whatever can only be justified by its being shown that the construction of such building is unfavourable to a reasonably economical introduction of a better system of attendance. Such, indeed, appears to us to be in truth the reason why the committee would necessitate our taking it for granted that this system of nursing is to be continued at Netley.

Lastly, it had yet to be determined whether the new institution would be adapted for a clinical school to the Army Medical Department—a school where medical officers and their attendants were to be trained and kept in readiness for service whenever and wherever they might be required, and a school in which such knowledge might be taught to the junior medical officers of, and candidates for admission into, the service as would tend to prevent the recurrence of such calamities as are well known to have taken place during the late Crimean War. Now, whatever the Victoria Hospital might be as a mere invalid depot, it must be admitted on all hands that, for purposes of clinical instruction in military medicine and hygiene, it would turn out to be in this—as in other points when viewed as a hospital—a *tremendous failure.*

We cannot conclude these observations without intimating the assurance of our belief that not a single opinion expressed in the report of the "commission" could have been intended to reflect upon the members of the "committee." Looking at the question from that point of view from which it was necessary for the "commission" to regard it, it arrived at conclusions at variance with those of the "committee," and it has felt it to be its duty not to conceal such difference of opinion. But we are sure nothing could be further from the "commission's" intention than to disparage, in any way, the labours of the intelligent and zealous public officers to whom the selection of the site and plans of Netley was entrusted, and who have afterwards, with perfect consistency, defended their selection.

Source: "Netley Hospital," *Leeds Mercury* no. 6837, 21 August 1858

Some time ago, we called attention to the Report of the Royal Commission on the Sanitary State of the Army, in which, amongst other important matter[s], those causes which had led to the high rate of mortality in hospitals during the late war in the East were fully exposed. The report showed that there is, in England, no general hospital system capable of being made the basis of general hospital administration during war, and that to the want of such a system at home were to be attributed most of the disastrous results which rendered the hospitals at Scutari little better than pest houses.

To avoid similar disasters in future, the royal commission advised the establishment of general hospitals at home. Some time before this, government had determined on erecting a large hospital for invalids on the banks of Southampton Water, upon a plan which has created perhaps more discussion than that of any other building in Great Britain in our time. We learn, amongst other things, from a large Blue Book just laid before Parliament by the Rt Hon Sidney Herbert and his brother commissioners, containing a number of reports on the site and plan of the Royal Victoria Hospital, that this great hospital for containing 1000 invalids is being constructed on a plan directly at variance with the best experience and with the principles of construction laid down in the report of the royal commission itself. We learn that the hospital is unsuitable for the sick, that it cannot be administered as a general hospital, that it cannot be used for clinical instruction, that all its outbuildings and offices have been constructed in duplicate, that, in short, it is fit for nothing but to be a kind of lodging house for a certain class of invalids at an enormous cost to the country. The British Army is therefore still without a general hospital. The point is one of great importance to the public service. There seems to have been no reason why such a plan as that of the Royal Victoria Hospital should have been selected in the first instance, excepting merely as a piece of perverse ingenuity. At any rate the evil has been done, and it will now be the duty of the government to provide suitable buildings for a model army general hospital elsewhere. Otherwise, we may have at any time to bear the disgrace and the burden of another great catastrophe like that of Scutari.

The royal commission has clearly shown that such a hospital should consist of separate buildings or partitions, having wards with windows on opposite sides, with the means of thorough ventilation by the windows; that these buildings should be connected together by corridors for the purpose of administration and of exercise; that over the entire hospitals should be placed a governor with absolute power to provide for and regulate the entire administration, that there should be a proper hierarchy of officers, attendants and nurses; that the wards should be of sufficient size for the purposes of clinical instruction and economical administration; and that, as the practical result of all, medical and other officers and attendants should be as thoroughly instructed in the organization and duties of general hospitals that the whole staff might be, if necessary, transported to the seat of any foreign war. Such is the result aimed at by the royal commission. There cannot be a moment's doubt that the Royal Victoria Hospital at Netley is quite unsuitable for a training establishment of this kind, and that the country, as usual, will have to pay for official stupidity by providing another building more suitable for the wants of its noble army at home and abroad.

Source: "Netley Hospital,"[58] *Saturday Review* 28 August 1858:206-7

Before the fall of Sebastopol, Lord Panmure bethought himself of providing a suitable building for the reception of sick and wounded men from the army, to replace the miserable casemates at Chatham, where at present a grateful country receives its invalids, if not with open arms, at least with open arches, neither so roomy nor so comfortable as those under the Adelphi[59] in which the youthful thieves of the metropolis find nightly shelter. The intention was a good one, but, like other good intentions with which a certain place is said to be paved, it appears likely to lead to very sorry results. Unfortunately, ministers cannot build hospitals by putting on wishing caps. Like all other War Office proceedings, the project in question had to begin from below, and to work its way up to the top, commencing with the now happily defunct Army Medical Department, and receiving there that mark of incapacity which it is likely to carry on its forehead in all time to come. Between the Barrack Department and the Army Medical Department, the matter was so managed that one of the dampest districts in England was selected. Then the banks of a tidal estuary were pitched upon with, as it appears, ten square miles of mud exposed at low water, on which to place the new building. To complete the folly, in a district with a gravelly soil, where there happen to be some two or three acres of clay land, this is the spot chosen where the hospital is being reared.

The plan is as bad as the site. It is incapable of economical and efficient administration; it is constructed on bad sanitary principles; and

58 Cook gave as Nightingale's title of the article, "Peel's Life Pills or the Elixir Vitae" (*The Life of Florence Nightingale* 2:438).

59 An area in London between the Strand and the river, where thieves gathered under the arches.

altogether it will involve the country in an enormous and unnecessary annual cost. Public opinion has never ceased from the first to raise its voice, in and out of the House of Commons, against such a wasteful and worse than useless expenditure of money, but, with a perversity peculiar, as we have hitherto believed, to the sister isle, the War Department took no steps to inquire into the allegations until the building was all raised above the ground. After the evil was done, a committee was appointed (on which were several members of the original committee which selected the site and planned the hospital) and most diligent inquiry was made to ascertain how the evil could have been prevented. A few amendments were introduced into the plans, but, unlike Mahomet and the mountain, the building could neither be got away from the shores of Southampton Water, nor could the ten square miles of mud by any means be got away from the building, and there they both are until this day, "to witness if I lie."[60] In an unlucky hour, Lord Panmure referred the matter anew to a commission of which Mr Sidney Herbert is chairman. It so happened that the Royal Commission on the Sanitary State of the Army had just completed its labours, and this new commission—deeply imbued, as it appears, with the undeniably correct principles of hospital construction and administration propounded by the royal commission—made short work indeed of Netley. They completely scattered it to the winds, and sent their report and criticisms to General Peel as a *bonne bouche* [tasty morsel] shortly after his accession to office.

The new minister appears to have been in what, in the language of nurserymaids, is called "a great taking" about it. And he therefore called together the old and defunct original committee, to whom he transmitted Mr Sidney Herbert's confidential report, and this committee, apparently also in a state of great alarm, called to its aid geologists, chemists, engineers, medical men and quasi-sanitarians, of whom experience shows that a certain proportion are always ready to help anyone out of a scrape. These very learned and benevolent individuals forthwith responded cordially to the summons of the committee, and the result of the whole is a Blue Book of some two hundred pages, containing an account of the descent, birth and early rearing of Netley Hospital, with a tremendous castigation of all those who have presumed to think that there is anything illegitimate in it. The

60 From Thomas Babington Macaulay, Horatius, in *Lays of Ancient Rome*, stanza 65.

bantling was, at that time, as we ascertain, only five feet above ground, and these learned men not only find no reason why it should not be allowed to grow to its full height, but think that those who ever maintained any idea to the contrary may fairly be charged with child murder. To their verdict are prefixed General Peel's instructions, as a kind of charge to the jury. He states fairly enough the objections raised by Mr Sidney Herbert's commission, and he asks for a delivery *upon* them, but, at the same time, he asks, in the most unmistakable manner, a delivery *from* them.

When a minister asks for excuses, we may be very sure they will be found. Indeed, it is wonderful what may be done in this line. For £1000 of public money (the inquiry from first to last has cost but this) a minister may have on very short notice 200 pages of excuses. We are reminded of the grain of mustard seed, which indeed is the least of all seeds, but it becomes a great tree, and birds live in its branches.[61] The excuse upon which Netley could be continued was the least of all excuses, but 70,000 pounds sterling have been lodged in its branches, and voted by the House of Commons this year, and about half a million will, it is supposed, be the aggregate vote of many years before it is completed. As for the quality of the apologetic argument, we must ask our readers to judge for themselves by the following specimens.

Of the referees to whom government committed the task of procuring what was wanted, we have one gentleman, an army medical officer, who informs us he has been at Madras and has come home in charge of invalids, and that *therefore* he is qualified to judge in England of the climate suitable for Indian invalids. We may say at once that this cruelly ill-used word *therefore* is required to play an entirely new part in this report. It is ignominiously made simply equivalent to *à propos de bottes* [without rhyme or reason]. Another gentleman among the referees—and this time it is a civilian geologist—tells us that the whole of the banks of Southampton Water, on which Netley is situated, are of gravel and are self-draining, but that just where the hospital is being built there are two or three acres of clay—not "London clay" but "brick-earth." The "*therefore*" to this information is supplied this time by the Netley committee. It appears to be that among any given hospital sites, where we have all England to choose from, three acres of clay are to be sought for in the midst of miles of gravel. Another authority,

61 In Matt 17:20.

a chemist, detects sulfurated hydrogen gas in the mud opposite Netley, but informs us that, although the sewage of Southampton is *not* to be detected in the water of the estuary at Netley, yet he is told that this sulfurated hydrogen is imputable to "ships' sewage"—the "ships" being some poor innocent barges occasionally moored opposite the hospital site—and he appears to believe it. We have another who attaches great value to the ages recorded on the tombstones near Netley as a proof of the longevity and health of its inhabitants, yet we are told that the population is all emigrant, and that the people who die there are not those who have lived there. "Therefore" Netley is healthy. The same gentleman is much in love with both the climate of the locality and the proposed construction of the hospital, yet he tells us that the former is only fit for consumption, and the latter is deficient both in light and air, in both of which assertions we believe him to be entirely right. "*Therefore*," say the Netley committee, the site is a good one, and the hospital structure excellent. Defend us from our friends! What worse has Netley's worst enemy said than all this?

Again, we have a fine sentimental flourish about the "Medicina Mentis" [mental medicine] and the sovereign cure which the soldier is to find in the "view" from Netley Hospital! We are aware that the sailor can hardly recover out of sight of his sea and his ships. We have also heard an old saw (the proverb is somewhat musty) that one man's meat is another man's poison. Here the soldier is to recover by the sight of a ship, as the sailor, we suppose, is restored by the sight of a camp. Would it not be advisable to bestow Haslar Hospital upon the military invalids, and to send the sick sailors to Aldershot? Another of these gentlemen announces the singular proposition that in planning a hospital we can only consider what is best for the majority. Such being the principle, we would ask for *what* majority? For fifty plus one out of every hundred, or fifty plus two? And how many are to die from not having the best chances afforded them for recovery? Is it to be forty-nine, or only forty-eight out of the hundred? In order to enable us to understand this curious principle, we should at least have the percentage of patients given whose recovery is *not* to be considered in building a hospital. What should we think of a surgeon who told us that he did not profess to consider that his operations were to be performed in a way to benefit more than the majority of his cases?

Again, the committee is asked how the patients are to be nursed in these uncommonly inconveniently sized wards, and it is answered that they are to nurse each other. And finally, we have a host of local

Southampton authorities to tell us that the climate is the most perfect in the world. It is an *elixir vitae*—the only certain panacea—a kind of specific. It is like Parr's pills for long life—it is a Morison's college[62] for the cure of all kinds of diseases, none of which, unfortunately, as these authorities admit, have ever been sent to them for cure, but they hope they will be. When the new hospital is built, they believe a whole town will spring up for wealthy patients to come and reside in for the benefit of their advice and their climate.

And who is to "pay the piper" for all this? The poor soldier. His grateful country is, as we have seen, about to remove him from the casemates at Chatham to the mud banks of Southampton Water. And in case he should recover his health too quickly after returning from India, he is to be consigned to a climate where there is not much chance of restoration, and where he and his comrades may learn an occupation by which doubtless they will hereafter be able to earn a living in any part of England—viz., nursing each other.

One of the reasons we have heard assigned for the high mortality from consumption among the Guards is the excessive care taken of the men when they come into hospital. They are not sent home to die when they are past recovery, but they are kept in hospital to die there, out of sheer humanity, and hence the Guards are most unfairly charged with the high rate of mortality attributed to them! We merely mention this as a hint to future defenders of the army. When they are taunted with the great loss among troops serving in India, as evinced by the statistics of Netley Hospital, they will perhaps be able to point to its beautiful situation, the care and comfort bestowed upon the men, and the long time they are kept there lingering before they die, as a convincing proof that the whole averment is a mere calumny. Now we confess we had rather see the soldier live happily than die comfortably. We think, upon the whole, that it would be cheaper for the country. We agree with Mr Sidney Herbert that possibly the Barrack Department may have made a mistake in planning a barrack when they intended to plan a hospital, and we think the least expensive plan, after all, will be to build a hospital where the men may recover and go out quickly.

A recent Parliamentary paper informs us that a large hospital is about to be erected at Aldershot. Why not make this building fulfill

---

62 Thomas Parr and James A. Morison, who were not medically trained, sold vegetable based cure-alls. Parr was said to have lived to 150. Morison called himself a hygiest.

the conditions required by the royal commission above named? Why not make it serve for a model general hospital on the pavilion plan adopted by that commission, and for an army medical school? Aldershot is high and dry and, as it appears to us, would answer these purposes both in construction and site which, as the Netley committee itself proves, will not be answered either by the site or structure of Netley Hospital. In conclusion, we must express our disapprobation (we would we could say wonder) at the method of dealing with a great public question exhibited by the report of this Netley committee. It is one of the disgraces of the present time that a *soi-disant* [so-called] science can be obtained to any amount to throw its weight into any scale. And we are sorry to say that this report shows how a government which requires help out of an ugly difficulty at any cost may obtain it by such an agency.

Editor: It seems that Nightingale asked Robert Rawlinson[63] both for advice on her articles and to act as intermediary with the editor of *The Builder*, George Godwin, whose opposition to Netley has already appeared (see p 235 above). He obliged on both scores, as the next letters show. Rawlinson sent her comments, which she incorporated as footnotes in the first and third articles. When she had the articles printed as an appendix to the 1859 edition of *Notes on Hospitals*, she removed the footnotes. It is likely that Rawlinson sent the articles in to Godwin, for the proofs were sent to him (Nightingale was ill at Malvern at the time).

Source: From five letters to Robert Rawlinson, Boston University 1/1/7-9 and 12-13

17 July 1858

Knowing your enlightened views on the subject of hospital construction, and the interest you took in *The Builder* at the time of its discussion of the Netley plans, I have thought that you might consider it useful to make some more remarks in that paper on the recent controversy about Netley Hospital. I put the enclosed at your disposal, subject to your alterations, if you judge such desirable, or to your doing, in fact, whatever you think best about it. . . .

The printed paper was presented by Mr Herbert privately to General Peel, being our answer to the defendants of Netley.

63 See the biographical sketch in Appendix A.

Great Malvern
17 August 1858

If you still think that the question of the general improvement of hospitals can be raised with profit, and that *The Builder* would take in two or three articles, will you take the trouble to glance over the enclosed,[64] and if you think it useful, to alter or add to it in any way you think fit? Any succeeding article ought to be illustrated with woodcuts of what ought to be done and not done, which I would gladly furnish.

I have been so impressed with the idea that hospitals, in their present condition, are a curse and not a blessing (and I am so little likely, I believe, to recover enough to make any great improvements myself) that I should feel a real consolation in thinking that you and *The Builder* would lend your powerful aid to this cause. . . .

If this paper is too little architectural for a *Builder*, perhaps you would kindly have it returned to me, as I think I should make some other use of it.

Gt. Malvern
31 August 1858

Thank you very much for what you have done—I think the tracings will do very well as indications. You and I should make some further criticisms even upon those we have recommended, if adopted exactly. I have no copy of the manuscript I have sent you. But, to the best of my recollection, the foreign hospitals I mentioned were Lariboisière, Beaujon, Vincennes, at Paris; St Pierre and St Jean at Brussels.

I have two letters to thank you for. All that you say is admirable and what you propose (the pamphlet) I must consider—the plans you allude to I must get. Jebb's I have. The internal arrangements of hotels, etc., upon which you make such a just crusade, are too common everywhere [signature cut off]

15 September 1858

I think I had better see the proof before it goes to press (for *The Builder*) if you would be so very good as to send it me to Great Malvern. Because I rather think *Infantry* Barrack should have been put for "Cavalry Barrack" in one place [signature cut off]

64 Presumably this is the article which appeared next in *The Builder* on the following page.

Gt. Malvern
22 September 1858

I trouble you with the proof, because I have not *The Builder*'s address. I am so driven with business today that I can do no more than thank you for all the trouble you have taken and for your plans, which I liked very much.

I hope to see you when I return to London next month. I have corrected the proof. I have made no alteration in your remark on artificial ventilation in the note. I hope your note will not be taken for an approval of it.

I should like to know the death rate in the American lunatic asylums. When buildings require artificial ventilation, it betrays an original defect in construction, when nations, a poverty in fuel. The Paris hospitals, otherwise so superior to ours, are *never* fresh.

Source: "Sites and Construction of Hospitals," *The Builder* 16,812 (28 August 1858):577-78, reprinted as "Sites and Construction of Hospitals," in *Notes on Hospitals* (1859):89-93

< > indicates words added in the reprinting in *Notes on Hospitals*
[ ] indicates words omitted from the original *Builder* text

We propose to devote two or three additional papers to a discussion of general principles on which hospital sites should be selected and hospitals constructed.

The sanitary history of hospitals may be summed up in very few words. There are hospitals on very bad sites; there are hospitals on comparatively good sites; but there is hardly an instance, in this country at least, of both hospital and site fully embodying those sanitary principles which are essentially necessary for a rapid recovery of the sick and maimed.

The one paramount sanitary condition which ought to be observed in all hospitals is that of having *pure and dry air* both within and without the walls of the buildings. The medical profession generally, and the public, have been so much in the habit of considering that medicine is some kind of occult force, by which disease is to be expelled from the human body, that it seems to have been thought sufficient, for all purposes of curing and healing, that the sick man and the doctor should merely be brought together, in any locality or under any conditions whatever. It used to be <thought> [considered] that human beings could live in any sort of place and under any circumstances.

And it is too much the fashion, even now, to consider that the sick ought to recover anywhere. Hospital trustees and committees <conclude that> [consider] they have done all that is requisite when they have provided "the very best professional advice and assistance that can be obtained," and so the enormous mortality in hospitals has come to be considered as unavoidable, merely indicating the "percentage of mortality inevitably resulting from disease."

It appears to us that sanitary reformers have too much overlooked the influence of hospital statistics upon the mortality of particular towns. It is true that the startling increase produced in the mortality of a registration sub-district by the accidental position of the union workhouse in it is well known. But it does not seem to us that the question has always been considered, whether much of the high mortality of particular towns is not due to the bad sanitary state of local charitable institutions.

Towns, as everybody now knows, are more unhealthy than the country. But is it recognized that hospitals in towns follow the same law? That, other things being equal, a hospital in a town ought to yield a higher mortality, fewer permanent recoveries, a longer duration of sick cases, and <therefore> a greater current expense to the administration, than a hospital in the country would do for the same number of cases? Again, "hospitals," says a great living statistical authority, "are adapted to an intermediate state of civilization." But the question of how much hospitals, in their present condition, increase the mortality among the poor of this "intermediate state of civilization" has scarcely been touched. We can only state the question and pass on. The importance of an inquiry as to what is the relative mortality in hospital practice and private practice among the poor (considering, too, that cases supposed incurable are never received into hospital) cannot well be overrated.

To return to our main question, we state broadly that "town districts" should be avoided for hospital sites. Air of sufficient purity is not to be obtained in towns. Every existing town hospital ought therefore to be removed into the country, if it be possible to do so. At a moderate distance from towns land is much cheaper than in close-built places, and there are many large hospital establishments covering considerable areas of ground in crowded and valuable parts of towns and cities which might be removed to the country, not only with incalculable advantage to the sick, but with great pecuniary gain to the hospital establishment. Even in so vast a place as the metropolis, a few casualty wards where accidents might temporarily be seen, rooms for the examination and the reception of cases and suitable vehicles for transferring them to the country would be all that would be necessary to effect the reform.

The single consideration that the welfare and speedy recovery of the sick must be considered as the main object of all hospitals ought to determine the removal and reconstruction of any unhealthy hospital, provided there be the pecuniary means of doing so, and if these are deficient, every exertion should be made to obtain them.

The foundations of every hospital should be laid in dry ground, which should be covered by concrete, or the building should have an arched basement, preventing the soil from having any communication with the floors above. Basements, enclosed and connected with the wards by staircases, are inadmissible as affording ingress for damp air from the sub-soil to the air breathed by the sick. A gravelly or sandy sub-soil, well drained, is the best. Clay sub-soils are unsuitable in proportion to their power of retaining moisture. Made ground, or ground covered with decaying organic matters, such as sweepings of streets, old burial grounds, etc., should be sedulously avoided. One of the most ill-advised proposals for building a hospital which perhaps has ever been entertained is that of extending one of our great metropolitan hospitals over St Clement Dane's burial ground,[65] which has for years been a public nuisance to the metropolis.

The vicinity of marshes, wet ground, damp valleys, river estuaries and mud banks should be avoided. The choice of the position of the new Royal Victoria Hospital, at Netley, with its ten square miles of mud, is singularly unfortunate. The natural configuration of the ground should admit of the buildings being protected from prevailing cold winds. The local climate should be dry. There should be a good supply of pure soft water.

Wherever "accident wards" are required in towns, care ought to be taken to select a healthy district, not closely populated, with no nuisances nor other local causes of disease in the vicinity.

The great principle to be kept in view in the selection of sites and climates is that recovery from sickness in the vast majority of cases depends perhaps more upon pure air and pure water, with suitable

---

65 King's College Hospital, which took over the St Clement Dane's Workhouse, was situated between the churchyard and a slaughterhouse, in a very poor, crowded area of London; for more on which see p 503 below.

diet, than upon any medical treatment, however skillful. The same remarks apply to surgical cases, in many of which there is a greater susceptibility to the influence of external causes than is to be found even in medical cases. The idea which ought to be uppermost in the minds of hospital committees, of architects and of medical men is that of *pure air*. Better leave the sick and maimed at home unless this be realized. The aggregation of a number of helpless sick and maimed under one roof, in a given space, without attention to this requisite, may be at any time, as it has often been and now is, nothing but manslaughter under the garb of benevolence.

The proof of this on a colossal scale was the mortality at Scutari, which actually reached in the month of February 1855, just before the sanitary commissioners commenced their labours, the incredible rate of 415 percent per annum.[66] And this when the character of the cases sent there from the Crimea had improved so much, that the general mortality of the army had diminished, notwithstanding up to this time the fearful and increasing death rate of the Scutari hospitals.

In the Peninsula, as we learn from Sir J. McGrigor,[67] the general hospitals had actually to be broken up, in consequence of the terrible rate of mortality within them.

Suppose a site already occupied by a hospital in which the condition above named, as first in importance, viz., that of *pure air* cannot be obtained. What is to be done? Ought we to go on receiving sick in such a building with the certainty that a number will be hurried prematurely to their graves, year after year, who would have recovered if the building had been in a more healthy place? Rather than admit so fearful an alternative, would it not be better to consider the question of removing the hospital altogether? Hospital sites in the midst of increasing populations are far more valuable for almost any other purpose than for hospitals. Why not sell them and remove the establishments into healthy districts, leaving only a few accident wards and offices for out-patients, and provide the means of transporting hospi-

66 A footnote in the original publication, by the editor or Rawlinson, quotes from the royal commission report and Nightingale's evidence. It ends, "The whole of the evidence by Miss Nightingale is so clear, so important, so terrible and so full of warning and instruction that we wonder it has not been republished in a separate form."

67 Sir James McGrigor (1771-1858), director general of the Army Medical Department 1815-51.

tal patients to the new hospitals? Even medical schools ought to yield to true sanitary requirements. The sick ought not to be permitted to suffer in order that any medical school, however good, may prosper. Medical schools would, however, prosper far more in the vicinity of good than of bad hospitals. The processes of nature by which the sick recover would be seen in operation, instead of the processes of foul air by which the sick die, which latter, it is to be feared, forms a considerable proportion of the experience of some hospital students at the present time.

Having obtained a good site, how is that site to be used? In other words, on what plan is the hospital to be built?

The fundamental idea of all hospital plans ought to be this: to have pure, fresh air in every part of the building. Fresh air is the sine qua non [without which nothing]. Unless a building can be so planned that the sick shall breathe air as fresh within its walls as they could do externally, they will suffer in a ratio corresponding to the degree of impurity.

All surgical operations, all medical treatment and all nursing are subsidiary to this great central point in hospital construction and management. We again assert that it should never be forgotten for a moment, by hospital committees, by architects and by medical officers, that on the purity of the air of a ward depend, in a great measure, the recovery or death of the sick and maimed, the usefulness or injury arising from the hospital, the duration of cases, and, consequently, the hospital economy: whether, in short, a hospital planned, erected and supported by “voluntary contributions” is to be a blessing or a curse to civilization. And when we consider that (in the words of the statistical authority already quoted) [“each individual requires a gallon of pure air every minute”;] that <“a man> [he] cannot forego <his> [this] supply of air so many minutes as he can forego food for days,” is it a subject for wonder that pure air should be the main condition, as of health, so of recovery?

In the infancy of knowledge, when Christian benevolence provided for the sick and destitute, and where it also was the sole foundation of the work, hospitals were built in situations and on plans which were far from realizing the intentions of their founders. Mere shelter, food and attendance were to be afforded to as large a number of sufferers as possible. In times of pestilence, the buildings would be crowded to excess, as we have seen in the case of the Irish workhouses during the famine of 1847. And who can tell how much of the dire loss of human life in the Middle Ages and during the great Irish calamity alluded to was due to benevolence misdirected?

One of the most striking illustrations of the results of absence of knowledge on these subjects is afforded by the experience of the Hôtel-Dieu at Paris. By the statutes of its foundation "all applicants" were to be "admitted." It had 1200 beds, and towards the end of the last century these beds used to receive at the same time from 2000 to 5000 sick. During epidemics as many as 7000 sick have been in the building at one time. From 20,000 to 30,000 sick passed through the hospital every year, about 25 percent of whom were carried to the cemeteries. In the other hospitals of Paris the mortality was about 12½ percent of the sick.

The excuse for the enormous mortality of the Hôtel-Dieu was the same as that which is put forward by ill- and even by many well-informed persons at the present day for the high rate of mortality in civil hospitals, and, during war, in military hospitals, viz., that only the worst cases were sent there, and that they were sent there only to die.

The frightful overcrowding and bad ventilation, with the absence of every sanitary precaution, were, however, the real causes of the catastrophe in the Hôtel-Dieu, just as the frightful overcrowding, the want of ventilation, defective draining and want of cleanliness were the real causes of the catastrophe at Scutari.

Both catastrophes led to great discussion and inquiry on the part of benevolent and intelligent men. In the Crimea the Sanitary Commission was the result; in the case of the Hôtel-Dieu, it resulted eventually in the introduction into France of the greatest improvements in hospital construction and management which have taken place up to the present time. In these cases great good came out of great evil. From the Scutari case it is also hoped that great permanent improvements will arise in military hospitals, and it will be well if the experience of our own civil hospitals should lead to similar results.

Let anyone conversant with the phenomena of disease go into a badly constructed, and, consequently, ill-ventilated ward, and look at the sick. Unless his senses are dulled by perverse education, he will detect that peculiar musty smell which always indicates more danger to the sick than there is safety contained in the long list of benevolent and eminent physicians and expert surgeons who attend in the wards.

Let him look at the languid powerless character of the patients and ask himself the question, what would be the effect of fresh air upon these poor sufferers? Let him ask if nurses, or doctors, or medical students are ever seized with fever, and he may elicit some facts which will astonish him.

Let him go into the surgical wards and ask whether wounds heal kindly, whether operations succeed, whether hospital gangrene ever appears, whether erysipelas is common, whether purulent ulcerations and discharges are apt to take place?

In the new surgical part of the Edinburgh Infirmary he will be answered that "hospital gangrene is never out of the wards <if full>." In the double wards of Guy's Hospital, in London, he will be told that they are only fit for medical cases. In the Scutari hospitals, he would have learned that out of 44 secondary amputations, 36, or upwards of 80 percent died, that in one month there have been recorded 80 cases of hospital gangrene!

To questions concerning the appearance of hospital fever among patients and attendants, the inquirer will also be answered too truly in the affirmative, and very likely he will be told at the same time "that it is nothing more than is to be expected, considering the kind of cases received into hospital." This was the reply at Scutari; this is the general reply as to all casualties of the kind occurring in bad hospitals, civil and military. In fact, Nature alone is to blame, according to these authorities, or else "contagion" is the cause.

Nature is never to blame. If the cases be bad as possible, all the more necessity is there for care in placing them where they may have a moderate chance to recover. To place patients in musty wards is simply to kill them, with the addition of torture.

The great army surgeon, Sir John Pringle, knew this quite well when he asserted that hospitals were amongst the chief causes of the mortality of armies.[68] We may safely extend this remark, and say that badly constructed civil hospitals and other charitable institutions increase the mortality of [town] districts.

We may take this for granted that no hospital ought to yield a [an annual] mortality on its [total numbers of] sick <treated> of 7 to 10 or 11 percent [per annum], as is the case with our existing metropolitan hospitals. A certain percentage of deaths is inevitable, but not a percentage such as this.

Again, the whole doctrine of contagion, in the case of fevers, may be said to rest on no stronger foundation than the observation of facts

---

68 Pringle, *Observations on the Diseases of the Army in Camp and Garrison* viii.

in badly constructed and ill-ventilated hospitals, where emanations from the sick play a corresponding part to the emanations from cesspools and other nuisances in producing fevers out of hospitals. Both classes of emanations may become fatal or remain innocuous, but all depends on the extent to which they are diluted in pure atmospheric air. A few fever cases in a crowded, ill-ventilated ward may spread fever, but in a well-ventilated hospital, with plenty of cubic space, they certainly will not. The mortality in some of our best-constructed fever hospitals is enormous, and indicates of itself how much they stand in need of improvement.

When fever, erysipelas or gangrene spread<s> in any hospital, such an event is no proof of <"contagion">? ["inevitable contagion"] or <inevitable "infection"> ["infection]. On the contrary, it is Nature's method of teaching men that her laws are being neglected. If a medical officer, or nurse, has fallen victim to the disease, we may be quite sure that the disease is not to blame, but those who failed to observe and to obey the laws by which the disease is infallibly prevented from extending itself.

Hospital sites and plans should be selected in strict conformity with Nature's laws, and not till this is done will the outcry against hospital contagions cease. [We propose in a future number to consider further some of the main principles of hospital construction.]

Source: "Hospital Construction: The Ground Plan," *The Builder* 16,814 (11 September 1858):609-10, reprinted as "Construction of Hospitals—The Ground Plan," in *Notes on Hospitals* 93-99

"Hospitals," wrote an eminent French physician of the last century, "are a curse to civilization."[69]

"Hospitals," said Sir John Pringle, "are <among the chief causes> [the chief cause] of mortality in armies."[70]

---

69 No such quotation has been found, but the five papers on hospitals published by Jacques Tenon in 1788, *Mémoires sur les hôpitaux de Paris,* convey that message (available in translation as *Memoirs on Paris Hospitals*).

70 "Among the chief causes of sickness and mortality in an army the reader will little suspect that I should rank the hospitals themselves, though intended for its health and preservation, and that on account of the bad air and other inconveniences attending them" (Pringle, *Observations on the Diseases of the Army in Camp and Garrison* viii).

It is not sickness, nor defective medical treatment, nor bungling surgical operations which the great surgeon blames for the mortality. The medical treatment may be of the most perfect order, and yet be of little avail, if the buildings are bad or are overcrowded. Given a crowded, ill-ventilated hospital and we are sure to have a high mortality; given the Hôtel-Dieu, with its thousands of sick lying five and six in a bed, as was sometimes the case seventy or eighty years ago, and it is quite certain that a fourth part of all sick and wounded who enter such a hospital will be carried out of it to the cemeteries. Given a hospital for fever cases, in which there are four ranges of beds between the opposite windows and no sufficient means to prevent the stagnation of air by changing it frequently, and we need not be surprised that, even in this temperate climate, we have a mortality of 10 and 11 percent on the cases treated.

(In our last <section> [article] we gave the mortality of hospitals as 7 to 10 <and> [or] 11 percent. So stated, the mortality appears much less than it really is. The deaths on *cases treated* may be fairly stated at 7, 10 and 11 percent. When the element *per annum* is introduced, it must refer of necessity to the number of beds constantly occupied by sick. And, if we apply this test to the hospitals whose deaths to cases treated we have given above, we find the *annual* mortality mount up to <85, 134> [85, 110], <110> [134] percent. This estimate, however, depends to a great extent on the rapidity with which the cases pass through hospital, as well as upon the mortality on the cases treated. The mortality on the cases treated in the metropolitan hospitals varies between 4½ percent and nearly 16 percent. Even this enormous mortality is a trifle when compared with the mortality in the metropolitan lunatic asylums. It varies from 9 to 10, 20, 25, up to nearly 42 percent of the cases which enter their destructive precincts. Surely there is "something rotten in the <state> [tsate] of Denmark."[71])

Can we avoid by any structural arrangements such excess of mortality? This is the great question to be decided by hospital architects. Experience replies that there are many illustrations of masses of sick who, having been treated in the open air, have escaped with few deaths, of large numbers treated in properly constructed tents and in small wooden huts who have also recovered. Even the famine-stricken fever population of Ireland exhibited a marked contrast in the small mortal-

---

71 Shakespeare, *Hamlet*, Act 1, scene 4.

ity of cases treated under hedges, in the open air, as compared with the same class of cases treated in workhouses and in hospitals. In like manner, in the large, but at first overcrowded, badly drained and badly ventilated hospitals at Scutari, the mortality rose as high as 42.7 percent on cases treated. In the wooden huts of the Castle Hospital above Balaclava, which only held from fifteen to thirty patients each, the mortality was under 3 percent of the cases treated. In the large overcrowded and badly ventilated hospitals of the Peninsular army, the mortality was so great that they had to be closed, and the sick to be subdivided amongst a number of separate buildings. The old idea that fresh air was dangerous, and that warmth must be obtained and preserved even for smallpox and fever patients, has been done away with. A smallpox patient will have more chance of recovery if placed on clean straw under an open shed and covered with blankets than in many private rooms or in most hospital wards. Smallpox cases have been so treated, and without loss.

After the pestilential hospitals at Scutari had been cleansed, ventilated and regulated according to the plans and under the directions of the sanitary commission, the deaths among the sick there did not much exceed the deaths among healthy guardsmen at home.

The lesson taught by all experience is, therefore, that large hospitals, as generally built and managed, are destructive of human life, unless extraordinary precautions be taken, and that it would be safer, as a general rule, in the absence of such precautions, to treat large numbers of sick in the open air. But we *must* have hospitals, and it is only by subdivision of the sick among a number of separate buildings, by relatively large cubic space and by ample ventilation that we can make hospitals furnish a minimum rate of mortality and a minimum duration of cases.

Large, rambling, low-roomed buildings, like old mansion houses, are utterly unfit to receive sick. Their wards, or rather their badly constructed, ill-arranged rooms, are hardly adapted for the smallest families of healthy people to live in, much less for numbers of helpless sick people to recover in.

Given a building like Netley Hospital, with 500 sick confined to bed under one roof, in a series of cells communicating with each other by corridors and staircases, and we have not our own intelligence to thank if the sick are not carried off by hospital epidemics. There *is* a certain ratio between the number of sick placed in a building and the amount of mortality. We know that, of the sick who were treated in the Crimea, almost exposed to the elements during the frightful winter of 1854-55, not above one half so many in proportion died as perished in the great hospitals at Scutari during the same time. In the Crimea, the sick were aggregated, twenty or thirty together. In the hospitals at Scutari, there were, at one time, crowded under one roof, upwards of 4000 sick, wounded and healthy men. The subdivision of the sick and wounded should therefore be made a primary object in all hospital construction.

To what extent should this subdivision be carried? We apprehend that the point must be determined by the twofold consideration of uniting the greatest advantages as to health with the greatest facilities as to administration and economy.

And, first, we would lay down the principle that no hospital should be more than two flats in height. By such a construction, the sick are spread over a wider area; the walls are not so high as to interfere with sunlight and ventilation of neighbouring pavilions; the accumulation of hospital miasms in upper flats is avoided; access to the wards is easier for patients and attendants; and the whole administration is much facilitated. "It will cost a great sum for land to build a hospital with only two flats," will say the hospital economist. No doubt it will cost more money to accommodate a given number of sick in a hospital of two than in one of four flats. But the question has been discussed and decided, notwithstanding, that the hospital of two flats is better than one of additional storeys, and many hospitals of two flats have been built. Those of St Jean and St Pierre at Brussels have each two flats, and land is dear enough in Brussels. In this country, also, land in towns has been used for building hospitals of two flats high. But even admitting the argument of the expensiveness of land as being entirely valid, the conclusion is certainly not that hospitals three and four flats high should be built in towns, but that hospitals should be built in the country where land is less expensive. It is little else than a breach of trust to build great lofty architectural structures merely to flatter the bad taste of committees or governors, or to place the hospital in a close unhealthy neighbourhood to suit the convenience of medical attendants, when the object of the whole ought to be recovery of the sick.

The number of sick which may be safely placed under one roof will, to a certain extent, be determined by the local position of the hospital, by the amount of cubic space allotted to the patients and by the state of ventilation. In the most recent hospitals, the number varies considerably. Thus, in the Royal Marine Hospital, which is at present being erected at Woolwich, 84 sick are to be accommodated under one roof.

In the proposed hospital at Aldershot there will be arrangements for about 100. In each of the hospital blocks at Beaujon, in Paris, there are arrangements for 60 sick. In the magnificent Hospital Lariboisière at Paris the number is 102 per block. At the Hospital St Jean at Brussels it is about 88.

Too great a subdivision of sick must necessarily incur an increase of cost in administration and nursing. On examining the experience of all these hospitals, we are of opinion that from 100 to 120 sick may be safely and economically treated under one roof, provided the ventilation and cubic space be sufficient, and the structure and communications of the building be so arranged as to facilitate the administration and nursing.

The next important question is how to arrange buildings so as to have pure air outside and inside the structure.

The air must be "moving air" in mass. The motion of the air in any room should never exceed a velocity of two feet and a half per minute, and should not be at any time much below this rate. There must be no "stagnation." It is a great error to imagine that, because buildings are erected around a large court, therefore they are airy enough. A court with high walls round it does one thing with certainty, it stagnates the air. All closed courts, narrow *culs de sac*, high adjacent walls, closed angles, overshadowing trees and other obstructions to outer ventilation should be sedulously avoided, at whatever cost. Plan the building so that the sunlight can strike as large a surface of it as possible, and so that the air may move freely over the whole external surface.

Figures 1, 2 and 3 represent arrangements of buildings at present occupied for hospital purposes, which ought to be carefully avoided. It may be considered certain that, wherever such arrangements exist, injury to the sick is so constant that, were it practicable, all the angles should be opened to admit of the circulation of air.

The simplest form of structure for ensuring light and ventilation is to build hospital wards in a straight line, Fig. 4, with windows on both sides, i.e., back and front, the lengthway of the ward being the lengthway of the building and the administration in the centre. By such an arrangement as this, however, no more than four wards could be obtained, if the building were two storeys high. For small hospitals not exceeding 120 sick, this plan would be economical and efficient. The direction of the axis of such a building should be from north to south, a little inclining to the east, which would ensure the sun shining on both sides every day of the year, and would also protect the wards from northeast winds.

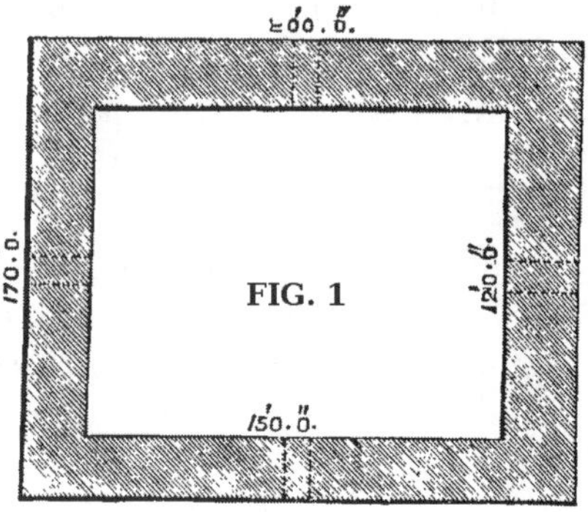

FIG. 1

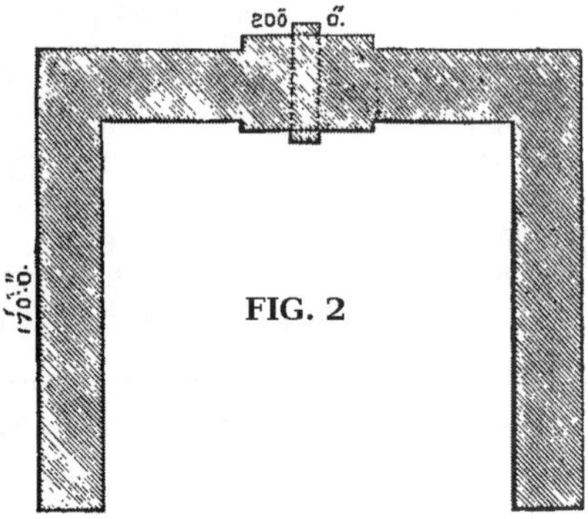

FIG. 2

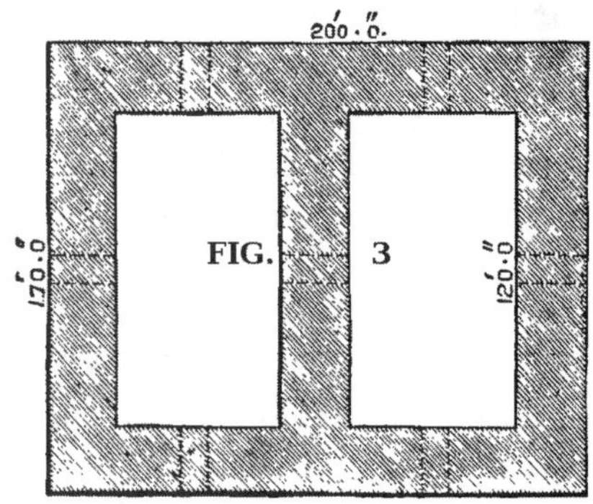

FIG. 3

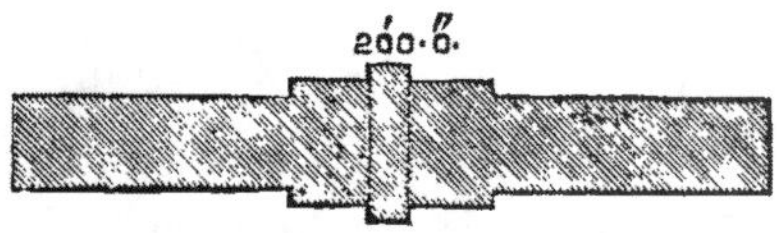

FIG. 4

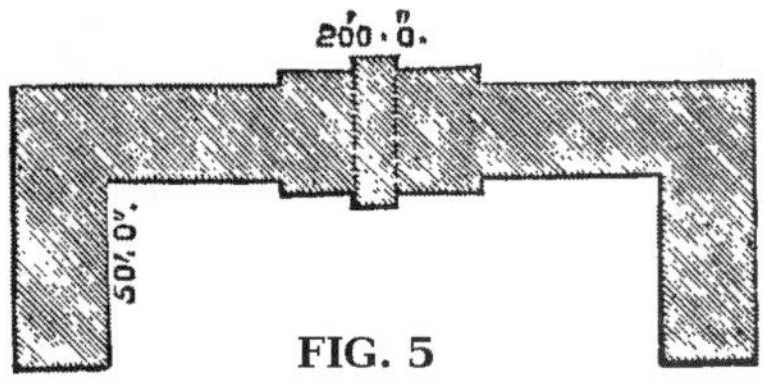

FIG. 5

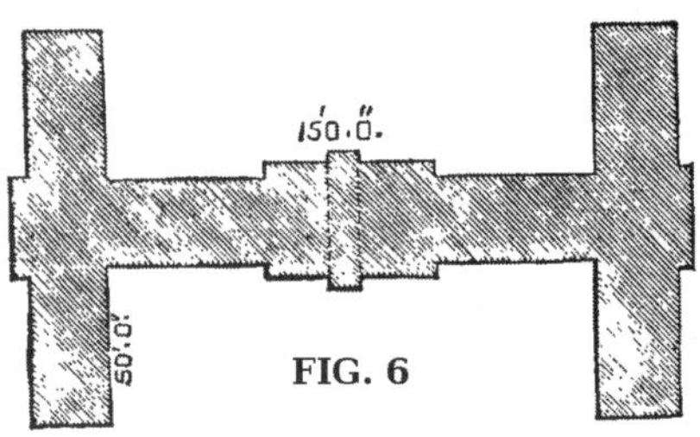

FIG. 6

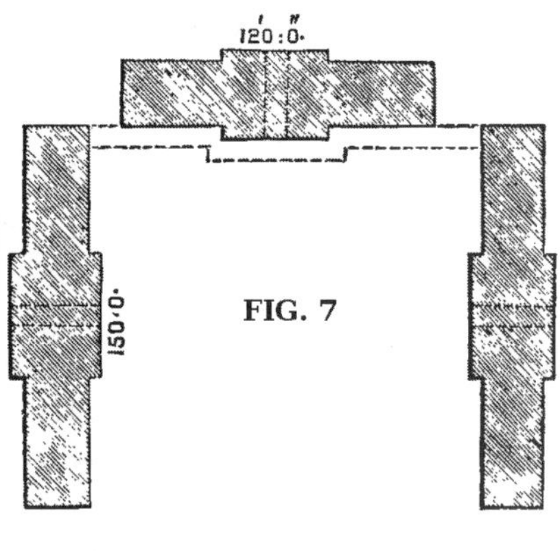

FIG. 7

One staircase would suffice for a hospital such as this. If it were carried from the bottom to the top of the building, and ventilated above the roof, it would cut off entirely one set of wards from the other, which is all that is necessary to prevent the possibility of any intermingling of foul air.

By adding projecting wings at the ends of such a line of building, as in Figs. 5 and 6, additional ward space might be obtained. But additional staircases also there must then be at the ends, and such a building would have the disadvantage of a closed angle, although this would be of less consequence if the wings were very short in proportion to the length of the front.

A much better arrangement is represented in Fig. 7, in which the wings are entirely detached from the centre and connected with it only by an open corridor on the lower floor. This is the plan adopted in the great military hospital at Vincennes, and is a very good one for hospitals of a certain size, for the open angles permit air to circulate freely round the building. All of these plans, however, have the disadvantage of not admitting extension beyond a certain limit. The only plan which allows as much extension as can be necessary in any single hospital up to (say) 1000 sick (beyond which hospital management becomes very difficult), is the plan adopted in the hospital at Bordeaux [of which we gave an engraving in our volume for 1856], or, still better, that of the Lariboisière at Paris. In that fine hospital, each block, containing 102 sick, constitutes a separate hospital. There are six of these blocks, which are arranged parallel to each other on two opposite sides of a square. And there are four blocks containing the administrative and other offices. The kind of arrangement is represented in Fig. 8. [(In an early number we shall give a detail plan of this hospital.)]

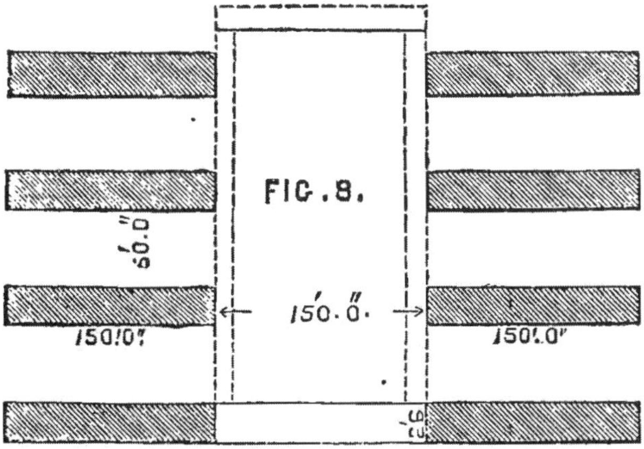

All the blocks are joined together by a glazed corridor along the lower flat, and by an open terrace above for convalescents taking exercise. In such a building, for the sake of sunlight, the axis of the wards should run nearly from north to south, and the distance of the blocks from each other should be about twice the height of the side walls.

We have given these illustrations of the arrangement of hospital buildings to show the more recent improvements in this important matter. Whether any of these or any better arrangement be adopted in building a hospital, it should be kept in mind that the great objects aimed at are subdivision of the sick, free ventilation outside and inside the buildings, abundance of light and windows on opposite sides of the wards, the heads of the beds being between the windows.

A hospital for 1000 sick ought to have none of its offices in duplicate. It should have one kitchen, so situated that the diets can be easily carried to any ward, and in the shortest space of time to all. The kitchen should be separately ventilated, and should not be under any part of the building used for sick. The laundry should be at a distance from the hospital, and in no way connected with it. The offices of the administration should be conveniently situated, not only for facility of access, but for efficiency of superintendence. This point was quite lost sight of in the Netley plans, in which, if the unfortunate governor happened to be wanted at the two extremities of the building successively, he would have to walk half a mile, while with such a plan as that of Lariboisière, he could in the same time walk all round the buildings.

No sewer <or> [nor] drain should pass under any part of the hospital where there are sick. Sewers and drains should be outside, and free even of the external walls; there should be means of ventilation in abundance; there should be means of inspection and for flushing. The water supply should be of the purest and softest description. It should be laid over the whole building, hot and cold. This arrangement, together with that of lifts, saves the service of at least one attendant to every thirty sick. For water supply, there should be a water tower and tank placed centrally, affording water under high pressure. The mains should be of cast iron, varnished; the service pipes should be of wrought iron; there should not be any cisterns, but the supply should be constant. Fire cocks, or "hydrants," should be placed at short intervals. Each supply tap should have a waste sink underneath it, and these should be placed so as to save labour. Water closets must be external, but near the wards, and under such arrangement of plan as to prevent any possibility of atmospheric contamination. There should be not less than one closet to each ten patients. [Lavatories should also be in like proportion. Warm, cold and shower baths should also be easy of access on each floor.] All staircases and passages should be wide, light and airy. This is a most important consideration in hospitals. The steps should consist of stone, but they may be covered with wood, as in some of the French hospitals. Stone is essential to prevent accidents from fire. All hospitals should have convalescent wards, supplied with dining and day rooms. In the pavilion structure these can be placed under a separate roof. Casualty wards and small wards for special cases should be placed in a separate part of the hospital.

The square within the hospital and the spaces between the pavilions should be laid out as garden ground, with well-drained and rolled walks and shaded seats for convalescents.

It is of great importance to provide places of exercise under shelter for patients, to be appropriated to that purpose alone. Such recreation and winter airing grounds may be comparatively large, and yet of cheap construction, if roofed on the Crystal Palace plan. The country can alone offer all the necessary facilities for the establishment of such valuable aids to hospitals. [In a future number, we shall discuss the structure and the arrangements of hospital wards.]

Source: "Hospital Construction: Wards," *The Builder* 16,816 (25 September 1858):641-43, reprinted as "Hospital Construction—Wards" 99-108

<In the two first sections> [In our former papers] on this subject, we have considered the question of sites and general arrangement of hospital buildings. We now proceed to discuss the question of ward arrangements with reference to light, ventilation and administration.

Without entering into any scientific discussion as to the effects of light on organization, it may be taken as proved that light exercises a peculiar influence on the two elements of form and colour. And, as both of these properties in living bodies are intimately connected with the *reparative* processes, we may safely consider it as certain that light is essential to the recovery of the maimed and sick. Experience in the more southern climates of Europe has determined the erection of houses for invalids in localities exposed to the full glare even of a southern sun, with which the rooms are flooded through a greater proportion of windows than would be considered safe by some of our medical men in colder climates. Very many of our civil hospitals would enable experiments to be instituted as to the injurious effects of absence of light on peculiar classes of disease. But the only experimental evidence we have hitherto obtained is that given by Sir James Wylie[72] in

72 James Wylie (1768-1854), a Scottish doctor who joined the army medical service in Russia, became its director and personal physician to three tsars. He was knighted when he accompanied Tsar Alexander I on a trip to England.

regard to certain hospitals and barracks at St Petersburg. In some of these hospitals there <were> [are] rooms without direct light, and the sick and wounded treated in these dark chambers yielded only a fourth part of the recoveries when compared with patients treated in the light rooms. Nearly twice the number of invalids, it was also found, were received from the dark side of the barracks as from the light side. Dr Edwards, who has paid particular attention to the effect of light upon health, has given equally strong testimony to its preventive and curative efficacy.

Altogether apart from scientific elements, common sense would lead us to anticipate such results. Now let us see how light is treated by some popular physicians and ignorant nurses. In nine cases out of ten, a physician will draw down the window blinds and half shut the shutters, while an ignorant nurse will probably shut the remainder of the shutters—especially if it be a bright day—and draw the bed curtains. We have the positive testimony of a well-known London physician, given in his report to the Netley committee, that "whenever he enters a sick room, he takes care that the bed shall be so placed that the patient shall be turned away from the light."

<Note. To show the want of acquaintance with the influence of light on recovery evinced by otherwise intelligent members of the medical profession, it is only necessary to quote the following passage from page 125 of the report on Netley Hospital, 1858: "In the sick chambers of private patients medical men generally enjoin that the bed should be placed in any other position rather than opposite a window." We are glad to know that there are medical men who entertain far more just and enlightened views as to the influence of light on disease.>

After this, we cannot blame army medical officers for not knowing much about the matter. An acquaintance of ours one day, passing a barrack, saw the windows on the sunny side boarded up in a fashion peculiar to prisons and penitentiaries. He said to a friend who accompanied him, "I was not aware that you had a penitentiary in this neighbourhood." "Oh!" said he, "it is not a penitentiary—it is a military hospital. There is a great horror of light on the part of certain army medical men. I suppose," he added, "the medical officers are afraid the light will alter the shape of the men." Not a few civil surgeons, also, treat light as if it were an enemy.

In the teeth of all these popular fallacies, we assert that every sick ward should be capable of being flooded by sunlight, and, consequently, that the windows should bear a large proportion to the wall space in all hospitals. Experience appears to prove that window space should not be in a much less proportion to wall space of a hospital than one to two.

The next important question is the <quantity> [amount] of air required in a hospital, and how best to renew it.

[In a former article, we stated the amount of air absolutely required for the *chemical* purposes of healthy respiration to be a gallon per patient per minute. This measure, however, by no means represents the amount required for a continuous preservation of health.]

The great and constant movements going on in the atmosphere prove that the amount of change which nature has provided for healthy existence is unlimited. The test of the ventilation of a sick ward is the comparative freshness or impurity of the air. The interesting experience of Lariboisière appears to prove that about 4000 cubic feet per bed per hour are required to ensure this.

There are two ways of maintaining the freshness of the air of a ward:

First, by so constructing a building that Nature will renew the air, if left to herself, which is by far the best plan.

Secondly, by artificial ventilation—never to be used except as a *pis aller* [last resort].

If the hospital is badly planned, or if fuel be dear, artificial ventilation comes into beneficial operation, for it admits of economical warming, but it never *freshens* a ward like pure natural air from without. Every intelligent physician and nurse knows the value of freshness in the air of a ward. It is better oxygenated, and, perhaps, contains more ozone. But whether or not this be so, it is quite certain that a condition of ward air is secured by open windows, and by open fireplaces for warming, which is never obtained by the best ventilating machinery, especially if warm air be thrown in by it.[73]

Architects must therefore well consider how in every corner of wards, passages and staircases air is to be kept constantly *flowing*, not air passing in a stray or in a strong current, but air gently moving. This can only be done by having wards of a certain height and breadth, and by having a window for every two beds, the windows opposite.

We shall afterwards discuss the questions as to the size of wards and the proportion of window space, but in the meantime we lay down a principle of construction applicable to all wards, of whatever size.

73 A footnote here with Rawlinson material gave further remarks on warming and ventilation in France, England and the U.S., and argued for English open ventilation.

Few greater mistakes can be committed in hospital construction, as far as light and ventilation are concerned, than placing the windows at *one end* of a ward, or even at both ends, with beds ranged down the sides, their heads to the dead wall. No greater mistake, we had nearly said, could be committed. But there has been a greater in the case of Netley Hospital, where not only has this most objectionable principle of construction been adopted, but also that of covering the windows in on one side by a glazed corridor.

In a hospital similarly built, we asked the medical officer how his sick, who were men in the prime of life, recovered? His reply was, "I do not know how it is, but all my cases linger." The reason why the cases lingered was obvious enough. For, in the first place, the air of all the wards communicated by the corridor, and, in the second place, wards and corridor were so arranged that thorough ventilation was impossible.

In another such hospital we expressed to the medical attendant our surprise that every ward was so uniformly full of sick. He replied that it did not arise so much from fresh admissions as from the fact that, when he got sick into the hospital, he could hardly get them well again.

Our military buildings have been and are most unfortunate in their arrangements. The unhappy Netley Hospital has been copied in its wards and corridor arrangements from such places as Chatham Garrison Hospital, Woolwich Hospital, etc. In fact, there are few military hospitals in which the error does not exist in one form or another. It was hardly to have been expected that, given the same directors, Netley should have escaped the same fate. A great mistake and a lamentable misfortune is Netley Hospital. But let us hope we have seen the last of such fatal blunders in hospital building.

Having alluded to military hospitals, we may say a word about regimental hospitals. We have visited several of these establishments, and certainly we can but consider their style of construction as extraordinary. They generally resemble a small ill-planned village residence, belonging, perhaps, to the attorney or the doctor. There are usually a narrow passage, a narrow staircase and small rooms in which the sick are stewed up: these rooms have a window or two here and there, as if each building had been an especial victim of the window tax. Buildings of this class have not such a thing as a proper ward. They have merely little bedrooms, and everything else upon a little scale. As for light and ventilation arrangements, these have not attracted much, if any, attention on the part of the adapter. We hope that there may be some regimental hospitals on a better plan. We speak from a knowledge of such as we have seen, and judging from these, we should say that a minimum of accommodation has been provided at a maximum of expense.

Besides arranging for light and ventilation, all hospital plans should provide for the greatest economy in administration consistent with healing of wounds and recovery of the sick. There should be facility of superintendence and nursing. The wards should be of such a size, and, if possible, so arranged that the head nurse may have all her sick under her eye at once. This is especially necessary for night watching. A single attendant can easily perform the duty of night watching for many bad cases, if the beds are so placed as to be seen from a single point. The head nurse's room should have a window looking into her ward. It is highly important that patients, who must necessarily be in various stages of sickness or convalescence, should feel that they are continually under the eye of the head nurse. It is, of course, most economical to have one ward to each head nurse. The ward, therefore, should be large enough to occupy her whole attention, but not too large to render its ventilation difficult. Small wards cannot be overlooked with sufficient strictness, unless, indeed, a head nurse is to be set apart for each—an arrangement which would enormously increase the expenses of nursing, without benefiting the patients.

A head nurse may adequately superintend a ward of from thirty to forty patients. But, if we are to be guided by the results of recent experience in hospital building, we should say that a ward with thirty sick, or thereabouts, is, upon the whole, the best for sanitary reasons, and this number of thirty we propose to fix as the ward unit for a hospital.

<Note. It is important, for the purposes of discipline, to isolate as much as possible the nursing staff of each ward. The head nurse should be within reach and view of her ward both by day and night. Associating the assistant nurses in large dormitories tends to corrupt the good and make the bad worse. Accommodation for the assistant nurses of each ward separate should therefore be found in each pavilion. This may easily be done in the roof over the front part, and the great staircase of each pavilion. In doing this, care must be taken that the night nurse shall have quiet to sleep by day. She should have a room to herself.>

Much has been said about the benefits of small wards for from six to ten sick, about the greater comfort and privacy of such wards, and the greater facility for ventilation which they afford. It is simply an error to assume that small wards afford any such advantages. Privacy, in a hospital, does not extend beyond any two adjacent beds. As regards complete ventilation, the effect of angles in retarding an even flow of air has not been sufficiently considered. Direct experiment, made in the wards of the Lariboisière Hospital, has proved that the amount of air circulating along the centre of a ward is two or three times as great as it is near angles. Such a result might have been inferred. But the important practical point never seems to have been comprehended, that the difficulty of ventilating a given cubic space occupied by sick bears a direct ratio to the length of the corridors and to the number of cells or "wards" into which that space is divided. Unnecessary rooms, angles or cupboards should be omitted in any structure. There should be no dark corners in any part of a hospital ward. Every recess or angle not easily overlooked is as injurious to hospital discipline as it is to hospital ventilation.

Each pavilion should have a staircase, wide, roomy, well lighted and ventilated from above. The gradients of the steps should not exceed a rise of 5 inches to 12 inches tread, to enable patients to ascend and descend with facility. There should be as little passage space as possible, and none of it should be dark. The head nurse's room should be situated, as already described, with one window opening down the ward, and a window looking into the open space. There must be a separate scullery for every ward, adjoining the nurse's room, but having a separate entrance and a separate window to the open air. A lift will be found an essential means of convenience as well as of economy. Each ward should have bathroom, lavatory and closets. On the male side there may be other necessary conveniences attached. The best situations for these will be at the ends of the wards, opposite the entrance. They should be separated from the wards by a partition wall with a half glass door. There should be a small lobby, lighted by a large window at the end, and from this lobby there should be doors opening right and left—one to the bathroom and lavatory, the other to the closets, etc. The ventilation and lighting of these places should be ample and independent of that of the wards. No ward requires more offices than are here enumerated. There should neither be small wards nor dining rooms attached to the large wards.

A ward for sick should not, as a rule, contain convalescents. This class of patients, under a proper system of hospital construction, should always have separate accommodation. Small wards for casualty cases, as already stated, should be built separately and be separately administered.[74]

In applying these principles it is necessary, first, to ascertain what ought *not* to be done.

---

74 Another footnote here with Rawlinson material argues against convalescent hospitals in favour of convalescent houses.

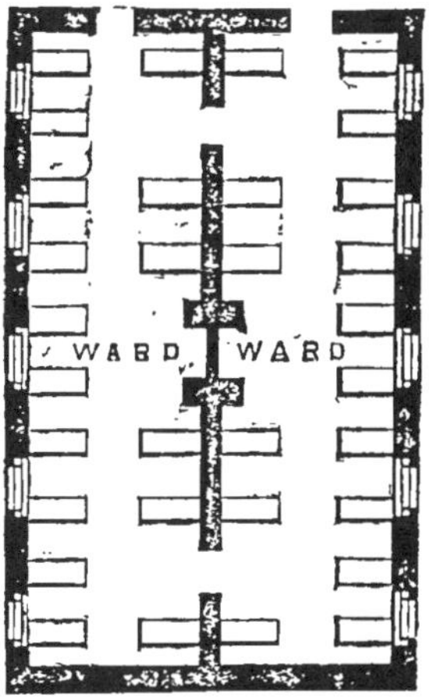

Fig. 1.

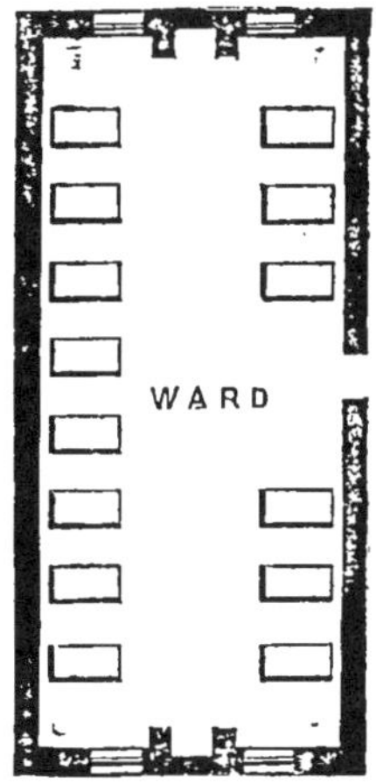

Fig. 2.

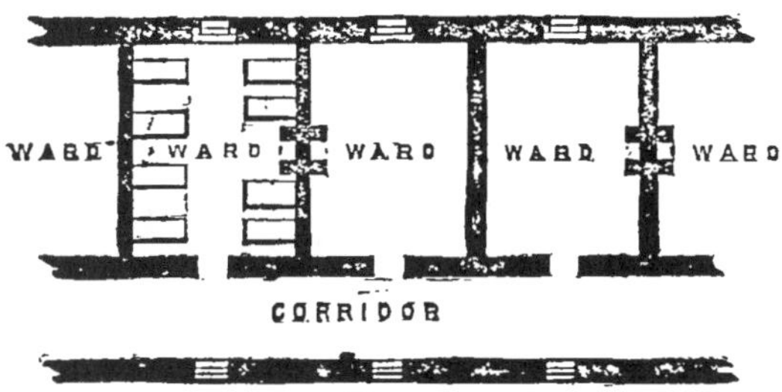

Fig. 3.

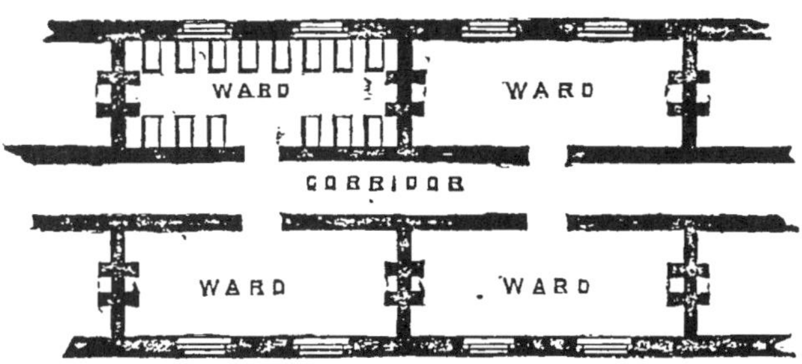

Fig. 4.

Figures 1, 2, 3 and 4 represent common errors in hospital ward construction, which ought to be carefully avoided. Figure 1 represents the arrangement in King's College Hospital and in the new wards at Guy's, London. Figure 2 is the ward arrangement usually carried out in buildings which have been adapted for civil hospitals. It was designedly adopted in the military hospital, Portsmouth, as also in many other military hospitals. Figure 3 is the arrangement in a few ill-constructed foreign hospitals, as, e.g., in one at Rotterdam. It exists at Chatham Garrison

Hospital, and is to be perpetuated at the new Victoria Hospital at Netley. Figure 4 shows the kind of arrangement in the wards and corridors in the old Royal Marine Hospital at Woolwich. These diagrams do not pretend to extreme accuracy; they simply indicate the arrangement.

These plans should be avoided for the future in hospital construction. They are contrary to every sound principle of sanitary construction, and can only be kept free from hospital epidemics by the greatest possible care, hardly even with that.

We shall next state what ought to be done in applying the principles of hospital construction we have laid down.

The best principle of hospital construction is, as <has long been> [we have long] urged, that of separate pavilions placed side by side, or in line. The former is preferable for large hospitals, for the reasons stated in our last paper. [See p 609 *ante* [above].] The distance between the blocks should be double their height. There should be two flats in a pavilion, and one ward to a flat.

The hospital should be erected to form a square, the basement storey of the pavilions being connected by a corridor, and the whole of the basements erected on arches. The wards should hold from twenty to thirty sick; each bed should have from 1500 to 2000 cubic feet of air space allotted to it.

The following table exhibits the proportions of a ward for thirty-two patients. The first column gives the proportions of such a ward in the Lariboisière Hospital, the second the proportions adapted to a larger cubical space, such as is given in our best hospitals in this country:

	1		2	
	Feet	In.	Feet	In.
Length of ward	111	6	128	0
Breadth	30	0	30	0
Height	17	0	17	6
Wall spaces between end walls and windows	5	0	6	4
Breadth of windows	4	8	4	8
Breadth of wall space between windows	9	2	11	4
Height of windows	13	0	13	6
Cubic space per bed	1760	0	2100	0

It is undesirable to increase the width of any ward beyond 30 feet, because the distance between the opposite windows becomes then too great for efficient ventilation.

The proportions of a ward for twenty patients might be 80 feet long, by 25 feet wide and 16 feet high. This would give about 1600 cubic feet to each bed.

One window at least should be allotted to every two beds. There are hospitals with a window to each bed. The windows should be double, or be glazed with plate glass, to prevent loss of heat. Tripartite windows, like those of Middlesex Hospital, are useful for ventilation. The ward walls should consist of pure white polished Parian cement, or some other equally white non-absorbent substance. Grey-coloured cements should be avoided: they never look clean; they give the ward a sombre appearance; and they hide dirt. The best ward flooring is oak. No sawdust, nor other organic matter capable of rotting, should be placed underneath hospital floors. The joints of the flooring should be well fitted together, so as to be impervious. Floors should be beeswaxed, or oiled and polished. The general baths of the hospital should be separated from the pavilions, but connected with the corridor. They should contain hot and cold water, sulphurous, medicated, hot air, vapour, shower and *douche* baths. The kitchen should have walls and ceiling of Parian cement.

There should, as stated, be a head nurse's room and scullery attached to each ward, and store presses in each ward.

The bedsteads should be of iron. The ward furniture should be of oak. The arrangements for water supply and drainage were discussed in a previous article. We have also pointed out already the best position for closets, lavatories, ward baths, etc.

The ward construction, now described, is that which, up to the present time, experience has shown to be best suited for fulfilling all the requirements of ventilation, light, cheerfulness, recovery of health and economy in this country. It is embodied in the plan, Fig. 5.

One great advantage of the proposed system of construction is that it admits of any arrangement of the pavilions on plan which is consistent with light and ventilation. Hospital establishments so constructed may be added to without difficulty and without altering, or indeed without interfering with any of the existing pavilion buildings.

The principles of hospital construction which we have now laid before our readers are a tacit condemnation of the majority of hospitals in the three kingdoms. It may be thought by some of our readers that we have expressed our opinions somewhat strongly. We have considered it necessary to do so because, as we have shown, large hospitals are even now being built in defiance of the most ordinary sanitary principles as to site and plan, and men have been found to defend

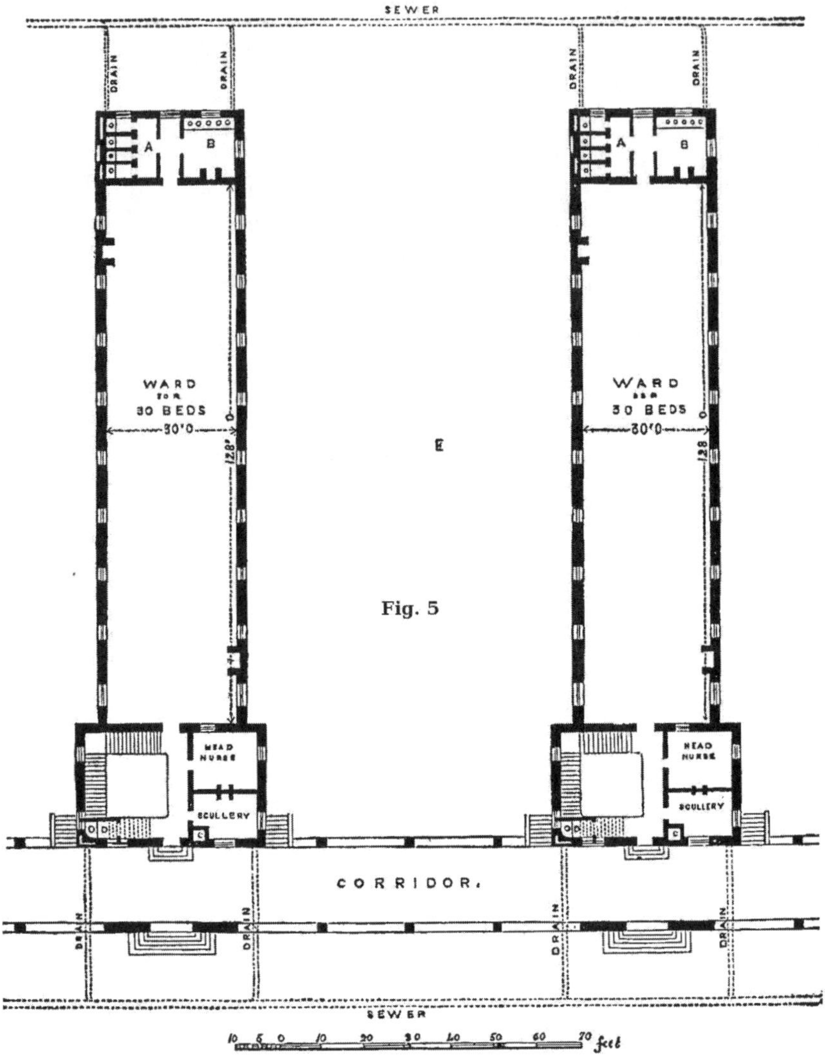

Fig. 5

A. Ward Closets
B. Band and Lavatory
C. Lift in Scullery
D. Private Closet
E. Ornamental Ground
Ward Windows to be 4 ft. 8 in. in the clear

these errors. Another opportunity is now afforded of retracing our steps. The noble bequest of Mr Morley[75] for the foundation of a con-

75 Atkinson Morley (1781-1858), a wealthy hotel owner and governor at St George's, left £100,000 in his will for a convalescent home; he had been Nightingale's landlord when she lived in Burlington St.

valescent establishment in the country near London may be a great practical advance in the right direction, and it behooves the governors of St George's Hospital to take care that an institution of such importance is constructed so as to realize the benevolent intention of its founder.

Most of the great hospital and charitable institutions in this country were suburban at their foundation; the rapid growth of our towns in modern times has encroached so much upon space once country that gardens and fields have been absorbed and are now covered by bricks and mortar; and hospitals are surrounded by the screaming and roaring traffic of railways, street cabs, omnibuses and wagons. It is due to the benevolent founders of our great charitable institutions that their humane intentions should continue to be realized by removing the sick and maimed to pure air and quiet. It is due to poor suffering humanity that any plans adopted should be the most perfect modern intellect can devise, and it is no less due to the cause of charity that there should be the best and most economical form of hospital nursing and management.

The following is a summary of the principles of hospital construction contained in this and preceding papers:

1. Never erect a general hospital within the precincts of a town or in suburbs likely to be built upon.

2. Remove all large hospital establishments out of town, or from populous suburbs, as soon as possible.

3. Build all hospitals in the country, on areas of ground sufficient to admit of extensions of the buildings, and to prevent other buildings from being erected within such a distance as shall interfere with a free circulation of air and with quiet.

4. Select a dry and mild climate.

5. Give the preference to a porous self-draining sub-soil, and avoid ground saturated with organic matter, especially old graveyards.

6. Build all hospitals on arches, to admit of a free circulation of air underneath the ward floors.

7. Let the plan be simple and have as few closed angles and corners as possible.

8. Do not provide for more than 120 patients or beds under one double pavilion roof. If the hospital must contain a larger number of beds, increase the number of pavilions, but on no account increase their size. Connect the pavilions by corridors running between the ends, and no higher than the ground floor.

9. Plan any hospital with no more than two flats, containing, in a single pavilion, two superimposed wards. Provide for convalescents and "casualty" cases in pavilions separate from the ordinary sick.

10. Provide for no more than thirty-two beds in a ward—sixteen on each side, with a window to every two beds.

11. Let the window spaces be, as near as may be, in the proportion of one to two of the wall space. The windows should reach from within 3 feet of the floor to within 1 foot of the ceiling.

12. Wards should not exceed 30 feet in width.

13. Each bed should have from 1500 to 2000 cubic feet of air space. In very exposed and airy situations the smaller cubic space will suffice, but where, from the nature of the ground, there is not likely to be much horizontal external movement of the atmosphere, the larger the internal cubic space is the better.

14. Trust for pavilion ventilation to open windows and fireplaces. Artificial methods are, in this climate, unnecessary with proper construction.

15. Place water closets, ward baths and lavatories at the far end of a ward, opposite the entrance, and, in addition to ventilating them, cut them entirely off from the ward by a separately ventilated and lighted lobby.

16. Restrict the ward offices to a nurse's room and scullery, with a lift.

17. Let staircases be wide, roomy and thoroughly ventilated up to the roof. Construct the stairs and entrance lobbies of stone, and cover them with wood.

18. Make hospital floors of oak, and walls and ceilings of pure white polished cement.

19. Supply hospitals with water at high pressure, and lay it on, hot and cold, over the whole of the buildings.

20. All sewers and drains must be outside and detached from the walls of the buildings. Provide for their ventilation at a distance from the wards, and also for their inspection and flushing.

21. Provide garden ground for exercise with properly drained and gravelled walks, sheltered seats for convalescents, and, where practicable, a promenade covered with glass for use in bad weather.

Other matters of detail regarding kitchens, washhouses, rooms for hospital administration, etc., can be best decided on according to local circumstances, but none of these should ever be under the same roof with the sick.

The public hospitals of any country may fairly be taken as a standard of the knowledge and care of the governing body, or of civilization amongst a people. Commercial wealth, political freedom and education ought to enable the inhabitants of Great Britain to set an example in this respect. Life is of more value in the British Empire than in any other part of the globe, and the means to secure it to the latest periods [(the full three score and ten of the psalmist[76])] ought to be sought out and put in practice. Let us reform our hospitals now and, as we improve our cities and towns, they will be less required.

Source: From a letter to Douglas Galton, ADD MSS 45759 ff9-11

Great Malvern
28 August 1858

Soyer's death is a great disaster. Others have studied cookery for the purposes of gormandizing, some for show, but none but he for the purpose of cooking large quantities of food in the most nutritious and economical manner for great numbers of men. He has no successor. My only comfort is that you were imbued before his death with his doctrines, and that the Barrack Commission will now take up the matter for itself.

1. Then you saw the paragraph in yesterday's *Times* about Grant's kitchen;

2. How has the gas kitchen in the Wellington Barracks succeeded? Would you ask the soldiers? and make your conclusion?

3. Do you know an intelligent, conceited, little clerk of poor Soyer's, called Warren? I conclude he could be heard of from Mrs Soyer, 15 Marlbor' Road, St John's Wood.

4. Possibly Warren could point out some man who was taught by Soyer and follows his methods. Do you not think it would be very important to have such a person to teach the men to cook?

Also, I was thinking of asking Alexander, the director general, to collect opinions of army medical officers as to the respective merit of each form of cooking apparatus used by the army. (Gibson, of Aldershot, has given a very decided and useful opinion against Grant's.) But I remember a mischievous little fellow, Mouat,[77] whom you saw at

76 An allusion to Ps 90:10.
77 James Mouat (1815-99), first doctor to win the Victoria Cross.

Shorncliff, and who used to declaim against Soyer as "all humbug" in the Crimea.

If Warren, the clerk, could recommend a cook, it would be perhaps better to have the opinion of such a man on the products of each form of cooking apparatus, before making your report.

Source: From an undated letter to Sidney Herbert, Wiltshire County Record Office, Pembroke Collection 2057/F4/67

[c1858]

Army Medical Contagion.

Your *Canterbury* report is gone in—but none too soon—fever had broken out in the barracks. In a very proper report, the medical officer referred it to the right (and very obvious) local cause, viz., the abominable drainage. The deputy inspector, *Mouat,* comes over, and to please the commanding officer, refers it to "*contagion*"! "The men had caught it in the town"!! But, with marvellous inconsistency, he recommended an improvement in the drainage. Why so? *Either* let us have contagion and cordons—*or* local causes and sanitary improvements.

The whole matter was referred to your commission. And very sharp I should have pulled up Mr Mouat, if I had been sanitary councillor (in the future office).

I know that Dr Sutherland has told you all this and the Croydon business. But could you not say something about it (in your own pointed way) in your article, to the effect that, had logic prevailed, Canterbury *Barracks* would have put Canterbury *town* under quarantine, and Croydon *Barracks* would themselves have been put under quarantine by the Croydon *town.* But fortunately common sense stepped in, and saved us from the effects of logic, and from such a catastrophe in the *un*improved Scutari hospitals to have been (proportionately) double what it was in the regimental tents of the Crimea exposed to *every* kind of want and hardship. And this is surely enough.

So much for the general question. But now that "Anonymous"[78] has started this particular point, I mean to set to work tomorrow with Smith's big Blue Books and work out (by the process of exhaustion) taking Smyrna, Abydos and all of the hospitals, *how much* the total deaths, now stated to the House of Commons, exceeded month by

78 A letter to T.G. Balfour identifies the author of the "anonymous pamphlet" as Dr Alexander Browne; letter 27 December 1858, Add Mss 50134 f69.

month *all* and *each* of the conflicting statistics which Anonymous states to be exaggerations and which are really *under*statements of the truth.

If you do write a note upon any of these subjects in your article, please let me see it before it goes to press. I think, if you notice the Guards' attack and its result (not forgetting the man who died of "old age" at sixty), this pamphlet might form a suitable pendant—in a note.

Source: From two letters to Thomas Alexander, of the same date, Columbia University, Presbyterian Hospital School of Nursing C45-46 and C-31,[79] typed copies Wellcome RAMC 474/1

9 September 1858

With regard to your draft letter, I have thought over very attentively your conversation with Dr Sutherland last night. It is to be considered that you are asked to make arrangements for a thing whose arrangements you disapprove. Also, to construct a scheme of government for a thing which is entirely new, viz., *an invalid establishment*—the invalids and the sick from among the invalids never having been before under one roof. To do this will require a great deal of consideration. It seems to me that what you want for your information is:

1. Present number of invalids at Chatham;
2. Present number of sick in Fort Pitt from among invalids; the same for Yarmouth;
3. The total average invalids;
4. Total average sick from among invalids.

Then: (No. 1) average number of men *not* confined to bed. (No. 2) average number of men confined to bed. On No. 1 to scheme a plan of government and *discipline*, on No. 2 to scheme a plan of government and MEDICAL *and other attendance*. For No. 2 will be a hospital and No. 1 will be a lodging house, although under the same roof.

Then to find the number of medical officers required to visit invalids in St Mary's Casemates, and who perform no other duties. Or the number of medical officers *who would require* to give their whole time to visiting St Mary's Casemates.

On these data I would frame my scheme. Note, I have never thought of the subject before. But it seems to me that, for the *invalids*, one medical officer might inspect 100, and from two [to] four orderlies do for each flat. The two ends on each flat for *sick* I would mount

79 C31 appears to be the enclosure referred to in C46.

exactly on the footing of a hospital. But it would be impossible to frame any scheme till you have the foregoing data.

As far as getting Netley abandoned goes, I would send your draft letter as it is, for I think it will frighten the War Department. But this would hardly be fair.

On the whole, I think that, under your administration, there may ultimately be the greatest blessings to the poor soldier that ever were, even through the means of Netley. For you will take care that your medical officers report to you all the incipient pulmonary cases from everywhere. And these will, if sent down to Netley, derive the greatest benefit.

Meanwhile, it is necessary to consider it as an invalid establishment and to consider it as the *invalids* being the *rule*, and the *wounded* from foreign wars the *exception.*

I enclose what I have been thinking about the organization of Netley for your consideration. But, as there may be, and most likely is, error in it, I shall make no attempt to found any scheme of organization upon it (as it might prove wrong or extravagant) till I hear from you.

[Enclosure]
The more I think and inquire into the probable working of Netley Hospital, as originally designed by Dr Smith, the more difficult does the problem become. The present practice at Chatham appears to be as follows:

1. There are two establishments, Fort Pitt [and] St Mary's Casemates, in each of which a different discipline has, of course, to be carried out.

2. When a ship arrives with invalids, the bedridden are carried to Fort Pitt, and the convalescents are marched to St Mary's Casemates. Both detachments, according to the rules of the service, are considered to be "in hospital." (The invalids at St Mary's are passed through Fort Pitt for the sake of registering their cases.) Fort Pitt therefore contains a certain proportion of bedridden sick and a certain proportion of convalescents, not bedridden, the bulk of the convalescents being at St Mary's.

The sick and convalescents at Fort Pitt are under hospital discipline, which is not a disadvantage, seeing that the bedridden must always be a large proportion. The convalescents at St Mary's, on the contrary, are not under hospital discipline but are under a kind of regimental discipline under the adjutant. And any defaulters at daily drill are liable to be sent by the medical officer to Fort Pitt.

According to Dr Smith's idea, embodied in Netley, this simple and rational plan appears set aside. And, as all invalids and sick are to be placed in the same building, he must have intended one of two things: either all the *sick and invalids* were to be subjected to hospital discipline, with its medical officers, orderlies and nurses in due proportion (thirty-three medical officers, 100 orderlies, other servants—plus divisional medical officers). With the sick and dying mixed up in the same wards with convalescents and men in health, a principle contrary to all humanity as well as to all discipline, he would have committed an atrocity and an extravagance he never could have contemplated. Or he must have separated the sick from the convalescents and healthy and treated them by themselves in separate wards.

The Chatham experience has fully shown that there are two distinct classes of cases, requiring two distinct kinds of discipline and management. And as both of these classes are to be placed under the same roof at Netley, it will be necessary, for the sake of economy, to place them under different discipline. The sick with their orderlies, medical officers and nurses would, I think, be most economically and humanely administered in a part of the building specially provided for them. And the convalescents, not requiring constant medical attendance, might be put under a different scheme in another part of the building.

If this be not done, there would in all probability be a great outcry at the enormous and unnecessary cost of carrying out hospital arrangements for (say) 1000 sick, of whom only 150 *are* sick in bed. The disadvantage of such a division of sick from convalescents would be at the same time enormous. Because you would have, in fact, a barrack and a hospital under the same roof. If the thing had to be done again, the most economical as well as the most rational way, as it appears, would be to have a building separately organized as a hospital for sick, and the great Netley establishment to be confined to convalescents and men able to walk about, placed under special but *not* hospital discipline. It is not likely, however, you will ever get a separate sick hospital—and the problem therefore narrows itself into this: how best to obtain hospital accommodation and arrangements in one part of Netley, and invalid depot discipline in another. The end wards might be used for sick and cut off by doors from the remainder of the building, or a flat, which holds about 150 beds, might be set apart.

The subject is a very difficult one. And, so far as I can see, the practical objections to Netley as an invalid depot (altogether apart from its site and structure) are as great as they are against it as a general hospital. The country has been landed in an irretrievable mistake—and a very expensive mistake for its pocket, too.

Editor: Nightingale and Galton began to work jointly on plans for regimental hospitals in 1858, with the correspondence immediately below. The result, in 1862, was two sets of generic plans, one for hospitals of 60 beds, the other for 120 beds. As the correspondence shows, Nightingale gave great attention to the best fittings and materials. Galton evidently followed up as the package sent out to stations around the world gave precise details of the size needed, often with brand names or suppliers. An article in *The Builder* reproduced his memorandum "forwarded with the plans for the guidance of commanding royal engineers in the erection of regimental hospitals," with the plans for the 120-bed hospital. Galton further explained: "You will see that in these plans I have embodied the principles Miss Nightingale and you contend for." Thus the cubic space was 1200 per bed in temperate climates, 1500 in tropical climates, with superficial area from 85 to 100 square feet, respectively. Other specifications were:

* the site should be airy and well drained;

* no drains of any kind should pass under the buildings;

* the building should lie north and south, so as to secure the morning and evening sun upon ward windows;

* wards should never be more than two storeys in height;

* there should be circulation of air under all wood floors;

* there should be no basement under the wards, except to isolate them from the soil, and then well ventilated and drained, and not to communicate with the wards;

* walls limewhited;

* floors should be of hard, durable, non-absorbent wood;

* doors should have glazed panels, to allow wards to be overlooked;

* large wards to be warmed by open fireplaces, provision made for admission of fresh air to backs of stoves.

There are further details about flues and lavatories, earthenware water closets, soilpipes, wastepipes, traps, sinks and shelves. There are specifications for the scullery, kitchen, roasting range, gas lighting, foul-bedding store, washhouse and deadhouse, detached lavatories and water closets for convalescents and orderlies. If the building was to be built in a malarial climate, the sick were to be placed in an upper storey only. Additional thickness of walls and double windows were specified for cold climates.

Galton explained that one such hospital had already been erected at Hounslow and one at York Barracks, but as they were the first constructed, there were some defects in details, "which have been lessened in the plans now issued."[80] Again, Galton was following Nightingale's principle of starting small and gaining experience before generalizing plans.

Source: From a letter to Sidney Herbert, Wiltshire County Record Office, Pembroke Collection 2057/F4/66

Gt. Malvern
19 September 1858

In order that you may see that I have not been quite idle in your absence, I send you a few newspaper articles on Netley.[81] (These are not all.) In the next debate on Netley, I should like some MP to get up, unroll these, and a great many more, and remark upon the beautiful unanimity of the British press and the *common* sense of the public.

Please return me this curious literature, as I have no other copies of my works. I hope you will come here and look at this place—a very handy place when one can't go abroad—and I don't at all "want *not* to be seen." But I hope you will not dispute my coming to London, too.

Among other things I have to do there is this. They want a regimental hospital for sixty men for the hut camp at Woolwich. And they are so obliging as to say that Galton may furnish them with plans. I want it to be a model of regimental hospitals for unborn ages. It is a fine opportunity. We have the plans sketched out, but cannot go on with them till we all meet in London. Galton's draughtsman has sent down the first draught to me here.

Source: From a letter to Douglas Galton, Add Mss 45759 ff14-15

Gt. Malvern
23 September 1858

Your Mr McKenzie has sent me the plan and section of the regimental hospital proposed. But this, too, I have said had better stand over (as to discussion of any alteration in the plan) till your return.

---

80 "Official Plans for Military Hospitals," *The Builder* 20,1035 (6 December 1862):872-74.

81 See p 271 above.

Source: From a letter to Sidney Herbert, Wiltshire County Record Office, Pembroke Collection 2057/F4/67

[after 25 September 1858]

I send you the third article I wrote in *The Builder*, because it contains the *canons* of hospital construction, and is therefore more suited to the practical Cheetham than the Liverpool papers, which contain only its *defects*. Moreover, it is the only one not out of print. . . .

There are one or two things in the Netley appendix you have which I think we have rather altered our minds about, as concerns at least a small hospital.

Source: From a letter to Elizabeth Herbert,[82] Wiltshire County Record Office, Pembroke Collection 2057/F4/67

Gt Malvern

28 September 1858

Would you tell Mr Herbert sometime that Neison[83] has read a very mischievous paper at the British Association at Leeds, reproducing in full his fallacies about overcrowding having nothing to do with consumption, and condemning the conclusion of Mr Herbert's report? I have written to Farr about it because, if not answered, the matter will do us much harm. To be as short as possible, Neison adduces the Registrar-General's statistics as to overcrowding. Someone in the Registrar-General's office has totally mistaken the question of overcrowding and has produced great mischief to our cause, on account of these population tables being quoted as authority. Thus: . . .

Dotted circles, registration districts, of which the population is given by Registrar-General. Black circles, actual densely inhabited parts. Now *Greenhow*[84] compares the density within the dotted circles and *not*

---

82 Mary Elizabeth Herbert (1822-1911), wife of Sidney Herbert, friend.

83 Francis G.P. Neison (1847-?), statistician. In his paper, read 23 September, he argued that overcrowding did not intensify pulmonary disease, although it did so for zymotic diseases, and generally dismissed the conclusions of the royal commission report: see "On Phthisis in the Army," *Transactions of the British Association for the Advancement of Science* (1858):189-94.

84 Edward Headlam Greenhow (1814-88), lecturer on public health at St Thomas'; he published statistical analyses of disease, notably *On the Different Prevalence of Certain Diseases in Different Districts in England and Wales*, 1858.

within the black ones, and shows that, inasmuch as the Manchester one is much less densely peopled than the Liverpool one, and yet has the same mortality from phthisis, therefore density does not influence phthisis, *therefore* overcrowding is rather a healthy thing, the real fact being that the density for Manchester and Liverpool is very nearly the same.

Neison seems to have done the same thing. But the worst part is this: surface density has in reality nothing to do with the matter, and Mr Herbert never said it had. It is density *in rooms.* Our barracks have a smaller surface density generally than any town or perhaps village population in the kingdom, but they have generally a far higher room density. And this it is which does the mischief.

Dr Farr ought on public grounds to correct this public error, as far as the Registrar-General's statistics are concerned. And the best way would be for him to address a correction to Mr Herbert, as chairman of the royal commission.

I am going up to London on Saturday, because I don't want them to do anything about some regimental hospital plans without me.

Source: From six letters to Sidney Herbert, Wiltshire County Record Office, Pembroke Collection 2057/F4/67, and an undated memorandum 2057/F4/69

4 October 1858

Dr Sutherland is writing to you. And I think he will give you reasons why it is *not* essential to the progress of the business that you should be troubled to come up to town *just now.* All that is necessary can be sent down to you. I am very sorry to trouble you either with the reply to Neison at this time. Nor do I think there is any great hurry about it. You can consider it later. But Farr and Sutherland met here this morning. And they concluded that two things were necessary:

1. and least important, that Farr should make a statistical indirect attack on Neison's figures at the Liverpool meeting—for which we have furnished him with barrack and other data;

2. that some sort of official reply should be made by you, sent to the different late royal commissioners for their adhesion, a copy sent by Balfour to the *Times* for insertion, and another to Owen,[85] the president of the British Association meeting at Leeds, for insertion into the annual volume of their *Transactions with* Neison's paper.

85 Richard Owen (1804-92), doctor and paleontologist, later Sir; president of the British Association for the Advancement of Science in 1858.

I enclose what Farr and Sutherland suggest for your reply. These are merely heads and very diffuse. If you, in your own terse way, could some time write a reply of this kind (which Sutherland tells me you think is needed), it would set the question at rest. We would have it put up in type. . . .

Neison's paper reminds me of Lardner's famous paper which proved incontrovertibly by figures that the *Great Britain* could never cross the Atlantic. The Bristol people answered it by sending her across the Atlantic.[86] And Neison's paper will be answered by your curing or at least diminishing consumption in barracks.

5 October 1858

I send you the leader with Guy's answer to Neison.[87] It is good—much what we would have said ourselves—if taken not on the statistical but on the sanitary ground. It will bring Neison out and there will be a "row." . . .

The barrack commission are in their vanity very angry. Because all the military newspapers attribute your excellent system of ventilation to General Peel.

6 October 1848 [1858]

Neison has not only made the mistake you mention in your note, viz., of estimating the population of the great city of Wilton as extending over a larger area of Salisbury Plain, but he has confounded together *surface* overcrowding and overcrowding in *cubic space*, which are quite distinct things, e.g., the Metropolitan Model Lodging Houses exhibit a larger amount of surface overcrowding than perhaps any part of the metropolis. But they have a much larger amount of cubic space than the working classes usually have. And they are well ventilated and otherwise rendered healthy. Hence, in spite of their surface overcrowding, they are the most healthy part of the metropolis.

Neison's whole inquiry is simply a stupidity and nothing more. But he has some countenance for it in the fact that the Registrar-General's densities of population refer (not to inhabited areas but) to empirical

86 A reference to the successful crossing of the Atlantic by the world's then largest steamship, *Great Britain.* Dionysius Lardner, however, claimed to have been misquoted, that he had said that the voyage was practicable, but if the first attempt failed it would cast doubt on the enterprise (*Steam and Its Uses, Including the Steam Engine* 118).

87 William A. Guy (1810-85), professor of hygiene at King's College Hospital.

boundaries of all kinds. To correct Neison thoroughly, therefore, it would be necessary to show that the Registrar-General's method of estimating densities was incorrect.

If you think it necessary to take this line in the reply, we had better consult Farr, and get him to give an explanation. We have been going into the barrack part of it to which you allude. And we find on a superficial examination:

1. that the largest surface area in barracks is possessed by the Cavalry and Household Cavalry;
2. that the Infantry are somewhat more crowded on square area;
3. that the Guards are most crowded of all.

As regards cubic space we find:

1. that the Cavalry have much the largest amount;
2. that the Infantry come next in order;
3. that the Guards have least cubic space of all.

Next, as to the external ventilation of barracks, we find:

1. that the barracks of the Cavalry Household Cavalry Infantry are generally free from surrounding buildings and mostly in the open country, thereby exposing them to the free action of wind;
2. that the Guards barracks are so constructed and situated as to be extremely deficient in external ventilation.

Lastly, that the existing ventilating arrangements of barrack rooms are very nearly equally deficient in all arms of the service.

We have not as yet accurate statistical data. But if you think it necessary, they can be obtained from the returns. In regard to the reply, you will see by the "leader" sent yesterday that Dr Guy has confuted Neison generally. Perhaps you would think it better to wait till we see if Neison replies to Guy, which he probably will. And then your reply will be the more victorious. . . . Dr Balfour has just been here and says that he was requested by the editor of the *Medical Times* to write a leader for next Saturday in reply to Neison. He has done so and sent it in.[88] From what he says he has taken very much the same argument as Guy—only he has shown up Neison more completely from his better knowledge of what the commission really said. I will send it you. (It is of course *un*official.)

Balfour says that the warrant is gone to Balmoral for signature and will be gazetted in about ten days, that they have made some alterations not of great importance.

---

88 Presumably the unsigned "Mr Neison on the Causes of Consumption in the Army," *Medical Times and Gazette* 9 October 1858:374-75.

8 October 1858

Surface density has nothing to do *per se* with disease, but the conditions to which density gives rise. Distinguishing surface density from density in cubic space, the surface density of towns is not known, *in itself*, to exercise any influence whatever upon health. But wherever there is surface density, there are in unimproved towns sanitary defects which give to surface density its power of producing disease—defective cleansing, drainage, etc. Even Neison assumes (what is contrary to fact) that, in towns of all densities, these defects are to the same amount. Thus just as the effect of overcrowding depends within limits on defective ventilation, the effect of surface density depends on the accompanying sanitary conditions. No correct vital statistician would ever adduce surface overcrowding or overcrowding in cubic space as *per se* forming an element in his calculations.

It is consistent with experience that two-storeyed houses may be so crowded as to give a higher surface density than that of five or six-storeyed houses. Into such a comparison the width of streets is not made to enter.

We can get out accurately the statistics of overcrowding in the Guards. The barrack returns in the royal commission report (imperfect as they are) show that the overcrowding is greatest in the Guards, in cubic space. And the numbers of barrack flats shows that the density is also greatest in surface. The barracks at Chatham are only occupied about six weeks by the same men. They don't, like the other barracks, enter into the system of rotation.

The infantry barracks, hitherto examined by the barracks commission, comprise the most overcrowded in the U.K. The average space in the Irish infantry barracks is much larger. Until the average is corrected for the Irish barracks, we cannot get the proportionate overcrowding for the infantry generally. With this proviso, the deficiency of accommodation at 600 cubic ft. per man stands as follows:

Household Calvary	7+ percent
Infantry Barracks } *excluding* Chatham}	25 percent
Foot Guards	26 percent

so that, exclusive of Chatham, but including all the other worst barracks (which are the southeastern ones), the infantry are still 1 percent better off than the Guards—*all* the Guards' barracks being taken and *not* the best infantry barracks. We are however going to ascertain the amount of cubic space in the three classes of barracks accurately—and will send it you. . . .

The Regulations have traveled *as far as* Robertson (purveyor-in-chief) at the War Office. There they have stuck. He "can't understand them at all." To us it sounds like finding out where the hitch is in the Atlantic telegraph. But I am not sure that the bottom of the Atlantic is not a less hopeless place than the bottom of the W.O. The diet tables have also stuck, in the same manner and at the same place. The council has stuck, but *not* at the same place.

25 October 1858

1. I *am* glad you did not answer Neison, because now we shall have all his say out, and be able to answer it in a lump. Neison believes man to be solely influenced by what he *does*. He is quite guiltless of all physiological, climate or sanitary knowledge—was himself a working man and thinks work the only element in our lives and healths.

2. *The* pamphlet which Neison asks after *is* the pamphlet I sent you last night.

3. The *Guards* are about to build a general hospital for the three regiments on the site of one of their regimental hospitals in Westminster. Nothing is settled yet. They would be very glad to receive hints, *provided* they may have all the credit of them (which you have no objection to) and provided they are not lectured officially. We were only waiting for you to come home to ask you to ask them to put the plans onto your hands, when, if you would send them to us, Sutherland and I would do our best. They are quite incapable of doing it themselves. But it must not be *official*.

4. I have gone through all the figures in Smith's Blue big Book today. And the result is simply this (a result which I must say has astonished even my old mind). In the six months October 1854 to March 1855 there are 735 deaths (unaccounted for—not included in *any* of the medical mortality statistics which have yet been presented to Parliament) which agrees (within 2) with what Smith says himself. Smith—regardless of exposure, as it seems—has plastered on with a trowel upon those six months thus:

Oct	211
Nov	9
Dec	151
Jan	239
Feb	122
Mar	3
[total]	735 upon Scutari and sick transport promiscuously.

This, if calculated into the rate of mortality, will raise it considerably *above* what Farr calculated and the "Anonymous" complains of. I must say I feel inclined to do it—heartsick as I am of the subject. If you feel inclined to put a note to your article. . . .

Further, the "Anonymous" has taken the head roll of burials from February, which I stated expressly to be for Scutari *alone*, and substituted it for the medical returns which are for Scutari *and* Koulali (the most unhealthy of all the hospitals[89]) together. See p 362 and p 391, Table IV, Report R. Commission, add the Koulali deaths to the burials at Scutari and, so far from the mortality having been overstated, it has been understated by 124 deaths.[90]

5 November 1858

There are 73,000 letters in thirty-two pages of *Westminster Review* type and 54,000 letters in what you have written already or about twenty-four pages of *Westminster Review.* (I assure you I have not done this by counting like a "learned pig"). The consequence I am very sorry for. We do not find any "medical heresies," or anything which require reconsideration, except Mr Chapman's space.[91]

If we could see the whole at once, I think we should be able to consider better what must be left in and what cut out. As it is, I incline to resuming about twenty (written) pages of controversy with Neison into three or four, and curtailing the rest as little as possible. I wish we could see the second half before suggesting any curtailment in this, however.

We have got the Aldershot statistics from Alexander. They are very favourable and (when calculated) may be inserted in this article, we think, with good effect as an illustration. Mortality from phthisis about 2 per 1000 only.

I have taken advantage of your condemnation of anonymous newspaper writing to indulge in an unrestrained course of the same of a vicious nature. As it is only in *The Builder*s, however, I am not incurably outrageous, I shall send you the course. (They attacked us on contagion.[92])

---

89 Dr Sutherland, in his evidence to the royal commission on 17 July 1857, said that the sanitary defects were "the most serious" at Koulali. U.K., *Report of the Commissioners* 2:334.

90 Quoted in Nightingale's own written evidence to the royal commission, in *The Crimean War* (14:961).

91 John Chapman (1822-94), editor of the *Westminster Review.*

92 This is possibly a reference to E. Headlam Greenhow, "Preventible Disease," *The Builder* 16,821 (30 October 1858):722-23, to which Nightingale responded in the next issue.

I *did* not agree with you about anonymous writing. But the *Times* has put itself so completely in the wrong that I think most people will agree with you now. However, the *Times* never can give up anonymous writing. In a mere mercantile speculation, which such a paper is, how could it?

Mr Neison, before the British Association, he calls in question the propriety and probable efficiency of certain recommendations made by the Royal Commission on the Sanitary State of the Army, the object of which is to diminish the risk of the British soldier to consumption and other chest diseases by diminishing the overcrowding and increasing the ventilation of the soldiers' dormitory. He attempts to show, by reference to the mortality statistics of towns and districts, in which the density of population varies, that, while there is a certain ratio of increase in the proportion of deaths from zymotic diseases and consumption corresponding to the increase of density, the proportionate increase from the latter disease by no means follows so rapid a rate of increase as ought to be due to the increase of density, if increase of density were really so powerful an operative cause of consumption as he supposes the royal commission to have stated. And he argues that, inasmuch as the mortality for phthisis and other diseases of the chest forms by far the largest portion of the soldier's mortality, and as his statistics show that density of population is not followed by anything like so large a proportion of deaths from consumption as exists among soldiers, that therefore the commissioners have arrived at an erroneous conclusion as to the cause of consumption in the British Army, and that therefore the measures for reducing the overcrowded state of barrack rooms recommended by the commission will not be followed by the anticipated results as to health.

In the first place, Mr Neison has entirely mistaken what the report really does say on the subject. The term *overcrowding*, when used with reference to health, always implies certain sanitary conditions as to ventilation, cleansing, drainage, etc., and it is so used in the report of the royal commission. It is nowhere stated in the report that consumption is occasioned simply by overcrowding.

The following passage contains the comparison between the army and civil life:

> It may be stated that, in civil life, insufficient clothing, insufficient and unwholesome food, sedentary and unwholesome occupations and the vitiated atmosphere of unhealthy dwellings all contribute to the propagation of this class of diseases ([FN] pulmonary). But in

> the army it cannot be alleged that the clothing, the food or the nature of the occupation in itself are of a character which would justify the imputation that they are among the predisposing causes of the excessive mortality of the soldier by pulmonary disease. If therefore it can be shown that the soldier in barracks breathes a vitiated and polluted atmosphere, it follows that, of the four predisposing causes above enumerated, the last is the one to which the excessive liability of the soldier to this class of disease may be chiefly attributed.
>
> The facts above stated lead us to the conclusion that the ravages committed in the ranks of the army by pulmonary disease are to be traced in a great degree to the vitiated atmosphere generated by overcrowding and deficient ventilation and the absence of proper sewerage in barracks.

After describing the overcrowding and ventilation of the barrack rooms, the report proceeds as follows:

> The result is that the soldier sleeps in a fetid and unwholesome atmosphere, the habitual breathing of which, though producing for the most part no direct immediate effects, probably lays the seeds of that pulmonary disease which is so fatal in the British Army.[93]

To remedy these evils, the commission recommend that 600 cubic feet of space be allotted to each man in his barrack room and guard room—and that a commission be appointed for "the thorough ventilation of barracks, the diminution of overcrowding, the abolition of cesspools and the formation of proper drainage and sewerage, and an abundant water supply.[94]

It will be observed that the report nowhere states overcrowding *by itself* as being a cause of consumption, and that it nowhere prescribes increased space *by itself* as the remedy—so that Mr Neison's assumption, both as to the causation of phthisis and the means of preventing it stated in the report, is entirely gratuitous. In the course of his reasoning, Mr Neison has confounded together two kinds of overcrowding, viz., overcrowding *on surface* and overcrowding *in cubic space*, which have quite distinct sanitary relations.

Surface overcrowding, together with neglect of sanitary precautions, has been long known to predispose to zymotic and pestilential diseases.

93 From the *Report of the Commissioners* 1:xv-xvii.

94 This last paragraph is a paraphrase from the *Report of the Commissioners* 1:xxx-xvii.

Mr Neison's statistics on this point have merely confirmed the observations of all writers on the public health. Overcrowding in unventilated cubic space, if it take place even in a solitary house on the hillside, may predispose to asphyxia, consumption and zymotic diseases generally. Even if the report had asserted that overcrowding *per se* in barrack rooms was the cause of consumption, it would be no answer whatever to state that consumption was not observed to increase in proportion to *surface* overcrowding.

For, as already stated, the two things are quite distinct. The report nowhere states that surface overcrowding is connected with the prevalence of phthisis *in the army*. And it is hence no reply whatever to show, even if it were correct, which it is not, that surface overcrowding *in towns and districts* and consumption do not go hand in hand.

But when Mr Neison meets the allegation of the report that overcrowding in cubic space, *together with* defective ventilation and other sanitary defects, predispose to phthisis, by an attempt to prove that surface overcrowding does *not* predispose to phthisis, or at all events that it does so in a minor degree, his conclusion is simply a *non sequitur*. He first mistakes the meaning of the report, he then assumes a meaning which the report was never intended to convey, and he then contradicts what he assumes and in so doing has given himself a greater amount of unnecessary labour.

N.B. If you agree to this or to something like this, it might be set up in type and circulated among the members of the late royal commission.

Editor: Malta was a major base of operations for the British Army, with large numbers of wives and children living there as well as soldiers. It was a stopping point en route to India. Nightingale herself had visited Malta in her days of travelling pre-Crimea. (Her ship also landed there on the way to the Crimean War, but she was too seasick to get out.) By the time of this correspondence she would at least have had a basic familiarity not only with the physical location but the garrison's many uses.

Malta has already received much coverage in the section on *Notes on Hospitals* in this volume—for the Valetta Military Hospital, see Plan 7. However, that hospital was never built, as a result of cutbacks in the War Office budget.

Source: From a letter and an undated note to Sidney Herbert, Wiltshire County Record Office, Pembroke Collection 2057/F4/67 and /69

10 November 1858

Malta is to have a new general hospital for 500. Plans have been granted for 300. They are come to England for approval. Mennie[95] has them in his hands. Burrell has seen them. He says they are atrocious. They must be bad indeed, if my old Burrell says so.

It is eminently legitimate for you to ask for them, because you have recommended a general hospital at Malta. Both Burrell, Sutherland and I are well acquainted with the intended locality at Malta. Would not you ask for these pestilential plans to be submitted to you?

Note on Malta Hospital.

1. So far as we can judge, the proposed site is better than the Floriana site, first proposed.

2. It would be a great advantage to have Lieutenant Brooke, R.E., in this country while the plans are being drawn and considered.

3. In order not to lose time, would you ask Colonel Owen for a plan of the whole *plateau available for the hospital and its grounds,* including the area which it is proposed to purchase? This will enable us to consider in the meantime the plan of the building.

The plans now returned, and which please send back to us, do not give the available area with sufficient clearness. The plan we want is the one which gives the available area coloured.

Editor: Major sections of Nightingale's massive *Notes on the Health of the British Army* are reproduced in *The Crimean War.* A few sections seemed to fit better here, as looking forward to new administrative procedures for hospitals, barracks and data collection to track epidemics in them.

Source: From *Notes on Matters Affecting the Health, Efficiency and Hospital Administration of the British Army.* London: Harrison 1858:323-31, 525-26, 545-46

Illustration of the imperfect Nomenclature of Disease.

The importance of using a more elaborate and specific nomenclature of disease is shown, from the consideration that the "febris c.c." (common continuous fever) of the British military hospital, a term including typhus, typhoid fever, relapsing fever and febricula, indicates neither the origin of the disease nor the kind of treatment,

95 R.O. Mennie, surveyor of works at the War Office.

inasmuch as it is made to include every kind of fever, together with drunkenness. We want a new heading, "drunken fever," to separate these casualties from fevers arising from other causes. All apoplexies, almost without exception in our army, might be styled "drunken apoplexy." A formal posting of the drunken statistics might exercise a salutary influence. In the proposed nosology of Dr Farr, we find the disease termed "alcoholismus," which includes "delirium tremens." This last is made to appear in army statistics under "diseases of the brain." But the terms which are used, e.g., in the Sardinian Army, and copied from our own civil Registrar-General's Office (with the addition of some diseases incidental to camps), *do* indicate both the origin of the disease and the mode of cure, and the mode of prevention. General La Marmora[96] was visited, in consequence of a request from home, by one of our sanitary commissioners, who was able to discover, from private returns, the absence of vegetable food, or the peculiarities of the encampment, as the remediable cause of the disease.

Another example of want of definition, still stronger than that of febris c.c., which includes tipsy headaches, is the heading "all other diseases," which has been seen to occupy 50 percent of a given register. This is *Hamlet,* with half of the "part of Hamlet left out."

If classification means assigning a place to each object, this is not classification.

Necessity of a Statistical Department for the Army in general. Colonel Tulloch's Materials.

It is essentially necessary that we should have an Army Statistical Department. Hitherto all that has been done for the army in this way has been done by the able Colonel Sir Alexander Tulloch, at first as a labour of love. From him should now be obtained,

1. A summary of the results of all his statistical inquiries into the mortality and diseases of the army.

2. A comparison between the mortality of *(a)* officers, *(b)* privates and non-commissioned officers, at the several ages specified in his reports, *(c)* distinguishing cavalry and infantry, *(d)* distinguishing results in England and Wales, Scotland, Ireland, foreign or colonial stations.

3. Taking each station, as West Coast of Africa, West Indian islands, East Indies, Mediterranean, etc., a statement of *(a)* What the mortality of the army is collectively at each of such stations, *(b)* what

96 Alfonso Ferrero La Marmora (1804-78), commander of the Sardinian troops in the Crimean War, later prime minister of Italy.

mortality of the native population and of the troops at corresponding ages, where this is known. Now, is it not a fact that the mortality of the British soldier exceeds the mortality of the civil population in many of those stations abroad?

Looking at home, and comparing the mortality of the soldier year by year, in ordinary times and in epidemic years, with the mortality of the civil population, is not the mortality of the soldier excessive? To what extent, we ought now to know, is the mortality of the army excessive? How many in the 1000 perish annually in excess of the mortality experienced amongst healthy classes of the community?

It has been attempted, in the preceding section, to give an accurate, though short and imperfect, answer to this. The mortality of the general population, as has there been shown, embraces the mortality of vagrants, of nearly 1,000,000 paupers (vide [see] Poor Law Returns) and of all the weakest and worst people in the country, as well as the healthy and vigorous. If such classes as the former were excluded, would not the mortality of the residue be greatly below the general average? Now, in the army, is there not a double selection constantly at work having a direct tendency to reduce the percentage of mortality?

The tests of health which the recruit has to undergo, before he can become a soldier, exclude all labouring under actual disease, such as consumption, and some of those predisposed to disease.

Again, if a soldier becomes consumptive, he is discharged or pensioned, in many cases before he is cured or dead. Now, what is the annual rate of mortality per 1000 among soldiers so discharged or pensioned, during the months after discharge: 0-3, 3-6, 6-9, 9-12?

It is to be feared that this is very high, from the imperfect data given at p 259, Sanitary Section. Now, if the strength of the invalided, one year after discharge from the army at home, and the deaths among them, were added to the strength and deaths of the army from which they are drawn, would not the mortality be raised considerably higher, as has been shown for five years, 1849-53, in the same sanitary notes?

What kind of diseases are, then, so fatal to the Guards, the Infantry and the Cavalry at home? If it is consumption, is not consumption the effect of bad ventilation chiefly? If it is fever, is not fever always preventible? What are the causes to which the bad sanitary state of the army is attributable? and how should these causes be combated?

At home, the Line suffers twice as much from consumption as men in civil life at the same ages. It suffers more than twice as much from zymotic disease. Now, there is no *à priori* reason for this. The mere statement of it would excite inquiry into its causes and their remedies, if generally made known.

Comparison of the Mortality of the Line with that of the Civil Population

Annual Rate of Mortality, Per 1000 Living from *All Causes, Zymotic Diseases, Chest and Tubercular Diseases,* and *Other Causes,* amongst the *English Male Population* (1848-54), and amongst the *Infantry of the Line,* Serving at Home (1837-46)

	Annual Rate of Mortality per 1000 living	
Causes of Death	Males aged 15 to 45 in England and Wales during the seven years 1848-54	Infantry of the Line, serving at Home, during the ten years 1837-46
All Causes	9.7	16.7
Zymotic Diseases	1.9	4.9
Chest and Tubercular Diseases	4.5	9.2
Other Causes	3.3	2.6

The deaths in England and Wales (1848-54) are taken from the Registrar-General's 18th Annual Report, p 150; and the deaths in the Infantry of the Line from Colonel Tulloch's Report of 1853, p 62.

Now, recurring to the latest date of Colonel Sir A. Tulloch's valuable reports, which is, we believe, 1853, and the last date in which referred to is 1846—recurring to the non-arrangement for their regular publication, we would ask, is there any *annual* medical and sanitary report whatever published, containing summaries and analyses of the reports of the medical officers of the army?

Why cannot what is done with apparent ease for Civilians, be done for Soldiers, in whose case the facilities of Registration are so much greater?

If the causes of death among 2,600,000 people in London can be printed *weekly*, on the Tuesday following the week, and if the births and deaths for the whole of England and Wales can be printed *quarterly*, within a month of the end of every quarter, could not classified returns of the attacks of sickness, and of the mortality of the army, be published periodically, with equal punctuality?

Does not the organization of the army offer the greatest facilities known for statistical registration? Could not the *mean strength* of each regiment be determined by monthly musters? Could not the *mean number* of *sick* from fever, consumption and other causes be determined by the same method?

Were the *strength* thus determined compared with the *deaths* by the various causes, and with the *attacks of sickness*, a complete view would thus be obtained of the main results of the sanitary or fatal influences to which the regiment had been exposed. If these results could be collected for *one* regiment, they could be collected for every regiment. This follows necessarily from the army organization.

The practical utility of such information would be greatly increased by its embracing the whole army, and above all by its being collected and analyzed immediately, the object being for the secretary of state for the War Department to be able to see the movements of the health of the army as clearly as the movements of time on the face of a clock.

The great utility of partial returns, published many years after the events have happened, after the men to which they relate are dead or have been discharged, has been shown by Sir A. Tulloch's Blue Books. Would not complete returns of the whole facts for every portion of the army be still more useful than these partial returns? Would not recent information, punctually supplied, be practically of greater use than the retarded, almost posthumous returns which have hitherto been published in England?

The difference in the efficiency of a healthy and an unhealthy army has been practically illustrated in the most terrible manner by our late Crimean campaign, where more than half the infantry was sick in hospital at once, part of the remaining half was told off to attend upon them, and the remainder only was capable of trench and fatigue duty, and of keeping the position.

It is unquestionable—and our experience of the way in which, in civil life, mortality can be, and has been, reduced, need hardly be referred to—it is unquestionable that the mortality and sickness of the army in peace may be reduced to one half, at most, of its present excessive amount. It is a thing beyond all doubt to be done. The degree to which this would affect our system of recruiting, our system of pensioning, the well-being of our men can scarcely be calculated.

One question remains: are vital statistics made a branch of medical education? Are the medical officers examined on this subject? To what extent have published works of army medical officers assisted Sir A. Tulloch in his statistical researches? Twenty years hence it will scarcely be credited that a time has been, so late as the year 1857, when there was nothing analogous to our civil General Register Office in military organization.

Main end of Statistics.

The main end of statistics should not be to inform the government as to how many men have died, but to enable immediate steps to be taken to prevent the extension of disease and mortality.

It is therefore of paramount importance to have special reporting for special occasions, e.g., the yellow fever breaks out in consequence of the locality or overcrowding of a barrack, or dysentery in consequence of monotony of diet.

If the government had known, week by week, that scorbutus was ravaging the army in the Crimea, the very first appearance of the disease in the weekly states, with a reason why the disease had appeared at all, would have led the government immediately to have sought for the requisite supplies to arrest it. If the medical officer waits till the time of reporting comes round, all that is accomplished is that the government know that they have lost a certain number of hundreds of men in a way which might have been prevented.

In France, in the event of an epidemic breaking out in any part of the army, the facts are noted, day by day, to the "Conseil de Santé" at Paris, who notify them, day by day, to the minister for war. It is therefore to be concluded that, from the above considerations, that:

1. Whatever statistical system be adopted should be uniform, and in every case where there is likely to be any doubt as to the precise meaning of a nosological term, it ought to be defined.

2. Whatever period is laid down for sending in the statistical reports, these periods should be departed from at the first appearance of any epidemic in the army. And the progress of the disease, with its *causes*, the means adopted to arrest it and the success of these means, should be reported, day by day, to the War Department, wherever practicable.

3. An officer should be attached to the Army Medical Department, with suitable assistance, to enable him to make up the army statistics with due accuracy. (One form, made up at home, should be the same as the Registrar-General's form.)

4. There being already an authorized and official form of registration for the mortality in Great Britain, it is in the highest degree important that the form used in the army should be the same.

5. The registration of disease and mortality would come under the Statistical Department of the Army Medical Department, for all medical and sanitary purposes, while the mortality might be very well transmitted to the Registrar-General's Office and published quarterly. (It appears to follow, from the proposal to transfer the statistics of death from the War Department to the Registrar-General's Department, that the same form of registration should be used.)

6. The forms required for such a purpose of army medical statistics as are here proposed, are

I. Weekly regimental state, showing strength (the regimental medical statistics should be kept on the same form as that used by the Registrar-General of England)

1. Zymotic diseases under their various heads
2. Mortality from these
3. More prominent diseases of other classes and mortality from these
4. All other diseases
5. Total admissions during the week
6. Total deaths during the week
7. Percentage of admissions from zymotic disease to total admissions
8. Percentage of deaths from zymotic disease to total deaths from disease
9. Admissions and deaths from wounds.

(This return to show the *causes* of zymotic disease and mortality in connection with 1 and 2.) Return, as already proposed, to be made up by the principal medical officer and sent home week by week, to the War Department, and also to the commanding officer.

III. General Hospitals

III. General Hospitals. Defects.

A great amount of mismanagement, failure and suffering resulted in the late war from the want of some supreme officer, who should be held responsible for the health and efficiency of the hospitals at the base of operations.

Suggestions.

The only way to prevent similar occurrences is to determine:

1. That a governor be selected and named by the secretary of state for war, by whom the other officers, heads of departments in the hospital, should also be named. In the event of a vacancy occurring on service, the commander of the forces to make a provisional appointment, subject to the approval of the secretary of state.

2. That all officers of engineers, sanitary officers or others employed on the application of the governor to carry on duties connected with the hospital be under the authority of the governor while so employed.

3. That all the labour required to carry out plans approved by the governor, under the directions of any department, be obtained or hired by the governor or by his written directions, and not otherwise.

4. That the government and control of the hospital be vested in the governor, except so far as relates to the medical and surgical treatment of the patients by the medical officers.

5. That the governor of a general hospital, whether he be a military or medical officer or a civilian, be considered and assume the functions and be vested with the powers of a civil governor.

6. That there be attached to the hospital one or more military officers of the Adjutant-General's Department, subject to the authority of the governor, to conduct the discipline of convalescents, when necessary, and to see that they are properly equipped when they proceed to join the depôt.

7. That all orders or requisitions of the principal medical officer, or of the steward, for supplies for the hospital shall be ineffective unless countersigned by the governor.

8. That the hospital be not dependent upon the Commissariat for any supplies, but that the Commissariat honour the drafts of a treasurer, countersigned by the governor, for the expenses of the hospital, including the pay of the officers, attendants and others attached to it, and that the governor be held responsible for the due and proper disbursement and application of the funds.

9. That the duties of the purveyor be equivalent to those of the steward in a civil hospital.

10. That no contracts for supplies to the hospital which the steward may propose to make be concluded until approved and countersigned by the governor, unless when made at a distance from the hospital by written instructions from the governor, by whom, in that case, they must subsequently be countersigned.

11. That all contracts for supplies contain a clause authorizing the steward to purchase in the market, at the cost of the contractor, any supplies which the contractor may fail to deliver in terms of his contract—if they are immediately required.

12. That all transport by sea or land required by the steward for the purposes of the hospital be obtained or provided by the governor, as also the transport required by the principal medical officer for stores strictly medical. . . .

[The last two paragraphs of the report:]
The sanitary improvements in barracks, hospitals and garrisons need not be delayed, but might be at once proceeded with, and special provision should be made for this work. So far as is known, certain improvements could be carried out with little difficulty and small cost, but others would require the execution of more perma-

nent works. Every barrack, hospital and garrison should be examined with reference to the sanitary condition, and all experience has shown that it is essentially necessary that the examination should be made, the nature of the sanitary works and their extent determined, and the works themselves executed, under the direction of persons competent to deal with special sanitary defects; otherwise the recommendations and suggestions made will be so unwise, and the cost so extravagant, that the whole thing will be brought into discredit.

The army mortality can be and ought to be brought down to 8½ per 1000. Of this there is no doubt; the model lodging houses, where 300-700 persons are congregated in a close space under good sanitary conditions, afford a convincing proof of it, if any such were wanted. (The model lodging houses were built for health and show a rate of mortality little more than one half of that of London. The common lodging houses were built for disease, but, under sanitary inspection, showed, in 1854, one sixth of the rate of cholera mortality in the whole metropolis. The barracks are built for disease and show twice the rate of mortality from consumption, more than twice that from cholera and fever, and nearly twice that from all diseases, which is shown by the civil population.)

It will be found that the repair of men is more expensive than the repair of buildings, and that these buildings may be put to rights at a cost equal to that of the treatment of the sick who come out of them.

Source: From a letter to T. Graham Balfour, Add Mss 50134 ff65-67

Christmas Eve [1858]

Many thanks for the pamphlet and also for the promise of the statistics.

I think, having referred to the passage to which you take exception, that our difference is merely one of words, viz., that between vital and sanitary statistics. By statistics bearing upon the health of an army or any other body, I don't mean statistics which prove that one station is healthy and another unhealthy, or one town healthy and another unhealthy. Those are vital statistics.

In no one published document with which I am acquainted is there any indication of statistics having been used in the manner I desire. I could only deal with published documents. And I have seen none, either in the army or out of it, at all up to the mark. The council of the new Army Medical Department will have to organize and carry out, for the first time, a system of sanitary statistics, i.e., bearing upon the health of the troops totally different from any I have ever seen.

And it was to the necessity of such a system that my remark was applied. Vital statistics are a basis without which we can do nothing; sanitary statistics indicate the direction in which we are to work—this direction has never yet been given us. Vital statistics are only of use in the practical application of hygiene insofar as they subserve the latter. And not until we have a complete system of sanitary statistics *in* the army shall we be able to administer the laws of health with that certainty with which we know they are capable of being administered.

A Contribution to the Sanitary History of the British Army

Editor: *A Contribution to the Sanitary History of the British Army* is a short, seldom-read and greatly underestimated paper by Nightingale. It takes up the great issue of Crimean War hospital deaths just after the completion of her major analysis, *Notes on the Health of the British Army*, and the first version of "Notes on Hospitals," both late 1858. Published in January 1859, *A Contribution* was, in part, a response to Andrew Smith's two-volume report on the war hospitals, *Medical and Surgical History of the British Army*, published in late 1858. Quite apart from its failure to recognize the enormity of the losses or make any attempt to propose improvements to save lives in the future, Smith's work contained puzzling new figures on deaths in sea transport. Nightingale here offered an intriguing account, discussed earlier in a letter to Sidney Herbert (see p 319 above).

In this new, short paper, Nightingale gives a brief step-by-step account of the Crimean disaster, stressing inadequacies in food, shelter and clothing, given the fatiguing workload and fierce winter conditions the army faced. Individuals are not blamed by name (as many were in *Notes on the Health of the British Army*) but "three things" said to have "all but destroyed the army . . . ignorance, incapacity and useless rules" (see p 349 below). From the analysis it is clear that the errors went well beyond those made by the Army Medical Department, all the way up to the army high command and the War Office:

> It appears a mere truism to insist that an army taking the field should be provided with supplies, transport, clothing, shelter and appliances for the sick and wounded. And yet the army in the Crimea almost perished for want of these [see p 351 below].

Oddly, the only people who were faulted by name were several post-war authors whose statistical analysis she thought got the causes of death wrong, especially by making "contagion" the culprit and downplaying overcrowding and bad ventilation as causes of disease and death.

The paper reports only a small number of figures, focusing on three major tables with associated charts. These are Nightingale's now-famous polar area charts, which first appeared in the (privately circulated) *Notes on the Health of the British Army*, where they were swamped by other data and analysis. Here they are prominent.

The basic death data were taken from Smith's (official) figures, reworked by Farr into deaths by "strength," or numbers serving. Two of Nightingale's charts are of particular interest for permitting both comparisons over time (highlighting the declining number of deaths after the sanitary and supply commissions set to work) and comparatively: one measures the Crimean War rates against those for the Manchester men of similar ages, the other against soldiers in army hospitals in peacetime in and near London.

Nightingale was mightily proud that, in time, with reforms brought in, the death rates at Scutari and Koulali were brought down. By the end of the war they were no greater than those of peacetime army hospitals in and near London, and no greater than among similar civilian men (in Manchester). These were the points to be made in her two innovative black-and-white polar area charts, and to which she often referred.

A Contribution also serves as a major rebuttal to the extraordinary accusations of Hugh Small, who wrote in *Florence Nightingale: Avenging Angel*, that it was her "negligence and arrogance" that caused the loss of the army, and that she suffered from "repressed guilt" as a result of this supposed fact (126). Small makes his points about guilt, repression and high death rates repeatedly, citing "complete mental and physical collapse" (3), "failure" (199), "shortcomings" and "blamed herself" (119), "blunder" and "failure" (121), "extreme anguish," "blame for the disaster" and "shame" (123) and "breakdown" (125). Far from blaming herself for the loss of the army, however, *A Contribution* shows that Nightingale attributed it to "very glaring disobediences" to the laws of health, suggesting a causal chain beginning with inadequate nutrition, and matters clearly the responsibility of the Army Medical Department.

Small also mistakenly and repeatedly described her hospital, the Barrack Hospital at Scutari, as the hospital with the highest death rate, for which he cited no data—and no such data are known to this editor. Yet, as the 1859 paper makes clear (as does *Notes on the Health of the*

British Army) the "Scutari" rates are for four to six hospitals combined: her Barrack Hospital, the General Hospital (under the superintendence of H. Tebbutt and under Nightingale's overall jurisdiction), the Palace Hospital, Stable Hospital and two ships. For some months these data were combined also with those of the hospital at Koulali (see her Table 3) under the superintendence initially of Mary Stanley, then Mary Francis Bridgeman, with the Irish Sisters of Mercy mainly as nurses—and not under Nightingale's jurisdiction at all. Nightingale never blamed Stanley, Bridgeman or the nuns for the high death rates at Koulali, for they were no more responsible for the unsanitary conditions at their hospital than Nightingale was at the one to which she was assigned. She was well aware that the sanitary defects at Koulali were even "more serious" than at Scutari (see p 320 above), and reported as such by the head of the sanitary commission, Dr Sutherland.[97]

The French statisticians did not make this mistake, but show the rates as having combined data from Scutari and Koulali.[98] The source for all of them, ignored by Small, was Andrew Smith's official report, *Medical and Surgical History of the British Army*. Smith did not pay the death rates serious heed, and indeed buried them in the second volume (Table I, 2:480). However, these data have been available in print since 1858, and on-line in more recent years.

Small is far-fetched in his faulting of Nightingale for failure to collect death statistics herself (121), although he did acknowledge that it might not have been her job (122). Yet, as *A Contribution to the Sanitary History* shows, the British Army was already collecting a massive amount of statistical data—with conflicting figures by source. The prospect of one further data set helping at all is hard to imagine, as is the willingness of doctors to submit data to yet another collector, no less than the nursing superintendent working under their orders. One has also to imagine Nightingale having had access to a printing press to produce

---

97 John Sutherland, evidence 17 July 1857, United Kingdom, *Report of the Commissioners Appointed to Inquire into the Regulations Affecting the Sanitary Condition of the Army and the Treatment of the Sick and Wounded* 2:334.

98 Jean-Charles Chenu, *De la mortalité dans l'armée, et des moyens d'économiser la vie humaine, extraits des statistiques médico-chirurgicales*; Gaspard M. Scrive, *Relation médico-chirurgicale de la Campagne d'Orient du 31 mars 1854, occupation de Gallipoli, au 6 juillet 1856, évacuation de la Crimée*; Léon Le Fort, "Guerres de Crimée et d'Amérique," *Gazette hebdomadaire de médecine et chirurgie* 2e série t. 5 (17 July 1868):449-53.

forms and staff to administer them. The difficulty with British Army statistics was not failure to collect yet another set, but utter failure to analyze, publish and learn from the existing data in a timely fashion.

Far from feeling guilty over the death rates of the Crimean War hospitals, Nightingale was proud of the results when the reforms were brought in. The polar area charts clearly mark the arrival of the sanitary and supply commissions, after which the death rates began to drop. By the time the army left for England in 1856, it was in a "more healthy state and with a lower amount of mortality" than when it set foot in the East, or at any time at home (see p 345 below).

Nightingale was puzzled by Andrew Smith's publication of some new statistics on death rates during transport, showing them to have been higher than those previously reported, and this puzzlement is the subject of a letter to Sidney Herbert (see p 319 above). She had already dealt with the great disparities in numbers by source, and here again tackled the subject. She reported the "remarkable fact" that Smith's reports of deaths in transit from the Crimea to Scutari, from 1 October 1854 to 28 February 1855, totalled 883, or 177 more than in the returns of deaths officially made by surgeons on board the ships. Either the surgeons made erroneous statements at the time, or the statistics were later "dressed" to account for 177 deaths, "which we adopt as the more probable hypothesis." The statement that the director general of the Army Medical Department deliberately fudged figures in an official report is an astonishing accusation, yet it seems that no secondary author has ever noticed it. Nightingale used these and other discrepancies to argue for a statistical section within the Army Medical Department, essential "before anything like sanitary progress is possible" (see p 342 below).

Nightingale's devotion to scientific explanation is succinctly stated in this paper. Mortality rates are determined by laws of nature, the "laws of health," which can be ascertained by research. The same laws govern life and death in civil and military hospitals, so that lessons learned in one sphere can be applied in the other. She asked "how it was that our noble army all but perished in the East," and why "hundreds of millions" of people perish before their time "by pestilence" (see p 346 below). Her classic (coloured) polar area chart shows the relatively small number of deaths from wounds soldiers faced, as compared with deaths "from the whole tribe of diseases" to which they were exposed, the "other diseases" category; and the far greater number of deaths from "preventible" diseases, namely, "fever, cholera, diarrhea, dysentery and scurvy." These last were the "scourge of camps and armies" now as plague had been in the Middle Ages. (The pathogens causing those diseases were not identified until many years later: typhoid fever in 1880, tuberculosis in 1882, cholera in 1883, diarrhea in 1885 and dysentery in 1898.)

Nightingale's summary on this point is another cogent answer to Small, who asserted that she never had another good thing to say about the hospitals after she came (supposedly) to blame herself. Rather her charts showed, she said, that when the necessary changes were made, the death rates were nearly the same as those of military hospitals at home (see p 351 below).

She explained that Chart 1 showed, initially, the bad side, or the results "by neglect of the laws of nature," while Chart 2 showed "what we may expect from their observance." She further argued the applicability of the same information in towns, for "Nature is the same everywhere, and never permits her laws to be disregarded with impunity." Bringing in improvements in towns would show the same good results as had been achieved at Scutari (see p 349 below).

Nightingale at this time used Farr's distinction between preventible "zymotic" diseases—fever, diarrhea, dysentery, cholera and scurvy—and "non-preventible," mainly chest and respiratory diseases and, notably, consumption, the name then most used for tuberculosis. In her analysis in *Notes on the Health of the British Army*, however, she treated respiratory diseases as the product of bad air from poor ventilation, or as a condition that was decidedly preventible (see p 347 below). The case she made on the great number of deaths from "preventible" diseases could, in short, have been made even more strongly if the two categories of disease causes were combined. Nightingale, in time, stopped using the term "zymotic" as a type of disease.

Statistics were key to achieving enduring reforms in soldiers' health, yet during the first (disastrous) year of the war, "there was hardly a single trustworthy statistical return produced," and statistics had yet to be "applied to the solution of problems" on the health and efficiency of the army (see p 352 below). Better statistics would be a major point in her next papers.

Nightingale examined the claim that the siege of Sebastopol had been undertaken by an army unprepared for lengthened military operations. Nothing had been organized for sheltering, clothing or feeding the troops: "No scheme of diet or ration appears to have been intelligently considered, and no transport was organized either for bringing supplies or for carrying away the sick" (see p 348 below). Again, these enormous errors go well beyond the responsibility of the Army Medical Department, and even in some respects past those of the army command to the national government at home.

Source: Florence Nightingale, *A Contribution to the Sanitary History of the British Army during the Late War with Russia.* London: Harrison and Sons 1859

London
January 1859

The statistics of sickness and mortality of the British Army during the late war with Russia have been and are likely to continue a subject of discussion. Various conflicting accounts of these have been from time to time given to the public, and recently two folio volumes of a report on the medical history of the war, prepared by the late director general, Dr Andrew Smith, profess, among other things, to give the vital statistics of the Crimean Army in a complete state. The public is therefore in possession of all the information it is ever likely to obtain on this great national question, and in the following pages it is proposed to give briefly the sanitary results of the whole, with the lessons deducible from them.

With this view, Tables 1 and 2 have been prepared by Dr Farr, from Dr Smith's tables given in the work referred to. Table 3 has been also prepared by Dr Farr from other official documents presented to Parliament.

Table 1 represents, month by month, the total mortality in the Army of the East, and the ratio of primary admissions into hospital, from the time the Expeditionary Force arrived there until the evacuation of the Crimea. The numbers in the first column are the same as those given by the late director general in his report, Table A. The ratios of the deaths and admissions to force per 1000 per annum are calculated from the monthly ratios given in Dr Smith's Table B (*Medical and Surgical History of the British Army*, Vol. 2, Tables A and B, page 252). The annual ratio has been preferred to the monthly ratio because the annual ratio is the unit adopted by statisticians in all civilized countries.

Table 2 was prepared also from the director general's Tables A and B, with the addition of the calculated weekly strength of the army. The first column gives the calculated monthly strength. The next three columns give the total deaths from zymotic diseases, wounds and all other diseases, and the next three columns give the annual ratio of mortality per 1000 strength for each month, due to each class of causes. The data have been arrived at by an obvious calculation from the Army Medical Department figures.

Table 3 is an analysis of the weekly states of sick and wounded in the hospitals on the Bosphorus from 1 October 1854 to 30 June 1855. It has been framed on three separate official documents:

1. The following abstract of weekly states, by Dr Lawson, deputy inspector general, contained in the Report on the Hospitals of the Army in the East (Cumming-Maxwell Report) which give the mortality from 1 October 1854 to 31 January 1855:

Date	Officers					Men				
	Remained	Admitted	Discharged	Died	Remaining	Remained	Admitted	Discharged	Died	Remaining
1854										
1 to 7 October	70	3	..	1	72	2,277	61	403	67	1,868
8 to 14 October	72	23	9	2	84	1,868	307	295	46	1,834
15 to 21 October	84	12	20	..	76	1,834	386	151	29	2,040
22 to 28 October	76	8	47	..	37	2,040	350	370	56	1,964
28 Oct. to 4 Nov	37	11	2	1	45	1,964	952	384	52	2,480
5 to 11 November	45	34	10		69	2,480	850	469	36	2,825
12 to 18 November	69	49	4	3	111	2,825	1,045	557	94	3,219
19 to 25 November	111	9	..	..	102	3,219	438	144	67	3,446
26 to 2 December	102	10	5	..	107	3,446	436	315	70	3,497
3 to 9 December	107	..	12	..	95	3,497	263	388	70	3,302
10 to 16 December	95	..	8	1	86	3,302	299	521	85	2,995
17 to 23 December	86	..	2	1	83	2,995	1,321	402	130	3,784
24 to 30 December	83	1	35	1	48	3,784	1,091	770	108	3,997
1855										
31 Dec. to 6 Jan	48	16	6	1	55	3,997	1,044	367	249	4,425
7 Jan. to 13 January	55	18	13	..	60	4,425	727	444	277	4,431
14 to 20 January	60	16	8	1	67	4,431	667	346	270	4,482
21 to 27 January	67	29	30	1	65	4,482	1,243	984	274	4,467
28 to 31 January	65	29	16	..	78	4,467	619	127	165	4,794

R.W. Lawson, Dy. I. Gen., P.M.O., Principal Medical Officer's Office, Scutari, 1 February 1855.

2. The following return for February 1855, sent to the director general by Dr Cumming, inspector general at Scutari.

		Remained	Admitted	Discharged	Died	Remaining
February	Scutari	4,165	1,895	2,139	1,027	2,895
	Koulali	434	795	65	302	861
		4,599	2,690	2,204	1,329	3,756

3. The weekly states for all the army hospitals on the Bosphorus, from 25 February to 30 June 1855, furnished officially by Dr Cumming to the sanitary commissioners, an abstract of which is given in their report.

On these three sets of data, relating to consecutive periods of the hospital administration, Table 3 has been framed. The first column in the table gives the periods deduced for the sake of comparison from the returns, the second the number of days in each period, the third the sick population of the hospitals, which has been obtained according to the Registrar-General's formula, by adding together the remaining at the beginning and end of each week, and dividing the sum by two, a method which gives approximately the number of sick constantly in hospital, on which the mortality can be calculated. The fourth column gives the "cases treated" for each of the periods. The numbers in this column are calculated by the Registrar-General's formula, and are obtained by adding together the total admissions, the total discharges and the deaths, and dividing the sum by two, which gives approximately the number which has passed through hospital; and by calculating the percentage of deaths on this number, we obtain the ratio of mortality to the cases which have passed through hospital. The fifth column gives the total deaths of each period. The sixth column gives the mortality to the sick population, and the last column gives the percentage of mortality on "cases treated."

The numbers in this table have been adopted in preference to any others. First, because they were rendered officially upon the spot, without any other design than merely stating the facts. Second, because they were officially presented to Parliament, as a statement of fact. And lastly, because although they are certainly not accurate, they contain the best information which could be had at the time, without any subsequent alteration or rearrangement of figures made to account for deaths which these tables do not account for. Moreover, as will be presently shown, they do not exaggerate the losses of the army, as there are other returns, at least as trustworthy, which state the loss as being much higher.

There were three separate registers kept at Scutari. First, the adjutant's daily head roll of soldiers' burials, on which it may be presumed no one was entered who was not buried, although it is possible that some may have been buried who were not entered.

Second, the medical officers' return, in regard to which it is quite certain that hundreds of men were buried who never appeared upon it.

Third, the return made in the orderly room, which is only remarkable as giving a totally different account of the deaths from either of the others.

The monthly mortality in the hospitals, as derived from these three sources, is given in the first three lines of the following table. The numbers in lines 4 and 6 have been extracted from Dr Smith's *History of the War.* No. 5 contains the medical officers' return, including Koulali.

Deaths at Scutari according to:	Oct. 1854	Nov.	Dec.	Jan. 1855	Feb.	Mar.	Total
1. Adjutant's Head Roll Burials	266	368	667	1,473	1,151	418	4,343
2. Medical Officers' Returns, Lawson and Cumming	250	267	393	1,235*	1,027	421	3,593
3. Orderly Room Returns	219	291	536	1,360	1,076	416	3,898
4. Dr. Andrew Smith†	235	320	601	1,393*	1,084	421	4,054
Scutari and Koulali:							
5. Medical Officers' Returns, Lawson and Cumming	250	267	393	1,235*	1,329	555	4,029
6. Dr. Andrew Smith†	235	320	601	1,393	1386	555	4,490

* The Returns for January do not distinguish between the deaths at Scutari and Koulali. The Adjutant's Returns apply only to Scutari.

† Medical and Surgical History of the British Army, Vol. II, General Hospital Return, No. I.

This table contains two groups of returns. The first, with the exceptions noted, refers to the mortality in the hospitals at Scutari. The second group refers to the mortality in the hospitals at Scutari and Koulali. Beginning with the first group, we have four accounts of the mortality in the Scutari hospitals, not one of which agrees with another, except for the month of March, when the extreme difference between the returns sinks to 5. Except during that month, it will be seen that the numbers actually buried in the Scutari graveyard exceed greatly the numbers contained in any of the returns of deaths.

The difference may be to a small extent owing to the fact that a few corpses of those who had died on board transports, while the transports were in the Bosphorus, were buried in Scutari graveyard. But even making allowance for this, which must be far more than counterbalanced by the deaths at Koulali, included in the medical officers' and director general's tables in the first group, it must be evident at a glance that neither the medical officers' return nor that of the orderly room, nor the director general's table, at all account for the number of dead buried by the adjutant. Singularly enough also, the total Scutari mortality given by Dr Andrew Smith for these months exceeds the mortality reported to him by his own medical officers, by nearly 500!

On comparing the different official returns made by the adjutant and the medical officers, we are compelled to adopt one of three conclusions. First, the adjutant must have entered a number of burials of men who never died, a supposition in the highest degree unlikely. Second, that the medical officers officially made imperfect returns. Third, that the Army Medical Department, in order to square the returns, added deaths here and there to the transport and Scutari returns, to reduce the discrepancies and to account for the unaccounted deaths to the greatest possible extent.

In order to make this intelligible it is necessary to insert the two following monthly returns of deaths on board transport ships arriving in the Bosphorus:

	1854			1855		
	October	November	December	January	February	March
Medical Officers' Returns made at the time	15	162	226	262	41	7
Dr. Smith's Return, made up three years after‡	84	153	314	289	43	7

‡ Vol. II, p. 465.

With regard to the additions made by Dr Smith to the deaths in the transports, we have this remarkable fact, that, while the return of deaths made officially at the time by the surgeons on board from 1 October 1854 to 28 February 1855 amounted to 706, the numbers given by Dr Smith as having died on board the transports are 883. In this case we must adopt one of two conclusions—either that the surgeons made erroneous statements at the time, or else that the statistics were afterwards "dressed" to account for 177 deaths, which we adopt as the more probable hypothesis.

The presumptive evidence all goes to show that the adjutant's head roll of burials is nearest the truth, as exhibiting the approximate monthly mortality of the hospitals at Scutari, exclusive of Koulali. Anyway, the returns are in such a state of confusion that they make good, if anything can do so, the recommendation of the royal commission that the statistical element should be effectively introduced into the Army Medical Department, before anything like sanitary progress is possible. (An obscure pamphlet, circulated without a printer's name, reproduces nearly every possible statistical blunder on this and other points. It purports to be a defence of the defunct Army Medical Department, "By a Non-Commissioner," but it is more like a *jeu d'esprit* [flight of fancy].) It also follows that on Table 3 the Scutari mortality is understated. As already mentioned, the medical officers' returns have been made use of in framing this table. But it will be seen on comparing the monthly deaths given by the medical officers for Scutari and Koulali with the adjutant's return, which excludes Koulali, and the director general's return, which includes Koulali, that, were a table framed on either of the best last two sets of official data, it would afford statistical evidence as to the bad sanitary condition of the hospitals during the winter of 1854-55 far more condemnatory than any which has been given.

This has been done for the sake of comparison on the following tables, A and B.

[Table] A shows the annual mortality percent on the sick population of Scutari, from 1 October 1854 to 31 January 1855, calculated from the remainings in Dr Lawson's table, already given, and the deaths given in Dr Smith's tables. It very much exceeds the proportions that have been adopted in Table 3.

[Table] B represents the ratio of mortality to sick population and cases treated in the hospitals at Scutari and Koulali for February 1855, calculated on Dr Cumming's admissions, discharges and remainings, and the adjutant's head roll of burials for Scutari, *plus* the medical officer's return of deaths for Koulali. If this mortality, which is probably the correct one, had been adopted in Table 3, it would have raised the ratio of deaths to sick population from 415 to 454 percent per annum, and on cases treated from 42.7 percent to 46.7.

Mortality in the Hospitals of Scutari and Koulali
Table A: Scutari

Time		Mortality: Annual Rate per cent, per annum on the Sick Population
1854	October	139
	November	140
	December	208
1855	January	385

It is impossible to reconcile the discrepancies in these various returns. One thing is quite certain, that hundreds of our brave soldiers perished, in regard to whom neither the when, the where, nor the how will ever be known.

The following table has been prepared from the Registrar-General's weekly reports and from the data on Table 3, to enable a comparison to be drawn between the Scutari mortality and that in the civil, military and naval hospitals in the metropolis. This table completes the chain of evidence, and shows convincingly the enormous and unnecessary mortality among the sick in the hospitals of the East.

Mortality in the Hospitals of Scutari and Koulali
Table B: Scutari and Koulali

Time	Sick Population	Cases Treated	Deaths	Rate of Mortality per cent	
				Annually on Sick Population	On Cases Treated
February, 1855	4178	3112	1453	454	46.7

To make the figures which have been adopted in Tables 1, 2 and 3 more intelligible, they have been transferred to three diagrams, constructed of wedges arranged round a centre, each wedge representing by its area the amount of mortality for the period to which it refers.

The Diagram of the Mortality of the Army in the East consists of two parts, 1 and 2. Beginning with No. 1, the first monthly wedge of mortality is that for April 1854, about the middle of which month the British Army arrived at Gallipoli, in good health. It went to Bulgaria in June. The three small wedges for April, May and June show what the comparative mortality was for the first quarter of the campaign. The dotted circle represents what the mortality would have been for the whole year if the army had been as healthy as men of the army ages are in Manchester, which is one of the most unhealthy towns in England. It will be seen that the average mortality for the first quarter was less than that of Manchester. The army was in Bulgaria in June, July, August and during the first half of September. It will be observed that during this period the mortality rises immensely, far beyond, in fact, what it ever attains in Manchester.

		Mortality	
		Rate percent, per ann. on Sick Population	Per cent, on Cases Treated
Eleven London General Hospitals		82	7.6
Fever Hospital		110.5	11.3
Military and Naval Hospitals in London		39	2.4
Scutari and Koulali General Hospitals	during 4 months	203	19.8
	during 4 weeks	319	32.1
	during 4 weeks	415	42.7
Koulali	during 4 weeks	608	52
Scutari and Koulali, summer, 1855		34	2.2

The army landed in the Crimea on 14 September, and sat down before Sebastopol in the beginning of October. During the month the health of the army improved, but the mortality was still enormous. It went on increasing in November and December, until in January 1855 it exceeded the proportionate mortality from the Great Plague of London. It was very high in February, but declined in March and April. In May 1855 (Diagram 2) cholera appeared in its epidemic form, augmenting the mortality in June. The mortality thereafter subsided, month by month, until in March 1856 it had very nearly returned within the Manchester circle, which it did entirely in April, May and June of that year, so that the army left the Crimea for England in a more healthy state and with a lower amount of mortality than it had when it set foot in the East, *or* indeed than it ever had before when stationed at home.

The first question which presents itself is, what can have been the cause of this? Health is known to depend on the observance of certain laws. Surely, before a picked body of men in the prime of life could have been cut off by a mortality greater perhaps than that of any pestilence on record, there must have been some very glaring disobediences to these laws.

A corresponding picture would be presented to the eye if the mortality of certain towns were depicted in a similar manner of diagrams. We should find, when the town was newly built and its population small, the wedge representing its proportionate mortality small, simply because the laws of health are not so liable to be infringed among small sparse populations as in large dense populations. Were we to follow the history of the town as it increased in size, and sanitary precautions were neglected, we should find the wedges of our diagram getting larger and larger with time, every now and then projecting out into gigantic dimensions from periodical pestilences, until, in the course of years, the town might become almost uninhabitable, as has been the case with many ancient cities, or until, by the introduction of sanitary improvements, the wedges became smaller and smaller, as in the case of Ely, Croydon, Tottenham and other improved towns. A camp is a moveable town; a town is a fixed camp. Nature administers her laws in both with her most impartial hand. Our duty is to inquire of her what are her laws, and upon what conditions she has given us the tenure of this frail life of ours. And, having ascertained those conditions, it is our duty to obey them.

Let us now ask, how it was that our noble army all but perished in the East? And we shall at the same time learn how it has happened that so many hundreds of millions of the human race have by pestilence perished before their time.

The lesson is most instructively taught in the diagram representing the *Causes of Mortality* in the Army in the East. It is the same diagram as the former with this difference, that it exhibits, month by month, the mortality from the diseases and accidents of war occurring during the memorable siege. Each diagram represents the mortality from zymotic disease, from wounds and from all other causes.

It used to be a common idea that the great mortality in armies arose from wounds received in battle. The inexorable figures of the army returns have dissipated this prejudice forever. The small pink wedges projecting a little out from the centre of each of the two diagrams exhibit the total deaths from wounds in hospital during the Russian war.

Henceforth no soldier need be afraid of dying from wounds in hospital. The black wedges show the deaths which occurred in hospital, not from wounds, but from the whole tribe of diseases to which men are exposed, with five solitary exceptions—fever, cholera, diarrhea, dysentery and scurvy. Those pestilences, which are the scourge of camps and armies now, as plague and Black Death used to be of towns in the Middle Ages, gave rise to a mortality in the Crimean Army represented by the blue wedges. It was not by wounds, it was not by ordinary diseases, that the army well nigh perished. But it was by these five mitigable and preventible pestilences that the British force before Sebastopol was all but swept away. Expunge the blue wedges, and within what insignificant bounds would not that great calamity have shrunk! These diagrams give the history of the whole disaster. In June 1854, the zymotic deaths from the diseases mentioned are all included in the small blue wedge for that month. What a different fate for the army had its mortality from zymotic disease alone never spread beyond those dimensions!

In June 1854, the army, as already mentioned, went to Bulgaria, an undrained, uncultivated country, at all times suffering more or less from malaria, and consequently rendering its inhabitants, but especially strangers, remarkably susceptible to attacks of any epidemic disease which may happen to prevail, altogether apart from the occurrence of what are commonly called sanitary defects. Judging from the experience of the shipping, the influence of this malarial atmosphere extended out to sea. In such a region, part of the army was encamped in a district so unhealthy that it had attained the Turkish name of the Valley of Death. Cholera soon appeared, and, as if such a contingency could never have been anticipated, the supply of medicines and medical comforts available for the sick was wholly insufficient. The large blue wedges of July, August and September show the result.

The siege of Sebastopol opened in the beginning of October. The army was unprovided for carrying on any protracted military operations, and it soon began to suffer. The mortality from fever, cholera and scorbutus [scurvy] increased during November. In December and January these diseases threatened the entire extinction of the force. From that period they declined, until the cholera epidemic of May, June and July 1855 again augmented the deaths from zymotic disease, but to a very trivial extent when compared with what the deaths from these diseases were during the preceding year. Towards the end of the occupation, zymotic maladies almost disappeared, and the army returned home enjoying a degree of health unparallelled in the history of war.

The most cursory inspection of these diagrams will show that the whole question as to the cause of the mortality narrows itself into an inquiry as to what laws of health had been so violated as to lead to so great a destruction of life from five diseases only.

Scorbutus, which lay at the root of the disaster of the first winter, is a blood disease, the determining causes of which have been long known. Let men be underfed on salt provisions, imperfectly cooked and without vegetables or fermented bread; let them at the same time be exposed to the elements without sufficient clothing or shelter and to excessive fatigue, and the constitution will rapidly acquire the scorbutic taint. When this circumstance occurs, a touch of ordinary illness may lead to rapidly fatal results. Diarrhea, dysentery and fever followed in the train of scorbutus, but they were all essentially scorbutic diseases. It has been stated that the siege of Sebastopol was undertaken by an army unprepared for lengthened military operations. Nothing had been organized, either for sheltering, clothing or feeding the troops. No scheme of diet or ration appears to have been intelligently considered, and no transport was organized either for bringing supplies, or for carrying away sick.

An admirable basis of operations was secured by the possession of Balaclava, but it never appears to have been considered practicable to connect the base with the camp by a passable road. The fierce winter of the Russian steppe swept over the scene of military operations and found the men unsheltered from its blasts. Blankets and clothing were piled up at Balaclava, while men were perishing from cold and frostbite six miles off, without any arrangements for either obtaining or transporting that covering, for the lack of which they were perishing. The Commissariat had thousands of cattle, its own property, in Turkey, and the hills of Asia Minor teemed with stock, at some thirty hours' distance by steamship, and yet the department was unable to bring over its own cattle, or to purchase supplies, any amount of which could have been at once obtained. Fortunately, the Commissariat had at its disposal salt beef and biscuit; otherwise, the army might have perished from hunger. Unfortunately, it did not supply any other food, and the army all but perished from scorbutus. But this was not the worst; there was the greatest difficulty in conveying the salt beef and biscuit to the front, and, even when it had arrived there, there were neither camp kettles nor fuel to cook it with, although any quantity of wood and coal might have been obtained, as it afterwards was obtained, from the opposite shores of Asia Minor, by merely sending for it.

Another of the notable expedients of that time must not pass without record, that of sending out green coffee to men who had nothing whatever to roast or prepare it with. It was the crowning touch in that system of mismanagement which has lowered the prestige of England, and which almost cost her her fair name.

The destruction of life was in itself so awful that men forgot, for the time, the loss of national honour. And if the national honour was retrieved, and it was most nobly, it was done by the starving half-clad soldiers of Inkermann, and by the heroic sufferings which they endured without complaint during the winter which succeeded that battle of heroes.

As it has too frequently happened in the history of our wars, a remedy was found for the evil after it was done. Public indignation at home at last told upon official incapacity in the East. Government, or more properly speaking the people, took the matter into their own hands. They tore the official covering to rags, and at a great pecuniary cost to the country, they at last undid the mischief which a system of administration, avowedly founded on public economy, had perpetrated. Unfortunately, they could not recall to life the brave men who had perished. Two commissions were sent out, one for the army supplies, the practical result of which was that the troops were properly clothed and fed, the other, for executing sanitary improvements in camps, huts and hospitals. Both commissions arrived in the East on 6 March 1855, and at the end of the month they were at work in the Crimea. The coloured diagram, No. 1, shows what was the sanitary state of the army before their arrival. The coloured diagram, No. 2, shows what it became after that event.

No. 1 shows what can be done with any army by neglect of the laws of nature. No. 2 shows what we may expect from their observance. Similar diagrams might be constructed for towns in their unimproved and improved state, and even for single buildings, inhabited by large numbers of persons. Nature is the same everywhere, and never permits her laws to be disregarded with impunity.

The three things which all but destroyed the army in the Crimea were ignorance, incapacity and useless rules, and the same thing will happen again, unless future regulations are framed more intelligently, and administered by better informed and more capable officers.

The large diagram framed on Table 3 represents a year's *Mortality in the Hospitals of the Bosphorus*, from 1 October 1854 to 30 September 1855. The long wedge on the right hand of the diagram represents the mortality for the first half of October 1854, and each of the succeeding wedges denotes by its surface the mortality per 1000 of sick treated for the periods stated on them. The area within the dotted circle shows the average annual mortality on cases treated in the military hospitals at home, through which, it must be remembered, every man not fit for duty from any disease, however trivial, must pass. The army in the East sent only those cases to Scutari which could not be treated in the hospitals at the front.

Diagram Representing the Mortality of the Hospitals at Scutari and Koulali, from 1 October 1854 to 30 September 1855

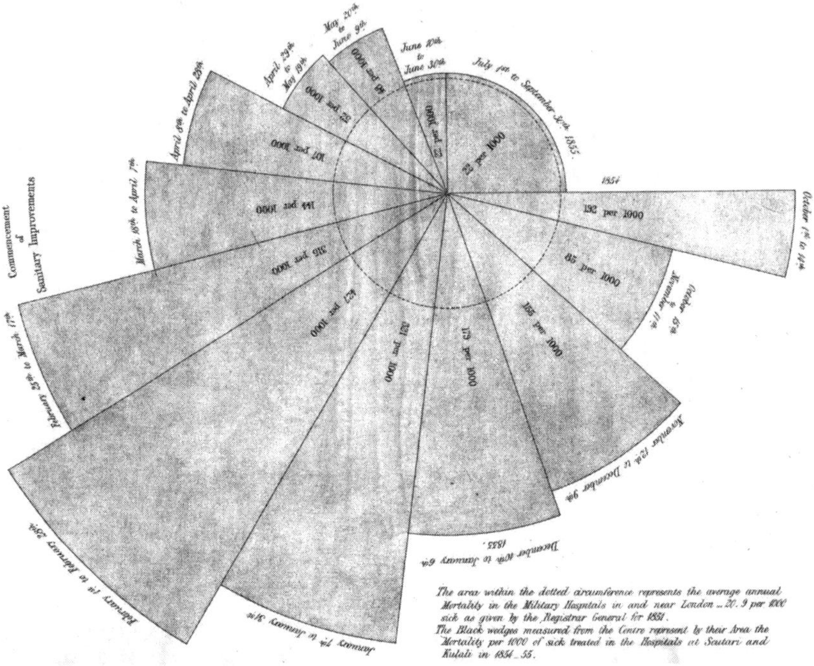

These cases were carried in unhealthy and defectively fitted transports, a distance of not more than 300 miles, and seventy-four out of every 1000 of them perished during the voyage.

The buildings at Scutari into which the survivors were received were in a very defective sanitary condition. And we now know, from the published correspondence of the Army Medical Department, that no steps of any consequence were taken to improve them (Report of the Royal Commission on the Sanitary State of the Army, Appendix LXXIX[99]). The hospitals were most defectively drained; they had no water closets and consequently the effluvia from the sewers pervaded all the buildings. All the hospitals were unventilated, and no steps were taken to remedy this defect.

---

99 Nightingale herself drew on this substantial appendix, consisting of 976 extracts of correspondence, in her *Notes on the Health of the British Army*.

The very first body of sick who were landed at the hospitals suffered an enormous mortality, as will be seen by the area of the wedge in the diagram for the first half of October, some time before the sufferings of the winter in the Crimea began. The mortality rose during November, December and January, until during the whole month of February 1885 it reached the unparallelled amount of 427 per 1000 of cases treated. (If, to the head roll of burials at Scutari the deaths at Koulali be added, the mortality in February would be 467 per 1000 on cases treated. The smaller mortality has been transferred to the diagram for reasons stated above.) During all this period, nothing was done to improve the sanitary state of the hospitals; shipload after shipload of sick were carried into them, and they became frightfully overcrowded. No adequate preparations were made by any of the departments, either for providing beds, washing, covering, food or comforts, and the nursing of the sick was at first wholly inadequate.

These deficiencies were gradually removed, although at the cost of breaking through all system, so that matters affecting the care, nursing and comfort of the sick were improved during the winter. In the second week of March 1855, the works recommended by the sanitary commission were begun, and were carried out as rapidly as possible. Windows were immediately broken to admit of the escape of foul air, and sailcloth flaps were at once placed over the mouths of the sewers to prevent the wind blowing through them into the hospitals; the hospital drainage was improved and flushed; the hospitals were cleansed, ventilated and limewashed; the numbers of sick were also reduced and nuisances were removed. From that time the sick had every requisite for recovery, of which they were destitute during the winter months, and the result is shown on the diagram by the successive contraction of the areas of the wedges until they have nearly the same area as that presented by the wedges of mortality in the military hospitals at home.

The first two diagrams represent what can be done by attending to the conditions required for preserving health among large bodies of men. The third diagram shows what may be done by observing the conditions required for the recovery of the sick in hospital.

It appears a mere truism to insist that an army taking the field should be provided with supplies, transport, clothing, shelter and appliances for the sick and wounded. And yet the army in the Crimea almost perished for want of these. It appears a mere truism to insist that sick transports should be properly fitted up and kept in a good sanitary state. And yet 74 out of every 1000 sick sent across the Black Sea perished, mainly from the state of the transports. It appears a mere truism to state that general hospitals should be provided with bedsteads, clean bedding, clothes, utensils, comforts and nursing, and yet, as everyone knows, the sick were crowded into buildings deficient at first in all these requisites.

The result of the whole experience in the Crimea and at Scutari, as well as the high rate of sickness and mortality among the army at home, have convinced all thinking men that military hygiene must henceforth become an element in the administrative arrangements of the army. This is the conclusion which has been arrived at by the Royal Commission on the Sanitary State of the Army, and it is amply confirmed by Dr Andrew Smith's statistics since produced. It was proposed by the royal commission as the basis of the required reform, and to found a school in which every medical officer, in addition to the specialties of his department, shall receive practical instruction in army hygiene and sanitary science. If any further proof of the necessity for this were wanting, we now have it.

The commission has proposed to reconstitute the Army Medical Department by attaching to it a council, the members of which are to be charged with the medical, sanitary and statistical service of the army. The commission has further recommended that a new code of regulations for remedying defects in the existing procedure, whether as regards troops or hospitals, should be issued by her majesty's government.

The practical part of the reform has been begun by appointing Mr Alexander as director general, and by the issue of a new warrant for the Army Medical Department, which will, no doubt, bring into the service men of the highest talent and character. It is to be hoped that the other reforms which are equally required will follow.

The organization of a statistical department has been proved to be essentially necessary for the public service, by the simple fact that, during the first year of the Russian war, there was hardly a single trustworthy statistical return produced. Besides, statistics have never yet been applied to the solution of problems connected with the health and efficiency of the army. And, indeed, the manner of conducting such inquiries is so little understood, even in civil life, that in the very latest contributions to sanitary statistics, as, e.g., in Mr Simon's and Dr Greenhow's Papers Relating to the Sanitary State of the People of England, 1858, and in Mr Neison's paper on the Health of the Army read before the British Association at Leeds, a want of acquaintance is evinced with the basis on which such inquiries should rest.

From this cause the former of these writers have, amongst other things, been led to assert that the great mortality from important classes of zymotic disease is practically unavoidable—a mistake they could hardly have been led into had they paid as much attention to facts as to figures.

(These writers have included in a statistical inquiry, from which momentous results are deduced by them, a sixth only of the English districts. They have dealt with all occupations collectively to show the effect of one, and they have ignored the influence of *age*. Their mistakes will, no doubt, be corrected in the Registrar-General's Report on the same subject, which is understood to be in preparation.) Mr Neison has, for similar reasons, called in question the causation of consumption in the army as stated by the royal commissioners, although the causes to which they have attributed the disease are the same as those to which a large proportion of the consumptive diseases prevalent in civil life is known to be due.

That comparison of *all the conditions* affecting health and life among groups of population, which must be settled before a single numerical result can be obtained, appears to have been almost overlooked in both cases, and the result of the figures is what might have been expected, viz., that the conclusions are in error on points of great public importance.

The new Statistical Department will have to make up the sanitary statistics of the army in a very different way from that followed in either of the papers alluded to. It will have, in fact, almost to originate the science of sanitary statistics, because it will have at its disposal all the necessary facts and conditions connected with a definite body of men, the history of every individual of which is at the command of the department. In this manner a trustworthy foundation will be obtained, on which, not only to build up sanitary progress in the army itself, but also in civil life.

Again, as regards the proposed Sanitary Service and the teaching of hygiene, there cannot be a doubt that the greatest benefits will flow to the army from both. The recently published correspondence of the army medical officers during the Russian War (Report of the Royal Commission, Appendix LXXIX) shows how very small a number of these officers was acquainted with even the elements of the subject. In the present (so-called) enlightened time, sound principles of hygiene are by no means widely spread even among the civil medical profession. To this circumstance it appears to be mainly owing that the belief in contagion as an unavoidable cause of death from epidemic disease is still so prevalent. This very doctrine is upheld in the *Papers on the Sanitary State of the People of England,* already cited, and it has been quoted, and most properly so if it were true, against reliance on sanitary measures for preventing certain forms of epidemic disease. (It is gratifying to know that the officers of health of the metropolis, as evidenced by their last annual reports, are pursuing a series of street-to-street and house-to-house statistical inquiries, involving *conditions* as well as *figures,* and that we may expect from their labours results very different from those arrived at by the mere men of figures. Again, we repeat, the most minute and practical examination of local and personal conditions is the very foundation of sanitary statistics.)

The only way of avoiding the baneful consequences of such doctrines is by teaching what the laws of nature really are, and how they are to be obeyed. Cordons and quarantine are the only logical preservatives from disease of which those principles can admit. To receive them in the army as a basis of sanitary procedure would be simply destruction. And to the tenacity with which similar views have been held by not a few of the army medical chiefs in times past, in spite of the growing intelligence of the age, may fairly be attributed part, at least, of the neglect of hygiene, which has added so much to the army mortality.

If disease ever appears to spread anywhere, *in* hospital or *out of* hospital, by infection or "contagion," no stronger proof of bad hospital construction or of neglect of hygiene could be adduced. And if this practical aspect of the subject were recognized and acted upon, we should hear little more of the spread of disease from person to person.

It is then, in the highest degree, necessary that sound practical views on army hygiene should be inculcated from the new professor's chair. If the reforms in army hygiene and hospital management advocated by the royal commission be faithfully carried out, and if the army medical officers so instructed are entrusted with the preservation of the health of the army to the same extent that they are now entrusted with the treatment of the sick, we shall hear little more of high army mortality, and of the great loss of efficiency from disease, and our general hospitals in war will cease to be what they have ever been, pest houses. They will cease to merit Sir John Pringle's condemnation of them, that they are among the main causes of mortality in armies.

TABLE 1

Deaths and Admissions into Hospital in the British Army in the East:

Date	Deaths in Hospital, including Bulgaria, Crimea, Scutari, Transports, etc.	Deaths to Force per 1,000 per Annum	Admissions into Hospital (Primary) to Strength per 1,000 per Annum
1854			
April	6	8.4	468
May	21	10.8	1,224
June	17	7.2	1,116
July	382	159.6	2,100
August	859	340.8	3,384
September	939	372.0	2,676
October	763	298.8	2,832
November	1,237	499.2	3,336
December	1,970	7212	3,888
1855			
January	3,168	1,173.6	4,176
February	2,523	979.2	2,760
March	1,409	561.6	2,316
April	582	223.2	1,716
May	594	202.8	1,944
June	1,042	318.0	3,396
July	540	152.4	2,832
August	672	181.2	2,760
September	485	121.2	2,004
October	199	49.2	1,380
November	243	52.8	1,176
December	187	32.4	1,332
1856			
January	92	21.6	1,116
February	43	9.6	924
March	50	10.6	972
April	41	8.4	840
May	29	7.2	720
June	6	2.4	432

TABLE 2

Table Showing the Estimated Average Monthly Strength of the Army; and the Deaths and Annual Rate of Mortality per 1,000 in each month, from April 1854, to March 1856 (inclusive), in the Hospitals of the Army in the East

Date	Estimated Average Monthly Strength of the Army	Deaths			Annual rate of Mortality per 1,000		
		Zymotic Diseases	Wounds and Injuries	All other Causes	Zymotic Diseases	Wounds and Injuries	All other Causes
1854							
April	8,571	1	–	5	1.4	–	7.0
May	23,333	12	–	9	6.2	–	4.6
June	28,333	11	–	6	4.7	–	2.5
July	28,722	359	–	23	150.0	–	9.6
August	30,246	828	1	30	328.5	.4	11.9
September	30,290	788	81	70	312.2	32.1	27.7
October	30,643	503	132	128	197.0	51.7	50.1
November	29,736	844	287	106	340.6	115.8	42.8
December	32,779	1,725	114	131	631.5	41.7	48.0
1855							
January	32,393	2,761	83	324	1022.8	30.7	120.0
February	30,919	2,120	42	361	822.8	16.3	140.1
March	30,107	1,205	32	172	480.3	12.8	68.6
April	32,252	477	48	57	177.5	17.9	21.2
May	35,473	508	49	37	171.8	16.6	12.5
June	38,863	802	209	31	247.6	64.5	9.6
July	42,647	382	134	33	107.5	37.7	9.3
August	44,614	483	164	25	129.9	44.1	6.7
September	47,751	189	276	20	47.5	69.4	5.0
October	46,852	128	53	18	32.8	13.6	4.6
November	37,853	178	33	32	56.4	10.5	10.1
December	43,217	91	18	28	25.3	5.0	7.8
1856							
January	44,212	42	2	48	11.4	.5	13.0
February	43,485	24	–	19	6.6	–	5.2
March	46,140	15	–	35	3.9	–	9.1

The Deaths under the heads of "Wounds and Injuries" comprise the following Causes: Luxatio, Sub-Luxatio, Vulnus Sclopitorum, Vulnus Incisum, Contusio, Fractura, Ambustio and Concussio-Cerebri.

When all is done, the great subject of extending sanitary measures to India will be left untouched. That subject must soon occupy the earnest attention of her majesty's government, and upon the spirit with which it is taken up will the ultimate fate of our Indian empire to a great extent depend.

TABLE 3

Analysis of the Weekly States of Sick and Wounded, from October 1, 1854, to June 30, 1855, in the Hospitals of the Bosphorus.

					Mortality	
Date	No. of Days	Sick Population of the Hospitals (mean of weekly numbers remaining)	Cases Treated (mean of Admissions and Discharges including Deaths)	Deaths	Rate per cent per annum on Sick Population	Per cent on Cases Treated
1854–Scutari.						
Oct. 1–Oct. 14	14	1,993	590	113	148	19.2
Oct. 15–Nov. 11	28	2,229	2,043	173	101	8.5
Nov. 12–Dec. 9	28	3,258	1,944	301	121	15.5
Scutari & Koulali						
Dec. 10 to Jan. 6, 1855	28	3,701	3,194	572	202	17.9
1855						
Jan. 7–Jan. 31	25	4,520	3,072	986	319	32.1
Feb. 1–Feb. 28	28	4,178	3,112	1,329	415	42.7
Koulali						
Feb. 1–Feb. 28	28	648	581	302	608	52.0
Scutari & Koulali						
Feb. 25–March 17	21	3,779	1,621	510	235	31.5
March 18–April 7	21	3,306	1,650	237	125	14.4
April 8–April 28	21	2,803	1,190	127	79	10.7
April 29–May 19	21	2,018	1,350	70	60	5.2
May 20–June 9	21	1,504	996	48	56	4.8
June 10–June 30	21	1,442	1,266	28	34	2.2

Diagrams of the Causes of Mortality in the Army in the East

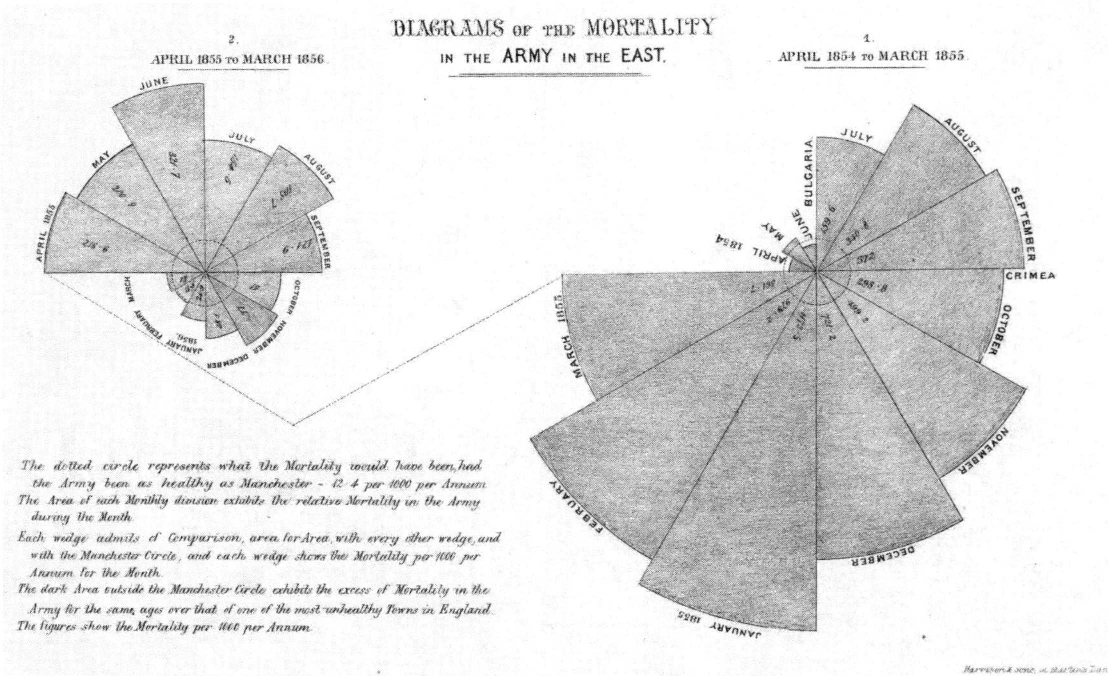

Diagram of the Causes of Mortality in the Army in the East

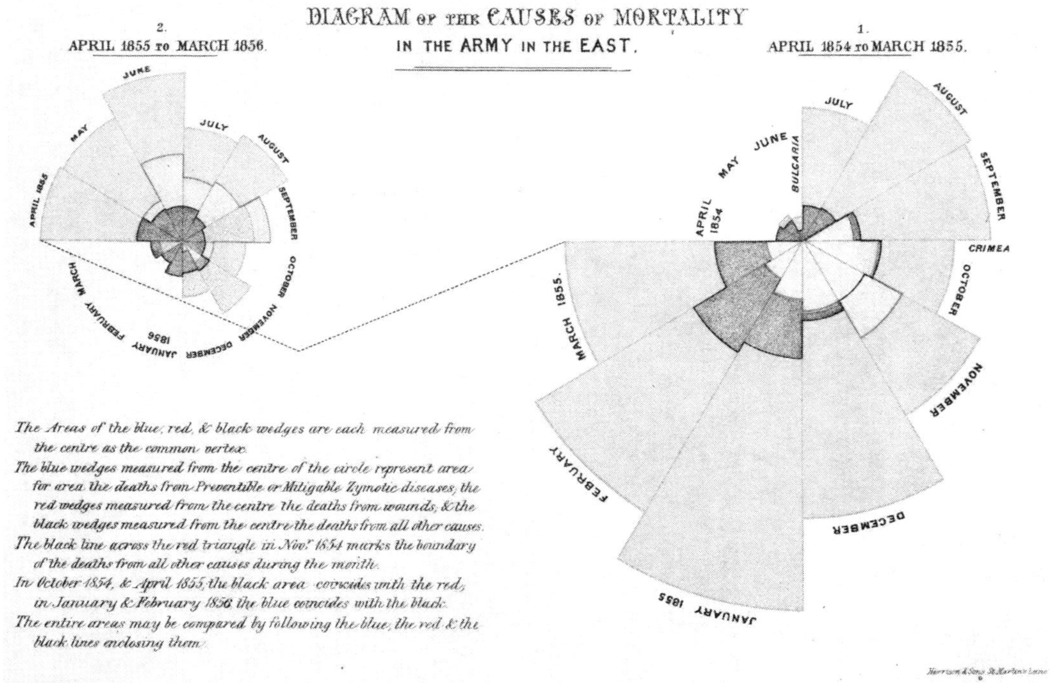

Source: From a dictated letter to John Richardson, signed by Nightingale, Wellcome Ms 5482/31

Great Malvern
8 January 1859

I have sent you a *Sanitary Contribution to the History of the British Army* that you may not think that we are doing nothing. I read *your* contribution to us at the Birmingham meeting last year and was delighted with it.[100]

Your letter [missing] is a treasure to me. It is so seldom that I receive that kind of wholesome criticism.

With regard to the question of a hospital governor, the army is under very different circumstances from the navy. At all the places where *you* have hospitals, you have everything required for hospitals. During war, the army has to organize general hospitals and requires a head for each, with absolute independent power to find everything. In peace, the principal object of having a governor would be only to prepare him for his duties in time of war. In fact, in time of war, without a governor, the principal medical officer would have to be invested with powers and responsibilities which would virtually make him a governor, if the hospital is to get on at all.

The army inspecting medical officers have also very different functions from any which can fall on the navy inspectors general, and except in special circumstances could not attend sick as you do in the navy.

The defects you mention at Haslar ought to be remedied. I think some few have recently been. The defect in the office of the captain, superintendent or governor there would be (in a military hospital) that he has another command and other duties and his interests are not wholly wrapt up in the hospital; if they were, I do not think he would be inclined to oppose the improvement of his hospital; it would keep up his responsibility.

100 Richardson, as well as deploring the "lamentable statistics of Crimean warfare," which showed a loss from disease springing from causes under control, made helpful comments on similar faults at home: "many of our barracks and public hospitals are badly ventilated, ill provided with the means of preserving the comforts and decencies of civilization, deficient in a supply of good water, situated near the deposits of the exrementitious matters of large towns, and surrounded by narrow lanes of the lowest kind of houses." He denounced the "misplaced parsimony in government in purchasing sites." John Richardson, "On Hygiene as a Branch of Military Education," *Transactions of the National Association for the Promotion of Social Science* (London: John W. Parker & Son 1858) 449-50.

I should like to write a great deal more in answer to your invaluable letter, but I am not able. Pages 11 and 12[101] are the only ones I will trouble you to read in the "Sanitary Contribution." Believe me, dear Sir John Richardson, with my kind compliments to Lady Richardson,

ever faithfully yours

Florence Nightingale

P.S. If you could send me any precise details about the sanitary defects of the Trinidad (?) Barracks (where your son is) mentioned by you, I think I could make use of them so as to have a practical effect.

Source: From a note to John Sutherland, Add Mss 45751 f133

[ca. March 1859]

Dublin Hospital. If the whole of central part [were] gutted, quarters and chapel removed, ward used for stores given back to sick, there would be the same number of beds (at 1200 cubic ft. each) as there are now (overcrowded), viz., 200 beds, the cost being:

1. Gutting centre building, putting up floors, opening windows, etc.
2. Building chapel, medical officers' quarters. But 500 beds are the amount required for a garrison of 5000.

Source: From a letter to William Aitken, Wellcome Ms 5471/4

Montagu Grove
Hampstead, N.W.
21 September 1859

You have heard, I dare say, from Sir James Clark that the scheme of the Army Medical School has taken a further extension and is to embrace the candidates for the Indian Medical Service as well as ours. The buildings (temporary) are actually begun at Chatham and we sent the proof of the scheme to press last week. Mr Herbert is really engaged in it. And I do not despair, though I dare say you do, of seeing it actually on foot next January and the professors appointed very soon.

101 These deal with organization of the Army Medical Department and implementation of the royal commission recommendations for reform (see p 350 above).

Source: From a letter to Sir Charles Trevelyan,[102] Newcastle University Archives, 35/11

12 November 1859

With regard to my *Notes on Hospitals*, I am glad that it affords you any suggestions. It was intended primarily for *temperate* climates. And if used in *tropical* climates, the following details should be added, which are known, of course, much better to Major Horsley than they are to me, but which have not been known to some English officers.

1. It is especially desirable in India to have but two flats, as also to subdivide the sick in pavilions, even to a greater extent than they should be subdivided in England, where from 100 to 120 sick may be safely placed under one roof, in India not above 60 to 80.

2. The roofs should be double and well ventilated between.

3. Not so great a window space is required as in Europe, but only enough to make the wards thoroughly light and airy.

4. All hospitals in India should be built on arched basements raised above the ground; basements may be used for stores.

5. Covered or shaded exercising grounds for patients especially necessary.

6. Walls should be double, with a current of air up the intervening space, or thick enough to prevent heat coming through.

7. Carry up ventilating shafts from the ceiling of each ward above the roof, one shaft at each corner at least. An additional shaft or two along the sides according to the size of each ward.

8. Cubic space must not all be *above* the beds, as Napier has erroneously supposed. 1500 cubic feet of space are too little (for India) per bed; 96 square feet of superficial area per bed also too little for India; 120 sq. ft. superficial area per bed should be a minimum.

9. Verandahs and jalousies[103] will of course be employed in India. But a regulation should be made that verandahs are never to be occupied, either by sick or well.

10. A convalescent hospital, governed and organized separately from *the* hospital, should be made to which to send the men, *after* they leave the wards, *before* they rejoin their regiments.

---

102 Sir Charles Edward Trevelyan, governor of Madras 1859-61; Nightingale knew him from the Crimean War, when as assistant secretary to Treasury he made arrangements for her expedition.

103 Blinds or shutters with slats facing upwards, to keep out rain, but let in air.

Source: From a letter to Samuel Smith, Add Mss 45792 ff100-01

Hampstead, N.W.
24 December 1859

There is a framed print (at Embley, I believe) of Winterhalter's "Queen, Prince Arthur and Duke of Wellington,"[104] which was sent me by the queen for "her wounded soldiers" at Balaclava in the spring of 1856. I have great fears of this being mislaid or otherwise appropriated. I had intended it to be placed in the first army general hospital completed in England, thinking that it would be Netley, but it seems likely that Netley will never be more than an invalid depot.

I now put the print under your charge (in order that it may *not be confounded* with my property but) that it may be sent, with a notice what it is, to Aldershot (or Woolwich) (or Chatham) General Hospital (whenever any one of these is ready), as Dr Sutherland, who is *au fait* [acquainted with the facts] as to the buildings of the army, shall advise.

Source: From a letter to Douglas Galton, Add Mss 45759 ff28-29

Hampstead, N.W.
28 December 1859

Mrs Herbert told me that you and Mr Herbert had agreed upon a plan for day rooms for the Wellington Barracks. As she is not very correct in her memory, would you tell me whether anything, and if so, what, is going to be done?

And remember, please, that I hold myself bound about the furnishing. I should like to see the plans.

Source: Notes, Add Mss 45825 ff115-24

[c1859[105]]

Heads of Specification for Woolwich Hospital

Total Beds	650
Venereal Cases, to be placed by themselves	320
Beds for other diseases	330

(1) The venereal cases require ten wards of thirty-two beds each, or some similar accommodation—the principle being that they are

104 From the famous 1851 painting by German painter Franz Xavier Winterhalter. Nightingale's uncle Samuel Smith assisted her on financial matters and correspondence.

105 These notes were dated by an archivist as c1865, but would seem to fit with the planning period for the hospital.

segregated. Each of these wards should have offices the same as any other, viz., wardmaster's room and scullery, and at the opposite end, bath, lavatory, etc. The exercising ground should be apart from the other division of patients.

Some of these cases will be medical, some surgical. Let the medical officers arrange this as they think best. But let them not put these cases in the other division, whether medical or surgical, of the hospital.

(2)	Itch Ward	12 beds
	Scullery and bathroom, etc., separate	
(3)	Offensive Ward	2 beds
	Scullery, etc., separate	
(4)	Noise Ward	1 bed
	May be contiguous with (5)	
(5)	Lunatic Wards	2 beds
	Two, one bed in each	
(6)	Invalid Ward	6 beds
(7)	Operating Ward, adjoining the Operating Theatre	1 bed
	Total Beds required	650
	Total Beds provided for as above	344
	Beds to be provided for in other pavilions	306

Conclusions:

1. The wards to be raised off the ground with ample ventilation beneath.

2. The pavilions to be two storeys high.

3. A space between the pavilions double their height.

4. Axis of pavilion to be north and south, a little to the east of the north.

5. Query. In these climates, is it not found better for sunlight, shelter from winds and discipline to accept, for the exercising ground, something of the Vincennes plan, instead of letting the men exercise in separate slips? There should be but two exercising grounds for a military hospital—one for the venereal and one for the other cases.

6. One surgical ward of thirty-two beds must be provided on the ground floor for accidents.

7. Three medical wards on the upper floor for severe cases (of thirty-two beds each) must be provided.

8. All the administrative offices will be wanted the same as in Malta Hospital. But some, such as baths, kitchen, etc., will require to be larger—the number of patients being double at Woolwich.

9. Hot and cold water laid all over the building and lifts are necessary everywhere.

10. Kitchen should be near the centre.

11. Connecting corridors should be one storey high—with footway above, covered in and roofed with glass slabs, supported by pillars.

12. Flight of stairs for each pavilion.

13. Oak floors to wards with watertight joints. Spaces between ceiling and floor to be filled up with some inorganic substance to prevent sound passing through. Floors should be waxed or varnished. If a varnish of sufficient tenacity not to break could be procured, it would be best. Experience about this *can be had* from Christoph, at Berlin, 11 Mittelstrasse.

14. Plate glass on double windows—especially on the north or northeast sides.

15. Water supply is very bad and will require special filtering arrangements. N.B. It is utterly unsuitable for surgical dressings. For all such purposes, and also for drinking, the water will require to be distilled or boiled. Query, could not better water be obtained in the neighbourhood of the hospital?

The number of N.C.O.s (thirteen) wanted for administration is to me quite unintelligible. It is indeed putting the stores before the patients.

It is *more* than they have asked for, even in their "Purveyor's Code." Three of the largest hospitals in Great Britain are going to send me a list of their servants. We shall then see: I hope we may be able to make a scheme for military hospitals of reasonable economy. Till then, I suppose this accommodation must be provided as you have done it.

1. Administration.

(1) We think the accommodation for N.C.O.s and orderlies amply sufficient.

Ground floor.

(2) Also for admitting patients.

(3) Also for offices of governor, P.M.O. and registrar. (One W.C., instead of two, would have been enough.)

(4) Also for orderly medical officer's quarters and paymaster's office.

(5) Also for linen store, etc. (One question: could hot and cold water be laid all over the administrative block? For the women's quarters it would be almost essential. I suppose it is intended to be so, by the baths.)

Question 2. The more I see of English people, who will not go out for a cold in their head, though they will be starved to death in a Crimean campaign, the more I feel that a covered way for the officers from the administrative block to the hospital is essential, other than underground. I have received ample information now about Lariboisière and Vincennes. And it all tends to this—that Vincennes construction is much better for supervision and administration than Lariboisière.

Upon all these quarters I would observe that, if I were any one of these officers, male or female, I would much rather have my *rooms on the* inside *and my* passages on the outside so that, from my rooms, I lose the view, but I gain the supervision of the hospital. But I suppose there are objections to this.

First floor.

6. We think P.M.O.'s quarters good. But why does the "store" open out of his bedroom? And what is it for?

7. Also the governor's quarters.

8. Also the captain of orderlies.

9. The dispenser's are too good. Better give him two rooms on one side the passage, with door through. Then the two rooms on the other side will make a separate quarter.

10. Nurses' quarters good. A very small scullery and sink will be wanted. Why not turn one of the upstairs W.C.s into one? There are three. Dr Sutherland does not like the darkish unused space in nurses' dormitory. I don't see how it can be helped.

Question 3. Would it not be better to put the officers' kitchens in the basement, and their servants' rooms in the first floor, where kitchens are at present? I had as lief [willingly] have my kitchen in my bedroom unless it is intended for merely toasting meat on the end of a fork.

Basement }
Upper floor } sufficient

2. General Plan. Basement.

(1) Very important that kitchen and dispensary should have enough light. This must be decided.

A military hospital must be a place for curing sick and not for being married in. Even in civil hospitals, you don't provide for your nurses and matrons being married. There is always danger of old fogies being appointed to the offices in a military hospital, as if it were a place for being comfortable in. I quite agree that the question of married soldiers is a much wider one than can be thus disposed of. But a military hospital is not the place to begin in.

One of the cook's rooms has no windows.

(2) There are four water closets taken out of the coal store. According to scale, this would do for forty orderlies. Are there so many?

(3) Is it intended that the dead shall be carried down the end stair to the basement, thence to the dissecting room and deadhouse, again

out into the hearse, to be backed inwards for the purpose? Are not the turns too many and too sudden for this?

(4) Is the itch ward in the basement? query, given up? We think it quite good enough. All that itch patients need is to be locked up and bathed and scrubbed. Give them baths, a communication, etc., and it will do quite well. There must be some gross mismanagement or miscalculation about their number. Dr Burrell says there ought never to be more than ten at Woolwich, at the outside. But we can't help it.

1. *Prisoners. Ground Floor* will do very well.

2. *Itch Ward* (if this *ground floor* one is decided upon) will do very well. A nurse's room is not needed for them. But you might put one of your N.C.O.s there to sleep. . . . A W.C. sink is not wanted. A scullery sink is.

Bath for Itch ward. *A bath (or even two)* is certainly wanted. Bathing is an essential part of the cure—one before the friction, one after, that each case, which ought only to be in twenty-four hours, takes two baths during that time.

3. *Lunatic Wards.* Are the delirium tremens cases, if any, to go into these wards? Each of these cases is better in a single ward.

1st floor (a) one dark, padded, room there must be, (b) a portable bath there should be, if possible. Apparently there are two (two-bed) wards. This is not a point for me to decide. But I believe single lunatic wards are considered best. Harmless cases may be in one large ward, but *two* is a bad number, I believe.

W.C.s at end of Wards. We fear the 3 ft. passage is too narrow. A 3 ft. door will do. But, if possible, the passage should be *3 ft. 9 inch.* wide at least.

Dust and Linen Chutes will do. Chutes should be ventilated.

Operation Ward. I approve—under protest—that it is all an arrangement for neglecting the patient. Give the nurse a window into the ward at least.

Offensive Ward distribution proposed very good.

1. Would you give them a folding door? I think not.

2. They must have a *bath.* But a portable one would do.

Total accommodation shown for patients is as follows:

1st Pav. Prisoners		28
Itch		12
Others		96
Lunatics		5
2nd	32 × 4	128
3	28 × 2	56

4	20	20	
5	28 × 2	56	
6	32 × 4	128	
7		128	
	[Total]	657	This is enough.

Hospital walls and ceiling, including skirting, beading, angles. For coating: one man with unpolished Parian at 1500 cubic feet £2.13.5. For coating: one man with composition (at 1500 c.f.) £3.6.11. For coating: one man with polished Parian cement (at 1500 c.f.) £5.10.1. P.p. 2/6 per yard.

Source: From a letter to Sir Charles Trevelyan, Newcastle University Archives 35/11

10 January 1860

No. 12 of your Medical Board's report cites an opinion of mine that 2000 cubic feet of air per *hour* should be given to each patient. This will not do for India. They are now giving even at Paris from 4000 to 5000 cubic feet per hour per patient. (The expression refers only to artificial ventilation—which is always undesirable—and therefore matters the less.)

Practically, you will find 2000 cubic feet of *space* per patient not too much at Madras with unlimited (natural) ventilation.

Source: From a letter to William Farr, Wellcome Ms 5474/17, typed copy Add Mss 43398 f169

2 April 1860

Imprimis [in the first place]: Mr Herbert will speak to Sir B. Hawes[106] about your being *mis*informed (to any extent you like) at the W.O., as to their estimates and accounts. And any day that you like to call upon Sir B. at the W.O., he will "put you in communication" with the necessary *mis*informants.

2. He, Mr Herbert, will speak to Milner Gibson[107] about putting Sutherland on to the commission for the International Congress (in order to hedge Simon[108]).

106 Benjamin Hawes (1797-1862), under secretary for war 1857-62.

107 Thomas Milner Gibson (1806-84), Liberal MP, president of the board of trade 1859-66.

108 John Simon (1816-1904), later Sir, was a leading "sanitarian" and former medical officer of health for the Privy Council Office, later on the staff at St Thomas' Hospital. For background on Nightingale's negative views of him see p 502 below.

3. He does not feel "a call" for the Royal Society at present—he says he is too busy, but he hopes (when less busy) that "the call" will come.

4. He would be very much obliged to you to write up his new Army Medical School in *The Lancet*, because he expects a "row" when the estimates come on (three weeks hence) and wishes to be able to quote from the civil medical papers. And as he has supported us (*anti* commander-in-chief), we ought to support him.

5. He looked over all your Indian commission papers, was not at all staggered by the expense, is to write to Dr Balfour to desire him to fill up the forms you send (for returns of Indian *Queen's* troops) and to desire him to call for extra assistance for doing so. But, as this is more Sutherland's business than mine, I shall leave him to tell you all about it, and to return your little portfolio.

6. Sutherland, in looking over your disease list for my hospital statistics (*prospective*), asks you the following questions, upon which I ask, why did not you ask them yourself when Dr Farr was here? To which the answer is not so clear.

Source: From a letter to Sidney Herbert, Wiltshire County Record Office, Pembroke Collection 2057/F4/68

14 April 1860

No answer. You are going to have a sanitarium at the Cape for the "sick and wounded" from China and India of from 600 to 1000 beds, with a regular transport service from India and China to the Cape. About half will be serious cases. And the D.G. [director general] says it will be "a second Scutari" (he does not mean in disorder but in importance).

The D.G. intends to bring forward the proposal at a W.O. meeting on Monday(?), present the C.-in-C. for organizing this general hospital (or sanitarium) upon the new "Regulations," *qua* governor, *qua* nurses, etc.

Of all this, you will say, you need not inform *me.* My point is this: the D.G. does not seem clearly to understand (even with his "Regulations" before him) that the appointment of the governor is in the hands of the S. of S. (vide [see] page 40), also of the superintendent general of nurses (vide p 47). He says that, *since* the promulgation of the "Regulations," the c.-in-c. has appointed a governor to the Yarmouth Hospital, "who has done exceedingly *ill.*" The D.G. is anxious for the introduction of female nurses and is looking about for some, as if *he* were matron as well as D.G. (Mrs Shaw Stewart is now in England, serving at King's College Hospital. I have no doubt she would accept a temporary appointment at the Cape. And I think her much better suited for such foreign service than for home. It would also not compromise you to anything further.) But this is a point of minor importance.

P.S. Hospital huts for 600 are to be sent out from home to the Cape, and I should be rather glad (Mr Herbert volente [willing]) to have my "finger in the pie" of their structural arrangements. Galton is in France till Tuesday. All my information comes through Sir G. Grey (Cape).[109]

We have put up the D.G. to reading his own "Regulations." My object in now troubling you (among so many greater troubles) is that the Cape is a place where it is essential, in Sir G. Grey's estimation, to organize a really efficient general hospital, because

1. it is so far from home that constant reference cannot be made to home;
2. everything has to be organized there;
3. it is likely to be a large and permanent establishment, from the fineness of the climate and other reasons.

(How I should like to be going out to have the doing of the female part of it!)

Source: From three letters to Douglas Galton, Add Mss 45759 ff34-37, 39-40 and 41

24 April 1860

Private. I write to you these points to discuss with Dr Sutherland because he, I am quite sure, would forget them on his way down to you.

1. In a pavilion ward (in a country hospital) 75 × 25 ft. and 15 ft. high, would one of your grates warm sufficiently, instead of two common grates, which is what they propose?
2. The Plymouth females have been again applying for their hut.
3. I upbraided Mr Herbert for his circular about hospital repairs. He has just sent it me (the enclosed). Would you and Dr S. discuss it and return it to me?
4. Mr H. and I had some talk about separating men and horses in the Cavalry Barracks. He says the C.-in-C. says we always put our grooms

109 Sir George Grey (1812-98), explorer and author, governor of Cape Colony 1854-61. Nightingale's correspondence with him is in *Public Health Care* (6:186-89).

over our stables. I said, but we never have 150 grooms. He had nothing to say. And he said he did wish to try the separation.

5. I told him that the space in Sheerness Hospital wards had not been redistributed. He was as angry as he can be—would he could be more so!

6. He says that he had neglected to give the order about the Cape Hospital huts—but that he will do so this week, and that you will have the designing of them. (Perhaps you have it already.)

7. He says that [Prince] Albert is very anxious about the Guards' Barracks plan, and that he, Mr H., is going to take it himself to the prince as soon as it is ready. Do please criticize it very much and let us see it to criticize it, too. I would even furnish Mr H. with a short memo upon it. (For he does forget so.)

He says (1) that the expensiveness of it is owing to its being on the "pavilion" plan; (2) that there was no ground room for its being on two storeys, and that he did not know there was any harm in three and four storeys.

I don't want him to indoctrinate Albert with false principles. And I should be very glad if we could agree upon a memo. (The expensiveness is NOT owing to its being on the "pavilion" plan.)

25 April 1860

Private. If the Guards' Barracks plans are really in their revisal, yours, I am perfectly satisfied. But I don't want Mr Herbert to go to Albert with a lie in his mouth (I mean, saying that things are inevitable which are perfectly evitable). And, therefore, if you would incense Dr Sutherland tomorrow, I *may* see Mr Herbert before he goes to Albert, and should like to be able to tell him what *is* good and what is *bad*, or to write it to him.

Thank you very much for your letter. Please talk over these things more fully with Dr S. tomorrow. I have acted upon what you wrote.

27 April 1860

Private. Would you be so good as to send me back my copy of the circular for repairs of hospitals, with any observations you will be so kind as to make upon it? I wanted to go over it with Dr Sutherland and to remonstrate with Mr Herbert upon it on Sunday, if anything can still be done in the way of carrying out *his own* "regulation," which is quite opposed to it.

Source: From an undated note for Sidney Herbert, 2057/F4/69

[ca. April 1860]

Hospital Huts for CAPE.

We find, "from "information," that such things as these are provided for *by the Commissariat*, without any reference to the Barrack Department, and in such a way as our Commissariat only knows how. (The last huts it put up at Gozo[110] tumbled to pieces.)

Seeing the great importance, should not the greatest care be taken to have a good design for these huts, with every appliance? And should they not be referred to the Barrack Department? (Galton has heard nothing of them.)

Source: From three letters to Douglas Galton, ADD MSS 45759 ff44-45, 51-52 and 62-63

11 July 1860

C.W.M.[111] keeps writing against the Woolwich Hospital site in *The Builder*. *C.W.M* keeps amiably sending me his articles. *The Builder* has always stood our friend in all enlightened things, specially about Netley. It is a great pity to have an enlightened paper putting forth fooleries—which I should myself believe, if I were an outstander from the general character of the paper.

The whole gist of its argument is: Mr Herbert in office is different from Mr Herbert out of office. This I am not at all prepared to deny—*in administrative* things. But as the case of Woolwich Hospital site is clear, let me either answer it in *The Builder*, which always puts me in[112] (admirable paper!), or get a question asked in the House of Commons for Mr Herbert to answer.

Upper Terrace
Hampstead
1 September 1860

Private. I sent your plans and my remarks (on the D.G.'s remarks) last night. My remarks were *only for yourself.* If the D.G., or purveyor-in-chief, insist upon things which are obviously in their province, I think it would be wise to yield, e.g., if the D.G. wishes for "two operation wards," although it is manifestly absurd, let him have them. If the purveyor-in-chief wishes for a *bakery* and *washery*, he will probably work them well and let him have them.

110 A small island belonging to Malta.

111 A frequent, anonymous contributor to *The Builder*.

112 As well as the three articles on Netley in 1858, and one on preventible disease in 1859, it published three unsigned articles by her on St Thomas' Hospital in 1859 (see p 780 below).

Dr Gibson's remarks struck me as those of a man who wished to be beforehand with others in the reform, and not of one master of his subject. Mr Robertson,[113] on the other hand, although he is a man I know and despise, writes like one at home in his own matters. Neither, it is obvious, knows in the least what the working of a large general hospital is—Gibson has never seen one.

However, it is a great point that he does not object to large wards. Please refer back to me any counter objections the D.G. makes or anything (before Monday) which you think wants farther explanation.

10 September 1860

Hospital Orderlies. Could you get (*in writing*) from the Army Medical Department:

1. In regard to *all* hospitals—in carrying out the regulation number of orderlies, viz., one to ten sick and one to every fraction above ten—do they apply this to the number of sick in *hospital*, or to the number in each *ward*? e.g., to a hospital of fifty-eight sick (in the five wards of 24, 24, 8, 1 and 1) would they have six orderlies or nine? and what number of N.C. officers? One or two?

2. In regard to *Woolwich* Hospital, could you get a list, *in writing*, of the *officers* and ranks of their "twenty N.C. officers," of whom I understand nine are for the wards, eleven [for] administration. Unless you ask for their offices (or what *they are to do*), you will merely get a list of so many company sergeants, sergeants, etc. I want their ranks too—but what I chiefly want is a list as follows:

Fuel Store	1 sergeant
Pack "	1 ? etc.,

and *to how many wards* (or to how many patients) one sergeant or company sergeant as the case may be. . . .

1. The enclosed plan is the same as if, out of the (lavatory) end of the Malta ward, one half of it were converted into a ward. Amputation cases had far better be located in any large ward than in such an arrangement, where the scullery, W.C. and sink all open into a narrow passage with the ward doors opposite.

2. It would be almost impossible to carry a patient in from the operating theatre, i.e., to turn him round at right angles in a passage 4 ft. wide. The

113 James Brown Gibson 1805-68), director general 1860-67, biographical sketch in *Wars and the War Office* (15:1039); James Scott Robertson (d. 1895), purveyor-in-chief in the Crimean War.

door of an operation ward had better be nearly opposite that of an operating theatre or the turn must not be so sharp and the passage much wider.

3. The little pencil sketch is much better, viz., with the nurse's room nearest the corridor on one side, and the scullery, sink, etc., on the other, and the wards occupying the *farthest side*. But I cannot conceive any medical officer preferring two bad wards to one good one. If there were no partition, there would be one good ward with windows on three sides, capable of holding two operation cases, who would be much better so and together.

4. As the two lower storeys will be thoroughfares, the patients would be much quieter so than just over the said thoroughfare and the refuse cart coming to the basement.

5. There would be many ways of isolating the W.C. and sink besides that indicated. Anyhow I am afraid it will be expensive. But, anyhow, operation wards, if opening upon a little corridor, must have that corridor with windows opposite their doors—not other doors. I would just as soon put an operation case into the lavatory of the Lariboisière ward operation wards.

(This "prisoners' sick return" for a garrison of 5000 men—exclusive of the sick prisoners in the Woolwich common huts—is certainly a most extraordinary exhibition of Woolwich administration.) According to Dr Mapleton's statistics, you must provide for *eighteen prisoners and a half*. But I don't see how this will do, when, in another month, you may require accommodation for *twenty-nine*. Adjoining wards must be thrown together for prisoners, or cut off for other sick, as occasion may require. To keep a large ward always for them would be wrong.

Ought not these average monthly numbers to represent the monthly totals for a number of years? They have taken only the months for one year. This return may show an excessive number or too low a number.

Source: From a letter to Robert Rawlinson, Boston University 1/1/17

Hampstead N.W.
27 September 1860

I have only just read over Dr Combe's paper in *The Builder*,[114] describing a plan for a regimental hospital. There are some points in it which I do not like to pass over without writing to you. Perhaps you would

---

114 Dr Combe, R.A., "Plan Proposed for the Hospital of a Regiment," *The Builder* 18,920 (22 September 1860):606-8. Combe also published three papers in the *Edinburgh Medical Journal* that were highly critical of the royal commission report, defended regimental hospitals, and made sarcastic references to Nightingale, later published as a book, *The Army in Its Medico-Sanitary Relations*.

think well to write to Mr Godwin about them. I cannot enter into any controversy. But principles are at stake. And as there is an *appearance* of knowledge in the paper, I ought, at least, to state my opinion on the plan, in order that, at all events, you may not think that I acquiesce in it.

The *appearance* of truth consists in using pavilions with windows on opposite sides, and in stating broadly the obvious fact that care and discipline cannot be maintained in "small" wards. The *error* is in the proposed arrangement. For no one conversant with hospital construction would ever build a hospital in three radii with closed angles. There are new regimental hospitals about to be built in which the sick are to be *in line*, as they ought to be. In fact, Dr Combe's plan is only a bad version of these new hospitals, *plus* the radius at right angles.

2. Again, his ward dimensions are not by any means good. And he does not make the best of the "1200 cubic feet per bed" allowed by the new "Medical Regulations."

3. It is impossible to understand on what principles he has placed his W.C. in the middle of the length of one side, and his scullery opposite. The result would be that the scullery would become a mere gossiping place for patients and orderlies. And, whenever the wind blew against the side where the W.C. is, the foul air, incident to military hospital W.C.s, would be carried directly into the wards.

4. I am not able to go into the errors of detail in the offices. There are thirty separate apartments (or places) for ninety-two beds—or nearly one for every three patients. Of all things, avoid unnecessary holes and corners in military hospitals: additional places to clean (also to skulk in).

5. The large hall is an unnecessary expense.

6. The hospital sergeant is placed exactly where he ought *not* to be, viz., at the greatest distance from the wards. The hospital sergeant ought to overlook his wards *by day and by night.* Military hospitals are to cure the sick, not to be married in.

7. There are two wards of four beds each, which have only one window each, and are not ventilated enough for a dog to sleep in. Dr Combe, it is true, condemns the wards, but at the same time counts the beds into his "ninety-two beds." The first thing I should do in an old hospital would be to close them altogether. I have seen such (in a British military hospital) for ophthalmic cases (as he recommends), which were nests of disease, and of *ophthalmic* disease, too.

8. The administrative offices are so placed that, besides there being an entire absence of anything like architecture in them, they would increase the difficulty of administration.

9. I am no engineer, but I would ask you whether his drainage is not as original as it is unnecessarily costly.

10. I am told that his estimate of £100 per bed is nearly double that for which better (one-storey) hospitals have been already estimated for.

11. Lastly, Dr Combe appears never to have apprehended the idea of a "general hospital"; he considers it necessary to "agglomerate" sick together in order to realize a "general" hospital.

The pavilion structure was introduced expressly in order to make possible a general hospital without any one of the risks of "agglomeration." There are general hospitals at this moment with fewer sick under one roof than Dr Combe puts in his "segregation," which, he justly insists upon, will be effectually carried out in the new *Woolwich* Hospital—if by "segregation" he means the placing but a small number of sick in each building, and the isolating each building so as to form houses much *more* separate than the houses in a street are.

I am quite sure that Mr Godwin is not taken in by these *neo*-hospital constructionists. But I am very sorry that he lends the great authority of *The Builder* to them.

Upon another subject, I see

1. That Dr Combe, who is an extremely able medical officer, supposes that the new Woolwich Hospital is to be an "agglomeration" of "regimental hospitals." Such is not the case. It is to be a *general* hospital under the new Regulations. (An agglomeration of regimental hospitals is simply an absurdity.)

2. That, judging by the style, the same hand has several times supplied *The Builder* with a criticism on the Woolwich Hospital site. Once he proposed a site which would have required the repository where men are drilled to their duties, at Woolwich, to be abolished. He proposed another, past which the mortar practice takes place. He proposed a third, which Sir Thomas Wilson[115] would not sell, and now he objects to the site chosen, "because it is on clay," *which it is not.* It is, I am told, on the Woolwich pebble bed, clay mixed with shingle, to obviate even the risk of damp from which the whole building will be raised on a basement, mostly above the level of the ground.

It would have better serve[d] the public interest, had Dr Combe said where a better site was to be had. I merely mention this, because I have taken at least as much interest in it as Dr Combe has. I watched

115 Thomas Maryon Wilson (1800-69), 8th baronet, a landowner who tried unsuccessfully to get permission to build houses on his large Hampstead estate.

anxiously for every [illeg] *The Builder* might contain, and *found non[e]*, only helpless objection.

This letter is, of course, only for yourself (and, should you choose to show it to Mr Godwin, for him). Discussion always does good. I have no pretension to "lay down the law." Nor has Mr Roberton, to whom I see Dr Combe attributes my papers in *The Builder*.[116]

The Builder had already, and *has since*, enunciated sound principles of hospital construction. But, alas! it does not follow that principles, however sound, necessarily involve their being comprehended or applied in practice. I wish the present case were the only one I knew (of such failure) since *The Builder* first advocated hospital reform.

I think I shall follow your advice of getting out, as soon as possible, a manual of hospital construction, when, as I shall be obliged to make use largely of my articles in *The Builder*, I suppose Dr Combe will accuse me of plagiarizing Mr Roberton, a man I greatly respect and admire.

Thank you very much for your two parcels of books and reports. Your article on "water" I had not seen. Most of the others (by you) I have, yet not the Woolwich one, marked by you, they are the more useful to me. But I would return them to you, if you want them for presents. Thank you very much for the beautiful little compasses. . . .

Dr Combe invites criticism in express words. And I believe is very fairly open to it. He is on[e] of the best officers the department ha[s]. There are some curious little err[ors] about *orderly attendance* on sick. But don't think these are things for *The Builder*'s pages.

Source: Letter to J.H. Lefroy, Wellcome Ms 5479/22

Hampstead, N.W.
28 September 1860

Hospital Tents. I am very glad to hear of your report upon tents. In reply to your question, I have never seen a tent (or even a hut) where the sick would not have been better without a stove than with one. It is so difficult to prevent extreme variations of temperature with the stove that I have often seen severe rheumatic attacks from its use.

I would much rather warm my patients with hot bricks and plenty of warm clothing than with fire in a tent (or even in a hut). You will say that patients require the *air* of the tent sometimes to be warmed.

---

116 In a footnote to the article, Combe indeed credited Roberton with Nightingale's three articles on Netley; however, he was complimentary about her Liverpool papers (606).

In bronchitis, pneumonia and such things they undoubtedly do. But it is a fact that, in the exposed conditions where tents (and huts) are used, you do not have these complaints to deal with often. And cholera and such other diseases, which require instant warmth to the skin, may better be warmed by hot bottles, etc.

However, I am only giving my own experience. Doubtless, if a good stove could be contrived, it would be a great comfort. But you cannot carry these very ingeniously managed stoves with you in a campaign.

2. According to the new "*Medical* Regulations" (if you do not happen to have a copy by you, may I send you one?) with the places marked, there is now *no* hospital tent, but a marquee for *sick* and a bell tent for equipments. After taking all the best evidence, it was thought right to provide *no* means for warming in the "Regulations," and *no* transport for stoves. (This last was said to be impossible.) These things, it was thought, must be very much left to the medical officers. The same thing as to cooking apparatus. They will have to excavate or build kitchens on march. It will therefore not be necessary to consider the question of "warming."

3. The hospital marquees are very bad for want of ventilation. Three years ago we began drawing up plans for ventilation. It was never continued. I venture to enclose to you our beginning. Although it rather shows what is required than how to do it, it may be of some little use to you.

4. If you liked to send me your report (or any part of your report), I should be very glad to suggest, for your approval, anything which may have come within my own experience. And I promise not to be so long as I have been this time.

I have only just opened yours of the 22nd (!). The fact is, I have been unusually ill and busy. And they deprived me of my private letters. Anything that you send to 30 Old Burlington St. is, however, always forwarded within the day to me.

Source: From a letter to Elizabeth Gaskell,[117] Manchester University, John Rylands Library

28 September 1860

Your Captain P. Jackson (who is also "*my*" Captain P. Jackson) is, I am afraid, rather in a scrape about his Gibraltar "Soldiers' Home." You know, I dare say, that he is married—that it is of material importance

---

117 Elizabeth Gaskell (1810-65), novelist and family friend.

to him to be repaid the money (above £1000) which he has advanced to the institution. You know, I dare say, that he is not very businesslike—that he has taken, altered and fitted up houses (for the "Home") without any written agreement as to lease or tenancy—upon a mere verbal arrangement with an old man of seventy-three. But, *I* say, there were many businesslike officers in the garrison who did nothing; there was one unbusinesslike one who did it all. And we ought to help it out of its scrape. That its want was pressing in a place like Gibraltar, and that it has answered the want is certain.

There are many difficulties which no one knows who does not know the soldier as well as I do.

I believe we could get the War Office to take over the whole thing, paying all the costs, if some kind of *lease* security could be had. But then it would fall under the Barrack Department. And if a barrackmaster were to be seen in the place, not a soldier would come near it. I have often been told better "beg, borrow or steal" the money than do that.

Under these circumstances, I am going to "beg." I am going to beg £1000, of which I may perhaps get *half* from the War Office, as a grant. And I am going to beg from you. The W.O. will bring us in a few other subscriptions. And I hope you will be the War Office in Manchester. Perhaps Lady Coltman,[118] Miss Pilkington's friend, would give something.

I am so incapable now of writing any but the most urgent business letters that I ask you, as being Captain Jackson's first friend—not to *give* but to use your influence to make people give. The rent of the place is £144 a year. But, if the debt could once be cleared off, the soldiers are so fond of it that they will make it nearly self-supporting. It is only on this plea, viz., the success of the experiment, that I think we ought to ask for support.

Source: From three letters to Douglas Galton, Add Mss 45759 ff71, 72 and 92 from Hampstead

3 October 1860

I return Mr Abel's letter to be registered, which certainly it ought to be. Scientifically, no doubt it is correct. But he takes the main practical point for granted, viz., that the "proportion of lime" used will *always* be *slightly* below that required, etc."

Could you ask Mr Abel for a report on the practical steps to be taken next, viz., tanks, sizes, etc.?

---

118 Widow of Sir Thomas Coltman, a family friend.

Hampstead, N.W.
6 October 1860

1. Could you tell me exactly how the sending out of the Cape sanatorium huts is going on? Are they all to be sent out? Is the hospital to be made complete? Is it already complete? or how?

2. I should answer the minute you sent me by saying that, as the W.O. has great difficulty in meeting the cost of accommodation for all its *patients*, it cannot do so for "medical officers with large families." And they must send out a P.M.O. with a *small* family. . . .

4. Are the Wellington Barrack day rooms open yet?

5. Have you had Captain Hale's report of the Gibraltar "Home" yet? . . .

Please let me have another talk with you about *ward presses* and such like (for the Woolwich Hospital) before you come to that in your working plans. I have had a good deal of information and made a good deal of calculation since I saw you about them.

Hampstead, N.W.
31 October 1860

I thought the sixty-bed plan of the regimental hospital EXCELLENT, too. But, if it was the purveyor-in-chief who told you to put stores in the head nurse's room (be this nurse a male or a female), he knows nothing of his business. It is equally essential for the protection of the nurse from suspicion, and of the patients from plunder, that everything should be distributed openly in the ward itself or in the kitchen storeroom, whatever that be called. And the fewer storerooms the better, i.e., the less chance of wrong.

Source: From a letter probably to George Godwin, Wellcome Ms 5482/37

Hampstead, N.W.
30 October 1860

The only observations I have farther to make upon Dr Combe is in reference to the statement that he has (in *The Builder*) pointed out other sites for the Woolwich Hospital. All these were carefully noted at the time and examined.

And I beg to enclose to you the following statement [missing], upon the accuracy of which you may rely.

Source: From a letter to T. Graham Balfour, Add Mss 50134 ff88-89

Upper Terrace
Hampstead, N.W.
3 November 1860

Do you remember sometimes talking to me about your Caledonian Asylum at Holloway? I have lately had occasion to see something of the children. And the master, Mr Davidson, whom you know, is, I find, very anxious to become an army chaplain (Presbyterian). Do you know him well enough to say whether he is fit for that particular line? Could you ask the chaplain at Shorncliffe, Mr Young, whose letter I enclose, the same question? And could you tell me how, if he is fit, the thing is to be set about?

Is it by speaking to Mr Herbert? And are there any rules as to these appointments? I presume that a vacancy must be waited for. And, if so, it appears so uncertain that Mr Herbert may be out, in and out again of office before it comes. Do you know how these things are managed?

Source: From two letters to Sidney Herbert, Wiltshire County Record Office, Pembroke Collection 2057/F4/68, both from Hampstead

Hampstead, N.W..
3 November 1860

With regard to general hospitals. Certainly, it is of the utmost importance, as you say, to organize these in the *camps.* I only mentioned Woolwich, Cape of Good Hope, Portsmouth, Fermoy, Plymouth, Dublin, etc., because these could be done at once. And every day's delay is so much in the balance *against* the success of the scheme, because for it to work it should be two years at least begun before you go out of office. But Aldershot is undoubtedly the best place of all for a general hospital. Because it would give the additional practice of carrying out general hospital arrangements during field operations—of collecting and removing sick in ambulances—and seeing the whole machinery of field general hospitals.

Aldershot is the only camp large enough to do this properly. And the constant succession of officers through it is an additional advantage. But there is no hospital at present there which will do. The one planned (but not executed) would do, with a few improvements. Or a hut hospital might be put up which would answer temporarily, or for a beginning. Sooner or later Aldershot must be *the* great general hospital. Shorncliffe would do much less well. The hospital is very inconvenient—ought to be removed altogether—has no administrative rooms and no place to build any. If *one* model general hospital is to be tried, certainly Shorncliffe is not the place.

But poor Alexander wanted General Peel to try thirteen, and gave in the names. And I believe he was right, i.e., as to organizing *several* immediately. If you determined upon Shorncliffe as one, it ought to be examined with special reference to the required additions and organization. The wards are very small—for seven only, I think.

Your "Regulations" regard all agglomerated hospitals as to be organized as "*general* hospitals," but not all under a governor. If the expense of having a colonel to each general hospital as governor is feared, let the P.M.O. be governor in such a hospital as Shorncliffe, which has from 200 to 250 patients only. He is so, in fact, at present, as to all administrative and directing functions, but *not* as to any supply functions. The principal medical officer and purveyor are in fact twin governors now. (There would be an average of 1500 patients at Aldershot.) . . .

I understand that Dr Gibson is so convinced of the impossibility of going on as we are now that he is anxious that you should appoint "captains of orderlies" over *districts*, even where there are no general hospitals. And I should think that the discharged (good) sergeants major (stewards) of the late Medical Staff Corps (I could give you names of such) would make the best captains of orderlies (if a commission were given them), whether for districts or general hospitals.

10 November 1860

I think the Treasury papers, in re female hospitals, are very easily answered. Would you be so good as to get for us, from the purveyor-in-chief, the enclosed information? He, I know, possesses it. And it would enable us to give the answer to the Treasury, in case you wished to urge the thing. . . .

N.B. Gentlemen of the Treasury don't seem to know that, although you may take a bed in a civil hospital by the year (vide papers) you must not send "lying-in" cases to it ("*promiscuous*"), which constitute half the whole of the cases, at least, in soldiers' wives' hospitals. And there are very few of those murderous institutions called "lying-in hospitals" in England,[119] thank God!

---

119 The high death rate of maternity hospitals is covered extensively in *Women* (8:141-408).

Source: From six letters to Douglas Galton, Add Mss 45759 ff94-95, 96-101, 102-05, 106-07, 118-19 and 120-21, all from Hampstead

8 November 1860

Thank you very much for the cements.

I have not the least hesitation in saying that common plaster and limewash is better than the UNpolished cement, and that the first thing to be done with it is to limewash it. You may see this at Guy's Hospital. To hospitals which cannot afford a polished cement should be recommended plaster and limewash. But some of the poorest hospitals of Paris have now a polished cement in the kitchens.

Would scagliola[120] be cheaper? It would do. I think however that the *polished* cement (at 10d per foot) would amply pay itself in a few years by saving the cost of limewashing. But people never think of this.

I do not like the green colouring—I think the palest possible pink might have an advantage over white. If you could get a very nice glazed brick, with a flat surface and finely set joints, would it not do for the interior walls of poorer hospitals? . . .

Is Keane the patentee of these cements of Francis's? I want to make out what "*Keane's* cement" is.

13 November 1860

In re 60-bed hospitals, Dr Sutherland, on looking at the woodcut, is horrified to see that "the ward is too short and too wide." I cannot conceive how *his* misunderstanding arose—because he and I fully discussed this defect together, when the first plan came to us. However, that does not much signify. The question is, what is right? I hold:

1. That every bed space should have 8 feet in width (= length of ward). You say in your report "7 ft. 8 inch," but *less* than 7 ft. 8 inch it should not be;

2. That every ward of beds above twenty is much better for being 26 ft. wide, rather than 24 ft.

Dr Sutherland says, "Yes, but that gives more than the regulation cubic space of 1200 ft. and the medical officers will fill up [the space] with beds." If this be so, I have nothing more to say. I was always against so small a quantity as 1200 cubic ft.—for this very reason that it makes too *narrow* a ward. Your ward must not be *shortened* in order to give it width. But 24 ft. is too narrow for above twenty beds.

It is always a good thing if dressers, tables and, above all, if your fireplaces could be put along the middle of the wards. If the ward is only

120 Plaster made to look like stone.

24 ft. wide, the M.O.s will always object they have no room to pass, and will abolish the dressers and tables. Where it is a regimental hospital, and only one surgeon, I think myself the objection is futile. Can't he squeeze himself into a passageway between bed foot and table? But where there are many officers, it is a serious objection. And where there is a clinical school, an insuperable one. There really is not space enough. You must settle the matter in the way to have fewest objections.

But unquestionably, while 7 ft. 8 inch. is a minimum for each bed's width (*length* of *ward*), a ward of 24 ft. is a narrow one for the length. . . .

Your ward ventilation should be by shafts and inlets, and *not* by holes into the roof space, with a louvre along the ridge. . . .

60-bed Hospital:

1. The staircase is enormously too large. Depend upon it, the upper flat will thus be made by the doctors into their principal wards. Put a ladder in one corner and a lift in the other (for the stores) and make it *impossible* for patients to go up—unless indeed you mean to add another storey of wards for patients some day.

2. The height of the upstairs rooms need not be more than 10 feet, if not for patients.

3. Would it do to throw back the *centre* of the two-storey building four feet both ways, viz., orderlies' room and surgery and waiting room and staircase area? Would it save money? Or would it do to make the surgery and waiting room 10 ft. wide in place of 12? the object being to contract the staircase area.

4. There is a disproportion between the cubic space (and superficial area) of wards and administrative offices.

5. Certainly the W.C. sinks are ill placed (of the two-bed wards). Could not there be placed in a lighted and ventilated space under the stair W.C., W.C. sink, lavatory basin and portable bath? It is most objectionable to multiply these ward offices more than can be helped—and therefore all that should be absolutely necessary is that the tenants of the two-bed wards should have nothing to do with the ward offices of the twenty-eight-bed ward.

6. Two, not three, W.C.s for the twenty-eight-bed ward are said to be sufficient (in a regimental hospital).

7. It is a primary principle in hospital discipline that the hospital sergeant should not be allowed to keep any description of stores in his room. All hospital stores should either be kept *in* the ward in lock-up dressers or in the general storeroom. (I see presses indicated in the hospital sergeant's room. This is wrong.)

8. I don't like the great dark space in the two-bed ward, but don't see how it can be helped—except by the plan enclosed.

9. There must be windows from the nurses' rooms into the two-bed wards.

10. According to my calculation, eight orderlies would serve this hospital—according to Dr Mapleton's, eleven, or sometimes thirty!!!! Anyhow there must be sleeping room for seven, not for "five" orderlies.

17 November 1860

1. You must not have a window *over* your bath. (Of course it has a hot and cold water tap, though this is not shown.)

2. Sick men like washing at a basin set into a table, which allows them to put down their bit of soap, etc., and is much more convenient than an isolated basin and soap dish. The arm is a bit of foppery.

The table should be white enamelled slate—something to show dirt (which slate does not), the basins also white and set into the table in the usual way, the space underneath the table left open for the sake of cleanliness. (Each basin of course is meant to have a hot and cold water tap.) I think 35 inch. a good height for the table.

The flooring should be of good wood, oak, if possible. And I wish the French or Berlin polish could be tried. The former stands water best.

3. I like the kitchen range. Every boiler should be supplied with water separately. There seems a deficiency of means for cooking small quantities of anything. No gas. There seems to be only a double range of steam boilers and double ovens. But you have a cook-in-state now. I should consult Warrener. Ask him both about quantity and variety—whether the range is enough. Do pray provide for the poor wretches in the administration, who have been so basely deprived of kitchens.

4. I calculate one jack towel to every three men (to be changed every second day at least). Or would you give us four rollers to the three basins? (The towel must then be changed every day.) If the rollers are not close to the basin, the men will use the *nearest*, however wet and dirty the towel.

I should be glad to look over any the smallest particular you choose to send me.

5. I should prefer enamelled earthenware baths, such as you have put up in the Wellington Barracks, however costly. They keep in heat better and are the only ones fit for hospitals.

6. I should like to see the warming and ventilating plan for these ablution rooms.

20 November 1860

Woolwich Hospital.

1. I should like to know what the thickness of the plate glass is which can be put in for £300 or £400 more—I don't think plate glass of less than from ¼ to ⅓ of an inch makes any material difference in warmth. I should doubt their having this for the price.

When one knows this, then one would farther consider (one) nothing replaces the ventilation of double windows on winter nights. (Two) *plate glass* single windows are undoubtedly more cheerful. But I should like to know the above as to thickness before going further.

2. I forgot to say a bath must be *locked up* when not used—the lockable up place must include a window, chair and room for one (or even two) bath men. I had understood the bath was to be locked up with fly door—so as to separate it from lavatory.

3. I had heard of a "soldiers' home" at Woolwich, kept up for two years by N.C. officers and men after the officers had let it drop. I asked Dr Sutherland to find out about it. And he, I find, has written to you. I do think it *is* very important, if you will find it out.

9 December 1860

Did I tell you that, as far as regards a hospital in the situation of Woolwich, I have quite made up my mind in favour of plate glass against double windows. I had a long conversation with the superintendent of King's College Hospital about it—she invites you or Dr Sutherland to go to look at their windows, and to ask for her, Miss Jones, lady superintendent.[121]

She could not tell me the exact thickness of their plate glass. But I guess it is about an eighth of an inch—rather too thin I should think (for your large wards). But she says their (lesser) wards are always warmed enough with one fire—by means of the plate glass—and that they *can always keep a couple of inches open at the top* in all weathers. The window is a "fall," not a sash. She likes the tripartite windows, as at the Middlesex Hospital.

Double windows are difficult to keep clean. Orderlies find them difficult to open wisely. If managed unwisely, they are quite as cold as single windows. And certainly they do make hospitals *very* dull—they may be seen at St Mary's.

---

121 Mary Jones (1812-87), Anglican sister of St John's House, and matron at King's College Hospital.

17 December 1860

I quite agree with you about Miss Jones—to my mind she has done (quietly and sensibly) the greatest work in hospital nursing which has been done.

As to the dust chutes, however, I do not quite agree either with her or with you. King's College Hospital is small. In large hospitals, even not so large as Woolwich will be, it is absolutely necessary (and in many is actually done) to have dust chutes, which can easily be contrived so that nothing else *can* go down. No other plan will secure the punctuality necessary in a vast hospital where the dust cart comes to the door only once or twice a day. . . .

John Bull will do anything well and regularly where a machine is in question, and nothing without. Miss Jones's "iron boxes" are quite out of the question in a hospital of any size.

Source: From two letters to T. Graham Balfour, Add Mss 50134 ff90 and 96-99

Hampstead, N.W.

10 December 1860

I cannot forbear thanking you for your article on the spirometer,[122] as well as for your valuable statistical table. (Why do you not include in it the R. Artillery now?)

The results are still far from what we could wish, are they not? (twenty-six and eighteen days sick per annum for strong healthy men).

29 December 1860

In the proof which you have been good enough to send me, I miss

1. any statistics of barracks and stations
2. any regimental statistics
3. any "constantly sick" in each regiment, and of each disease
4. any quinquennial tables, either for regiments or for a whole arm of the service.

Perhaps these will come in the next proofs, or perhaps you have not the materials for them yet. Anyhow this should be stated. The few comparative summaries are very useful, but by no means all that is required to give materials for a sound opinion as to the health of the army. Summary tables are indeed comparatively useful only as affording a key to detailed statistics.

The desiderata I have enumerated are not, I know, all, but certainly they are essential to make a satisfactory beginning. No doubt they are

122 A device for measuring the volume of air breathed in and out of the lungs.

coming. If not, I would state, if I were you, that my material was defective, and the point in which it was defective. Because the first report will be taken as a model of what army medical officers ought to do in the matter. And a report in itself defective should not be sent out without explanation.

2. Is not entering into *causation* hardly a statistical matter? Also, I can scarcely agree in the conclusions: they seem to imply that hygiene, in strict logic, has little to do with the army's health. And they seem to ignore what has been done to improve the sanitary condition of the army. But statistics have "to do strictly with facts in figures." I would therefore extend the statistics so as to give a complete picture of the state of the army during the past year, regiment by regiment and station by station. Or I would state fully that you are aware of the defect, that the data are defective, and what the statistics will in future contain.

I have the less scruple in saying this because no one has ever felt or spoken so strongly of the great service rendered by the army statistical reports, far ahead of any documents of the day. And therefore I should like to see their author as far outstrip them. This proof is too much like the older ones, and does not quite come up to my idea (as it does not to yours) of what you might do, with good material, in giving a statistical report on the army.

Source: Notes, Add Mss 45825 ff103-14

[c1860]

Orderlies' Quarters. Take care as to what these men ask for. They never know what they want.

1. Supply of hot and cold water and use of lifts certainly makes the difference of one orderly's service to each ward of thirty-two beds. A ward so supplied could be efficiently served by three orderlies and half a nurse. A ward not so supplied would be inefficiently served by four orderlies. (This includes night duty.) Food, medicines, linen and fuel should all, *at fixed hours,* come up by the lifts into the wards.

2. I understand that they require "twenty-one N.C. officers' rooms." (I don't know what they mean by a "sergeant major." By the new Regulations, the captain of orderlies, a commissioned officer, has the control of all orderlies and N.C. officers. And the wardmasters are all equal under him. Assistant wardmasters, then, are only to be in hospitals where there are no nurses.)

Now a number of these N.C. officers should certainly be lodged in the little rooms off the wards, in order to ensure discipline, one certainly off each ward (where there are no nurses), one wardmaster for every four wards of thirty-two is amply sufficient—perhaps for every six, i.e., where there are nurses—where there are not, one wardmaster should sleep off *every* ward, though it might not occupy his time all day—there are no nurses) whether it takes his whole day duty or not, one certainly in each pavilion (where there *are* nurses), but probably not more than one. (Anyhow this diminishes the number of rooms wanted for N.C. officers.)

I never saw any medical officer who had any other idea but quartering all his patients together, and quartering all his N.C. officers apart, probably with their wives and children.

3. I think the governor should decidedly be quartered in the hospital. Otherwise he will sink into what a governor of Chelsea Hospital is.

4. A N.C. officer should certainly be all night on duty, perambulating the wards.

5. Two presses should be provided for every ward, *in* the ward, at the end nearest [the] nurse's room. If they can be perfectly dry, it is better for them to be built in the wall.

It strikes me that Dr Gibson has been the worst of all about this authority for the "instrument money."

Private. Dr Gibson's objections.

1. The end ward window cannot be given up. It is especially useful for night ventilation. But, by a little rearrangement of the W.C.s, the cross-ventilated lobby can quite easily be obtained.

2. The question of nurses' W.C.s is already decided.

3. It is objected that fireplaces in the centre of the wards would occupy space and would not ventilate so well as fireplaces in walls.

a. The wards are 24 feet wide, 14 feet of which would be occupied by the beds, leaving 10 ft. between. If the fireplace were 3 ft. 6 inch. wide, it would leave 3 ft. 3 on either side. Is there any practical objection to this?

b. The question of ventilation you have already considered—the question of sufficient draught along the flue is an engineer's question.

In Manchester, they are already planning central fireplaces to wards. (Is there any existing instance of open fireplace where the draught is carried underneath the floor?) As there must be flues in the wall, would it not be well, in the event of the draught under the floor not being sufficient, to provide the means of placing a fire grate under a window on each side of the ward? This would cost four bed spaces to each ward. . . .

A W.C. sink would be desirable for the operation ward—in place of one of the two W.C.s indicated—*and is quite necessary above stairs for the "offensive" ward.*

5. The accommodation for officers should be strictly limited to the accommodation for their *ranks.*

6. There should be a business office for the P.M.O. and clerk.

7. Under the new Medical Regulations, the purveyor is called "purveyor or steward." And there are two rooms allotted to him in the first floor plan.

8. How singular it is that there should be less discipline in a military hospital than in a civil hospital. If "irregularities" take place, can they not be prevented?

Kitchen. In the latter all the cooking is done for all classes, except for married men outside. According to Dr G.'s scheme, there must be fourteen kitchens; there should be different cooking ranges but not different kitchens, which multiplies confusion and "irregularities," instead of preventing them.

9. Whether you have apothecary or dispenser and give him one or two rooms, his sleeping room should be near his dispensary.

10. If sick officers are to be accommodated, it should be in a separate building or pavilion, or in the centre of the administration.

11. The nurses' quarters are more than enough, as (wherever possible) they should sleep and eat, each in her little room off her ward. The superintendent must have a storeroom, servant's room and sink. There is ample space for this. The wardmasters must sleep in the little rooms inside their own pavilions, with the exception of those in charge of the orderlies' rooms. There must be rooms for N.C. officers (five).

In a hospital organized with nurses, there are no assistant wardmasters. One wardmaster for each pavilion is enough, unless in the convalescent and venereal wards, where the medical officer might desire to have one sleeping off each. . . .

12. The proportions adopted give 3 ft. 4 between the beds on the wall space, and 6 ft. between the beds measured across the window.

Private. Mr Robertson's Objections.

1. I see that it is better that each hospital of such a size as this should have its own general washing establishment. But I understood this was decided against. Unless a general washing establishment is within 200 yards of a hospital, it is quite necessary to have the little washhouse (here contrived) for washing bandages, wringing out very soiled sheets, etc. (before sending them away). Otherwise these things will be done in the ward scullery, a most objectionable practice.

It would be better to have even this little washhouse in a separate area of its own than where it is. I presume there must be a N.C. officer in charge of it. Therefore he must have a separate room.

There is plenty of space in the basements under the wards for a teasing room for hair beds, also a stove for stoving hair will be required. The best place for the dirty linen room would be at the far end of the corridor, whence the linen could be removed in a cart.

2. I should have thought storage for 500 or 600 tons of coal quite too much. But this is entirely a purveyor's question. Would not 200 tons be enough? A ward store is required, also one for coke. The straw store should be at a distance.

3. The scullery of the kitchen is more convenient where it is (in the plan).

The purveyor-in-chief should give an estimate of the cubic contents of his stores.

I agree that a bakery would be a very good thing, not however to train bakers but to make good bread. It must of course be at a distance from the hospital.

A "purveyor or steward'"s office, apart from his receiving room, will be required for keeping his books.

4. There is ample space in the basements of the pavilions for any extent of storage.

5. Two rooms, as quarters, have been provided for the steward or purveyor.

A room will be required for the servant of each officer.

One kitchen is enough for the whole establishment.

6. There appears reason in what is said about the boiler. One boiler establishment, if placed in the centre, sufficiently large to provide steam for the kitchen, sculleries, baths and ablution rooms, and also for supplying distilled water, might be best. In this case, the kitchen basement distribution would have to be reconsidered.

Don't have any committee. Confound committees! I have only now seen the *top-flat* plan.

With regard to orderlies, the amount of accommodation required for them must be settled by the D.G. With regard to "boardroom," the situation is bad, necessitating an extra staircase all to itself to clean. With regard to nurses, the extra accommodation would be only in the way. The two storeys already provided are quite enough, if one or two additional rooms are given on the same floor.

The bath is dark and will not do.

The nurses' quarters in fact should consist of:

1 Clean Linen Store

1 Mending Room

1 Linen Nurse's Room

2 Matron's Rooms and Store Closet and Servant's Room

1 Sick Nurses' Room and their Attendant's Room.

The dormitory it is as well to have, because nurses might be put to wards where they could not sleep.

As the whole question of offices, together with that of sick officers' quarters, has come up again, would it not be better to reconsider the whole administrative block, instead of patching it up, adding to or altering it?

Sleeping accommodation for nurses. Nurses' quarters. One head nurse can very well superintend fifty or sixty patients, provided they are in two adjoining wards. Wherever the patients are "*sick*" or *severe cases*, she should sleep and eat in her little room off her ward. But medical officers are not always particular in classifying their patients. Sometimes indeed it is impossible.

It may be found desirable to attach also nurses to the regular convalescent and venereal wards, on account of the decency, order and absence of wrong which is thereby secured. Nurses of such wards should certainly not sleep in their little rooms. It is useless, for they are not wanted at night. And it is ridiculous to spoil such cases by overcare.

Sleeping accommodation must therefore be provided for these nurses in the *female* quarters. Considering the variable nature of military hospitals, all the female staff might have to sleep in these quarters. Why not then, when building these, provide a few more compartments, so as to take in *all*, if necessary? After all, it is only eleven for 660 patients. This is not providing for everything "in duplicate."

The little rooms off the wards must be there. *Whoever* is in charge of the ward must have a day room off the ward. And a wardmaster, if not a nurse, *ought to* sleep there.

All French military hospitals are now served by "sisters" [Roman Catholic nuns]. They do about half as much for the patients as our nurses do and require just twice the accommodation. For, *besides* the day rooms off the wards for their use (quite necessary), they have twice the "communauté" [community] accommodation we ask for. (I don't consider the little room off the ward as a question of female nurses at all. It ought always to be there, whether the hospital is served by men or by women.)

Source: From a letter to T. Graham Balfour, ADD MSS 50134 ff100-101

20 January 1861

I have first to thank you for the two pairs of "*breeks*," which are being used for a pattern and shall faithfully be returned.

I return your proof with many thanks. I like this one much better than the last, because it is statistical. I cannot still keep regretting that the first year's statistics of the army should not be what we both desire and what your own royal commission[123] intended. Even now, could you not give us (if not statistical) at least regimental tables, with admissions, deaths, constantly sick *and diseases*? Facts, not comparisons, ought to be the heading for all statistical work. We cannot have all the facts yet; let us have what we can.

I do not like the prospect for this year's report. Again, as you have a sanitary branch now, its report should be separate and the statistical report should not intermingle causation. Even you are not quite correct about the dates of sanitary improvements. They were already actively begun early in 1858 throughout the London district. Still I do not say you should notice these, but it is lending your powerful confirmation to error to notice other presumed causes of improved health and not to notice these.

I do not think your report would be "dry," or rather the drier the better. Statistics should be the driest of all reading. (I remember hearing one of the cleverest women I ever knew, and a good historical writer herself, say that a full chronology of dry dates was to her the most interesting, the most passionate,[124] of all reading. I am conscious of the same feeling in reading a column of dry and full statistical figures.)

But, in reading your report, I am conscious of receiving a wrong impression, because your details are *not sufficiently* "dry or full" or sufficiently extensive. My conception of the future army medical statistics does not, after all, I believe, differ essentially from yours. Nor does yours from that of the statistical commission (in essentials), whose recommendations ought, we both agree, to be followed, or the fullest reason given why they cannot be. You will think me very disagreeable.

---

123 Balfour had been secretary of the Royal Commission on the Sanitary State of the Army.

124 This oblique reference to "passionate" feelings for a list of dates seems to the origin of the description of Nightingale as the "passionate statistician." Who the clever woman was is not known.

Source: From three letters to Douglas Galton, Add Mss 45759 ff139-42, 165 and 171-74

14 January 1861

Burn. Mr Herbert told me yesterday that he had sent the Woolwich sketch of organization for a general hospital to you, and that I was to have it from you. But lest he should forget, as he goes out of town today, I tell you myself. . . .

As to the Woolwich new hospital, I agree with you not to run any risk. But I think, before the pavilions are finished, you will know whether it is a risk. All that Jebb said to you he has said to me—and I am not convinced. He says, have wards side by side along a corridor, because it is so dangerous to have damp courts between pavilions. That is as much as to say that it is more dangerous to separate towns by streets than to build without streets at all, in a compact mass. No streets are so short or so low as yours. Yet we have seen sunny streets. And I had much rather live opposite than alongside my neighbour. However, all I say is, wait till just before the finishing of your hospital to decide this question. Then you will see. After all, your second corridor need not be more than 4 feet higher than the lower storey of wards.

I have had a sketch of yours for a female hospital above a fortnight. But the fact is, I told Sutherland that it required a delivery one-bed room for lying-in women, and told him to ask the D.G. about it, which he has only just done. D.G. says "yes."

3 February 1861

Mr Herbert sends me the weekly returns sometimes—I see (about your grates): Surgeon Black, 2 Battalion, 11 Ft. [Foot Guards], Portsmouth, temperature exactly the same in the rooms with yours and with the old ones. Now this shows the complaints were stuff. They did not complain with the old ones. Yours with less fuel give same heat. Indeed the thermometer (58° to 62°) is too warm for *well* men, I conceive.

6 February 1861

I am considerably stumped, not to say *floored*, by my D.G.'s figures. He says "the nurses' rooms have only 500 cub. ft. each." Do you make your height then, when you build, 4½ ft.? The rooms are 12 by 9, and I had an idea they were 14 ft. high. Is that 500 cub. ft.?

He says that, for a hospital of twenty-four beds, he wants a matron, with "separate" rooms, two nurses and a cook, all to sleep on the premises. I see one ward [of] eight beds, one ward [of] twelve beds. Does that make twenty-four?

My idea of a hospital of that size is to have a midwife sleeping off the "lying-in ward" (*by no means* with "separate accommodations," else you will have a fine lady), one nurse *under her* to sleep off the other ward—where there will often be children—and one woman to come in and do the cooking and sleep away from the place.

We might wish things otherwise, but a soldiers' wives' hospital *must* be a rough place. Unless you have a confinement every day, there will be days and days when there will not be a helpless patient in the place. And even in a civil hospital, it would be thought quite preposterous to have a constant staff of four for a hospital of twenty.

The midwife ought to (and does) do so much of the messes [meals] herself that many people think it unnecessary to have a cook at all (they only have a charwoman to come in). *I don't.* But the D.G.'s Hibernian estimate is curious. However, I have sent to Robertson to know what they *do do.* And then I will consider and let you know.

One thing we must bear in mind. For common decency and humanity, there ought to be soldiers' wives' hospitals wherever there are soldiers. And if you mount these "en prince" [as for a prince] you won't get them, that is all.

I don't approve, in general, of patients being employed as helpers. But in this case, if you can't do with one midwife, one nurse and one woman to come in by the day, with the help of the patients themselves, who *will* always be getting themselves admitted to be with their sick children (and quite right too), why, you don't deserve to have a hospital. And if you serve them à la Gibson, you won't have one. . . .

Colonel Lefroy has written me a long letter about the horrors of not having married women's quarters everywhere. He instances Corfu. Did you have a letter from Sir J. McNeill to me about Corfu forwarded to you by Mr Herbert? I will send (or show) you Colonel Lefroy's letter. But I don't see how things can be gone on with (in that respect) much faster than they are.

Please to remember that you have never sent me the tracing (or lithograph) *and estimate* of the two-floored regimental hospital for Winchester, and now I want another copy for a convalescent hospital to be built near Ascot[125]—please.

---

125 The Ascot Convalescent Home, at the Sellonite establishment at Ascot.

Source: From a letter to Robert Rawlinson, Clendening History of Medicine Library, Kansas University Medical Center

12 February 1861

Enclosed is the long-promised tracing of the regimental hospital for £100 per bed (120 beds), which I think on the whole the best thing we have done. I need not point out to you that some alterations must be made for a civil hospital with women patients, that a better elevation might cheaply be procured by a little more relief, that, etc. You are quite at liberty to have the tracing copied, if agreeable to you. But I have no other copy.

I read and returned your Winchester report. Could you have a stronger fact than the death from fever of poor Mr Barton, the warden of the college itself? What do they want more? I have just heard a similar fact, where danger was succeeded by death as rapidly. Now for these mortal fevers among well-to-do people, living good and temperate lives, there can be but one explanation. Would to God that people would see it!

I don't think you could say more than you have done in your report. I thought Mr P. Holland's[126] Manchester letter exceedingly good.

Source: From four letters to Douglas Galton, ADD MSS 45759 ff189, 190-91, 197-98, 204-05

24 February 1861

I have a very few criticisms to make upon your Woolwich plans. But I have not got through the specification yet. Dr Sutherland has been so lazy. I hope to send you all back tomorrow.

26 February 1861

We have at last gone through both plans and specification (Woolwich). I think there is more to say about the specification than about the plans.

I should like, at all events, to see the specification again *after* it is printed, because there are some things about ward scullery sinks which I should like to make full inquiry about, which would take some days to get an answer, viz., as to the proper size of sink for thirty-two-bed wards, etc.

If you would walk up here today or tomorrow about 4 o'clock for a cup of coffee, we might talk over things with Sutherland. I should prefer tomorrow, because I am afraid I shall not be up today—*not* because

126 Dr Philip Holland, Burial Acts Office.

I shall have settled my sinks tomorrow. But *either* day you will find Urim and Thummim[127] here.

And I hope tomorrow to have done your female hospital at last.

4 March 1861

All landings, stairs and passages inside the *pavilion* doors should be covered with oak. The corridor may be of *tiles*, because the same argument about the patients' feet being cold would apply to the garden, and you could not line the garden with oak. But I would lay matting in the *corridor*. It can be dusted, when required. To matting or carpeting where the *sick* are *constantly*—or indeed inside the *pavilion* doors at all—I have the same objection as to kamptulicon.[128] They all accumulate and *hide* dirt, and some absorb foul air. And this you *can't* shake out, like dust.

Hot water pipes may be used for the corridor. Certainly rain may drive into the corridor and damp the floor. Hence tiles are best, *unless oak is cheaper*. You put your matting down the middle, where it is not likely to get so wet, and if it does get wet, you take it up and dry it outside. It is sufficient to open the corridor windows (in summer) right and left on hinges like French windows.

14 March 1861

As to Stuart's motion about the grates: do cite the experience of Wellington Barracks, two winters before any other grates were put up—if you have any favourable reports, ditto Woolwich and Portsmouth.

I saw a surgeon's report that the temperature was the same at Portsmouth with the new grates, although complained of as with the old. I would not dwell so much upon the saving as upon the ventilation effected in winter. I would dwell upon the *sweetness* of the rooms with those *sweet* grates.

Last winter was unusually severe. Still the exceptional winters must be met and might be met by a trifling alteration. This I would state.

Source: From two letters to T. Graham Balfour, ADD MSS 50134 ff103-04 and 105

1 March 1861

Again I sent back your last proof without a word, and for the same reason. But all I had to say was that in this, as in the others, I still miss that full statistical account of each corps and disease. In all stations

---

127 Hebrew for "revelation" and "truth."

128 A composite flooring, precursor to linoleum.

affected by special diseases, these should be specially made subjects of statistical comparison. I want to know what your "paroxysmal fever" are separately.

I think our old friend Farr's method becomes ridiculous under this treatment. Perhaps you wished to show that it could be so.

To compare small things with great, I make my probationer nurses send me, fortnightly from St Thomas', a record of their cases. And I had occasion to criticize their records in this way, viz., that they excited all my curiosity by some general remark, similar to that of the paroxysmal fevers, and then balked it, by telling me nothing farther in detail.

6 March 1861

I never meant to impute to you the intention of making the new classification ridiculous. I only hinted at the result. The abstracts do not seem sufficient to enable us to draw practical conclusions. Would it not be better, while giving the abstracts by classes and orders, in the manner you have adopted, to give separate tables for the more important diseases? For example, in the China return, most of the admissions are from miasmatic, enthetic, respiratory, digestive—these being the real groups to consider—should you not give a table of each specifying the diseases?

2. Is it not a pity to put three diseases, dysentery, diarrhea and cholera, in one line, as a constant heading, because there may be no cholera (when the heading contains it), and the fact whether there is cholera or not is in itself a most important fact.

Is there any great difficulty with the single exceptional deaths you mention? If the period has been a year, then you have a *per annum* by which to calculate the ratios. But if you have only a week or a month, then you have no *per annum*, and it is a fiction, most especially if it is a small corps. And I would not calculate ratios at all, but merely state numbers and time.

But 320, *if you have a whole year*, would make a fair number as a corps.

Source: From a letter to John Sutherland, Add Mss 45751 ff181-82

[ca. March 1861]

About floor cleaning. In preparation for the great event (of Woolwich Hospital) I want you to try at Netley *all* the experiments.

1. The Berlin lacquer, which I have always been bothering about. I don't want you to go to Berlin. There is a much greater and more *improving* trade carrying on of French polish in London than at Berlin.

Could you not consult the best French polisher here as to the best lacquer for hospital floors?

Bowood[129] and some other places I know varnish their floors and it stands for years. But I would tell my polisher *of all a hospital floor would have to stand,* viz., constant passing to and fro, carrying of heavy weights, even dragging furniture, which the Berlin lacquer does not stand, coal fires, which also it does not. The cleanliness (and the little labour of cleaning) of the Berlin lacquer is the beauty of it.

2. Then I would try (at Netley) saturating with mastic, saturating with beeswax and turpentine, the old-fashioned way (which I did at Harley St.), the French parquet, etc. The great misery of the French "frottage" [polishing] is its excessive labour, which I believe to be unnecessary. I have described a way of cleaning which I have known answer, in my larger edition of *Notes on Nursing.*[130]

Source: From a letter to Harry Verney, Wellcome (Claydon copy) Ms 8999/6

15 March 1861

I have not a copy of the army estimates by me, but the increase of £40,000 in the hospital is part of the grant taken for the new Woolwich Hospital.

Pray do not oppose our estimates. The fact is, the choice has only been between what we could least afford to spare. We have not had a single new hospital yet. Aldershot and Malta—we have given up both. And yet a large part of our mortality has been traced to our wretched hospitals. But there were more crying things still, such as married women's quarters, etc.

They were so alarmed at the size of the estimates that the commander-in-chief and others wanted to give up Woolwich Hospital. But Mr Herbert stood firm and said he would have it. The old Woolwich Hospital is the most beastly place.

Any improvement in this respect is economy, for the life of the soldier is the most costly article, and the artillery soldier the most costly of all our troops. We are greatly disturbed by the small fight which Baring makes, e.g., as to our new grates last night.[131]

---

129 Bowood House, Wiltshire, home of the marquesses of Lansdowne.

130 The expanded "library standard" edition, in *The Nightingale School* (12:701-02).

131 Thomas George Baring (1826-1904), later earl of Northbrook, then under secretary for war. Baring's answer to the question about barrack stoves was highly complimentary to Galton, as the inventor of the grates (Hansard, *Parliamentary Debates* 14 March 1861:1973).

Source: From a letter to Douglas Galton, Add Mss 45759 ff212-13

22 March 1861

I understand that Baring won't ventilate the barracks in summer because the grates are not hot enough in winter. I think Baring must be an army doctor. Why are the men to die of foul air in August because they say they are too cold at Christmas?

For the next nine months certainly let them breathe (by their shafts and inlets—which have valves to close) and then see how you can warm them in the next three. But on no account give us an iron-heated surface. At least in hospitals I stipulate against this in any improvements which you may consider necessary.

Source: From a letter to Elizabeth Herbert, Wiltshire County Record Office, Pembroke Collection 2057/F4/65

23 March 1861

Dearest, Thank you 1000 times for your splendid amms and rhododendrons and flowers. . . .

If S. Herbert should wish to act upon the idea of separating the ventilation from the grates—the rationale of the thing is this: ventilation is required all the year round, warming (by the excessively hot grates) only in the winter and only in such a very severe winter as the last. (It is not pretended that Galton's grates do not warm enough for ordinary winters.)

Ventilation can be carried out by the shafts and inlets alone, if properly managed—even in winter. The shafts and inlets can be closed to any extent—so that, at the worst, in the severest winter, it would be necessary only to close them for a time, while they would be in action all the rest of the year. Why give the men typhus in the summer because they *might* catch cold at Christmas?

The great advantage of the shafts and inlets is that the air is kept *constantly* moving in the room. The essence of ventilation is movement rather than quantity. Why make the ventilation of every day dependent on warming in exceptional seasons?

It is true that, in summer, when there is no fire, the *grate* inlet will supply air, but it is not requisite for this, because the shafts and inlets ought to give enough. The use of the grate is to warm *part* of the incoming air in *very* cold weather, allowing the ventilation to go on without interruption. But why, because partially warmed incoming air is good in a very severe winter, are we to have *no* air all the year round, and wait for that part of the ventilating apparatus which is adapted for winter?

Source: From a letter to Richard Baggallay,[132] Florence Nightingale Museum (LMA) H1/ST/NC1/61/5

3 June 1861

I agree with you that Lariboisière has built its pavilions too close. But what a difference between it and the Woolwich plan!

	Lariboisière	*Woolwich*
Height	55 ft.	31 ft.
Distance between Pavilions	68	62

In other words, distance is to height (in Lariboisière) as 13⅗ to 11, as 2 to 1 (Woolwich). In both cases, I reckon from ground floor ward, i.e., from what affects the patients, the light which reaches the *wards*. The construction adopted for Woolwich was the only one of which the ground admitted. But if you examine the plan, you will see that it obviates all your objections.

To all the pavilions, excepting the two right-hand double pavilions, the basement is a false one. Only in the latter is it used, and only in the small itch ward for *patients*.

The two outside double pavilions at either end have outside views, which none of the Lariboisière pavilions (for sick) have. Take the next double pavilion at either end, and one side of it has a distance of (not 60 feet but) nearly 300 ft. The single pavilions on the other side have also a distance of about 150 feet, owing to the short pavilion between them. In short, there is but one side each of two double pavilions which have *only* the distance of 62 ft.

The cubic space of the London hospitals was returned to us by the hospitals themselves. I have now St Thomas' return before me.

Maximum 1600 cub. ft.
Min. 800 " "

I most warmly re-echo your hope that you will improve upon the report. In fact, I believe every year brings such improvements that we shall be quite antiquated old "fogies" with our report in five years. Many thanks for the copy of agreement.

132 Richard Baggallay (d. 1870), treasurer, St Thomas'.

Source: From a letter to Douglas Galton, Add Mss 45759 f230

[ca. 21 June 1861]

Mr Herbert is inclined for your little commission for looking into the administration of hospitals. Will you urge it with him, if you are still of the same mind?

Can you send me the plans of the OLD Woolwich Hospital? It is for the purpose of making a scheme for the new governor, whom Mr H. SAYS he will appoint at once.

Editor: The hospital referred to in the next letter as the Devonport Hospital (strictly speaking, the Devonport, Stonehouse and Cornwall Hospital) was named, after the death of Prince Albert in 1861, the Royal Albert Hospital. When built, it had lock wards for both men and women syphilitic patients, and regular hospital wards for accident and eye cases. It became part of the National Health Service in 1948 and remained in operation (with further changes of name) until 1981.

According to a report by the hospital, Nightingale arranged the wards with the approval of Sir John Liddell. Certainly she saw the plans, was appalled by the whole approach and presumably sent comments to that effect. Evidently only insignificant amendments were made. A letter she wrote Galton stated that she and Dr Sutherland had never seen the "revised plans" (see p 411 below), meaning plans further and adequately revised.

Much can be read between the lines in the explanation of the ever-sympathetic journal *The Builder*: "The committee submitted the plans of the internal arrangements to Miss Nightingale for her approval, and valuable suggestions were made by her in reference to them."[133] Some of her key principles are evident: two beds only between the windows; care for ventilation and warming; lavatories, bathrooms and water closets at the ends of wards; washhouse and laundry in separate buildings. But significant defects remained, as is clear in Nightingale's exasperated correspondence with Galton. The hospital's architect was Alfred Norman (1823-93), but there is no surviving correspondence with him.

The combination of a general with a lock hospital Nightingale thought badly mistaken. She pointed out the objections of ordinary poor, honest people, who saw the government providing services to cure

133 "Devonport, Stonehouse and Cornwall Hospital," *The Builder* 20,1018 (5 July 1862):474.

prostitutes, who would then promptly go back into business. A letter to her brother-in-law makes her points succinctly, stating that she had been asked to make plans for a hospital at Devonport for ten prostitutes for the army, and fifteen for the navy, to be "comfortably accommodated in illness." Yet she and her colleagues had "to beg and sue to get hospital accommodation for honest wives of soldiers" (see p 408 below).

Nightingale was also asked to advise about nursing at Devonport, but would not, since she altogether disapproved of the building and its purpose.

The correspondence on Devonport predates the passage of the Contagious Diseases Act of 1864, which was intended to control syphilis in the army and navy by identifying diseased prostitutes and forcing them into treatment, with nothing commensurate for the men.[134] At the time Nightingale wrote her views on Devonport, these measures, in force in France and much of the Continent, were merely a proposal at the War Office. She naively assumed that such laws would never be adopted in Britain. The proposal, she wrote, amounted to "licensed vice," and the whole "national feeling revolts" against it (see p 405 below). She again put forward better alternatives to prostitution, proposing that the army permit more soldiers to marry, and provide healthier leisure occupations and amusements, such as with gardens, coffee and reading rooms.

Source: From three letters to Douglas Galton, Add Mss 45759 ff228-29, 232-37 and 238-40

20 June 1861

This defies criticism. There is no improvement possible.

If the object is to build a suitable hospital where people are to have a chance of recovery—and not to cover a particular bit of ground with buildings—what can one say to this but condemn it utterly? Even with this particular bit of ground—even with the condition of combining a lock with a general hospital—this is the very worst construction possible. And a different and better plan might be made even on the same piece of ground. Where you can't improve, you don't know how to criticize.

E.g., that there should be no closed angle in any hospital building is a first principle. Therefore this architect bisects the angle with an

134 Nightingale's opposition to the Contagious Diseases Acts is reported in *Women* (8:411-505).

extraordinary spike, and then he crams up the *two* angles thus formed with out-office buildings. Why? That there may be no closed angle.

2. Then, having made a gully for the wind to blow into, he places lavatories and W.C.s just where, when the wind blows in that direction, it will blow all into the wards.

3. For a hospital of sixty beds, of whom half [are] lock patients, what a ridiculous surgical establishment—nearly one third of the building.

4. Are the people in Devonport born triangular? or on an average how many are born so? or what is the meaning of these triangular wards?

5. Is the architect's ideal the profile of a revolver pistol? If you look at the block plan in this point of view, it is very good. But as he asks me my opinion, it is that I would much rather be shot outside than in.

As hospital principles are beginning to be well known, it would be quite enough to engrave this plan on the card of solicitation to stop all subscriptions. No patient will ever get well here, and as I don't approve of the principle of lock hospitals, I had much better let it go on.

Seriously, the plan is unimproveable, and if he wants me to criticize it, he must make one upon the (now) well-recognized principles of construction. You show him your regimental one and he produces this!!!!!

25 June 1861

It's no use. You know it's all wrong. They have improved the plan as to the few details in which they have improved it. That is all. The plan is radically vicious and can't be improved.

They have taken a piece of ground with no consideration as to whether it is suitable for hospital construction, and then they come to Miss N. and ask her to say that it is a good plan. I can't—I would not put a patient into it if they had made me a present of it. It looks now like an ill-fitting pair of trousers.

The only idea in the architect's head has been the portico and square of [the] building behind it—which is to make him a name, I suppose, by its beauty—and all the rest has been sacrificed. I said, of the former plan, it's all bad. And as they have preserved the form, I suppose they mean to preserve those radical defects, which under no circumstances can be improved. They must be removed. Of these are:

1. Kitchen under sick wards;
2. Washhouse and laundry within the building;
3. Deadhouse in the cellar!!!
4. Position of operating theatre interfering with the bad external ventilation, arising from angular form of construction.

N.B. Have they made the least calculation as to how many surgical operations they will have in a year? You see they have but two general wards—no surgical wards at all—only thirty general patients.

The operating theatre seems quite ludicrous. In a general county hospital of four times the number of beds, it was found that there was one female operation in fourteen months and two or three (men's) operations in a year. If this is the kind of proportion they will have, let them have a light room at the top somewhere. I am sure they have staircase enough for a Buckingham Palace, let alone a poor operating theatre.

5. The arrangement of wall and window space in the wards is as bad as possible. The beds will be *under* the windows and two in one corner. (You know all this has been settled long ago, viz., two beds at most *between* the windows and one bed at most in corner.)

6. A separate entrance could be obtained for the lock wards on a better plan.

But to combine a lock with a general hospital in this way is a radically vicious thing to do. You don't know what the honest sick poor say—I do. They say: yes, the wretches who bring disease upon our husbands and sons are cared for and cured, to be turned out again to pursue their vile trade again. And what does government do for the sick *wives* and children of soldiers and the sick *wives* and children of sailors? Why, they take more care of the prostitutes than they do of the honest wives. (This is true in India. And there is enough truth in it *everywhere* to make it worthy of notice that the honest sick poor say so.)

Now look at this hospital. The best end is given to these wretches. The honest *must* go into their end if they are sick. Because they can't help themselves. But what will they say? Depend upon it, it does not do to lower this tone of feeling among them. The only place to put your lock wards, if you will have them, is by themselves on that tongue of land which runs out. And build a high wall between. This is what is done in any honest seaport.

The sick poor say: the lock charity is the only charity which cures a person to be sent back to vice [prostitution]. Why? Because government cares about having diseased soldiers and sailors. It does not care about having honest soldiers and sailors. If what has been actually proposed in the War Office, viz., to bring in the French system of registration, medical inspection and treatment, licensed vice, as long as it is healthy, be done (which it will not be, because our whole national feeling revolts against it) I can conceive no completion of the system of lock hospitals which will more tend to debase our national character. I can tell you (I who have seen the French and British armies) what that is. I have not the least objection to this letter being shown to Sir J. Liddell, who I believe more than half agrees with me. And I will not sanction in any way your pair of trousers. . . .

Let me say that I am perfectly aware that (what I have related of) the tone of feeling of our honest poor is pretty exaggerated, that a great deal *is* done to reclaim these poor wretches. But I entirely agree with the honest wives in this: you cannot reclaim prostitutes; you must prevent prostitution. The last way to do this (or rather the best way to increase prostitution) is to provide means free of expense and ostentatiously handsome and comfortable for the cure of the disease it entails. If you were to provide means for the marriage of one honest soldier or sailor, or for keeping him honest, if unmarried, by proper occupation and amusement, you would really prevent prostitution more than by reclaiming ten prostitutes.

In civil life you don't expect that *every* workman who does not marry before he is thirty will become diseased. In military life, you do. Why? Because a workman may have occupation and amusement and consort with honest women. This is a horrible subject and people always say, a woman can't know anything about it. It is because I know more about the actual workings of the thing in the national mind and body than most men that I cannot hold my tongue.

I believe I was the principal means of putting a stop to the horrible proposition in the War Office above alluded to[135] (by procuring information from France of the effects of it there). I wish my life were beginning instead of ending. . . .

I think I could do something to inoculate the country with this view of preventing instead of cure. Every time you provide a hospital for sick wives and children, means for making marriage respectable, for making the soldier's life comfortable, you are doing something towards it. Every time you provide means for making prostitution comfortable, you are doing something against it.

135 Nightingale managed to delay the passing of the first Contagious Diseases Act, but not stop it. The bill was introduced without notice and passed without debate; some members thought that the bill concerned diseases of cattle.

2 July 1861

Your plan is better than theirs for a general hospital, inasmuch as yours is on the pavilion plan. But the fact is you and I are both in a fix, because they want to make us say that wrong is right. It is wrong to have the lock ward parallel to the sick ward. It should either be at right angles, though separate, as per scratch enclosed, or away altogether at a distance. The small wards in the sick wing are not good. One in the angle is specially bad. The stair and hall are very large for such a building. The patients' waiting room is too far from the dispensary.

I cannot advise about nursing in a building of which I altogether disapprove. But, with regard to the nurses' rooms, have they considered the following questions?

The number [of] *patients*, fourteen, which is Jack's mystical number, is objectionable because you must have two nurses to nurse fourteen. And you cannot have a head nurse, such as a head nurse ought to be, to preside over one nurse. Were this hospital a general hospital, it would be nursed with one head nurse *for the whole* (amply sufficient, if the sick were better distributed), one night nurse *for the whole*, with occasional assistance for bad cases from the two nurses for *each* ward. This is a very ample staff. But how are you to do in *this* case? Is the same head and the same night nurse to do for the *whole*? lock patients and all? Most objectionable, if so. Most extravagant, if not.

Is a nurse to sleep off the men's lock ward? A respectable woman ought not to be asked to do so. Still less a *dis*respectable one.

Men's lock cases are seldom severe, hardly ever dangerous. Real nursing they want in no case. A man, a N.C. officer he ought to be, to sleep off the ward, with men under him to clean the ward, and a woman to give superintendence (for lock men patients are *always* more orderly where there is a woman over them). This is what you want.

In military hospitals, we have entirely refused to put nurses to nurse these cases. In most foreign hospitals, they are locked up. And it is my opinion they ought to be always so. Treat them like itch cases. I never would sanction the giving a woman the trouble and charge of being the turnkey, in fact, to such cases.

I presume the upper storey is to be female. Female lock cases are different. They are generally severe, often in danger. They require the best nursing and closest surveillance from a very competent woman (and no surveillance I have ever seen prevents the appointments for further vice being made actually in ward). A woman's lock ward is a far sadder place and more hard to manage than a man's. But you won't get a head nurse *competent* to manage for these arrangements (which are made for the patients). *Such* a head nurse is, and ought to be, very highly paid.

Don't ask Sir J. Liddell about *this,* for I made the closest personal inquiry into the nursing at Haslar. And the character of the nurses there is notorious. I wish we were well out of this, or rather had never undertaken it. No one but a John Bull (and a seaport John Bull) would ever put the two sexes of lock cases on two flats of the same building, if as I suppose, this is the case here. Male and female lock cases ought to be on different sides, if under the same roof at all.

Source: From a letter to Harry Verney, Wellcome (Claydon copy) Ms 8999/31

12 July 1861

It appears to me so shocking that the government should be actually providing lock hospitals in order to enable its prostitutes to continue their profession, and will do nothing to prevent it, that I have thought whether private hands could do nothing.

It is a fact that I have been lately requested to make plans for a hospital at Devonport, where Lord Herbert's ten prostitutes and the duke of Somerset's[136] fifteen, are to be comfortably accommodated in illness, for the army and navy respectively. . . .

And this when we have to beg and sue to get hospital accommodation for honest wives of soldiers.

Source: From a letter to William Farr, Wellcome Ms 5474/42

Monday 22 [July] 1861

I am sorry that you have been ill. I go from hence to Hampstead on 1 August. Could I see you here before that? Any day would suit me except Friday and Tuesday week. And we would feed you, "sleep" you if you like.

2. I take for granted that a copy of the enclosed has been sent you. Would it be of any use to show it at the British Medical Association? Are you going to the Dublin Social Science meeting? The Dublin hospital authorities have asked me to urge the same hospital statistical scheme at that meeting. And I shall do so (in a letter).[137] Would you advise also in this?

---

136 Edward Adolphus Seymour (1804-85), 12th duke of Somerset, first lord of the Admiralty.

137 Nightingale sent a paper to be read to the August meetings of the National Association for the Promotion of Social Science, in Dublin, "Hospital Statistics and Hospital Plans" (see p 561 below).

3. I have completed all the inquiry which *I* can make as to the causes of death after operations (in preparation for a surgical statistical scheme). Will you look over here some day the lists of said causes obtained by me from the different hospitals, and say (1) whether you will make a scheme from them? (2) whether you would advise this being done in time for the Dublin meeting, (3) whether you would like to moot it at the British Medical Association, in which case I would send you these lists[138] at once.

Source: From an incomplete letter to Samuel Smith, Add Mss 45792 f232

[after 2 August 1861]

[Tell R.G. Whitfield] that he appears entirely to have misapprehended the Woolwich Hospital plans, for every objection he makes to them is answered by the plans themselves; in fact his own letter answers itself. [Tell him] that I will write as soon as I am able and show, point by point, how the plans exactly correspond to his requirements as put forth in his letter. [Tell him] that, meanwhile, I entreat him not to spread his statement concerning them till I can have shown him his error, not as to principles but as to the actual facts of the plans.

Source: From a letter to William Farr, Wellcome 5474/46

5 October 1861

I have got McGrigor,[139] and have looked him through but find nothing in him which will do for your paper. Indeed it is remarkable for so entertaining a book how little there is in it. But, if you wish for that period, why do you not look at a much more able work of his, his report in the sixth volume of the *Medico-Chirurgical Transactions*.[140] I

---

138 Nightingale included lists, "Nomenclature of Operations" and "Nomenclature of Complications Occurring after Operations," in the 1863 edition of *Notes on Hospitals* (see p 215 above).

139 A reference presumably to James McGrigor, *Autobiography and Services: With Notes and Original Correspondence*, 1861, republished as *Sir James McGrigor—The Scalpel and the Sword: The Autobiography of the Father of Army Medicine*, ed. Mary McGrigor.

140 James McGrigor, "Sanitary Condition of the Army," *Medico-Chirurgical Transactions* 6:463-82, quoted in *Notes on the Health of the British Army*, in *The Crimean War* (14:584-86).

made large use of it in the preface to my "confidential" report to Lord Panmure, which preface I have torn out and now send to you, as well as the account of Walcheren, where McGrigor succeeded Webb as inspector general, which I have torn out of the same (my confidential report) as these bits may save you some trouble in reference. Do not return them to me.

Source: From a letter to an unnamed recipient, University of California at Los Angeles #1

12 December 1861

I was sorry not to see you on Friday—the more as I have so little to say that it is scarce worth correspondence.

The matters now under consideration are matters for an architect, not for me. I can only say generally that it is better to keep the nursing staff of each ward separate, in one or more rooms attached to the ward, independently of the head nurse's room, for which there can be only one place, viz., at the entrance of her ward. Or, if this be not feasible, to have the night nurses together in one room and the day nurses in another—each nurse separated by compartments, in a top storey over the centre of the building.

The nurses' room on the basement storey will accommodate *two*—the question is asked in pencil. But it would be very undesirable to have one nurse from the accident ward and one from another ward in it—or to have a day and a night nurse in it. The night nurses must have a room or rooms to themselves.

To the special ward A the nurse's room would do, as indicated, *next* the ward, the scullery between the two nurses' rooms, but not opening into either but into the passage. The adding to the length of the ward, as indicated, would be an advantage. . . .

I can scarcely terminate this correspondence without renewing my protest with which it began, viz., against the immoral tendency of these lock wards. I have always steadfastly refused to help the War Office in this matter. And I am happy to say that the best army medical officers are now of my opinion. But no one knows so well as I the fatal effect it has upon morality to see government doing so little for the honest wives and children of its soldiers and sailors, and so much to enable these wretched women to resume their vile trade—by curing them of the disease which Providence has assigned as its punishment. . . .

You had far better have been rid of government altogether and built your own hospital—even for economy's sake.

Source: From four letters to Douglas Galton, ADD MSS 45760 ff47-48, 65-66, 94-95 and 96-98

11 January 1862

About Chatham, as a general hospital, there is no doubt that Chatham has advantages for carrying out the system. It is merely a question of money. Will Chatham be less costly than Devonport?

We thought of Chatham, and these were the pro and cons: Fort Pitt and the Garrison Hospital could both be placed under one governor, an advantage. Beds: Fort Pitt 241, Garrison Hospital 332. But both are so crowded that the numbers ought to be 128 + 172 = 300. Of course they will not enlarge either hospital. So call the two = 500 beds.

This is enough—but the hospitals are two miles apart and they will require duplicates of some of the inferior officers. The governor ought to reside at Ft. Pitt, but there is no room to build on (?). There is no room for nurses—hardly any for orderlies. Whatever room is wanted at the Garrison Hospital will have to be built.

These were the things which made us pause before making the two Chatham hospitals into one general hospital. Devonport is the only building I know (except Yarmouth) in the least fitted for a general hospital. Would Chatham be available at less money? Could you get for us the amount and class of accommodation at present existing at Ft. Pitt and at Chatham?

You will want house room for a governor, P.M.O., purveyor, paymaster (I would make one of each do for *both* hospitals together), captain of orderlies (with one subordinate to take the discipline at the other hospital), superintendent of nurses (same provision), nurses, N.C. officers, orderlies. If we had the most general reply to this most general question, I think it could be roughly determined whether any money would be saved by adopting Chatham, vice Devonport. But please still press on with the other estimates. My impression was that Devonport could be done with much less. But I never could get Sutherland to look over the plans with me at Hampstead. We have never seen the revised plans. So we are really not in a position to judge which hospital should be proceeded with.

The reduced plan is beautiful (Woolwich). Many thanks for it.

12 April 1862

Would you kindly send me up a complete set of the York Hospital plans, for Sutherland to lecture to me upon?

I congratulate you upon your complete success—I believe it to be the best hospital at present in Europe. But it is quite clear that the details of fittings must not be left to local ingenuity. You must have specifications for windows, locks, bolts, water taps and all such things. It will amply "pay" to have the sizes and method of fitting laid down. So much depends (for the sick) upon these small things.

Would you also tell me exactly the cost of the hospital? I hear £75 per bed for sixty beds. This is wonderful, if true.

Did you have a note from me about a "Finch" and porcelain sinks?

31 May [1862]

As to the regimental hospitals:

1. The position of beds in *small* wards and in "nurses'" rooms had better not be shown. It is not the best here. And the M.O. and hospital sergeant could find better. In the large wards, I would leave the position of beds as at present shown.

2. The hot and cold water taps in the portable bath place are not shown in plan. Ought they not to be? Generally the construction is very good—immensely better than any other system.

3. Have no *windows* over ward doors. This is a sine que non. Every ward must be ventilated *by itself.* It must have no community of ventilation with the administration. Generally, the construction having obtained this point of improvement, the small details and fittings have to be studied. These are as essential to convenience as the architecture is to health. And this is the next improvement to be made.

2 June 1862

Private. At the new Dalhousie Barracks, above 900 men sleep in three rooms (306 in a room), three floors one over the other, six rows of beds between opposite windows. And this "accommodation" is considered "perfect"!!!

A.M.D. will undoubtedly eventually do the sanitary service both for the field and for buildings at home. At present, however, knowledge how to adapt remedies, or whether a remedy suggested touches the evil, is still more scarce among A.M.D. than knowledge of evils. This ignorance [is] by no means confined to A.M.D. Very few civil M.D.s ever make good health officers. So, civil architects are, of all men, the most ignorant of sanitary construction.

Object: to find out special talent in A.M.D. and to train it in the *practical* hygiene, i.e., of finding suitable remedies. Chatham School may do this in about ten years. Indian Sanitary Commission is advising for India health officers (not necessarily M.O.s), to do the sanitary service apart from M.O.s, who are to do the regimental sanitary business.

2. Why should not a standing committee in W.O. do the business? Have such a committee (of heads of departments) before fitting out a

force—only no *standing* committee necessary or desirable. All you want is to make your departments individually efficient, to give them direct and energetic action. This is their contribution to the health and efficiency of the men. Bringing them together (except before an expedition) weakens, not contributes, to their force.

3. Final proposition. Without continuing the Barrack and Hospital Improvement Commission, although its instructions are not exhausted (if you can't continue it), make a requirement on the Barrack Branch that, *for the present,* all sites and plans of barracks and hospitals, and all structural sanitary improvements in existing barracks and hospitals, should be referred for advice to the sanitary member of that commission, who must be authorized by letter to undertake that duty.

And if a promising youth can be found in the A.M.D., let him be temporarily attached to Barrack Branch, and under the training of Dr S.

Source: From a copy of a note of the purveyor-in-chief, War Office, Buckinghamshire Record Office

11 April 1862

Cost of [horse]hair mattresses in our military hospitals per bed per annum. Interest on original cost at 5% [=] 2s; cleaning and remaking 2½d; loss of hair 2d; [total] £0.2.4½. "Cost of washing the cases a mere trifle."

Editor: The next few items concern plans for a women's hospital, the Woolwich Female Hospital, i.e., a facility for army wives.

Source: From a memorandum and three letters to Douglas Galton, Add Mss 45760 ff67-68, 69-74, 75-76 and 161

19 April 1862

Woolwich Female Hospital.

1. You require one fixed bath on the general side, not on the midwifery side. This applies to all.

2. Two basins on the general side are quite enough for ablution. You could thus transfer the fixed bath from the midwifery to the general side.

3. This would give you space in the midwifery lavatory for the portable bath and for an infant's bath (quite necessary to have at hand and immediate) in a place where hot and cold water can be obtained and the bath run off. The portable bath places at the end of wards not required. (These appear to be framed on the principle of the duke of

Clarence's tub, in which he was drowned,[141] being square deep places for people to bathe on their heads.)

4. It is desirable, though not necessary, for a linen closet to be within the hospital and not in the kitchen building. If it is put in the space left by removing the portable bath, now in the W.C. compartment, there must be a similar one for the other ward in the similar space. Or two moveable presses, one *in* each ward, would do, if this is not crowding.

5. I altogether condemn the "fever" ward. Besides putting the worst case in the very worst place in the whole hospital, it is putting her in a place where she must be neglected. The Lariboisière experience is altogether conclusive about this. The same reasons do not hold against the "delivery" ward. If you *will* keep the "fever" ward, call it the "spare ward." And let the engineer paint on the doors respectively: Midwifery Ward, *Delivery Ward*, General Ward, *Spare Ward.* (This is of importance.)

Note: I do not believe that you can serve a hospital of sixteen beds without a resident servant, i.e., a third person besides matron and nurse. And this third person ought never to be admitted from among the soldiers' wives *living out.* Otherwise you admit the brandy bottle, too, and the carrying away of unlimited quantities of provisions. This third woman, therefore, must sleep *in* the building—perhaps by a little rearrangement in the kitchen store space you could find room for a bed.

Chatham appears to have no need of light. It has no skylight in the roof of the passage.

It would be very desirable to put up one hospital first and let us see. Improvements always suggest themselves.

[ca. April 1862]

I corroborate all this, but I say still more strongly:

1. That my opinion that there should be no general stores, especially not the pack store in the hospital, has always been the same, and in this I agree with the purveyor-in-chief.

2. That there can be no good order in a hospital where the "nurse" is allowed to keep any description of ward stores in his (or her) room—these should always be kept in the ward itself.

---

141 During the Wars of the Roses, the duke of Clarence was stabbed and then drowned in a vat of malmsey wine, as described in Shakespeare's *Richard III*, Act 1, scene 4.

3. That the assistant steward (or N.C. officer) should sleep near the orderlies. If the wardmaster is in charge of the patients at night, he cannot be in charge of the orderlies.

4. That there should be a small window from the "scullery" into the ward, with a curtain inside the scullery, to be drawn at pleasure.

I like the plan, but:

1. It must not be considered a hospital for "seventeen," but for sixteen. The small lying-in ward is only occupied for a few hours.

2. A bed on casters (with a woman in it) must be easily wheeled out of the small into the large ward. I think this could be done under the present arrangement of doors.

3. It would probably not add much to the expense to make the opposite ward of ten instead of eight beds, which would also prevent the building from being lopsided.

4. Would it be better to turn the W.C. round as in sketch? This gives an end light to the ward. But the cross-ventilation of original plan is certainly better.

5. There are especial reasons in female hospitals for not letting any kind of stores be kept in the nurses' rooms, where there seem to be presses. In each of the wards, on the other hand, should be some lock-up place for brandy, linen, etc. For everything else there is ample storage near the kitchen.

The plan should now go to the director general and he should be requested to give his opinion in writing, founded on his experience of Aldershot—which opinion I should much like to see.

I can hardly see anything but mischief (in a hospital like this) in giving a third ward for epidemic children—they *must* be neglected, poked up by themselves. At the same time, it would be very undesirable if a medical officer were to turn the nurse's room into a children's ward.

W.C. for "general ward." N.B. The "lying-in ward" should be called the delivery ward and the large ward the "lying-in ward." The opposite ward should be called "general ward." The lavatory of the lying-in ward need have only two fixed basins, but it must have at least two moveable basins. Consider that there will always be eight little people in it who must be washed at least twice a day by the bedside.

According to this, the nurse would be under the conjoint authority of medical officer and ladies' committee. So far as I know, this is the best provisional arrangement which could be made. But it is not a desirable one for discipline. When a superintendent general of nurses is appointed, it would be advisable to introduce some modifications. The discipline of all women employed as nurses in the military service should devolve upon her, subject to the "Regulations for Nurses," which point out their and her duty towards the medical officer.

22 April 1862

2. I sent back your female hospitals with a note, but as a whole they are *admirable*.

3. I admired your sink very much—could you lay your hand on the Finch's note to me about these porcelain sinks and send it me back?

4. I send you Whitfield's pamphlet about the removal of St Thomas'.[142] They are in a terrible dilemma (their own fault). I recommend them to put up hospital huts, like yours, till they can build. They have actually nowhere to lay their heads.[143]

Hampstead, N.W.
23 August 1862

It is utterly absurd that plan for a swimming bath (for the Herbert Hospital). The conservatory can wait. It is not a bad idea. But it is a question of cost.

Source: From three letters to Douglas Galton, Add Mss 45760 ff163-64, 180-81 and 186

2 October 1862

I asked Dr Sutherland to ask you about the female hospital at Portsmouth. But I am sure he will forget. The Rev Sabin[144] says, if you will not give them the hospital you promised, will you allow £240, which will make the present wooden hut practicable? They have private subscriptions and ladies' gifts. And an Anglican sisterhood (very foolish) have been allowed entry by Lord W. Paulet,[145] and are, I verily believe, doing good. Pray talk to Sutherland about the hospital.

Lord Stanley told me privately (I don't know that he knows) that Sir G. Lewis is going back to the Home Office, Sir G. Grey to retire,[146] Lord de Grey[147] to have the W.O. But I am tired of hoping.

---

142 The pamphlet is not available, but an article quoting it extensively appeared in the *Medical Times and Gazette* (see p 785 below).

143 A paraphrase of Matt 8:20.

144 J.E. Sabin, formerly senior chaplain at Scutari.

145 Brigadier General Lord William Paulet (1804-93), commandant at Scutari when Nightingale was there.

146 George Cornewall Lewis (1806-63), secretary for war.

147 Lord de Grey (1827-1909), later 1st marquess of Ripon and viceroy of India. A close collaborator on both War Office and India concerns; he had been under secretary for war, to become the full secretary for war in 1863; George Grey (1799-1882), 2nd baronet, then home secretary.

I don't congratulate you on your new Engineer's Department. You have changed names, not persons.

Hampstead, N.W.
23 October 1862

Dr S. gave me a most splendid account of your Herbert Hospital. (Poor woman! I showed *her* [Elizabeth Herbert] your photographs of it. She is gone abroad today for the winter.)

He also asked me about the nurses' kitchen. Under me and Soyer the best way was to cook their food in the general kitchen. But then neither I nor Soyer are going to be superintendent. Would you ask Colonel Wilbraham to ask Mrs Shaw Stewart what she would recommend? Whether she would have a small kitchen in the administration block for nurses, well and sick (there must be some means of cooking for sick nurses). If so, this small kitchen apparatus might be in the nurses' day room, which will be very little used by them—or in the small scullery, which, if I mistake not, is near the sick nurses' room. Or whether she would have the nurses' food cooked in the hospital and carried to them in their little ward rooms? And if so, whether the general kitchen may be used—or whether one of the little rooms in the hospital could be set apart for this purpose?

Anyhow the nurses must have the means to make their own teas and breakfasts. Anyhow the superintendent, her maid, linen nurse or nurses, sick nurse or nurses, must have their dinners cooked. So that I think Mrs Shaw Stewart had better say what she recommends in *all* these things after her year's experience, which has somewhat modified her opinion.

3 November 1862

You will remember that you were so good as to say that, if Mr Sabin (Portsmouth chaplain) would state his case about the female hospital, you would see what could be done.

Here is his case. Has a formal application come before you? What shall we do?

Source: From eight letters to Douglas Galton, the first two of the same date, Add Mss 45760 ff220, 226-27, 228-29, 230-33, 234-35, 238-39, 263-66 and 270-71

2 January 1863

My "view" is that the gap of non-governorship between this and the opening of the Herbert Hospital is too dangerous and that, whatever government the new hospital wants, is equally wanted by the old—also that all difficulties of government will be enhanced by the ungoverned interval.

I was aware of the fact about the invalids. It is a disaster, but cannot be helped. You know that I would mesh *any* agglomeration of "regimental" hospitals into a general one, and give it a governor. And this is in fact what Woolwich will be. You want governor establishments ready to transfer to the seat of war, in case of war.

In regard to the Woolwich governorship, I am very sorry that I am too ill to see Lord de Grey *now*, as he so kindly proposes. But I hope in a few days I shall be able to do so.

If Dr Rutherford[148] is appointed governor pro tem [for the time being] (for which he is totally unfit—but then it is quite true there is nothing to do), his appointment must be carefully worded, *not* "till another governor be appointed," but "till the opening of the Herbert Hospital when another governor *will* be appointed." But even this I think so dangerous that I should prefer leaving Colonel Wilbraham in charge of both hospitals (with Dr Rutherford as his *locum tenens* [stand-in]) till the Herbert Hospital be opened, Colonel Wilbraham of course residing at Netley.

A good many questions will arise in the transfer for him to settle. Don't cancel his appointment to Woolwich. That is all that is necessary, if this plan is adopted.

30 January 1863

As you are rapidly putting up female hospitals, the question has come up again, how to organize the nursing. (I send you two letters, which please return, as to the appointment of a matron to the Chatham Female Hospital.)

About December 1860, Lord Herbert referred the question to me, and at his request I drew up a minute for the Treasury as to hospitals for soldiers' wives (which was sent in to the Treasury) and also a draft code of Regulations, which possibly may be in the War Office now. Could you find it?

Could you tell me in what state the question of female nurses for female hospitals is? How are they selected at present, and by whom? Who pays them? And in what way? Is the aid of local committees ad-

148 William Rutherford (1816-87), soon to be the British representative at the Geneva Convention.

mitted in providing clothing, extra nursing, etc., and in what way? The purveyor-in-chief would tell you all about this.

If you like to send me any information, I would gladly go into the question again of mode of appointment and organization, etc. I think it is important both to vest the choice of nurses in a superintendent general, and to admit the help of the ladies of the regiment in providing for the soldiers' wives' hospitals.

31 January 1863

You are quite right about "getting into great expenditure with your female hospitals." And it is high time it were put a stop to.

We considered all these questions at the time of framing the "Medical Regulations." The regulation is that the wives and children of soldiers, clerks, office keepers, permanent labourers, etc., are entitled to medicine and medical attendance if within one mile of the dispensary or hospital, but only for children under fourteen years, and not in labour cases at all, unless no other assistance can be had. None of these persons are entitled to any medical comforts, *nor to diets.* And one main reason for this is that, with such people, you have no control over the manner in which such issues would be used. (Medicine can be given, because it is not a popular article of diet.)

The poorest class of these cases is the very one which the ladies of the regiment, etc., should look after, and help with diets and comforts.

The origin of female hospitals was the way in which soldiers' wives and families pig together. Were it possible to give two rooms for a quarter, a hospital would hardly be desirable. Neither is it desirable where the number is very small. In large garrisons, however, you must have female hospitals. And having them, you must give their inmates diets and comforts. And of these you can control the use. This is simply a matter of administrative necessity. And, accordingly, the Medical Regulations enable the wives and children of soldiers (those, of course, only for whom quarters are provided) to receive hospital diets, etc., so long as they are in hospital.

I would request the D.G. to see that the Regulations are attended to. And I would charge all issues *not in accordance* with these to the medical officer.

In the event of any regimental or local committees, at stations where there are female hospitals, being desirous of obtaining admission to a vacant bed for the wife or child of a permanent labourer, there would be no harm in permitting it, provided such committee guaranteed a certain daily payment to cover all the hospital expenses, except that of medicine.

4 February 1863

It is most important that the right man should be selected for Woolwich General Hospital. But I referred the matter to Colonel Clark-Kennedy (through Lord Herbert) before. And I have all along urged that this should be done again. Accordingly as it could not, it appears, be done officially, I did it privately yesterday on my own responsibility. But I could not get his address at his house in town.

I again urge that you should ask him from yourself—but if not, that you should forward the enclosed note from me, which inquires simply about Colonel Wilford[149] in reference to this appointment.

He must be a clever man who makes out anything of a recommendation from my guarded notes to Captain Jervois.

5 February 1863

Confidential. I am reduced, by the position I am placed in, to say dogmatically and mysteriously, without giving my authorities, what my opinion is. And this is emphatically against Colonel Wilford. My reasons are (and they are strictly private) that he is wanting in tact and plain good sense, not progressive and crotchety. He is also as much *too old* as the other was too young. His great merits are not for me to descant upon. They are too well known. But he is not rendered by them more able to see the nature and scope of the duties of the office he wishes to fill.

Take my opinion for what it is worth, I can only say that, after much inquiry, I have no doubt myself of its correctness. The only way in which I can serve you farther is, if you choose to send in to me the names of the other candidates, besides Colonel Desborough, I will make farther impartial inquiries and let you know which I consider the best—rather than negative anyone. But I must not be asked for my authorities.

N.B. I think Colonel Wilbraham has performed his office to perfection. But I would not take his opinion of men *by itself*. . . .

All this is *strictly private.* I had much rather the opinions of responsible men were asked. But if you ask mine, it can only be of use by your considering it as confidential and not even *guessing* at my authorities.

18 February 1863

I heard yesterday from Woolwich that Major [T.S.P.] Field, R.A., has been appointed "acting governor."

---

149 Colonel Ernst Christian Harts Wilford, R.A., director, Artillery Studies, Woolwich.

It is now needless to enter into details. Major Field is a good staff officer and has not the *raging* religious views which so curiously tinge so many good artillery officers (I suppose it is something in the guns). It incapacitates them from governing well their [illeg], their sick men, among whom there are of course *all creeds*. (Some of the officers named in your list were by no means not of this class.)

I see by the new army estimates that only a governor is entered, so that I may say as follows: although Lord Herbert fixed the pay at £600, house, fuel and light, we understood him that it was not to be in addition to military pay, but that, in consideration of Colonel Wilbraham's standing, he was to be permitted to draw the half pay of his rank (about £200) and it is not too much for the appointment at Netley, which includes headship of the invalid depot, etc. But it would be an excessive rate of pay for the Woolwich Hospital governor, whether he be on half or full pay, and justly open to cavil, when compared with the duties now to be performed there. (Besides which, Lord Herbert never contemplated a hospital governor under the rank of lieutenant colonel.)

Would you communicate for me to Lord de Grey, who might otherwise justly think I had neglected his letter of the 7th [missing], which I received late on that (Saturday) night, but acted upon before it had been an hour in my hands. Sunday is, for inquiry at Woolwich, a *dies non* [non day]. So that I had exactly three days to do what I had been urging for three months, and been told that the Horse Guards would not consent to, and then was not told that they wanted done in three—three—days. (There was nothing in either of your letters—which I have by me—to indicate that three months might not be taken for the inquiry.)

One of the officers who employed himself in this so disagreeable a task is very much annoyed, first, at having been given his trouble in vain, and then at having been left, as I was, to learn by common rumour that the appointment had been made.

9 March 1863

The purveyor-in-chief, who is sincerely anxious to make the nurses answer, writes to ask what interpretation he should put upon "linen" (in the Regulations), whether it includes *clothing* or only sheets, shirts, etc., the blue clothing, blankets, etc. (in the latter case) going to the charge of the captain of orderlies.

My own opinion is that the blue clothing should, for the sake of cleanliness, always be in the hands of the "linen nurses," as it was at Scutari, while I would leave the heavy baggage, like blankets, mattresses, bolsters, pillows (but not pillow*cases*) in the hands of the captain of orderlies, if so desired. Perhaps they may object to giving linen room to such an extent to the women.

But would you object to take privately, through Colonel Wilbraham, Mrs Shaw Stewart's own opinion on it *and send it to* me. It is she who will have to work it practically. (The purveyor-in-chief is waiting for an answer as soon as possible.)

Source: From a letter to T. Graham Balfour, Add Mss 50134 ff112-13

20 February 1863

It is long since we have communicated. I have to thank you for your last kind letter [missing]. I venture to send you some surgical operation tables (Tables 1 and 2 which, with the kind assistance of Mr Paget of St Bartholomew's, I have been drawing up).

I have sent copies to the director general, explaining that they are intended not only to register cases but to enable results of particular operations to be better ascertained (statistically) than at present. If I linger on so long, I mean to write a paper on the subject for some meeting.

Source: From five letters to Douglas Galton Add Mss 45761 ff18-19, 43, 44-45, 126-27 and 128-29, the last two from Hampstead

4 June 1863

I don't approve of your cavalry horse arrangements at all. Because the horses in the loose boxes can't see out of window.

I do not speak from hearsay but from actual personal acquaintance with horses of an intimate kind. And, I assure you, they tell me that it is of the utmost importance to their health and spirits, when in the loose box, to have a window to look out at. A small bull's eye will do.

I have told Dr Sutherland. But he has no feeling.

20 July 1863

I send you back your official papers on female hospitals, also your private letters on the same, "of no use to anyone but the owner." I entirely repudiate all responsibility about the present Regulations as to the same. These hospitals will never work until they are all under one responsible female head or superintendent general. But this is no fault of yours.

22 July 1863

The arrangements and alterations proposed for Fort Pitt Hospital on the plans in these papers are sufficient. Wherever they are departed from (in the report of the board of officers) these departures should be disallowed.

Warm water for the baths should, of course, be provided from one common centre, the kitchen (?). The absurd proposition of the director general [Gibson] to reduce the cubic space for sick again reappears in these papers. Some time ago I asked if Lord de Grey should not tell the D.G. that the question is settled and *not to be reopened.* This interference should be put a stop to at once. If you have people who do not understand what they are about, they must be treated as if they did not.

When the hospital (garrison) is removed to Ft. Pitt, it will be necessary to have one or two receiving wards for casual cases at Chatham in the manner proposed.

24 September 1863

If we cannot have a polished white impervious surface of Parian cement, it is all "up." But Mr Mennie's minute is not satisfactory, because it appears that the proper cement was not used in the trial ward. But if the testimony of others is to be received, then we should obtain from it solidity and polish—but not whiteness.

I should be very averse to return to so primitive an expedient for hospital ward walls as plaster. Let us by all means escape scraping and limewashing. If you are personally satisfied that there is nothing else for it, then I would propose for your consideration whether unpolished Parian should not be used to give solidity and imperviousness, and the surface then painted of a light cheerful colour (varnished, if necessary), sufficient to receive a polish which will enable the surface to be washed, as has been done at Lariboisière. This would include the ceilings also.

The only question that ever occurred was whether Parian cement was not an improvement on this process. If it is not, then this process is the next best. As regards Aylesbury Infirmary, I have reason to believe that the first quality of cement was not put up there anymore than at the Herbert Hospital. It is a great pity.

26 September 1863

As to Parian cement, after consultation with King's College Hospital, I fear we must give up the white, and adopt the lightest grey that will keep a colour and try to tint it of a pale *giallo antico* [antique yellow], (ceilings of white plaster). If we cannot get the tint for the walls, then a strip of coloured enamelled slate to be carried round the wall between the ceiling and the wall, also making panels, the colour of the slate to be such as will lighten the grey. The grey Parian put up at K.C.H. was intended to be painted. But they had occasion to wash it and in the process it took such a polish that paint was unnecessary. And the ward can be used very shortly after the washing is completed.

N.B. The washing must be done (not with a whitewashing brush but) with a hard scrubbing brush. The soap must be (not soft soap but) white curd soap. Would you give authority for a trial to be made in one of the wards? at the Herbert Hospital?

The colour at K.C.H. has not altered after three years' use—so say the W.O. surveyors. But I do wish you would go to K.C.H. and look at the walls yourself, *with* Miss Jones, who is *the* practical person there. Dr Sutherland and I have both examined her on the subject. He differs with me as to her conclusions and *I* can't go to the hospital to see.

Source: From two letters to T. Graham Balfour, Add Mss 50134 ff114-15 and 168-74; typed copy of the second, Add Mss 45772 f261, both from Hampstead, N.W.

29 September 1863

It is long since I have heard of you. I have just been looking through the new annual report. It is an admirable work—by far the best we have had—and answers, I think, nearly all the promises made for it. I mean to write more fully about this when I have read it through.

What I come now about is, as usual, a begging excursion. Could you, and would you? give me the following data? I hope it will not cost you much trouble, excepting perhaps for 1862.

Mortality per 1000 per annum according to ages
Infantry of Line at Home

Years	20-25	25-30	30-35	35-40
1859				
1860				
1861				
1862				
Average of 4 years				

A similar table for Foot Guards at home
" " " for Household Cavalry
" " " for Dragoon Guards and Dragoons
" " " for totals for all these arms.

3 October 1863

Private. I have received your note, and need hardly say that I concur in it entirely. It would be impossible to do without you in the office—it would be impossible to fill your place in the Statistical Branch (it must be either you or Sir A. Tulloch). It would be unfair that this very fitness should stand in the way of promotion.

I do not think they would "promote a junior over your head" to the inspector generalship in the office. But I cannot see why the Treasury should not allow two inspectors general, under the circumstances, in the office. I will do my best to represent these circumstances. It shall not be my fault if you do not succeed.

But I need hardly tell you that my position in the W.O. is very different (and ought to be very different) now from what it was in Sidney Herbert's time. He and I worked together daily for five years. It is not to be expected that I should find two such friends. Nor indeed, were it otherwise, is my strength up to seeing one every day, as I saw him.

You ask for my "advice." I can only say, consider, you know the statistics can't do without you. And you know your claims shall be represented as strenuously as possible.

Source: From two letters to Douglas Galton, Add Mss 45761 ff168-71 and 201-02

Hampstead, N.W.
29 October 1863

I do not approve of these fittings at all—they are a great dissight to the ward and there is real danger of a delirious or melancholy patient hanging himself by them. If you wish to have some arrangement of the kind, I would recommend you either:

1. To have a plate in the floor, behind middle of bed, screw-in plate and iron rod. This may be seen at King's College Hospital. They have a wooden ledge or skirting on the floor to keep the bed a few inches from the floor. And the iron plate is outside this, so that the rod does not touch the wall. It bends over the bed. (Pray remember that in the venereal or convalescent wards you need nothing of this kind.)

2. *Or* you might have a Tollitur,[150] which is an apparatus that screws onto the bed and requires no fittings at all. This, too, may be seen at King's College Hospital. But this may be decided on any time.

3. There is a machine (like a bed table), a Staffordshire patent for moving a patient completely off the bed—not merely for enabling him to raise himself. This is to be seen, I believe, at St Bartholomew's

150 From the Latin, meaning to lift up.

Hospital. This, I believe, requires no fittings. I would recommend you to send someone to King's C.H. to see the plate in question, making an appointment to see Miss Jones. This is the only one of my three contrivances which requires a fitting. It is not unsightly, which the Tollitur is. But I cannot imagine that you require two, or even one, to *each* ward, or even to each *sick* ward.

Military cases are always less severe than civil ones. And indeed, in severe cases, I think personal human help better than mechanical—except in long incurable chronic cases, which you *don't* have in hospitals.

2. If you send someone to King's C.H., pray let him take the opportunity of seeing the Parian (*with* Miss Jones) "down her private staircase." They don't defend their great staircase, which was all run with iron mould from iron bedsteads. Besides this, there are great water marks in other places from a cistern in the roof. But she would like to show you what was the best *and has improved* (not got worse, as ours has) by time. . . .

Whatever you do, *don't* disfigure your Woolwich wards with those gibbets, which have, I am told, made Netley look like a madhouse.

Inkermann Day [5 November] 1863

You can't prove a negative. You can't order out a detachment of Guards and one of our men to prove that their sick are less well off than ours.

Some time ago, at the time of the first royal sanitary commission, it was actually shown that, where there were *plenty of* sick, a profit was made out of the /10 a day. It is really not our fault if there are not enough sick to make the *tenpence* a day afford them the good diets we give ours. It will be a very good joke if the Guards' sick wish to go into our hospitals to get our "butter." . . .

The diet scale, which has so enchanted the Guards' sick and their doctors, and which the "gold stick" and the "three colonels" "trust and beg" that you will deliver them from, was fixed upon in consultation with all the leading diet men of science, including Christison, and all the leading civil hospitals. And one of its objects was to get the men as speedily out of hospital, and as speedily convalescent, as possible. But (as I say) you can't prove a negative—you can't prove that the absence of the "butter" stops a man's convalescence. Though it *does*, for all that.

Source: From a note and a letter/draft/copy to R.O. Mennie, Add Mss 45798 ff220 and 221-23

2 February 1864

Miss Nightingale presents her compliments to Mr Mennie and begs to return the Indian barrack plans, by Captain Galton's desire, which she thinks admirable. She has no further criticism to make. She will return the hospital plans tomorrow.

3 February 1864

This hospital plan has come out remarkably well, but may be improved in the following points:

Plan A. bed space rather small—wall should project beyond bed on each side, corner beds to be 18 inches from wall, large end windows to be reduced to three feet in width, bath to stand out in floor of bathroom.

Is not the space for basins in lavatory too narrow? Change sergeant's bed as suggested: show walls double plan B, shift corner beds 18 inches from wall; other alterations similar to plan A. In both plans, show only one stair.

Elevation: show a shield in front of louvre sections required to show ventilating and other arrangements. Show a first floor, laid out for patients' dining, day and reading room, games, etc., ward stores, etc., orderlies' rooms, etc., and night orderlies' sleeping room separate.

Also, on the first floor of one block, waiting room surgery, pack store, office, clean linen store, bedding store, utensil store, as well as day room—in which case there should be two stairs. We want a set of sketch plans of first floors to show how all the accessories can be accommodated in the hospital blocks.

The block for convalescents should have day room and dining room, because the patients will be the greater part of the day in their day room—the ward being only used for sleeping room at night. The block for sick requires space only for ten out of twenty-four to have day room.

Source: From six letters to Douglas Galton, Add Mss 45762 ff26, 65-66, 67-68, 71-72, 86 and 117-19

3 February 1864

Perhaps you may like to see the enclosed papers about the Halifax Soldiers' Club. Please return them to me. You will see that they have subscribed and spent a good deal of money on doing works of construction which the W.O. ought to have done in the first instance.

Perhaps, another time when an institute is to be tried, the works may be done by you, and the subsequent expenses borne by the men, in the way recommended by the day rooms' committee. You will see, also, that the "*light*" allowance is not enough, and that the subscriptions go to provide more light.

29 February 1864

Lord Hartington: Army Estimates.[151] I should say *very* shortly (the House of Commons is not very logical).

Medical and Hospital administration. In 1854 there was a frightful breakdown, which was only repaired at the cost of millions. The country demanded it should not happen again. And it did not. Lord Herbert's commission in 1857 provided that it should not. But the measures recommended, of course, cost money.

What has been their result? The death rate of the British Army at home *was* 17½ per 1000, that of the Foot Guards being 20.4, of the Line Infantry 18.7, of the Dragoons 13.3, of the Household Cavalry 11. *What it is now?* (Refer to Balfour for the years '59, '60, '61, '62 and if possible '63. I have them before me. But he has not given them me, calculated according to *numbers.*)

Lord Herbert showed that H.M.'s Army Service was the *most unhealthy* trade among H.M.'s subjects *then.* What is it *now?* It is the most healthy. The British Army hospitals are now the best (among all armies). We may say, compared with our own civil hospitals, which have advanced like tortoises, they have made giant strides.

In 1853 there existed *no* hospital or sanitary administration or organization for time of war. And we saw the result in the colossal calamity of the Crimean War. In 1864 our hospital and *sanitary* administrations are the finest in the world. And we have already seen the result, as in the Chinese war and other war contingencies—so in time of peace at home.

May we see such results also *soon* in India and in our tropical stations! But, to do this, we must not cut down, we must build up! I enclose a more "solid" statement.

There is nothing in the world I should like so much as to have to do Lord Hartington's speech, and stand in his shoes on such an occasion.

4 March 1864

Private. Now that the immediate pressure of preparing army estimates is over, I am going, like the House, to put a few questions.

---

151 Lord Hartington (1833-1908), later 8th duke of Devonshire, then under secretary for war; he spoke frequently defending the government's army estimates.

Please to send me a copy of the Female Hospital Regulations. In today's *Times* is an advertisement for a matron midwife for the Aldershot Female Hospital. Now, whether this is contrary to regulation or not, it is contrary to common sense, and the W.O. ought to put a stop to it.

I say nothing of the fact that these are the people who have always abused me for taking any but soldiers' widows as nurses for soldiers, and now they are advertising for anybody. But, when they have been admonished in the Regulations to have matron midwives trained at King's College Hospital, it is rather too bad.

And more than this, they have actually offered to train a woman for the Portsmouth Female Hospital (as midwife) whom we had consented to take at King's College Hospital, and I had paid the £10 for her, when they have not got a midwife themselves. What "rum" doings are these? Oh! those ladies' and officers' committees!!

7 March 1864

The enclosed were sent me "to see," especially on a black March day. They are "seen." Of all *rum* things, H.G. [Horse Guards] things are the *rummest.* Set me down for slang but rum, rummer, rummest are the only words in the Queen's English to apply to the Queen's Army.

The W.O. (unfortunates) go into fight with flanks exposed (purposely, as it seems). The Cavalry attack them on one side, Foot Guards on the other. And smash you go. This is *rum.* Your reserve, the Horse Guards, is placed, or, rather, places itself, in so exposed a position that it gets shot at by all sides. This is *rummer.* Now for *rummest,* the royal letter of 1798, from which one learns that, before that date, the surgeons *did* all the Guards hospitals in everything for a certain pecuniary allowance.

This letter abrogates the past practice and gives the surgeons 12/ a day, instead of profits. This letter is put forwards now as the Magna Charta[152] of the household hospitals. The surgeons all swear by it, but nevertheless they have given up the 12/ a day long ago for the pay of the warrant.

The best cure for the present disastrous defeat would be for the W.O. to stick to the letter, including the 12/ a day. All the doctors would then find out the "admirable virtues" inherent in the new Medical and Purveyor's Regulations.

---

152 Magna Carta, or the "Great Charter." Signed by King John in 1215, it limited the ruler's arbitrary powers in favour of the rule of law.

There is nothing more to be done. Everybody has been beaten, except that, in two or three of the hospitals, the new diets are in use.

4 April 1864

This is as satisfactory as could be hoped. The experience of Parian cement shows that it will not stand alternations of heat and moisture—but it will make a good white surface (i.e., with good workmanship and favouring conditions and these conditions you have in the wards of the Herbert Hospital).

4 May 1864

When we say "thirty beds," we mean that there are thirty people in them for 365 days in the year, except during an odd night or two.

But see how unkind you are to these poor women. I understand from Chatham that at first the "thirty beds" *were* occupied. Why? Because the soldiers were admitted to sit in friendly conversation by the bedside. (Mind you, the very first rule of all proper lock wards is that no man visitor is admitted, on any pretence whatever, to the female wards, not even a clergyman other than the appointed chaplain.) It seems that you had the unkindness to enforce this rule at last at St Bartholomew's. And immediately the *occupied* beds fell to eleven (and have remained so). (This fact is answer enough, without another word, to all the *bosh* that is talked about these places being places of reformation.) They are just places for the encouragement of prostitution. And nothing else.

I quite agree with you that the report tells nothing at all. I send what it does tell, and also a way of improving the method of recording, in order that you may know how your money is spent. The following is the result of the table:

Days included in return	167	
Patients admitted	46	
" dismissed cured	23	
Remaining in hospital	9	(beds occupied)
Days spent in hospital by 46 patients	2307.	

Cost of 2307 days' occupation at 1s 4½d per diem = £25 per bed (say) £158.16. (Should you want to know *how much too much* you have paid, you deduct this sum from what you have paid.)

Proposed heads of Register for St B.'s:

No. of Case

Name (Married to be marked M.)

Age (last birthday)
Place of Residence
Date of Attack
" " Admission
" " Discharge
Result (Cured) (Relieved) (Otherwise discharged) (Died) (Transferred)
Disease (Primary/Secondary, etc.)
Duration of case in hospital stated in ____ days.

Annual Summary of Cases

Remaining on 1 January	Admitted	Cured	Relieved	Died	Otherwise Discharged	Remaining 31 December	Total Days Patients in Hospital

No. of Beds Occupied						
Max	Min	Average	1st Quarter	2nd Quarter	3rd Quarter	4th Quarter

Source: From four letters to Douglas Galton, Add Mss 45762 ff122-27, 156-57, 215-18 and 222, the last two from Hampstead

17 May 1864

The minute in Lord Herbert's handwriting 25 April 1861 contains the pith of the matter and is the only just and wise course. It was written at my own house and, to the best of my recollection, that is the *very* sheet of paper (my paper) which was written at my house. If a circular on this minute had been issued, great good would have been done and no complaint would have been possible. (Of course the line about the D.G. would have been left out.)

The embroilment begins with a proposal to issue, *not* this minute but one of date 9 May 1861, in which there occurs *for the first time* the following passage, and which I never saw till I saw it with wonderment in the circular:

> Every case to which such extras (beer, wine, spirits) are prescribed must be entered by the surgeon in the medical casebook, and the amount of extras daily given as well as his reasons for giving the same, also duly recorded (*sic*).

It is curious to trace back the history of this passage, or rather this gross blunder, in the original draft 9 May 1861; the direction is that the case be entered in the "casebook," an instruction in some sense conformable to the regulation . . . which directs that, when these extras are ordered, they are to be marked on the diet roll opposite the names of the patients—a very proper precaution and quite sufficient as a check. The term "casebook" has been used for diet roll. Then comes the word "medical" inserted before "casebook," a record of a totally different character, intended for registering the medical experience of the regiment, and in no sense as a check record. And to make matters worse, other words are added on the margin, "as well as his reasons for giving the same." And the result is a perversion of one of the most important statistical documents of the regiment—an altogether useless amount of writing, immense discontent on the part of the department, and relieving the D.G. of the responsibility which Lord Herbert's minute of 25 April 1861 directly placed upon him.

N.B. I was told that the pencil writing was mine. I never saw the paper. Besides, the handwritings are sufficiently distinct. Three ink notes are Lord Herbert's, two (including the word "medical") are Mr Robertson's, and the pencil note (as you can see at once by the word "issue") is either by the same scribe who wrote the text or by Mapleton or Godley.

What could Lord Herbert do after having written so clear a minute? In place of simply transcribing his minute, they put forwards a totally different one, based on a different administrative principle. There is only resemblance enough to mislead. (I don't at all wonder that Lord Herbert was misled.)

Clearly, what you have to do is to withdraw that circular of 20 May 1861, No. 683, and to substitute another based on Lord Herbert's original minute, i.e., provided a circular is still necessary. If there is extravagance in the issue of diets *beyond the diet scale*, it would be a fair case for requiring a full record of the circumstances. But you would hardly need to call for this, as every such case will be of sufficient importance to ensure its entry in the medical casebook. . . .

You will have heard of Sir A. Tulloch's[153] almost sudden death at Winchester, nearly the last of Sidney Herbert's *Crimean* friends. I hear that poor Lady Tulloch is quite "stunned" by the shock.

27 July 1864

We think this scale a prodigious improvement upon everything that has gone before it. And quite worth all the trouble it has cost. Of

153 Sir Alexander Tulloch, member of the supply commission with Sir John McNeill in the Crimean War.

course, if it were possible to give more fresh and less salt meat than even this scale gives, it would be better. And we may get it, as civilization advances on board transport ships. With proper care as to ventilation and exercise, there should be little scrofulous taint, if this scale is put into operation.

We think, therefore, it should be forwarded for trial, including the scale of rations for children under five years proposed by the committee. In Lord Herbert's time, all diet questions were referred to Dr Christison of Edinburgh—the greatest living authority on such subjects. It would be more satisfactory if his opinion were now taken. At the same time, the improvement in this scale is beyond a doubt. . . .

If you write to Dr Christison, let us draft the letter.

24 September 1864

We have been trying all we can to make out about the Bermuda epidemic. No one in the A.M.D. has been able to give any help; they know nothing but that the yellow fever is there.

In 1853-54, the Colonial Office referred the reports of the then epidemic to Dr Sutherland, before they were presented to Parliament. There is also a report of a slight outbreak in 1856. And there are returns made to the Barrack and Hospital Improvement Commission from Bermuda barracks and hospitals. Dr S. will make an abstract of the whole. But in the meantime we want you to know generally how the question is.

In 1853 and 1856, the disease began like ordinary epidemic attacks—a case here and a case there—sometimes miles apart. In '53, nearly every barrack had fatal cases among soldiers, women or children—215 soldiers and officers died. The general information as to the sanitary state of the island (during these previous epidemics) is tolerably full. And it shows just such a state of things as *ought* to precede epidemics—in fact, Gibraltar over again: a porous red earth sub-soil over coral limestone—no drainage, "every house its own cesspit, emptied when required"—water supply apparently from wells in the vicinity—overcrowded houses—want of cleanliness—obstructions to ventilation—and worse than all, bankrupt municipal authorities, who say it is out of the question to call upon us to improve, because we have no means." Tant pis pour eux [too bad for them].

Your most important consideration regards the barracks. The engineers, in the course of ages, have managed to transport to the hot, close, moist climate of Bermuda all the worst errors of construction which you found existing in the worse class of casemates and barracks at home, e.g., close position, double-floored casemates, barrack rooms and casemate rooms with small windows at the end some 40 feet apart; the largest barrack, for about 220 men, has all its rooms of this construction and communicating by window openings through the walls from end to end, the object being, as the engineer naïvely says, "to improve the ventilation." The windows are all casements, not admitting of opening at the top, commonly shut at night. *No* ventilation except in the large barrack referred to; in each (nineteen men) room of which the magnificent provision of 8 pipes, 2 inch. in diameter, carried through the roof, has been made. Overcrowding in all the barracks excessive for the climate, i.e., it was so in '53. But some troops have been removed since then. Even at the date of the returns, however, the men *in such rooms* as described had little more than 600 c. ft. each, or about half what the barrack structure and climate require.

All the usual defects in latrine drainage—drains exist, but bad and unwholesome. Officers' quarters bad—small single rooms, *in fours*, without thorough draught. And of this state Sir E. Lugard[154] says: "no means of guarding against yellow fever" he thinks it so perfect. And medical officers the only "means of prevention." The question is: is the assistant under secretary of state for the colonies and yellow fever to have his way, or Lord de Grey and the soldiers to have theirs?

The improvements required must be carried out partly by the authorities and partly by the W.O. As regards the first, you must make this the occasion of getting a complete report on the sanitary condition of Bermuda and the works required to improve it, just as you did in regard to Gibraltar. And the W.O. must be prepared to support the improvements as against the S. of S. for the colonies and for yellow fever, if necessary. Would not the best way be to refer the whole subject to the B. and H.I. Commission?

As regards barracks, what you want is something very like rebuilding. Only the building material is perhaps the worst in existence, viz., consolidated sea sand, used for everything, roofs included, through which rain *drips*. The unkindest cut of all[155] is that the bankrupt municipal corporators, who can't afford to improve their own house, have actually printed out that the barracks are unfit places for human beings to live in. . . .

---

154 Edward Lugard (1810-98), under secretary for war and the colonies 1861-71.

155 From Brutus' stabbing of Julius Caesar, in Shakespeare's *Julius Caesar*, Act 3, scene 2.

By the way, I heard from the H. Guards that, ever *since the 9th*, there has been lying a reference to your Barrack and Hospital Improvement Commission of the *Delhi boils* at the W.O. unanswered. I forget whether I wrote to you about this epidemic. I did to Sir J. Lawrence. I dare say he has used the "*charm*" against this already—which Sir E. Lugard says there is no using.

As regards Bermuda, the whole of the evidence points to one thing, viz., the evacuation of every barrack as soon as disease appears in its neighbourhood. Or if there be no civil population, as soon as the men on parade show the slightest "yellow" tendency—camping them on a dry surface not exposed to marsh air, of which there is enough in Bermuda—spreading the tents over a large area—a few men only per tent—a rigid attention to cleanliness and very careful attention to the quality of the water supply.

The wonder is how could man contrive to make such a narrow slip of an island unhealthy?

3 October 1864

I am sorry to hear of your uncle's[156] death. It is sorrowful to see the old swept off—but how much more sorrowful to see those in the prime of life.

Dr S. tells me that he has written to you "my (!) opinions" about the Herbert Hospital grates. I dare say he does not know them. For I have not got any—put your grates in the middle of the floor, if you possibly can. If you can't (but I never would give up striving to find a way), it does not much signify whether you put them *under* or *between* the windows, for economy of bed space. Either way you *must* leave room on each side for the patients to sit by the fire—consequently you can't have the beds up to the fireside (as in Dr S.'s plan of having the fires under the windows to save bed space).

It will be some compensation, if you really can't have your grates in the middle of the floor, that it will save those great transverse beams.

Source: Note, Wellcome (Claydon copy) Ms 9001/79

5 November 1864

It is ten years today since Inkermann. It is ten years yesterday since we landed at Scutari. It seems to me like three lives, though I have spent seven of those ten years in bed. It seems to me like three different existences in different worlds.

---

156 Hubert John Barclay Galton (1789-1864).

In that time I have won all and lost all three different times. The last three years have been quite as different to me (since Sidney Herbert and Clough left me) as if I had gone to another world.

Source: From a letter to T. Graham Balfour, Add Mss 50134 ff120-23

9 November 1864

Private. I am very much obliged to you for your kind note. The West India returns are most encouraging. And I would have used them, had not my argument, as to the want of capability in the Briton to adapt himself to other climates than his own been intended to include all classes, although tropical climates are alluded to in connection with soldiers specially.

The W. India mortality is much lower than the E. India mortality, thank God and you all! But I was obliged to take into account both elements, viz., "mortality" and "diseases," in estimating the India sanitary state, as one must in estimating the sanitary state of any race or people.

I mean my point was (the same as yours) to show that India miasmas, and India suffering from miasmatic diseases, are preventible. Now the very diseases which I have cited as proofs of the preventible unhealthiness of the W. Indies are still preventible in the W.I. And more than that, yellow fever *still* breaks out there.

Besides, W.I. regiments have now, have not they? short periods of service. And I want to show that Europeans can live in tropical climates, without being brought away, as you bring out a weak patient from a vapour bath. . . .

Short service, hill climates and other precautions have improved the health of W. India troops. But they are not fit to possess the country till they have expelled the "dragon" of miasma. (Vide [see] the picture of Apollo killing the dragon, who lies half in a marsh and half on the hillside.) . . .

I have just received a pheasant and two rabbits from Wilton. And while apologizing for the small present, I thought you would like to have them in memory of our dear friend, Sidney Herbert.

Source: From a letter to Douglas Galton, Add Mss 45762 f257-62

16 November 1864

The chief point in the new diet scale requiring explanation is the scale of substitutes to which the committee have agreed. Are the substitutes in the scale to be arbitrarily issued in lieu of the articles in the diet scale?

Perhaps you can ascertain this in the office. If so, then have nothing to do with it. If, on the other hand, it merely means that, e.g., when salt meat is issued under the scale, one lb. is to be considered equal to a lb. fresh meat, there would be little harm in it, but then, why have it at all? E.g., by no conceivable arrangement can flour, split peas, calavances [chick peas], and dhal [lentils] be considered as dietetic equivalents to preserved potato or compressed vegetables.

Again, the note at the foot of the scale of substitutes states that fresh bread should be considered a "desirable substitute" to be issued "whenever practicable," while the diet scale lays down the precise number of days in the week when fresh bread is to be issued. In fact, with the new diet scale, this list of substitutes is useless and seems to have been adopted in the first instance to supplement the deficiencies of a radically bad scale, which have now been swept away.

As this scale of substitutes at present stands, it would open the door to all sorts of irregularities in dieting. But if it must be kept, take out the words "fresh bread" from the footnote, and continue the footnote as follows:

> Every transport ship for troops and invalids must be provided with the articles required for dieting troops and invalids in accordance with the authorized scale. And it is to be understood that the articles in the scale of substitutes which are not included in the authorized diet scale are to be over and above the quantities and articles required for the daily issues under the authorized diet scale and that such substitutes are only to be issued when, from unforeseen circumstances, a departure from the authorized diet scale becomes necessary, or when the medical officers should recommend a change of diet.

Of course all this is on the supposition that it is proposed to use this scale of substitutes in the manner supposed above. But perhaps you would be good enough to inquire in the office.

2. In the new list of medical comforts the following articles are omitted, while they are included in the list of medical comforts contained in the "new Medical Regulations," p 113 (green book)

Coffee
Salt
Pepper
Mustard

3. The following is a list of substitutes taken from the Admiralty list which would comport with the new diet scale:

Flour ¾ lb. }
Rice ¾ lb. } equivalent to { ¾ lb. Biscuit

Fresh Meat { 1 lb. equivalent to ¾ lb. Preserved Meat
{ ¾ lb. ¾ lb. Salt Meat
Spirits ½ gill equivalent to Porter 1 pint
Coffee 1 oz. = Tea ¼ oz.
Fresh Vegetables ½ lb. = { Preserved Potato 2 oz.
{ Chollets [Shallots], Compressed Vegetables 1 oz.

Flour ½ lb. {
Split Peas 2/9 pint { to be substituted
Calavances ½ pint { one for the other
Dhal ½ pint {
Rice ¼ lb. {
Oatmeal 1/6 pint = Split Peas 2/9 pint

Before everything is finally settled and the scale issued, please let us see a printed copy of the proceedings, that we may have an opportunity of considering the whole carefully over.

Source: From a letter to T. Graham Balfour, Add Mss 50134 ff128-29

20 January 1865

Private. In your volume for 1862 (which, I assure you, is always in my hands—it is the sword and buckler to which I always trust, to do battle) have you observed that, at p 14, there is a misprint, the substitution of healthy civil population and of general civil population for each other, in the last two lines of the final table on that page?

Your report stood me in good service lately, when "the military," my esteemed patrons, made a private attack, which came to me from Lord Stanley, saying that all the improvement in the health of the British Army, not in India, was due to invaliding only. It shows how wise you were to put the deaths of invalids in your columns—and I was able to show what the improvement was, even including these.

I assure you I have not neglected in spirit your letter of 18 November, I mean to make another attack. But I thought it best to wait awhile. We have not a S. of S. now [de Grey] who will impose his will for good on the H.G. We expected better things of him. But there are many worse.

Source: From two letters to Douglas Galton, Add Mss 45763 ff32-33 and 41

7 March 1865

I don't know whether you remember a certain Rev C.B. Gibson, a Presbyterian chaplain, dismissed the Irish Convict Service because he wrote a book[157] establishing certain facts against that service, and in favour of Sir J. Jebb's.

Rather more than a year ago we made great efforts to have him made an army chaplain. For, quite independently of the above facts, he is a chaplain who obtains an extraordinary permanent influence over the men, which chaplains, I am sorry to say, in general do not. And this, though (perhaps because) he is very Irish and "gushing" and all that.

A semi-promise was obtained for "the Rev C.B. Gibson" then that he should have the first vacancy among army Presbyterian chaplains. It is said that "the War Office is about appointing two Irish Presbyterian chaplains."

The chaplain general told Lady Herbert, in a note (which she sent me) that he "had put down the Rev C.B. Gibson's name, but that there was no vacancy *then*." There is one now. If you think it desirable, Sir Harry Verney would wait upon Lord de Grey and restate what we know about Mr Gibson. I think I sent you a copy of his book.

15 March 1865

The Rev Gibson (Presbyterian chaplain) has applied for one of the *N.C.* [non-conformist] chaplaincies "so the Presbyterian troops at Sheerness, Warley or Shoeburyness," to which he has received an acknowledgment, signed Partington or some such word.

"Thankful for small mercies," he is greatly encouraged by this. But he wishes to know if he might be "allowed to select between the three places mentioned," though none has as yet been offered him.

Your, etc., Importunate Widow[158]

Source: From an incomplete letter to an unnamed recipient, Columbia University, Presbyterian Hospital School of Nursing C81

8 March 1865

Private. I will answer the last part of your kind note first.

You are perhaps aware that all barrack construction, new and old, comes now before a standing commission at the War Office, called the "Barrack and Hospital Improvement Commission," and founded by Sidney Herbert. In this way, I see pretty much all that is going on. And if at any time you saw anything wrong about to be done, and would send me a line, I could probably put you in the way of making an official representation.

157 Charles Bernard Gibson's two-volume *Life among Convicts*, 1863, which Nightingale bought and sent to Galton.

158 An allusion to Luke 18:3-5.

With regard to your barracks, however, the case stands thus, in the cavalry barracks the rooms are to be greatly improved, and all the present schools and recreation rooms are to be removed out of them and built elsewhere. The infantry barracks are to be extended on new ground, and the present barracks improved. Suitable recreation rooms will then be provided.

I am glad you mentioned it, because now I can be on the lookout to see that these promises are fulfilled.

The other matter (about the prohibition to form any temperance society within the battalions) I will today write about to the War Office. I don't say this at all in any sanguine hope.

Source: From two letters to Lord Stanley, Liverpool Record Office 920 Der 15/68

12 March 1865

Confidential. General Peel "is going to attack the Herbert and other military hospitals on army estimates,"[159] I hear. Now General Peel is as much more formidable an antagonist to us than Lord Panmure,[160] as a gentleman is more efficient than a "snob." Besides, General Peel has always behaved most generously to Sidney Herbert's memory, Lord Panmure most ungenerously. (I do not mean to weary you with saying how.) My object is: would you think well to say a little word for our poor new hospitals, if General Peel attacks them? in the sense of advocating the (at-present) received principles of hospital construction, as set forth in your India sanitary report.

21 March 1865

I take the liberty of sending you a copy of the last *Builder* and of asking you to read the article on the "Herbert Hospital,"[161] which is *not* by any of us.

Lord Panmure's attack in the House of Lords on the pavilion hospital system in general and on the Herbert Hospital in particular has damaged us with people whose action, not whose opinions, we want. And we can't afford to lose our patrons.

---

159 General Peel, in Hansard, *Parliamentary Debates* 12 March 1865:1782-88.

160 Panmure (Lord Dalhousie), in a long speech, both defended the Netley Hospital, building and site, and attacked the Herbert Hospital. He preferred the opinions of military medical officers to "hygienists," who had gone "too far" (Hansard, *Parliamentary Debates* 11 March 1865:1099-1107).

161 The Herbert Hospital, Woolwich," *The Builder* 23,1154 (18 March 1865):183-85.

Source: Memorandum, Wellcome (Claydon copy) Ms 9001/114-15

[13 March 1865]

Pavilion Principle. In 1856, a committee of the Army Medical Department, presided over by Sir John Hall, declared in favour of the pavilion principle. In 1857, the royal commission did the same. The "Herbert" Hospital is simply an embodiment of the principles of that commission. I would name, in addition to those I mentioned (as completed examples of recent construction), Bartholomew's, Rochester, South Devon and Cornwall Hospital,[162] Devonport.

Of our hospitals:

Herbert Hospital	650 beds
Hounslow Cavalry	60 "
York "	60 "
Hillsea	20 or 30 "

The first three it was necessary to build on account of the bad state of the old hospitals. The Hillsea Hospital is for new forts. Of old hospitals built on pavilion principle, there are:

Fort Pitt Garrison
Dublin Military Infirmary
Aberdeen Regimental and other small ones.

The pavilion principle means only the adaptation of the principle of separate buildings for sick, with windows on opposite sides of wards, and free ward ends. The Winchester Hospital is on this principle. So is old Bartholomew's (London) *in part*. *All* the best hospitals in Paris and Belgium are really built on it. The pavilion principle has been reaffirmed by Lord Stanley's commission (Indian). Our window space is the same as in the French military hospitals in their more brilliant climate. Light can always be moderated by blinds.

The War Office says perhaps we are to be attacked on the score of extravagance in construction. What appears extravagance in construction is nothing more than economical application of means and material. We have merely picked up ideas from various quarters and put them together, e.g., Parian cement, adopted from King's College and Guy's Hospitals and from evidence before the R. commission of 1857. It is necessary to enable the walls to be washed readily and kept sweet.

E.g., oak floors we get from Paris; e.g., ward offices—once admit that they are to be introduced into hospitals, we must have them of

162 A new wing was added to the South Devon and Cornwall Hospital, Plymouth, in 1863.

the best, e.g., baths, sinks, wash-hand basins (complained of by Lord Panmure) ditto. It is poor economy to save a few £.s.d. [pounds, shillings, pence] on these, when many thousands have been spent. We can find authority for all these improvements in existing hospitals. The cost of the new Hôtel-Dieu at Paris is set down at 40,000 francs per bed (including land). This shows how much more economical *we* are.

Source: From a letter to Harry Verney, Wellcome (Claydon copy) Ms 9001/118

14 March 1865

What night will army estimates come on? I was rather glad they did not come on last night.

Our defence against all accusation of extravagance is, besides the diminution of army *mortality*, the old regulations for hospital accommodation was 10 percent of the strength in barracks; a short time ago the regulation was reduced to 7 percent (by representation of the Barrack Improvement Commission) on inquiry by the Horse Guards, but the ACTUAL average now of sick in hospital to strength in barracks is *3½ to 4 percent.*

Upon this average we take our stand—as proof of what we have done. We think it wise to let the amount of hospital accommodation (required) be still 7 percent, for in time of epidemics it may still rise to that *for a few days a year.* But we have the time quite within our grasp when, in consequence of the improvement in barracks, we shall be able to say 5 percent is the utmost limit of what we shall want of hospital accommodation, even in epidemic times.

The fact is that, even now, if the number of occupied sick beds ever rises to 5 or 6 percent, it is only *for a very short period.* We are accused of extravagance because the new hospitals, Woolwich, Hounslow, York, Hillsea, are so much larger than will be necessary. Really it is not our *fault* if the number of sick has fallen so much that they can't fill their hospitals.

The Army Medical Department make requisition (for each of these hospitals) at the old percentage of 10, upon the strength of the garrison. They have now consented to 7 percent. And we mean to bring it down to 5. The Horse Guards have formally acknowledged this diminution. It was they who made inquiry of the "Barrack Improvement Commission" as to what it should be.

It seems very hard upon us now to turn round and say, you have thinned our hospitals, and ought not to have built them so large, when the Horse Guards and Army Medical Department themselves fixed the number of *beds* for all these hospitals (10 percent), and we have reduced the number of *sick* to 3½ or 4 percent.

Source: From a letter to William Farr, Wellcome Ms 5474/91

7 July 1865

I send you the *second* copy I have been able to lay my hands on, in order that you may get it noticed in the *Times* (which, I believe, was your intention) together with the Return of Deaths, etc., Queen's Troops 1856-64, which you called for (8 June, House of Commons). But the *Times* will not say anything right, unless you tell it how.

Source: From a letter to T. Graham Balfour, Add Mss 50134 ff130-31

29 July 1865

I hope that you have not judged of my interest in your (statistical report) pages by my delay in acknowledging your kindness. I read them with the greatest eagerness. I wish I could send you anything you would care for so much.

It is a most important chapter in army mortality. You have succeeded in showing that, in the French Army, certain conditions of levy and furlough may affect the law of mortality. This is a most remarkable point. A minute examination into the habits of each service would determine the conditions which bring about this difference in mortality law. I shall look forward for the appearance of your annual report with intense interest. . . .

You must not judge of me by the little you hear from me. We have been overwhelmed with business. I get weaker and weaker. But all the old associations are as strong as ever.

Source: From a letter to and an undated draft note for William Farr, Wellcome Ms 5474/92 and Add Mss 43400 f216

Hampstead, N.W.
2 September 1865

Private. There has been nothing in the *Times* (nor in any newspaper I know of) in reference to your reply to the Government of India. I think it of the utmost importance that you should have a short pithy paper, which would certainly force attention to it, at the Birmingham meeting.[163] Tell the object of your doing so. But always give Sir J. Lawrence[164] credit

163 The Royal Statistical Society met at Birmingham in September 1865; Farr was a vice-president, but did not give a paper at those meetings.

164 Sir John Lawrence (1811-79), later 1st Baron Lawrence, first viceroy of India.

for practical support (which he always gives) to us. Let your paper, while scattering people's illusions unmercifully, have a practical bearing.

The newspaper paragraph about the Herbert Hospital was written by the same hand apparently which informed us last year that the hospital was a ruin, and this year that it was to be given over for a barrack, which report was believed in, even by M Husson of Paris. The *fact* is that the building has been handed over to the purveyor-in-chief for sick.

I don't think I ever thanked you for your letter about the Herbert Hospital, so gracious and grateful to me. Yours are almost the only letters I ever had about Sidney Herbert which really soothe my wounded soul.[165]

Our dear friend Hilary[166] is dying painfully. The only wonder is how she lives through each twenty-four hours. But the suffering is much less acute and the wandering of mind much less painful.

[ca. September 1865]

I have heard a report that the people are going to convert the splendid Herbert Hospital, the best hospital extant according to all British and foreign authorities, into a barrack. Now I don't know whether this be true, but it has occurred to me that *The Lancet* has taken much pains with the barrack question already, and may possibly take more, that this is really a question to be inquired into. Could you give a hint at this without bringing me in? If there is any truth in the matter, I think a good deal should be said about pearls and swine.[167]

Source: From two letters to Douglas Galton, Add Mss 45763 ff96 and 99-102

15 November 1865

I return your *Herbert Hospital*.[168] We think it is now complete. It will do a great deal of good. And I want a GREAT MANY copies for myself—one is promised to M Husson of Paris—and I want to instruct *all* the hospital builders in England!!

The pictures at the end are very pleasing and will prove a great attraction. People do so like pictures. (I think them better than lithographs. But why can't the sun do distances?)

---

165 Probably his letter of 7 March 1865 wishing that Herbert had been in the House to reply to detractors: "to what heights might he rise?" (Add Mss 43400 f21).

166 Joanna Hilary Bonham Carter (1821-65), cousin and friend.

167 An allusion to Matt 7:6.

168 Douglas Galton, *Report to the Right Hon the Earl de Grey and Ripon, Secretary of State for War, Descriptive of the Herbert Hospital at Woolwich.*

We have made one or two little suggestions in the margins of the proof. Remember, I want a great many copies for myself, please.

28 November 1865

Private. Of course I flew at Dr Sutherland, in order to hear how beautifully all your arrangements at the Herbert Hospital worked—how well the governor administered, etc. When I heard his account, I thought they had been to *old* Woolwich by mistake. I can't well conceive anything worse. I am sure I am thankful M Husson, of Paris, is not now here to see.

How "gat" the governor[169] there? By accident, it seems—and because he has twenty children.

If, after all the pains (in sifting) which Colonel Clark-Kennedy, Lord Herbert and I took—we only got a Wilbraham—it is not very surprising that the H.G. only got a donkey—who is perfectly incapable of grasping your details, or bringing anything under your Regulations. But it is very mortifying indeed to hear, as I do from the whole A.M.D., that there is not a P.M.O. who would not have made a better governor—mortifying, because true.

Considering the immense interests at stake in making your new model hospital work, I think a little more trouble might have been taken at the beginning to secure the only points which could make it work.

The ludicrous misappropriations (which do, I assure you, beat all my experience of Scutari) may be put to rights. But the heads which could be guilty of such inventions will not be put to rights, ever, by a six months' course under Dr Courtly. I was quite ashamed that Messrs Ellis[170] and Chadwick should see our model hospital in such a condition.

However, there is one thing can be set to rights at once. If I understood them right, the sick are all placed in the south ends of the pavilions and the north ends more or less used for stores. Any such arrangement is perfectly destructive of government or nursing. I thought the advantage expressly to be secured by the double-pavilion Herbert Hospital plan was that part of it could be *occupied, governed and nursed* as well as the whole. This was a positive point aimed at in the construction.

That "peculiarly helpless creature," the British Army, seems to have been incapable of grasping this. With the present small number

169 The first governor was Colonel H.J. Shaw, replaced by a medical officer when he retired.

170 Robert Staunton Ellis (1825-77), then in England, sanitary commissioner for Madras.

of sick, they must take either *pair* of the end pavilions they like and fill them—make these the present hospital—cut off the communication so as to include library, chapel, day room, in the part of the building allotted for sick. And, if they *must* put stores in the wards, use the wards at the end opposite from the sick. This is not a matter of choice but of necessity, and should be done at once.

I should think the west pavilions, with their operating theatre, the best for the purpose. But again I say—how "gat" the governor there? Que diable allait-il faire dans cette galère? [what the devil could he do in this mess?] When hundreds of thousands have been spent on this model hospital, was it not worthwhile to take a little pains to occupy it properly? Or is its *occupation* to be a "model" too? Shall *I occupy this* house after *your* model?

You make me fit for Bedlam—which ought to have been your governor's destination—only he *must* be incurable.

yours distractedly
F. Nightingale

Source: From a letter to William Farr, Wellcome Ms 5474/98, typed copy Add Mss 43400 f103

[January 1866]

About your prison mortality paper, I have ascertained from the War Office that there is to be no meeting of their commission before Ellis and Sutherland come back. So I have kept your paper for Dr Sutherland to see *here* before it goes into committee.

Don't forget to send me a "Recensement" [census] *for my directeur de l'Assistance Publique at Paris, who asked for it. . . .*

My happiness was so bound up in those two guns we have got back from Bhutan. But Sir J. Lawrence won't give them to Lord Hartington. He will give them to me. And I shall mount them on the noble leads attached to this mansion. And I shall teach my cats to be artillery men. And I shall use them against all my enemies of Victoria Street and Pall Mall (including Dr Sutherland).

By the way, have you seen Surgeon Rennie's attack upon you, "Story of the Bhutan War" p 235, upon your "Nosology" "sunstroke."[171]

---

171 David Field Rennie, *Bhotan and the Story of the Dooar War.* On p 235 Rennie referred to Farr's nosology, acknowledging that exercises in the sun had an "injurious effect on some," but doubted that they were so inimical as represented.

Source: From two letters to Douglas Galton, ADD MSS 45763 ff144-45 and 148-51

15 January 1866

I have received with great pleasure your beautiful book on the Herbert Hospital. I wish you would send a copy forthwith to M Armand Husson, directeur de l'Administration Générale de l'Assistance Publique (Place de l'Hôtel de Ville, Paris) *from the War Office.* I told him (may I be forgiven!) that the War Office was languishing—dying by inches, in fact from its anxiety to send him this book (he came over in July to see the Herbert Hospital). Also to Henry Currey, Esq, 4 Lancaster Place, Strand (he is the architect of new St Thomas' Hospital). I think this would come with a better grace from the W.O. too.

I shall have many more people to send copies to, but I will profit by your kind offer to send them for me, if I give you a list.

26 January 1866

Female Hospital. With eager carefulness, and with all the tremendous force of intellect, I have spent a long and laborious life in going over Captain [Edward] Belfield's plan.

1. I entirely approve the pulling out the wards, like a book-tray, to the utmost length of ground, for the simple and undisputed reason that the more ground the sick (or for that matter, the well) cover, the better for them. For the same reason, I prefer the blue slip, where the "verandah" is open from end to end, to the kitchen block projecting it out and interfering with it (as underneath slip). But:

2. What you want a double cook and double kitchen for passes my genius to discover. You might just as well tell me that it would prevent the spread of the cattle plague into Scotland, if there were a queen for Scotland different from the queen of England. Do you mean to tell me that the cook will catch lying-in and convey it to the other ward?

And here you must put up with some improper observations. I have always maintained that the *lying-in* are, of all others, the most susceptible of the influences of foul air, and the kind of patients who most generate foul air among themselves, which is called "infection."[172] Therefore you cannot be too careful to prevent foul air. But here is the very best exemplification of the meaning of the word "infection," since no one, I believe, asserts that lying-in is caught by "infection." In large lying-in hospitals, such as the Maternité at Paris, where no case but of

172 The bacillus that causes puerperal fever was not identified until 1902; it is a streptococcal type and highly infectious.

lying-in is, of course, ever admitted, the destruction among the poor lying-in by fever is, or was, in my day, awful. Unwashed hands of a stupid doctor or nurse may certainly convey disease to and fro also between lying-in and fever wards.

But my genius was completely at a loss to understand Messrs the Cattle Plague commissioners, or to understand the Army Medical Department on lying-in wards and, generally, etc.

Would it do if the cook were to change her name when she cooks for the lying-in and call herself Mary Smith and Betsy Godfrey when she cooks for the other ward? I really know not what to advise you, as it is no use kicking against the pricks[173] (of the Army Medical Department). And if the D.G. tells you lying-in is catching, of course we must say Amen.

But, as this is to be a pattern female hospital, I would strongly suggest, for the sake of precedent, that you do not publish the plan till Wombwell's[174] menagerie comes back from Algeria. Let*him* fight the battle of infection with the D.G. *I* can't.

Editor: In 1866 Nightingale asked Douglas Galton to make arrangements for the matron and treasurer at St Thomas' Hospital to go over the new Herbert Hospital "steadily," seeing all the fittings.[175]

Myers, the Herbert Hospital contractor on floors, later worked on Nightingale's own floors, at Douglas Galton's recommendation.[176]

Source: From a letter to T. Graham Balfour, Add Mss 50134 ff132-35, typed copy Add Mss 45772

19 December 1866

Confidential. I think you know that there needs no apology for any communication from you to me—so old a friend as you are and associated with a work (and a time) so dear to me, that, though it is connected with much of disappointment and much of bitter sorrow, yet it is, if possible, more constant and eager an object with me than ever.

I need scarcely say that I agree in almost every word you say. But I believe that, under present ministers, I am quite certain not to be consulted about the future D.G. It would, however, grieve me so much to

173 An allusion to Acts 9:5.

174 Adolphus Ulick Wombwell, R.E., later Colonel.

175 Letter 9 May 1866, Add Mss 45763 f171.

176 Letter to Douglas Galton 26 August 1870, Add Mss 45764 f179.

be in the least degree disingenuous with such a tried and noble friend as you are, that I will tell you (QUITE confidentially) what has taken place, as far as I know it.

It being understood that, if the C.-in-C. proposed that Sir J.G. [James Gibson] should continue in office after his term had expired, the S. of S. would not consent—a kind of *unofficial* correspondence ensued. All that was done was to recall the steps which were taken to ascertain the qualifications of a number of men out of whom the D.G. could be selected in our good friend Alexander's time, and that one name was then considered second only to Alexander. The result was that it appeared highly probable that the office would be filled up on principles different from those which led to the selection of Dr Alexander.

I have consequently done nothing more. And I have really no precise idea who the coming man is likely to be. I will only mention that the name pronounced by all the Great Gods, excepting one, was Dr Logan's.[177] Now it is impossible for anyone to have a higher opinion of the character of another than I have of Dr Logan's. But I don't think his health or spirits equal to the task, which certainly killed poor Alexander. Dr Logan has perpetually said that his present office was too much for him. And what is that, in regard to strain upon mind and spirits, compared to the D.G.ship?

As I have said, I am quite certain not to be consulted farther than what I have already intimated. I need scarcely say that, except the one I have mentioned (and it is only fair to say that I have not had the slightest communication with him and I believe I never saw him in my life), I consider you as *far, far* away beyond all the others in point of fitness and capacity for the D.G.ship. And, I assure you that, should *your* appointment be the result, I shall congratulate *ourselves* as being very fortunate indeed (*not you*). And I shall look with greater hope than I have done for the last five years to Sidney Herbert's reforms being carried out.

---

177 Thomas Galbraith Logan (c1809-96) was the next director general of the Army Medical Department after Gibson, serving 1867-74; see biographical sketch in *Wars and the War Office* (15:1040). Balfour never got the directorship, but he did have a distinguished career, was honorary physician to the queen, a fellow of the Royal Society and president of the Royal Statistical Society.

Source: From a letter to Douglas Galton, ADD MSS 45763 ff272-75, draft partly in Dr Sutherland's hand ff270-71

20 December 1866

26. *Purveyor's* 1176. When you send me a publication of such absorbing and romantic interest as this, you cannot expect me to skim it over lightly—I must savour it slowly. I have read it thus all through and, what is more, I have compared it with *green medical*, and with Colonel Clark-Kennedy's report. I have also gone through it with Dr Sutherland.

We think them, the Regulations, very full and very good—very carefully and artistically drawn up. But we think the end rather too tragical: P 42. Reg. 197 we think ought to be expunged. The precedent is so highly dangerous, and would open a door for so many excuses that it virtually undoes the work done by the Regulations for equipping hospitals. Every hospital, whether at home, abroad or in the field, should be complete. There should not be the possibility of incompleteness, except from capture or destruction of the purveyor's stores. The principle of Reg. 197 was the very one which led to half the misery endured by the sick at Scutari. A man wants according to his wants—not according to what is in the purveyor's stores.

Suppose, e.g., soldiers going into the field have all the asterisked articles in the list; the steward depends on this fact, which he knows to be true. But the packs are thrown away or lost (an actual fact) and the poor men had no changes at all. We would abolish this Article 197 at any cost or inconvenience.

2. (I am progressing backwards) please look at p 36 Articles 167, 170. You see there is to be "a small lock-up case" *in* "each ward." You see that "nurses' rooms are not to be used for stores on any pretense whatever." We have always said that suitable press "for each ward" to hold the "medical comforts" and the supply of ward linen to be given for immediate use to the nurse.

3. P 12, Article 41. The principle in the first line leads to indiscipline. All employment of patients in the ward sculleries, in the "kitchen," as orderlies, etc., is a flaw in discipline. Patients should never be out of their wards except for exercise. Even after all we have done for military hospitals, the discipline among the patients is not equal to that of a ward of forty men in a civil hospital under one woman.

But I suppose the British soldier and sailor considers it as the Briton's right to see after his victuals in hospital. However, at least, I would give the "patient" the right "to attend," but leave it *optional.*

Source: From a letter to William Farr, Wellcome Ms 5474/116

3 March 1868

Private. I return you, with very many thanks, Mr Spencer Wells.[178] The figures are satisfactory, but they would be more satisfactory if Mr Sp. Wells could take a small house in the country, high and dry, and operate there. There are several points besides which should be noticed, such as the state of the patient, the *period* of the disease, the precautions taken during and after the operation, as compared with those which used formerly to be taken, and the period at which it used formerly to be operated upon. However, this operation is evidently entering the domain of operative surgery with a fair chance of good results.

About "M Husson's lucubrations," it is an extremely awkward thing for me to have to confess that I don't know whether I "have seen them" or not.[179] He wrote to me in October, saying they were coming. Since then I have received many hospital documents from Paris, "Comptes Rendus" and things, but nothing which at all tallied with what I supposed these "lucubrations" were to be. I put off writing to him, and now—could you let me see the "lucubrations" for a minute (I will return them by messenger) in order that I may know, before I write to M Husson, whether they are *not* what I have, or whether they are?

Editor: Dr Sutherland informed Nightingale in 1869 that the plans had come back from Portsmouth, where the commanding royal engineer had "adopted essentially the plan as amended by you and by us here." A few things were compromised, so that the superficial area allotted was only 75 sq. ft. instead of 80, for a "large saving" in cost. Her recommendations about fully private nurses' rooms were met: "partitions will be carried up to the roof in all cases." A letter Dr Sutherland wrote her the following day further stated that each room would have a window that opened and that good space for a sick room for nurses had been found.[180]

---

178 Thomas Spencer Wells (1818-97), gynecologist, probably his *Diseases of the Ovaries: Their Diagnosis and Treatment,* 1865, which reviews his ovariotomy cases.

179 Probably his *Statistique médicale des hôpitaux de Paris,* 1867.

180 Sutherland letters 1 and 2 October 1869, ADD MSS 45754 ff1-2 and 5.

Nurses' quarters at Netley became an issue in 1869 on the appointment of a new superintendent to replace Jane Shaw Stewart. Jane Deeble[181] was a widow with young children, who had evidently been promised, along with a high salary, space for her children as well as herself. But Nightingale, as she told Henry Bonham Carter, thought that "no child, in my opinion, ought ever to come within a hospital, especially a military one."[182] Dr Sutherland at that time did a critique of the new nurses' quarters, on which she commented, and sent it to Henry Bonham Carter.[183]

Source: Notes, Florence Nightingale Museum (LMA) H1/ST/NC18/15/34

3 September 1869

Proposed alterations for accommodation of nurses: Netley.

1. There will be no difficulty in dividing off the separate nurse's rooms—each with its window—each with its partition *up to ceiling.*

2. There will be no difficulty in dividing off the diminished linen store by a glazed partition so as to leave the proposed passage.

3. The room marked "linen nurse's room" has no fireplace, although they have shown one. It has no flue, and none can be carried up. This proposed appropriation cannot therefore be carried out. But instead of this, it is proposed to improve the whole accommodation as follows:

4. To break a door through the wall between C and A where the pencil marks are. This door to be the door into the nurses' and superintendent's quarter from the hospital corridor.

5. To convert the proposed linen nurse's room into a store opening directly out of the linen store, to continue the division separating the linen store from the "passage" through to the end as shown by the pencil mark, so as to cut the storage entirely off from the nurses (which is essential for their privacy and comfort) the door at C to be retained exclusively as an issuing door and half door with counters. In this way no orderly could ever come out of the corridor, unless for carrying in the clean linen and for heavy work. Of course the partitions shown at the end of the linen store cutting off the lobby would not be introduced. The end of the store would come close up to the main wall, and being lengthened in this way, it is proposed:

6. To convert the "store" close to the superintendent's bedroom into a linen nurse's room and not to disturb the partition with the red

---

181 Jane Cecilia Deeble (1828-1913), St Thomas' trained nurse, superintendent at Netley 1869-92; biographical sketch in *Wars and the War Office* (15:1034).

182 Letter 10 June 1869, Florence Nightingale Museum (LMA) H1/ST/NC18/15/11.

183 Sutherland memo with Nightingale undated notes, Add Mss 45754 ff17-18.

marks across it. There is no fireplace there at present, but there is a flue and a fireplace can be easily made.

7. Good reason should be shown for proposing to cut off two dark stores from nurses' dormitory (*day room*), an arrangement otherwise so objectionable.

8. The superintendent's office seems dark—but, as all the rooms are 15 ft. high, perhaps there is light enough.

9. The servant's bedroom being the passage to the kitchen is objectionable. A partition could be run up where pencil-dotted, so as to give her a room to herself. The door at B is, I understand, never used except by the superintendent. Otherwise the poor servant's domain would be intolerable.

10. The "nurses' scullery" to the far left of the plan belongs to one of the wards.

11. We used to think a *mending room* indispensable. But, I understand that at the Herbert Hospital, in order to simplify wages, rates and books, the linen is to be returned into the superintendent's linenry, *repaired* from the laundry. Possibly this is the case at Netley now. Otherwise we used to think the mending best done on the superintendent's premises in a room adjoining linen store.

Source: From five letters to Henry Bonham Carter, the first two of the same date, Florence Nightingale Museum (LMA) H1/ST/NC18/15/18-19, 23, 42 and 44, all from Embley, Romsey

3 September 1869

Netley. I wrote to you in great haste (to save this morning's post) about the Netley plan. But, I don't know that I have anything to add except that I will gladly see Mrs Deeble, if it will do the least good, either here or in London, "about the end of September," as you say before she goes to Netley. You shall keep me informed, please.

I hope she is a woman of some nous [mind]. *Nous* is wanted everywhere, but most of all, I think, in a military hospital—besides gentleness and firmness. Military officers are such queer things and have such queer ideas about nurses.

Netley. I thought it better to obtain some information from Major (now Colonel) *Ravenhill, who built the hospital*,[184] before sending you in my remarks on the plan. Here they are:

184 Philip Ravenhill, R.E., deputy director of barracks works.

I think, with the proposed alterations, the plan is a very ingenious and good one and gives no more than is absolutely essential for respectable women. Of course an adaptation must always be awkward. And one would not have made such a plan originally.

It is essential that all serving out of linen to orderlies should be over a counter, and (as it were) *outside* of the nurses' quarters—so that, on *current* business, the orderlies should have no business to be inside the nurses' premises. It is essential for decorum, comfort, everything—the more so, as I believe it is impossible to help (entirely) occasional, though more rare, calls to give out linen *at night.* The linenry ought by rights to be like a shop with private dwelling behind, entered by separate passage.

Perhaps you would say, when you send in your plan, with report, to the W.O., that such and such (giving a list) is the accommodation you consider required. But that, if this can be secured in some other or better way, *that* would be, of course, all you desire. Or something to that effect.

I understand that the W.O. is anxious to have your report in as soon as possible, in order to make arrangements to enter on the work at once. So I will send this off at once. Excuse haste.

10 September 1869

Draft letter. Furniture. It is obviously necessary that furniture should be provided. And I believe that the W.O. will assent to this.

1 October 1869

Private. Netley Nurses' Quarters.

About this troublesome business (now pray your good gods that I may be short!), I thought (as you seemed to anticipate) Mr Whitfield's letter so very objectionable, both as to matter and manner (objectionable because the W.O. would certainly say: "here is an old house surgeon, on the faith of a whippersnapper of an architect's boy,[185] dictating to us!!"

I do not say that it would be either fair or honest for them to say this. But they *would* say it. And it would be putting us into quite a false position with the W.O.) the more so as Mr. W. is quite right as to "cost" and "time," though unquestionably right in some points and probably right in others, that I felt no doubt as to not sending it to the W.O., and yet did not like to make no use of it.

185 Whitfield's son was a junior architect working in the office of the architect for St Thomas', Henry Currey.

I therefore took the liberty of sending the whole to Dr Sutherland. And he has retained Mr Whitfield's letter until he sees that the plan (expected up yesterday from Portsmouth) includes all the requirements. He takes note of Mr Whitfield's statements. He thinks it quite out of the question showing Mr Whitfield's letter at the W.O.: I am afraid that your reference to plan and cost will be reckoned an undue interference, if ever it gets into the Works Department for a similar reason.

Private. (N.B. Not Colonel Ravenhill, but the C.R.E. at Portsmouth,[186] is the responsible planner. And all that we can do is to see that the plan fulfills the conditions.)

Embley
7 October 1869

Netley. I am sorry the W.O. have not sent you the plans—I understood they would. Neither have they me. But orders have been sent that the quarters are to be ready for occupation by the end of this month. This then is settled.

There is no danger of national bankruptcy on *our* score. The estimate is £180, and they have added £20 for contingencies!!

Source: From a note to John Sutherland, ADD MSS 45754 ff14-15

Embley
Romsey
[10 October 1869]

Netley Quarters. Here are these dreadful plans again. (Yet I do not like to decide upon them without you.) Vide [see] *H.B.C.'s letter marked in red.*

1. You told me that all the nurses' bedrooms were to be divided up to the top. Only two are to be. I think this a very serious grievance. These quarters are not temporary, but permanent. These nurses are not probationers, but head nurses. I think it a very serious grievance also to move nurses 2, 3, 4, 5 for any slight illness into nurses' rooms 1, 6. (There is nothing annoys a respectable woman more than not to have a single spot she can call her own), then to move back nurses 1, 6, into the (late) sick room, without a possibility of any airing or temporary evacuation for thorough cleansing. This *makes me think* that we *must* have the place marked "Infirmary."

---

186 John William Gordon (1805-70), R.E.

I would let the "linen nurse" sleep in it, on condition that she evacuates for a sick nurse (our "linen nurse" *has* been a governess and, but for her nervous timidity, is just as fitted as Mrs Deeble to be superintendent).

The grievance in this case would not be the same as it would in the other case—because she would go into a spare compartment, which she might even retain if she wished it—at all events till there had been a thorough cleansing (a thing necessary even in a private house from time to time).

As for typhus and smallpox, *that* must always be removed out of the hospital at once, if possible, and nursed elsewhere..

Source: From a letter to Margaret Verney, Wellcome (Claydon copy) Ms 9003/125

22 November 1869

Here are the statistics you asked me for and if they will be of any interest to Lady Sarah Williams,[187] I shall be the more repaid.

Every year, in the Home Army—taken on the last four years for which returns are complete—we have 729 men alive who would have been dead but for Sidney Herbert's measures, and 5184 men always on active duty who would have been "constantly sick" in bed.

At the Herbert Hospital we have (unfortunately for the hospital) about 400 patients fewer than the hospital was built for, and 500 fewer than the "requisition" for sick accommodation was made for. And so, mutatis mutandis [with appropriate changes], with other hospitals.

Source: From a letter to T. Graham Balfour, Add Mss 50134 ff137-38

14 July 1870

I have read a good part of [your annual report] and am very glad to see that it not only keeps up to its high standard of usefulness but improves upon it.

I will venture only one question at present. Is the evidence about the "Contagious Diseases Prevention Act" any more conclusive than it was? Unless its efficiency in results is proved, it would be worthwhile to compare the saving to the army, if any, pecuniarily, with the outlay on the hospitals, would it not? so that it might be known exactly where they are in money as well as in figures.

It seems like old times to be writing to you.

---

187 Mother of Margaret Verney (1844-1930) and Maude Verney (c1846-1937).

Source: From two letters to Henry Bonham Carter, Florence Nightingale Museum (LMA) H1/ST/NC18/17/24 and 18/19

22 December 1870

Netley Night Nurses' Quarters. I do not see how, as you say, we can do anything but accept this. Nothing can have been so unreasonable as Mrs Deeble in all this, and nothing can be less perfect than these rooms for night nurses.

The window opening into the corridor looks straight across the corridor on the open sky. Otherwise I should say we were hardly justified in putting a night nurse into a room with only a borrowed light, and next door to a kitchen. There will be room for the beds being placed with the heads away from the division wall—which is a thick one, and not very permeable to noise or heat.

Otherwise, knowing, as we do now, Mrs Deeble's great want of consideration for the nurses, I should say that the position of a night nurse sleeping on a summer afternoon with, at her back, what *may* be a roaring kitchen fire, cooking for Mrs Deeble's boys and unable to open her window into the corridor, moreover, on account of the noise, was not a desirable one. As you say, two servant girls sleeping there are not so objectionable as one, but in that case, with Mrs Deeble's "slammerkin" [slovenly] girls (maids) "of sixteen," I should think they had actually better be sleeping together (without a compartment, I mean). Altogether, I fancy this must be the end, viz., that the maids should sleep there and the night nurses in the superintendent's late bedroom. But I don't see how you can do otherwise than accede and say that, if practical evils should arise, they can be dealt with afterwards, and that both windows should have cords for drawing them up and down at top.

I am so sorry about all your child misfortunes, but they seem to be pulling through them very well, thanks to your good management. And I hope Sibella's[188] will be the merest shadow of an attack. Pray give her my love and sympathy.

22 June 1871
7 A.M.

Mrs S. Stewart. I send you one of the many letters of this poor woman.[189] (Recently I have had quite a correspondence about saving

188 Sibella Bonham Carter (1837-1916), his wife.

189 Although Shaw Stewart had been forced to resign as superintendent of nurses at the Herbert Hospital, she kept in touch both with her successor and Nightingale, passing on information both ways.

the *nurses' quarters* at the Herbert Hospital—*for nurses.* The authorities at the H.H. (*not* the W.O.) wished to divide off part for some officers—in a way which would have made it impossible for nurses to live in them. We won.

And it is to this she alludes. (One letter by her on the subject to the W.O. was so admirable as to put poor Mrs Deeble's—on the same subject of quarters—to the W.O. in a very unfavourable contrast.) I sent this letter enclosed to Dr Sutherland for information, and enclose his reply.

If you could tell me at your very earliest convenience (remembering that she will write to me twelve or sixteen pages every day till I answer) what you think I had better answer to her.

Source: From four letters to Harry Verney, Wellcome (Claydon copy) Ms 9005/162-65

18 October 1872

Herbert Hospital Nursing. I am so very sorry to trouble you about this now. But the matter, I am told at the War Office, which they beg you to undertake, scarcely admits of a day's delay. You are aware that at the Herbert Hospital, Woolwich, nursing quarters were built expressly for our accommodation and according to our plan, that we occupied these up to the time of Mrs S. Stewart's resignation . . . that your committee[190] were then asked to undertake the nursing and that of Netley, that you did the latter, but postponed the former.

You are perhaps not aware that for the last two years I have had perpetually to defend these quarters—now occupied by only one acting superintendent (a nurse), two nurses, one of whom however we have taken at St Thomas', and one maid—against receiving sick officers or cadets (with their servants) in with our nurses, or against our nursing quarters, devised specially for women, being appropriated altogether as a cadets' hospital. During the last fortnight these attempts have been constant, unceasing and intrusive. The question about turning our quarters into a *cadets' hospital* came about a fortnight ago to the W.O. and Army Medical Department, and was *directly negatived.*

Then the Horse Guards attempted to put in (amongst our women) that poor Lieutenant Custobadie, who was dangerously hurt at the review. Of this the W.O. received no official intimation, but said they "will negative the proposal, *if* it comes to them." I was then, 16 Octo-

190 Sir Harry Verney was chair of the Nightingale Fund Council.

ber, strongly urged to "bring the whole subject to an end with the secretary of state." I was told to ask you, as chairman of our committee, to see Mr Cardwell yourself, also Sir Henry Storks,[191] and to state that your committee is under engagement at present to complete the nursing staff at the Herbert Hospital, that you are only waiting further experience, that in the meantime these attempts to bring young men into the nurses' quarters, and necessarily with them orderlies and other officials, would render it quite impossible to proceed, or even to continue the present nursing, and that it would be advisable for the S. of S. to decide whether female nursing is to cease, or not, and to take steps to prevent these intrusive propositions being made in future, if the work is to go on, because they are quite destructive of present or prospective efficiency. (I was asked to write myself to Mr Cardwell. But this I feel I cannot do.)

A few hours after this, 16 October, I received another note from the W.O. (marked Strictly Private) to this effect, that Lieutenant Custobadie was not to be placed in our nursing quarters, "which is so far well, but the point should be set at rest by the secretary of state's distinct interdict, or it will crop up again," and a hint that "the present question should be treated as affording a reason for settling it."

Yesterday, 17 October, I received a hurried letter, marked *Immediate*, stating that H.R.H. the duke of Cambridge had been himself to the nursing quarters, inspecting them and proclaiming his intention of appropriating them immediately in whole or in part for sick cadets or officers. And, a few hours later, a hint to take "immediate steps" to "urge in the strongest terms" (through Sir H. Verney) that it is a question of nursing and no nursing, and that, if the nurses' quarters are to be taken in this way, they must build new ones, that this cadet question has been "up" before, that they, the cadets, could easily have a ward to themselves (among the vacant wards in the Herbert Hospital), "or be treated like other people in their own quarters," that it is not a case of necessity to take the nurses' quarters for such a purpose, but that if they are bent on doing so, they must give up the nursing.

I also received another letter, "15 October," "Reference to the plan of the hospital, and to the number of patients now in it, will prove at once that either a ward (several are of different sizes) or several rooms (special small wards) can be at once assigned to this poor gentleman,

191 Edward Cardwell (1813-86), later Viscount, secretary for war; Sir Henry Knight Storks (1811-74), an ally from Crimean War days, under secretary.

Lieutenant Custobadie, or to sick cadets." Also, "Of all changes, that of bringing sick men, and their attendants who are not sick, into rooms set apart for women, and with one only door, staircase, passage, W.C. and sink and kitchen for them and the women to use in common, does seem the one against which common sense and common decency ought to give the protection of reference to the War Office before it is carried out. But, if carried out, the War Office ought to put the women out before it brings the men in."

I will refer this letter to Henry Bonham Carter before referring it to you for his remarks.

19 October 1872

Private. Henry Bonham Carter tells me that he forwarded my letter to you yesterday (about the nursing quarters at the Herbert Hospital), adding that he "thought there were difficulties in the way of our interfering—seeing that we had had no communication respecting Herbert except the proposal of 1868—suggesting that" you "should write to Mr Cardwell and offer that (he) Henry B.C. should call upon him, or the under secretary, neither of whom" he (Henry B.C.) "knows personally." I would only remark upon this that it is a very different thing if you, an MP, *see* Mr Cardwell and *see* Sir H. Storks (which was the course suggested to me as likely to prove successful at the W.O.), that your weight would be infinitely greater as an MP (of their own party) than as our chairman, and that in this respect it does not so much signify that there are "any difficulties in the way of our interfering," but that on the other hand in this respect Henry B.C.'s "calling" *might* be of scarce any use at all.

Three different friendly members of the W.O. (who are quite cognizant of the fact that we are not at this time directly concerned in nursing the Herbert) suggested the above course for *you* and thought that this would be quite conclusive, if you were good enough to do it, in the secretary of state's mind, for securing us the nursing quarters forever—against intrusion. We owe something too to these unfortunate nurses there now, continually threatened with having young men put into their quarters along with the women.

Sorry to trouble you. God bless you.

23 October 1872

The Chief Clerk's Statement. Herbert Hospital.

There must be some mistake. As to not being able to have nurses in a hospital like the Herbert, *because* the wards are called "*regimental,*" the patients are the same. But it is impossible, it was never intended, to "*train*" nurses at all in a military hospital. Nurses can only be *trained* in a large civil hospital where there are all ages and both sexes and where the one nurse is not the only *woman* in a man's ward. They are then transferred to a military hospital to learn its ways before sending them abroad.

To avoid misunderstanding on the subject, the Herbert Hospital was specially built for military nurses—it was one of several hospitals set apart for this purpose—it was not intended as a place for training, because the facilities for training do not exist in a military hospital. The arrangements of military hospitals are intended for (solely) *nursing*, but trained nurses would be naturally sent to see the details of military hospitals before being sent abroad. It follows from this that the larger the number of such hospitals, the larger will be the number of *practised* as well as *trained* nurses at the disposal of the W.O.

The N[ightingale] committee consider themselves as bound to train a reasonable number of nurses and superintendents if applied to (for military hospitals) by the W.O. to do so. Sidney Herbert's royal commission of 1857 (on which was Sir H. Storks) advised that there should be a certain number of such hospitals—at present there are only two, Herbert and Netley. Herbert Hospital, although under the administration of brigade medical officers, is not a "*regimental*" hospital in the sense in which the R. commission dealt with these for nursing purposes, its administration is essentially "*general*." It depends on the secretary of state to increase or diminish the number of such hospitals, but to limit the number to *one* (Netley), would be to diminish the nursing staff of an army in the field and to go back from the recommendation of the commission.

N.B. Netley nursing quarters will not hold one more nurse, as they are at present. Nor is there scope for more than one or two more. Nor would it be desirable to increase the number.

5 November 1872

Herbert Hospital. Your little pencil note of 1 November seemed to me disastrous. Because if Mr Cardwell replies to you *after* he has "decided," and that "decision" is against us, it will be difficult, if not impossible, *then* to have it revoked. The not having a complete nursing staff there is our ruin, one for linen, one for sick, to have all these fine quarters for! built for a complete nursing establishment for 650 beds.

I sent down to the Army Medical Department for advice. This [is] the context of the answer: unless we are prepared to back up the two women as representing a staff, we must either let them go, or we must provide a staff complete.

How to do this? For me to write out a statement of what was the original intention, and what we should propose (250 sick including venereal), address it to chairman (you) and let him forward it to the secretary of state.

This, their advice (to this Henry B.C. says "yes"). As the matter of nurses rests primarily by regulation with the director general of the Army Medical Department, perhaps it would be well, I am told, for Sir H.V. (you) or Henry Bonham Carter to see him (Sir G. Logan) and go into the whole subject with him, i.e., on the assumption that you will put in a complete staff. (H.B.C. says "in a year." Henry B.C. says "yes, best for *Sir Harry* to introduce the subject and let me, H.B.C., follow it up") with Sir G. Logan. In this way to obtain Sir G. Logan's views (he could give us great support with the War Office). All depends upon

1. whether you will undertake;
2. whether they will let you undertake the proper nursing of the Herbert Hospital. Henry B.C. says "we cannot think of such a thing *under a year*, but if principle agreed to, the time ought not to be of consequence."

In taking steps for such a proposal, there does not seem to be a day to lose. For if the secretary of state and his royal highness [duke of Cambridge] once turn our nurses out, we shall never get them in again. God help us. . . .

It is eighteen years today since we landed at Scutari and undertook the hospitals. It seems hard that this should be the day to turn us out.

Source: From a letter to T. Graham Balfour, Add Mss 50134 ff147-48

27 June 1873

I congratulate you on your work. It is a capital report: I give you joy. It suggests the great advantage of including in all official reports facts only, leaving discussions and opinions to the medical journals, and how careful we should be not to support anybody's peculiar views.

Burns well said that "Facts are chiels that downa ding."[192] You can't knock them over. Opinions, on the contrary, are the scriptural "fowls

192 Robert Burns, in "A Dream," actually said: "Facts are chiels that winna ding./An downa be disputed" [Facts are fellows that cannot be overturned, and don't . . .].

of the air,"[193] affording neither shade nor resting place. Plato[194] said all this very strongly more than 2000 years ago! But we have not listened yet. You, however, with your statistical facts, have done more than anyone to bring us back to common sense.

Take, e.g., the contrast between the Delhi paper and the Gibraltar work at p 50. In the Delhi affair the lieutenant governor, having no belief except in his own eyesight, finds that the whole place where the people suffered was foul beyond description, and that, moreover, all the filth of Delhi was emptied close to their wells. Is not this whole paper but a witches' cauldron, out of which there is nothing but "bubble, bubble, toil and trouble"?[195] But take the result of the Gibraltar work, p 50, there is no "bubble," simply looking, seeing and *doing*. And the work is Gibraltar drained and supplied with good water, and with an active sanitary police. And the result is last year's death rate (1871) 5.87 per 1000, and an average of ten years preceding of 8.45. Part of the south end of the rock still needs improvement, but this will soon be done, please God and you all.

Malta, which alas! has not decided after ten years to do anything but wait to try the result of next cholera, is pretty much as it was, is it not? All we should do in reports, is it not? is simply to record facts, no opinions.

It will be years before the health law of India is made out. It is scarcely made out yet for London.

Source: From a letter to John Sutherland, Add Mss 45757 ff197-98

21 October 1873

Herbert Hospital. Nursing Quarters. Do you know anything about this? I mean about what is in the letter marked "Confidential"? It is the continuance of a correspondence (which I showed to H.B.C.—you were abroad) saying that there was a probability now of its being decided once for all whether the nursing quarters now occupied by sick cadets should be permanently alienated to other purposes, that the present P.M.O. avows himself anxious to have a complete nursing staff, but if he cannot have this to have no nurses at all. Our secretary and committee are not the least anxious to fight the matter with the W.O. or to

193 Matt 6:26.

194 Plato, fifth-century BCE Greek philosopher.

195 As per the witches' brew in the opening scene of Shakespeare's *MacBeth.*

take any initiative with them. They say it would be different if Muir were D.G.[196] and if *I* would fight it with *his help.*

Do you know whether or what has been decided about the *sick cadets* or the *nursing quarters*? (It was said that on the removal of the sick cadets, if *we* did not reappropriate the quarters vi et armis [with force and arms], they would be made into M.O.s quarters.)

Source: From a letter to Harry Verney, Wellcome (Claydon copy) Ms 9006/92

6 May 1874

Malta. This question has been played with by successive governors, and amongst others by the one named.

We have had to fight every step. The dry earth was one of the dodges. One year's cost of it would lay down about 60 miles of pipe sewers. It would go far to pay the outlay for the entire improvements. It is quite true that the soaking of the rock is the cause of mischief. But this can be cured entirely according to the estimates for about £6000 or £7000.

The Admiralty and W.O. are going to divert half the *sewage* at their own expense immediately. And the local government should complete the work of the city improvements. The delay is entirely due to the authorities. It is just twelve years since the evil was pointed out, and they have quite lately had a new scheme, perfectly impracticable and dangerous, to do a small item of work at a capitalized cost of £50,000. We shall succeed, I dare say, in time in getting the work done. The dry earth was fully considered and pronounced, without regard to cost, quite impracticable by engineers on the spot.

Editor: The next letters concern hospitals at Gibraltar, a major base for the British Army, and one, like Malta, where many women and families lived as well as soldiers. Thus there are issues of a "women's hospital," largely for midwifery, as well as the usual hospital needs for the men. Nightingale strongly supported decent family housing for soldiers at the station. She was pleased that Balfour was to become principal medical officer at Gibraltar, as the next letter shows. By March 1876, with Balfour in Gibraltar, Nightingale was seeking ways to promote the building of a women's hospital there (the second letter).

---

196 William Mure Muir (1818-85), later Sir, in fact director general 1874-82; see the biographical sketch in *Wars and the War Office* (15:1040).

Source: From two letters to T. Graham Balfour, Add Mss 50134 ff150-51 and 154-56, typed copy of the latter Add Mss 45772 ff280-82

6 May 1874

No overwork or illness could prevent me from writing to bid you "God-speed." You have done admirable service at Netley, as everywhere, and the things you have done, which ought never to have required doing, show that you have been the first P.M.O. there who understood his work.

We are very sorry to part with you, but cannot be sorry that you are going to Gibraltar, as we wanted just such a man to do. . . . The local commissioners have just completed the arrangements for finishing the sanitary improvement of the whole rock.

You will of course specially see that the hospital improvements are completed and look well to the barracks and see that the drainage, ventilation and water supply are properly done. Under you I am convinced that Gibraltar will be about the healthiest spot in H.M.'s dominions. God speed you! . . .

Pray remember me most kindly to Mrs Balfour and also to your boy[197] whom I remember a baby.

13 March 1876

About your *Women's Hospital*, your unceasing efforts after the good *ought* to meet with support, and a question shall be asked, such as you propose, in the House of Commons, about it.[198] Will it not be well, too, to put in the same question a reminder about the new *married quarters* which ought to be built? Were they not to have built *married soldiers' quarters* for the whole strength? And *with* these did not Captain Galton and Dr Sutherland consider that a separate hospital was scarcely required? What do you think of this? What *they* proposed was, I believe, that each block should have a special end ward with appurtenances for any infectious cases, most ordinary cases to be treated in quarters. But, unless the quarters be built, a proper hospital is urgently required.

I suppose your answer will be that the quarters are farther off in the future than the hospital, and we must get the one first and strive for the other afterward. . . .

---

197 Also Thomas Graham Balfour, their only child (1858-1929), later Sir, a distinguished biographer and education expert.

198 The question was asked by Samuel Whitbread (1796-1876), Liberal MP for Bedford (see p 466 below).

Your energy must and will meet with its reward about the *sanatorium* at last. Windmill Hill[199] is a capital place. Has it not, however, in times past been scourged by epidemics in consequence of sanitary neglects? I heard with great satisfaction that it is now being drained and supplied with water, mainly I doubt not owing to your representations. I fear that they will scarcely go to the cost of a building yet. Would it be possible, during summer, for men to go under tents there? Or for wooden huts to be put up? People here however *will* generally consider it best if men want change to send them home. They say it is only five days' steam. But I hope for Windmill at last.

About the *water supply*: I understand, on inquiry, that your wise and strong representations and suggestions have been acted upon. They seem at the W.O. to be aware of your facts. And a report has just gone in which states that the Gibraltar water supply is to be improved. (This report made its appearance at, i.e., was sent as passed, to the Army Sanitary Commission.)

You have done wonders. Your representations should never cease. They will bear fruit: they do bear fruit.

Source: From a letter to Harry Verney, Wellcome (Claydon copy) Ms 9007/10

14 March 1876

You were so good as to say that you would ask Mr Whitbread[200] to ask the question for us in the House of Commons. I think it would be better to leave out the first two lines of your form of the question: on the other side of this sheet is the substance of what we want asked (I have consulted a man at the W.O. about it): whether it is the fact that in so large a garrison as Gibraltar no provision has been made for a hospital for the wives and children of soldiers, and if married soldiers' quarters for the whole strength are to be built?

Editor: Sutherland's reply was equivocal, that he did not think that whatever Balfour was doing would lead to results. The following day he queried how long there would be married men in the army needing married quarters.[201] Nightingale, however, pursued the matter, as

---

199 The British Army had barracks on Windmill Hill, Gibraltar; there was a "sanatorium" for convalescing officers there, but it had been abandoned.

200 Samuel Whitbread, who asked questions in the House of Commons for Nightingale on army matters, but apparently not this one.

201 Sutherland notes 15 and 16 March 1876, Add Mss 45758 ff19 and 20.

can be seen both in her positive letter to Balfour immediately below and her subsequent efforts to get the matter raised in Parliament. She drafted a question:

> Whether it is the fact that, in so large a garrison as Gibraltar, no provision has been made for a hospital for the wives and children of the soldiers, and if married soldiers' quarters for the whole strength are to be built, and whether any representation has been made on these subjects by the local military authorities.[202]

Correspondence resumes on other issues.

Source: From a letter to Douglas Galton, Add Mss 45764 f251

15 April 1879

Herbert Hospital Foul Linen Chutes: I have often wished to ask you whether these are worked, and *how* they are worked, and if so whether they work well. You know that our *foul linen chutes* at St Thomas' Hospital are not used at all, partly because they have no receptacle at the *bottom* for the linen, partly because they are too small, but chiefly because no one will be at the trouble to make them work. And all sorts of bad contrivances are used instead. Till lately, the dirty linen was removed out of the wards only *four* times a week. And I am sure much hospital disease was the consequence.

How work the Herbert Hospital chutes?

Editor: In the 1880s Nightingale again took up the issue of nurse training for men orderlies. At this point she considered that medical officers would require training in nursing, laundry and nutrition in order to conduct the training. It seems nothing came of this idea.

Source: From undated notes, Add Mss 45826 ff143-44, 147-50[203] and 222-23

[1880s?]

Suggestions for Report. Netley. If the Army Hospital Corps is to be entirely under the Army Medical Department, it is manifestly necessary that the army medical officers should train the men of the hospital corps in their several duties. And therefore that the young medical

---

202 Undated draft question, Add Mss 45758 f18.

203 A similar draft is headed "Question (to Dr Longmore) about Netley" at ff101-06.

officers themselves should receive some form of instruction at Netley and Aldershot or elsewhere, so that they shall be able to instruct the orderlies in the methods of taking care of the wards, methods of preparing diets (cooking), methods of the general charge of the hospital (ward management inclusive) and above all instruction so as to qualify them for teaching the men to nurse.

Nursing. A. It is a matter of primary importance that the medical officers should be able, not only to teach the men to nurse, but to train the head nurses, i.e., the N.C. officers, the wardmasters, the sergeant major (the chief of the nursing) to carry on the instruction of the men in the same way as the "sisters" (the head female nurses) in civil hospitals train the probationers and staff nurses under them. The medical officers must be taught all the duties of nursing. (For who is to teach the orderlies all these things, if the medical officers do not?)

... At present we *have no* wardmasters. Neither captain of orderlies, wardmaster or sergeant major know anything at all about nursing.

Q. 3696. Teaching the nurses to manage helpless patients in the ward is the head nurse's work, and not the medical officer's. Most medical officers do not know how to do it themselves. They *must* be taught and taught how to teach the sergeant majors. As a matter of fact, medical officers at Aldershot did not give clinical instruction to the hospital corps men, even when the order to do so had been issued. . . .

Medical officers never look after the Army Hospital Corps men—how they are carrying out medical orders, nor how they are nursing. (Nor is this their business in a civil hospital, but the business of the head nurse.) But the wardmasters, the N.C. officers must be taught to be head nurses—by the medical officers. . . .

Netley and Aldershot must both teach. Take care that the sisters at Netley do teach the men (not doing what they like themselves and leaving the orderlies to do what *they*, the sisters, don't like to do). Do the "sisters" see to the beds themselves? It is said *not.* Then the sisters must have had a thorough training themselves. Nurses who have only had a year's training at Netley have not. There are many things they do not know how to do by the bedside, much less teach to orderlies how to do.

Trained women cannot be *substituted* for medical officers to train the men. Also, how can the medical officers know whether the *women* are good nurses or not, whether the *women* are well *trained* or not if they, the medical officers themselves, know little or nothing about nursing, and have never been taught, as in the case at present? To *substitute* trained women for trained men, or to *substitute* women for medical officers to train the men, is equally impracticable, however valuable the women as ward sisters and as teachers (of what is taught by the sisters to the nurses in civil hospitals) to the orderlies.

Netley. As the great fault of the Army Medical Department is want of discipline (the young medical officers come from the hospitals in London where they have had professional training but no discipline), whilst they are at Netley, what attempt is made to train them in discipline? as well as in the special matters which army surgeons are supposed to require? What distinct military supervision is there by means of their own officers? What one head over the teaching? head over the professors, who directs the studies, who sees that the young medical officers are systematically trained in the various departments of hospital organization? How far does Netley admit of it? How far is the whole time of the officers while there occupied in one form of training or another? in the washing establishment? in the cooking, purveying?, nursing? etc.

What functions of hospital administration are they taught? as to cleaning wards, washing linen? disinfecting hospital equipments or clothing? How are the medical officers taught as to what extent men are capable of physical exertion? as to the hours during which men can be continuously worked? What charge of orderlies do the medical candidates have?

Orderlies *eat.* There should be a free hospital ration, not accommodation, of sixpence a day, *plus* barrack ration. There should be no temptation for the orderlies to eat the patients' diets.

Orderlies *drink.* How can they help it? In Egypt, even where they had no fatigue duties, they had only 3½ hours in bed out of the twenty-four. The doctors say the Army Hospital Corps are not more drunken than "other soldiers." One might as well say, civil hospital nurses are not more drunken than their patients. The thing is that nobody who nurses in a hospital should drink at all.

There is *no professor of nursing, no organization of night nursing.* There is a law of human energy, of course, a law of nursing power. But *the laws of nursing* power are *not known.* There should be a professorship of hospital administration, hospital construction and hospital nursing.

2. Professor of surgery and his assistant to deal with equipment of field hospitals, and by *models* at lecture *and by practical pitching in the Netley grounds* to show the M.O. *a field hospital at work* in tents, in which in summer a certain number of cases might be treated. (In summer, sick might be treated in tents at any large hospital with actual advantage from a sanitary point of view.)

3. As regards *nursing training*, the course of the Army Hospital Corps must be made *thorough*, and the young medical officers must be put through it. And they must be examined in it at the end of term. They must be taught the organization of night nursing, the laws of nursing power and human energy. There should be a professorship of nursing and hospital administration (*not* necessarily a *separate* professorship).

Cooking in the same way should be explained. The young medical officers should know how to make certain dishes and should make them, and have marks at the end of term for it. *Laundry* to be visited and explained to the young M.O.s. *Ward management* to be taught (as to the orderlies) and questions given in it.

4. Organization of foreign medical services, German, French, Italian, etc., and their field hospital system taught by military surgery professor. M.O.s to be examined in it at end of session.

5. Examinations for all medical officers at the end of three years' and of ten years' service on *hospital administration and* NURSING as well as on professional subjects, promotion to surgeon with five years increase of pay and to surgeon major's rank to depend upon these.

6. Further course. If the orderlies are to be efficient, teaching must go on through all their service, and the senior sergeants must instruct the men every week and go over minor points. The medical officers must examine *them* once a month and explain and lecture.

7. In every garrison, scientific meetings once a month for all the medical officers.

Netley. Candidate and orderly in ward, sister doing nothing, waiting in corridor hernia case. Sister was doing nothing. Professor Longmore dates from Crimean War—has seen nothing since. Instructions for nurses may be good, but no personal practical training. They have not got the cases. Their cases can all walk about. Most of them dress themselves if they have dressings to do, not confined to bed.

Our wars are all at a distance; by the time they [the soldiers] get to Netley they are well.

Abscess of liver incurable—they are discharged. Ague, phthisis: these are the cases.

Netley tide's running out, and Netley's stranded, fixity of tenure its ruin. Professorships should be for seven years. No one will work up for the post if it's in the running—men will work up for it not a question of Netley, but of human nature.

Ophthalmoscope.[204] Netley. Ophthalmic professor of Charing Cross Hospital.

Source: From a letter to Thomas Crawford,[205] Florence Nightingale Museum (LMA) H1/ST/NC1/82/4

29 June 1882

Private. I have been turning over in my mind what you were so good as to ask me, viz., about a proposal to allow one or two night "sisters" for special cases at the Herbert Hospital. And I cannot forbear troubling you with these few remarks or rather questions:

I think I understood you that there are very few serious cases in the Herbert Hospital, and most of them, I suppose, are among artillery "*invalids.*" But, taken as a whole, you would perhaps say that the great building is rather a sick barrack than a hospital. Its pavilions are so separated that a nurse cannot have more than sixty-four sick on one floor. And she might have only thirty-two (or even twenty) on a floor.

Would it be possible so to arrange the cases that the one or two or three bad cases requiring (occasionally) night nursing should be in the same ward or floor? Systematic night nursing, I understood you to say, was not at all required. (And indeed I know that, at Netley, where there are so many more "invalid" bedridden cases, the night "sister" has often nothing to do all night: the patients are "all asleep.")

What you propose is simply to detach a nurse for special duty, as the medical officer should judge needful. The "partitioned room" for the National Aid Society's nurses is no doubt in the nurses' block, which is too far away for effective work. I hardly see how you can have night supervision from there. But a telephone to Miss Caulfeild's[206] room would bring her at once.

In each pavilion there is a nurse's room and scullery in line. Could one of these rooms be given up to the night nurse? If you detached two nurses for the night work, could one of them be on duty and the other at hand in this room?

---

204 A lighted device for eye examinations.

205 Thomas Crawford (1824-95), director general of the Army Medical Department 1882-89; see the biographical sketch in *Wars and the War Office* (15:1040).

206 Anne Ellen Caulfeild (c1845-1937), lady superintendent at the Herbert Hospital; nursed in the Egyptian campaign of 1882 and was awarded the Royal Red Cross medal.

What occurred to me after thinking over what you had said to submit to you and to ask you was this: would it be possible to have the bad cases on one floor of the same pavilion? If so, could the night nurses have one of the ward rooms *for the time*? (with a telephone to the superintendent's room?). But if the bad cases were in different pavilions, might it not be necessary to have a similar arrangement for each?

In the great difficulty of having one woman alone at night in that great building, with perhaps two bad cases requiring her care in different pavilions—and in the great unwillingness to leave those bad cases without trained female night nursing, *if it is desired*, pardon me if I have submitted these things *for your consideration*, merely. And thanking you for your most kind visit which I trust will not be the last. . . .

I am so very sorry not to be able to see you.[207] I have quite knocked up and am obliged to put off all appointments. Nothing else would prevent me from what I so much wish—I still hope to see you at some future time.

Source: From an undated note, Add Mss 45826 ff53-55

[1882-85]

Nurses: [We] should be very wary of recommending the employment of female nurses, i.e., the placing of female nurses in the hospital wards. She cannot remedy the defects of the Army Hospital Corps. And if they are not efficient and well-conducted nurses, it would lead to grave scandals.

But before recommending any extension of the training of Netley, very full evidence ought to be taken from the medical officers themselves who had the opportunity of seeing the nurses as to what were the qualifications of each of the nurses in Egypt. The mere general report from the Army Medical Department ought not to be taken, but questions should be asked of the individual medical officers who had the nurses under them.

The proposal to cure the orderlies' want of training only by having "trained female nurses" resembles much the case of disinfectants. Don't remove the evil, but order a disinfectant. Don't improve the orderlies' training, but have nurses to act as disinfectants.

It is much more to be feared that, in other than *large* hospitals (such as Netley, Woolwich, Aldershot, Portsmouth, etc.), the nurses, if

207 It seems that Dr Crawford called on Nightingale unannounced, so that the two possibly exchanged notes rather than meet; his reply is the same date, Add Mss 45772 f1.

introduced, will be dragged down to the level of the orderlies than the orderlies be dragged up to the level of the "trained nurses." Not to mention the probability of scandals where nurses are put down in twos or threes, which would discredit the whole system.

Nurses: great danger half-trained woman will fall into discredit. If the trained woman is indispensable, the trained man is so, too. Neither must cause us to dispense with the other. Or they will all come to grief. So hamper the D.G. as that he can't take any woman who comes. Make such a Code of Regulations as won't take in anybody.

Let the D.G. have a printed form to answer all applications:

How many years have you served?

What training have you had?

What is your education?

Medical certificate of health.

You may dictate your own terms.

Nursing is a profession. You must stand out against social pressure. A.H.C. organized to crush out nursing, weak idiotic man becomes a nurse.

Source: From a letter probably to G.J.H. Evatt,[208] Columbia University, Presbyterian Hospital School of Nursing C148

23 January 1883

Private and Confidential. You have talked much and wisely about the necessity of teaching, if the A.M.O.s [army medical officers] are to have all the administration in their hands (to them) administration. Could you write me a few lines suggesting what questions should be asked to elicit *what* administration is or can be taught at Netley, including nursing, cooking, ward management, etc., and suggesting *what* and how the ideal course of administration should be taught. *What* would be your course of administration? and could it be taught at Netley?

The field hospital course would have to be taught at Aldershot. How?

We have also said much about nurses and the undesirability of SUBSTITUTING trained women for trained men, or of considering that the SUBSTITUTION of women for medical officers, to train the men, is desirable. Besides, how can the M.O.s know whether the *women* are good nurses or not, if they themselves know nothing about nursing, and have never been taught, as is the case at present?

---

208 George Joseph Hamilton Evatt (1843-1921), later Sir; army medical officer, then at the Royal Military Academy, Woolwich.

Could you send me such questions as you think desirable for the D.G. to obtain answers to from the medical officers in Egypt as to the nurses (trained women) who have been or are serving there (a) as to their work, descending to particulars such as giving enemas [and] opium, changing helpless men in bed, washing backs in bed, preventing bedsores, dressing wounds, accuracy in reporting to medical officer as to results of treatment, including stools, urine, etc.; (b) as to capability of training orderlies, etc.

Source: From a letter to an unnamed recipient, Columbia University, Presbyterian Hospital School of Nursing C149

27 February 1883

I think your scheme of the "Army Hospital Flower Mission" most admirable. I wish it "good speed" with all my heart. It will do a great deal of good. I wish I could see my way to doing as you ask, but I never like to give my "name" where I cannot give my work, and I think it would be putting myself forward.

With regard to my writing to Sir Henry Ponsonby,[209] I do not know him personally, and after taking some advice I find it is feared that he will say that he has so many things to lay before the queen that he cannot do this.

Source: From a letter to Harry Verney, Wellcome (Claydon copy) Ms 9010/8

19 February 1884

I was in hope that you and Dr Evatt would have settled it together. Here is the question, which for various reasons I will tell you when I see you, he wishes put, if you approve. . . .

To ask if in the field hospitals detailed for service in the approaching campaign any increase of the Army Hospital Corps staff would be made for the purpose of providing for washermen, sanitary police, watermen and other subsidiary services of the hospital of which the want was so much found in the Egyptian campaign.

Source: From a letter to John Sutherland, Add Mss 45758 ff183-84

5 October 1884

Malta. Private. I have no doubt that you have been consulted about the following, and shall be very glad if you will kindly tell me what you have advised. "Mr Bell, a very gentlemanly, middle-aged architect,"

209 Sir Henry Frederick Ponsonby (1825-95), private secretary to Queen Victoria.

went out in August in the same ship with one of our sisters who was returning to her post in Cairo Military Hospital.[210] "He has been sent out to *Malta* for a few weeks by government to visit a site (which has already been settled upon) for a new military hospital, and to draw the plan of it, with *every modern improvement*, so that it may be the most *perfect* hospital possible."

Mr Bell says "that it is to have a training school for *female nurses* attached to it," but we "can't help thinking he must be mistaken on this point. All that I am telling you he of course told us in confidence." "The hospital is to contain 240 beds only." Not enough, I should have thought. He thinks the building will be commenced early next year. "Mr Bell has been getting *our opinion* upon several points with regard to his plan of this hospital."

N.B. Our sister is quite first-rate as a hospital sister, but not as a sanitarian. I hope that *you* have given your best advice.

Gordon Boys' Home, 1885-90

Editor: Nightingale knew the famous "Gordon of Khartoum," General Charles George Gordon (1833-85), and was involved in supplying nurses for the Egyptian expedition that attempted to rescue him.[211] After Gordon's 1885 death in Sudan, much consideration was given to a fitting memorial to him. The first proposal, soon dismissed, was for a hospital in Port Said, Egypt (the first two items below). The *British Medical Journal* objected to it, calling the town small and not suited to a hospital. It hoped that any hospital built in Egypt would not be for the treatment of the English only, but open to Egyptians and others, as Gordon had lived much of his life for and died for the Egyptians. Egyptians themselves did not "repair to Port Said, but Cairo and Alexandria."[212]

The lord mayor of London asked Nightingale for her opinion and any "suggestions" she might make on the memorial. As was her custom, she undertook to comment if sent the plans and a sketch. No such

210 Sybil Airy (c1841-1918), awarded the Royal Red Cross for her service in Egypt; later matron, Royal Victoria Hospital, Bournemouth.

211 Related in *Wars and the War Office* (15:964-1019); correspondence with him is in *Society and Politics* (5:490-503), that on the Gordon Boys' Home (5:242-56).

212 "What Is the Best Site for the Gordon Memorial Hospital?" *British Medical Journal* (4 April 1885):709.

material is evident in her files, and in any event the Port Said project was abandoned.

The memorial that did proceed was a boys' home, effectively for homeless boys, such as army orphans. This was an appropriate choice, as Gordon himself for some years had taken boys to live in his home, an old rectory at Gravesend.[213] Strained correspondence on the appointment of the first matron for the Gordon Boys' Home, Lydia Constable (c1840-?), a St Thomas' trained ward sister, and Nightingale's protest of her later dismissal, has already appeared.[214] Here the correspondence relates the formulation of plans and choice of site. The architect finally selected was William Butterfield, who had designed the Winchester Infirmary. Here he appears in a bad light for disregarding the building committee's injunctions and his own promises. A letter to Galton refers to "Butterfieldian evils" (see p 487 below). There are letters to Gordon's cousin, Amy Hawthorn.

Nightingale had yet again to remonstrate for the provision of a bedroom, sitting room and private toilet for the matron. The home was in due course built at Chobham, near Woking, Surrey, opening in 1887. Temporary quarters were provided by the War Office at Ft. Wallington, Hampshire, for residents between 1885 and 1887.

Source: From a letter to Harry Verney and a draft letter to the lord mayor, of the same date, Wellcome (Claydon copy) Ms 9010/66

18 March 1885

Gordon Memorial Hospital. You see that the proposed hospital is to be for 100 beds, that the site is given by the Suez Canal Co. and confirmed in perpetuity by the Egyptian government, that the building is to cost £11,000!!! and to be erected in four months!!! (possible, but not at all right). I only remind you of these things, as you are now on the committee.

Proposed "Gordon Memorial" Hospital at Port Said.

[I am] very much honoured by the lord mayor's request for my "opinion" and any "suggestion" "in regard to it." To give any "opinion" at all worth the lord mayor's having, I should see the sketch *plans*, if the lord mayor will be so very good as to let me see them. And if possible a sketch plan of the site, giving the points of the compass also, and

---

213 Doreen E. McLellan, comp., Gravesend Local History Pamphlet No. 3.
214 In *Society and Politics* (5:242-56) and *The Nightingale School* (12:511).

perhaps the prevailing winds. Also, if I might ask, what kind of estimate? and what the time for the building? To have a real hospital on a good plan built there "on the great highway between two worlds" is truly a national object and worthy of a *national* memorial by England.

I should be truly glad to contribute my little best in the way indicated by the lord mayor.

Source: From four letters to Amy Hawthorn, Add Mss 45776 ff134-37, 192-93, 201-04 and 208

4 July 1885
7:00 a.m.

Private. Pray "mention the subject" of the Gordon Boys' [Home] "privately to Colonel Geary when he comes to see" you tomorrow, as you kindly propose. I must tell you that the member of committee who spoke to me was not one of the seven whose names he gave me (which you will see in the *Times*) as forming the sub-committee, which is to report in about a fortnight on plans for beginning: Lord Napier, Sir John Cowell, Mr Walters, Sir Dighton Probyn (Prince of Wales), Mr Sutherland, Admiral Grylefield, Sir Henry Gordon,[215] I think they are.

I am not sure that these are so set as they ought to be for beginning *immediately*, but he is extremely anxious about it. He showed me all the papers. Have you seen them? General Higginson's[216] plan to have a camp, which will cost £12,000 (but cannot be done even for that), 480 boys at £20 a year = £10,000 a year. As the men of business say, where are we to get £10,000 a year? £10,000 a year represents a capital of a quarter of a million. How is a quarter of a million to be had?

There is now £20,000 all told. It is thought that £100,000 might have been raised if all had been unanimous at first, that now, if a plan could be begun at once with hardly any expense, a considerable sum, though nothing like £100,000, might still be raised.

The "rent of two or three cottages" might certainly be "paid out of" this poor little £20,000. But it was thought that government has so

215 Robert Cornelius Napier, 1st Baron Napier of Magdala (1810-90), r.e., field marshal and former commander-in-chief in India; John Clayton Cowell (1832-1911); Sir Henry Gordon (1818-87), older brother of Gordon; Dighton Probyn (1833-1911), v.c. and major general.

216 George Wentworth Higginson (1826-1927), later Sir, Grenadier Guards, whom Nightingale knew from the Crimean War, and with whom she worked on soldiers' institutes.

many buildings at its disposal, buildings and cottages, that something might be granted which could be arranged for boys at once, at almost no expense. This advantage of its starting under you and Colonel Hawthorn[217] would almost outweigh all else.

It was thought that there would be no difficulty in some gentleman *giving* fifty acres for a future camp, since good farming land is not required—nor desirable, since it should be near Aldershot, but it was said that it would be desirable to be near some port. To begin with a schoolmaster, a good sergeant, a carpenter, a sailor, a farmer—all village ones—would be perhaps all that was necessary. Carpenter, mason, smith and ultimately quartermaster, surgeon to teach ambulance work. [A] commandant would of course be necessary.

Sir R. Loyd Lindsay would, I am sure, have given the land, but then, you see, he is against trades. The barrack which it was mentioned that government might possibly lend was that of the Oxfordshire, near Oxford. That was what they meant by barracks "in the country." The cottages mentioned were at Shoebury (Soldier's Wives Quarters, I believe). But I merely report this to you as an answer to your question. No peculiar advantage was attached to them, indeed none at all.

It is noble of you to be willing to give the inestimable advantage of your help at the start. I am glad you will not live *in* Chatham. All that you say about the neighbourhood of Chatham Barrack for the Gordon boys must of course be attended to and "rent for cottages" should be paid "out of the fund," if nothing else can be done. All that I can do will be to report what you are kind enough to tell me when you have the information.

I am sure that the thanks of the nation will be due to you and Colonel Hawthorn if this Gordon Home can only be started under your auspices. God speed the plans. In great haste. . . .

The sub-committee is to report in about a fortnight.

Claydon House
Winslow, Bucks
18 May 1886

Dearest Mrs Hawthorn, I am so glad that you are going to see the Gordon Boys' Home with Miss Augusta Gordon.[218] Thank you for the

217 Colonel Robert Hawthorn, R.E.

218 Mary Augusta Gordon (1822-93), sister of General Gordon.

most interesting packet you so kindly sent me a few days ago. I was so glad to see it. . . .

I should so very much like to know what you think of the management of the Gordon boys—whether they appear to you to need a (motherly) matron's care. So much that is wrong, not to mention so much that is unhealthy, takes place among boys under the best discipline—where there is no motherly woman. And some boys get depressed and others become tormentors—some are devourers and some devoured. And whether you think they are subdivided enough. Or are they all together? And do they live enough in the open air? And do they look happy and look you in the face? Are their quarters in the fort dark or unairy?

I suppose no animals or pets can be kept in their present quarters? for them to look after. And how do you like the look of the N.C. officers? and the apportionment of schooling and workshop work? But so much will suggest itself to you that would not to me.

Sir Harry Verney is going up to London tomorrow (Wednesday) to attend the meeting of the Gordon Boys' Home at 20 Charing Cross from 11 to one. Afterwards he will be at his brother's, 38 Upper Grosvenor St., till Thursday morning. He may possibly write to trouble you (after the meeting) to make some inquiries for him at Ft. Wallington.

9 September 1886

I want to know what your view of the last meeting of the Gordon Boy's Home is. "Field Marshal" Lord Napier, in direct opposition to some of his committee, wrote to the home secretary accepting, *on their "unanimous" behalf*, the grant of the "permanent use" of the "Woking Male Prison" for the Gordon Boys' Home, as you know. Had this been allowed to pass, some of the committee would have resigned. I wonder what you think.

The experience we have gained during the last thirty years goes to show that health, morals, discipline, have to be obtained in huts or small pavilions, not in a huge building containing 300 cells (and which it is said would hold 1000 boys), however well rearranged and remodelled. The youthful Sir Harry (then about eighty-five) went up to London yesterday by the first train, without his sandwiches or telling anyone but the pony, attended the meeting (where he was chairman), and a copy of Lord Napier's letter was read, and then on to Woking to see the prison.

Colonel Beaty Pownall (I wonder what he thinks about it) will have told you how Sir Harry told the meeting that the committee were *not* "unanimous." General Philip Smith[219] backed him. General Higginson I believe, wrote a letter in favour of the prison. However the Noes had it. And Mr Tennyson[220] offered to go off to Lord Napier and ask him *viva voce* [out loud] to withdraw his letter, which offer was accepted. We have not of course heard the result.

Arrived at Woking, the youthful Sir Harry called a cab, but perched himself on the box of the cabman, in order to "see better." The cabman turned out to be a soldier, a R.H.A. [Royal Horse Artillery] man, who was in the Martinière with Sir James Outram,[221] and side by side with the *Shannon* Naval Brigade (in which Captain Verney[222] was) in all its work in that Lucknow campaign. "They tossed their guns about as *we* couldn't do," says the R.H.A. man. He also told Sir H. a good deal about Woking Prison. Coming back in the train, he, Sir H., found a gentleman of those parts who knew him and who extolled Woking Prison with its houses round for matron, chaplain, doctor, etc., just what Gordon would have deprecated. "But," says he, "for your purpose you want a pony and you get a white elephant."

I have asked to write a penny pamphlet with a sketch of Gordon and an appeal to the troops. But we must know more! *Are* we to have this prison and its fine officers' houses?

2. Could you kindly tell me what is the scheme of work? Is it for one or two years training? or what? Do the committee then intend to place the boys "out," as Gordon did, according to the character of each? I can never find a committee man to tell me. Are you not rather afraid of the Aldershot proposal to raise £22 per regiment (£20 would require 800 sixpences). Would not the men give more freely if it were not asked in that way?

Colonel Robinson, A.A.G. [assistant adjutant general], at Aldershot is working the matter well. Please tell me your mind.

---

219 G.A. Beaty-Pownall (d. 1905), secretary of the Gordon Boys' Home; Lieutenant General Philip Smith (d. 1894), Grenadier Guards.

220 Alfred Tennyson (1809-92), poet laureate; he wrote the epitaph for Gordon at Westminster Abbey and promoted the home as a memorial.

221 General James Outram (1803-63), 1st baronet, famous for the campaign in Oudh against the Sepoy Mutiny, or First War of Independence. The 1858 taking of Martiniere College, a school for half-caste boys and girls in Lucknow, was crucial in the British defeat of the uprising.

222 Edmund Hope Verney (1838-1910), later 3rd baronet, oldest son of Sir Harry Verney; the *Shannon* was a 51-gun steam frigate sent with reinforcements to help put down the siege of Lucknow.

One man at the meeting yesterday said we must succumb to the prince of Wales,[223] if he was *for* the prison, but Gordon would not have done this. I cannot imagine, but you will know better than I, any plan that Gordon would more have disliked than the palatial prison and the grand officers' houses round.

10 December 1886

Gordon Boys' Home. I believe the Woking Prison *is* entirely abandoned. But they are not beginning to build as yet at Bagshot, because the government has as yet only offered a twenty-one years' lease, and they say they must have more to build.

I mentioned to two of the committee the grievous want of hospital accommodation, and that, even if they had a nurse, they had not a place to put her in. Both said that a house ought to be taken as near as possible for patients and nurse.

Next Wednesday is committee day. I shall try to remind them.

Source: From a letter to Douglas Galton, with his comments, Add Mss 45766 ff82-87

30 May 1888

Gordon Boys' Hospital plan. This plan (rough) has been just sent me, though I understand the hospital is all but quite finished. I think—I hope the *wish* is not father to the thought—it must have been submitted to you. Can you explain it to me (Butterfield's)? (It is not as General Higginson, with whom I had a long interview, told me. You know perhaps that I am commissioned to find them a matron.)

Ground Floor Kitchen and Scullery.

Surgery?

Matron is to patch up *out*-patient boys in surgery and attend to their little ailments. *Ablution room* opposite. Is that for *out*-patient boys? Surely not for *sick* boys *upstairs*? **DG:** Ablution room is for boys not in bed.

Staircase: Is there a big window over staircase? **DG:** Yes.

Otherwise a long cross vestibule with four doors and no window and *cupboards,* left of *entrance,* prevent cross-ventilation from east to west right through. **DG:** I did not know of cupboards.

Large Room to South 19.6 × 12 said to be matron's bedroom. She does not want so large a bedroom, and she *does* want a *sitting room.*

223 Edward (1841-1910), prince of Wales, the future Edward VII.

And she, the trained nurse, ought to sleep on *ward floor upstairs.* **DG:** Yes.

Bedroom a very nice room × two windows to south. But what does she want with a bedroom near 20 ft long? Matron must have a W.C. **DG:** None.

And I should have thought one for surgery. **DG:** She ought to have sitting and bedroom, but that idea was [illeg].

Upper Floor or *Ward Floor* Ward to left 20 × 24.8 × 11 very awkward, so nearly square. Three windows, unless I am blundering, to N.E., and W. will get *none* but *east* sun (see projection south of west), said to be for ten boys (General Higginson said for six). Where are *sick* boys to *wash*? **DG:** In the ward.

Small room at right angles, to west, 12.9 × 8.8 × 12 opposite W.C.s, which have all the southern sun. This, I was told, was to be the "infectious" room, and when not occupied by an infectious case, was to be occupied by the "slavey," a girl at "£10 or £12 a year."

If the sick boys are *not* bedridden, *she* cannot control their tricks. If they are, the matron, who is the trained nurse, ought to sleep on their floor. (But this is not a nice bedroom for a *matron.*)

There ought to be an *inspection* window onto the large square ward. (*Night* and day inspection altogether deficient.) But if an "infectious" case is to be there, an inspection window is of all things to be *avoided.* (General Higginson was not quite sure whether this room was to have more than a "borrowed" light.) Anyhow the window can be only N. or W. (unless I am blundering).

Staircase. I take for granted by window over staircase and another at the other end—sweeping ventilation from end-to-end of passage. Perhaps it is intended to shut off "infectious" room and W.C. (one) opposite and slop sink with passage window when there is an "infectious" case? But *is* it a *fit room* for "*infectious*" case? and ought not the door to be nearer the big window, if for infectious case? *Matron* is to be a *trained nurse,* to take entire charge of hospital, with a "*slavey*" to cook, etc., to take charge of *general* health of all boys—and prevent illness and treat little ailments without doctor, to take charge of *new arrivals* who are generally ill) and of their dormitory, to supervise *general* kitchen and soldier cook and introduce healthy variety, broths, economy, and good dishes, and fruit, to supervise *laundry,* where boys are taught to wash, but without a laundress!! This is, in brief, what she is to do.

She cannot, therefore, be always in hospital. After much search, I have submitted a matron (who has been with us ten years) to General

Higginson; she would take it under *conditions.* She must have a *competent woman servant* who is to cook for hospital—not under thirty—who can be trusted with boys of from fourteen to eighteen, especially if she is to sleep on that floor at night and when matron is about on her duties. And this woman must have a bedroom. Matron ought to have a *sitting room.*

Could *room upstairs* be made *fit for matron's bedroom* for *maid* be taken off the south room downstairs, this to be the matron's *sitting room*? It would be far better if the matron and maid could sleep in *upper or ward floor.* Ward to south beautiful ward, 19.9 × 12 by 11, best room in the place, two windows to S., one to E. (unless I am blundering). (General Higginson says for four boys.) But difficulty of inspection or supervision?

W.C.s good over entrance, window I presume between them, and windows *in* each to S.; good broad passage, swept by air, I presume, from end-to-end. Slop sink window ditto, I presume, south or west. But I do grudge their position with all the S. and W. sun. And it would make such a beautiful bedroom for matron. (All on the N. side the passage I don't like—do you? square ward, infectious room, etc.) *Where is the "slavey" to sleep when "infectious" room occupied*?

Ground Floor. Back door under staircase. Back door quite necessary to admit *out-patient boys* to surgery and ablution room is at front door. **DG:** They would come in at front door, I imagine.

And to admit boys, who are taught to assist in the hospital, and the delivery of supplies. But for discipline it will be a very easy descent for the sick boys on upper floor down the staircase and out by the back door. This makes it the more imperative to have a trustworthy maid to matron.

Matron may have boys to tea. She *must* have a sitting room adjoining rooms upstairs. But it does not seem possible. And, after all, *where is the woman* who sleeps in the empty infectious room *to sleep when that is occupied by an infectious case*—the time of all others when the *trained nurse* is most wanted upstairs at night?

These are the difficulties about which I must ask you. (There *must* be a laundress under the matron. But as she would not sleep in hospital, I need not trouble you about that.) If you would kindly return me these sheets, WITH YOUR KIND REMARKS, it might save you trouble.

Source: From a letter to Arthur Clough,[224] Boston University 5/19/12

4 June 1888

Don't vilify my character by saying that I would have recommended poor Mrs Axton for Gordon Boys' Home matron. The woman I have recommended was trained by us at St Thomas', has served ten years in our work in different posts. I have taken her character "confidentially" from her authorities. I have talked with her for four hours, written for five or six hours more about her to the Gordon Boys' authorities, making conditions and otherwise—and besides had plans and criticized them of their little hospital. And with all feel by no means confident. That is the worst of it.

ever dear Arthur

your affectionate Aunt Florence

Source: From two letters to Thomas Wentworth Higginson, Wellcome Ms 5483/48, and Clendening History of Medicine Library, Kansas University Medical Center

8 June 1888

Private. Many thanks for your most kind note and its enclosures, with General [Henry] Tyndall's answers to questions.

Is it to be understood that you kindly wish to give the "southern ward upper floor," 19.6 by 12, for the "matron's bedroom"? This should be for the present only, as being the best ward or room in the hospital, it would doubtless be for the patients most ill, the north ward being very inferior to it. Query, will this north ward have much sun, except from the east window? That the "present surgery," "ground floor" (is that the room next the kitchen, 10 × 15 or the larger room to the south, 19.6 × 12, ground floor?) is to be given as the "matron's sitting room *and surgery*," "dispensing with a complete surgery and receiving room *for the present*."

If there are "wretched lads," poor fellows! by which I understand boys with something serious the matter with them, yet not confined to bed, for her to have charge of, the room 10 × 15 would be, would it not? rather close quarters? But as you speak of the "so-called matron's room downstairs," I conclude it is *this* room to the south, 19.6. × 12?

"Sister" Constable shall go "on a visit of inspection to the hospital" and to see the home, "as soon as possible" after I have received your kind directions, if they are to this effect, and she shall do as you say.

224 Arthur Hugh Clough, Jr (1859-1943), son of Arthur Hugh Clough and Nightingale's cousin, Blanche (Smith) Clough.

10 June 1888

Gordon Boys' Home. *Matron.*

Sister Constable will be at Waterloo Station on *Tuesday* morning in time to catch the 7:35 A.M. train there to go to Sunningdale, where the F. Verneys[225] will meet her and take her in a fly to see Gordon Boys' Home and Hospital, returning to Sunningdale at 11. She will then come here, according to your kind wish, and "report" to me "quietly" "what she thinks of it."

I am sorry her visit there will be so hurried. On account of its being the Ascot week, she was advised to put it off till next week. But if you mean to come to a "formal" decision at your Wednesday's meeting, she must, at least, as you wisely stipulated, have seen the "Home" and hospital first.

I wish she could have spent some more hours there and seen the boys' dinners served, etc., the sickly lads. But when will you or your "Home" committee see her before your Wednesday's meeting? Shall it be on Tuesday afternoon at Cockspur Street? I will keep her here till any hour you may appoint for her to come in the afternoon, if you wish it. And when will you take her character from her matron, Miss Vincent, at St Marylebone Infirmary, Ladbroke Grove Road, W.? independently of us; I trust before Wednesday.

I have just ascertained that "she will have to give one month's notice" (this "one" month is a concession) "to the committee" at St Marylebone Infirmary, "and stay the month, and should have *at least* three or four weeks' holiday, before she undertakes a new post," if you engage her. They will "miss her work" at St Marylebone Infirmary "extremely."

Unless you could put off the proposing her at the meeting of the general committee on Wednesday, how are the most necessary steps to be gone through? on Tuesday? (It was "impossible" to arrange her going to the Gordon B. Home on Monday—tomorrow.)

Have I met all your wishes as nearly as was possible?

I have sent S[ister] Constable a copy of General Tyndall's kind answers to our questions—also a copy of the "matron's duties," as laid down by you. As you will see her so soon, I will not trouble you with more. May the Home's best interests be served. . . .

---

225 Frederick William Verney (1846-1913), youngest son of Sir Harry Verney and a close friend of Nightingale's; his wife Maude (c1846-1937), née Hay Williams; their country house was at Sunningdale, near the final location of the Gordon Boys' Home.

I have troubled you with the hours of S. Constable's visit to Gordon B.H. on Tuesday, as you kindly wished to "warn General Tyndall."

Source: From a letter to Douglas Galton, Add Mss 45766 ff94-95

19 June 1888

Could you kindly look at this letter of F. Verney's to General Higginson, which he has sent to me to look at and post? It is the *second* subject in the letter to which the *little sketch* refers.

I had called his, F.V.'s, attention to it. But I must have your "imprimatur" please, before it goes. Could you return it to me by bearer, with your verdict? if you will be so good. I am going to send you the hospital plans as you kindly allow. . . .

Very many thanks for your criticism, which I have forwarded to F. Verney. I am so thankful I sent to you.

I did not mean to do dishonour to my "*education*" by supposing *this* was the proper thing. But the boys are behaving badly. Their habits are not decent. And it would be desirable that something should be done, if it could be sanitarily done.

Source: From a note for Frederick Verney, Add Mss 68889 ff150-51, and two letters Add Mss 68886 ff63 and 70-71

14 June 1889

They, the building committee, *with D. Galton present,* had a meeting last week, in which all but your important evidence came out!! Mr Butterfield had disregarded all their injunctions and his own promises and made the contractor go right against them. And there is no recourse except to cashier B., which Colonel Hamilton won't.

30 June 1889

I want very much to hear what you alone can tell me about G.B.H. . . .

Private . . . I don't think it would do to have in a civilian sanitarian. None of them know half as much as Douglas Galton. When I saw him last, some two weeks ago, he said, and almost told me to tell you: "It is no use doing anything now. All the things are *made* for this new block. It would save no expense to alter it now. But Butterfield says he will do nothing *after* this block. And then will be our time to alter, renew, reform, modify." Valeat quantum [take it for what it is worth].

25 July 1889

Gordon Boys' Home. *Private.*

Your messenger and letter arrived quite in time yesterday, and I pitched into Sir Douglas Galton, though I had a great deal of worriting business with him, with all my might, like a man. First of all, he will certainly come to the *annual inspection* at the Gordon Boys' Home, on August the first, as you desire—and he will talk to *Rev Mr Pine,* and Mr Trevarthen of Red Hill[226] as you order. He went in to a most unusual rhapsody for him, as he is the greatest frondeur [rebel] I know, about you and your work at Gordon Boys' Home (and how they were indebted to you) really, seriously.

2. He was really and properly excited about the "no alteration" proposed in *opening the windows in the dormitories.* I do hope his just rage will not "fade as a leaf,"[227] but that he will do something. He seems quite disposed to do so. He approves the Sherringham ventilators. He does not approve the ventilation over the doors, which, he says, will only let in the staircase foul air. He says the staircase foul air can only be carried off by a tube going out at the roof. And that perhaps they will not do.

3. He is rather despairing about the ventilation of the workshops, especially of the shoemaker's shop. Are the windows the same as those of the dormitories? He thinks not. He thinks that they can't open them because of the draft, and he says how uncommonly difficult it is to ventilate tailors' and shoemakers' workshops. But perhaps he will look into this.

4. With regard to your question about dimensions of dormitories, windows, etc., for young men and boys, in buildings erected during the last ten years, he says (like the man who wrote a chapter on snakes in Iceland: "There are no snakes in Iceland") "there are no buildings erected during the last ten years." But the dimensions, etc., which he did give me, I do not quote, because they are against us. They are in fact worse than those of the Gordon Boys' Home.

5. He did write a tremendous letter to Colonel Beaty Pownall about the abomination which you discovered. I think he is a great deal more aware, thanks to you, to the Butterfieldian evils, and Gordon Boys' Home backslidings, than he was. A good deal may be gained by pitching into him from time to time.

---

226 John Trevarthen (c1837-?), secretary of the Farm School at Red Hill, Surrey, established by the Philanthropic Society for Delinquent Children.

227 Isa 64:6.

Source: From a letter to Amy Hawthorn, Add Mss 45776 ff269-70

13 January 1890

I think the way of solving the difficulty about *Gordon Boys' hospital* books is, if you will be so very good as to add this to your fund, and take the trouble to choose the books and dispatch them to the hospital, and say nothing about me, please.

Editor: The Gordon Boys' Home became the Gordon Boys' School in 1943, to become Gordon's School in 1990 when it admitted girls.

Correspondence on other issues resumes, beginning with a tribute to Douglas Galton in 1893, for an unknown purpose.

Source: From a draft tribute to Douglas Galton, Add Mss 45819 ff156-59

29 June 1893

Sir Douglas Galton's title to public honour lies in the thousands of lives he has saved (*not* killed), military and civil, in the health he has restored to tens of thousands and will to generations yet unborn. He is the pioneer of SANITARY military engineers. He has served for twenty-thirty years in great public offices and since his retirement has been and is at the call of great public bodies and private individuals and has always put his great experience at the disposal of his benevolent and active genius, where his disinterestedness equals his ability, which is saying a great deal.

As a youth, he passed the highest examination on record at Woolwich and belonged to the Royal Engineers. At that time we were almost in black darkness how to *prevent* disease. And a well-known R.E. nobly said, in 1857, "I know how to build so that it shall not tumble down, but how to build so that it shall be healthy I know *not*." Sir D.G. had to teach himself the application of sanitary practice to engineering to buildings and to works. And well he did it—in the nick of time, the "acceptable day," the "day of salvation."[228] For, On the return of the troops from the Crimea, where they had died in the first year like sheep or like heroes, not from guns or the bayonet, but from disease, preventive disease.

Sidney Herbert had devoted himself by two royal commissions, one for the British, one for the Indian Army, in his powerful position with crown, Cabinet and Commons, and lastly of secretary of state for war,

228 An allusion to 2 Cor 6:2.

to remedy these frightful evils up to his death in 1861. And he left us a legacy in the Army Sanitary Commission to carry on his work. Sir D.G. is one of those who was and still is on that commission, which now embraces Indian affairs, civil and military—one of those by whom the extraordinarily high death rate of our army at home has been so greatly reduced—and by whom sanitary improvements have been started all along the line, civil and military.

He has other titles to honour. After having been secretary of the Railway Department of the Board of Trade from 1854 to 1859, he was "assistant" inspector general of fortifications 1859-62. Then he became "assistant" under secretary of state for war 1862-70 (i.e., financial secretary for W.O.), then director of public works and buildings, 1870-75. I do not know what "assistant" means—he was always called "financial secretary" for the War Office.

After twenty-one years of the most energetic public and professional life, he continued the same ceaseless and enlightened activity in many different forms—sent for by great public bodies, not only at home but in America, Paris, Antwerp, Vienna, etc. He distinguishes himself for hospitals, schools, county councils, sanitary institutions, for all objects connected with the improvement, the well-being and the health of populations. He built the great Military Herbert Hospital at Woolwich. He was chairman of committee of the International Congress of Hygiene in 1891.

He has been member of the Army Sanitary Commission (formerly, under Sidney Herbert, called "Barrack and Hospital Improvement" Commission) from the beginning, which embraces the Mediterranean stations, and in India the *native* populations as well as the troops.

He now appears as one of the most active members of a county council and one often applied to for his advice and support in these and other bodies.

Editor: In 1893 Nightingale was approached by a distinguished American doctor, John B. Hamilton (1847-98), United States Surgeon General 1879-91, editor of the *Journal of the American Medical Association* 1893-98 and an expert on yellow fever. The concern he raised with her—the need for army doctors to get practical training in the field—has to be gathered indirectly, for the paper he left her to read, which he never published, is not extant. Nor could a letter by him in the *Times* be found, although the first item below refers to one. Nightingale's remarks, such as to the "evil in our machinery for war" are hardly specific. The question she succeeded in getting asked in the House of Commons, however, makes the problem clear, for its answer, recorded in Hansard, *Parliamentary Debates*, refers to the provision of "practical experience" in the field for medical officer (see p 492 below).

Source: From a letter to J.B. Hamilton, Columbia University, Presbyterian Hospital School of Nursing C221

10 November 1893

Strictly Private. I beg to acknowledge your note of 1 November as also your letter in the *Times*, which I had carefully read.

I am sorry to be obliged to concur with them both, as far as my knowledge extends. The thing is, how to get an inquiry into these facts, as you say. And I have delayed my answer till, by questioning people, I could propose something to you. If you could kindly make a clear, concise sort of statement, showing what is wanted, stating the danger of the present system, the need and necessity of reform in the particular branches, it should then be submitted to Sir Redvers Buller,[229] and supported in every way that was feasible. This, if it commends itself to you, should be done as soon as possible, I understand.

May the highest success attend your exertions in remedying so great an evil in our machinery for war.

Editor: Hamilton's reply to the above letter said that "no assistance" was to be expected from Sir Redvers Buller, who, with Lord Wolseley, then commander of the forces in Ireland, was to blame for the state of affairs.[230] Nightingale's next letter invited him to visit her the next day (16 November 1893), "if you do not mind seeing a great invalid who is now entirely a prisoner to her room, but who still sees people on pressing business."[231] The two evidently met, when Hamilton left a paper with her at that time.

229 Major General Henry Redvers Buller (1839-1908), then chief of staff.

230 Hamilton letter 13 November 1893, Add Mss 45812 f55. Nightingale knew Wolseley from her work on the Egyptian campaigns of 1882 and 1885, in *Wars and the War Office*.

231 Letter 15 November 1893, Columbia University, Presbyterian Hospital School of Nursing C222.

Source: From a letter to J.B. Hamilton, Columbia University, Presbyterian Hospital School of Nursing C223

18 November 1893

Private. I return you with many thanks your valuable paper. And could you kindly let me have the typewritten copy (with ample spaces between the lines) that you were so good as to promise me by Tuesday morning?

It is very much desired that you should write an article for *The Nineteenth Century* or the *Fortnightly*, giving the sting of that paper. But you may perhaps object to this? Also, could the director general bring about as regards Aldershot at least some part of what is so desirable in the paper I return?

(Lord Ripon is not now available, as being in the Cabinet.) These are the things which are said to me. I hope next week to have more to say.

Source: From a letter to Douglas Galton, Add Mss 45767 ff101-02

21 November 1893

I was so very sorry to see you so overtired and anxious the last time you were so kind as to come.

1. You were so good as to speak of seeing me on Thursday or Friday about Dr Hamilton's business. I have another engagement for that time, but I might make it either Thursday afternoon OR Friday afternoon, if I could know at once which day, IF *either*, you could kindly give me in the afternoon. (I am very busy this week. And so are you.)

2. Dr Hamilton is going to send me *this morning a typewritten copy* of the paper I partly read to you. And I will forward it to you at once, if you will allow me, and tell me *where*. He is quite ready to write in *The Nineteenth Century* or *Fortnightly*, as you advised, *if* it can be accepted.

He is printing in pamphlet form his original letter in the *Times and* the manuscript I read to you for our distribution. I am afraid he expects a great deal too much of my strength. But, as you say, the state of things he describes "drives one mad," that is to exertion. At all events I can do nothing for him *this* week. For I have work which must be sent in by end of week. . . .

Dr Hamilton's question was to be asked by Mr Plunkett last night.

Editor: D.R. Plunkett, MP for Dublin University, asked the war secretary if he had taken any steps to secure army medical staff opportunities for acquiring practical experience in field duties, the want of which was a weak point in the present system. The answer was short, and evidently not satisfactory, that "steps will be taken" for a two-week course the next summer.[232]

Source: From two letters to J.B. Hamilton, Columbia University, Presbyterian Hospital School of Nursing 224A and 225

30 November 1893

Private. I have not been idle, nor, I am sure, have you, about your admirable "Suggestions," which I have heard pronounced as giving the whole case *unanswerably.* There seems however no opportunity of getting a "day" for it in the House of Commons *this* session. There is nothing coming on about the army, is there? The thing is now to get public attention drawn to it in view of the next session.

The thing is now, and these are the questions asked me with reference to the forthcoming pamphlet, is it to be *published*? Who is publishing it? It is feared that, if it is published, *The Nineteenth Century,* which likes something fresh, would not insert your article. If you mean to publish it then *the thing* would be to get it reviewed?

But the pamphlet might be *given* about, I am told, without detriment to the article being received into *The Nineteenth Century.* Anyhow it could not come out till the January number.

It would be as well, if you are kind enough to send me some copies of your printed pamphlet for distribution, that it should be as soon as possible, because the Christmas holidays are so near, when no man will work.

Pray believe that I wish the highest success to this important movement. I am sorry to seem so dilatory, but I have much work on my hands and am much interrupted.

9 December 1893

I am glad to hear that you are making progress. You truly say that we shall in the end get all we want, but that it will be a long and uphill fight. We await your promised article for a magazine, and Sir Douglas Galton will try and get it into *The Nineteenth Century* for January. But, for this, your manuscript should be ready by the middle of this month. I wish that you knew Sir Douglas Galton, and he would be very glad to know you and would be helpful. (You know that he was for years at the War Office, that he is on the Army Sanitary Commission, and is I suppose the first military SANITARY engineer of the time.) His address is. . . .

232 Hansard, *Parliamentary Debates* 20 November 1893:1281-82.

Will you not leave your card upon him with a message, if he is not at home? He is a very busy man and is often not in London for more than a week together, besides being sometimes at his Worcestershire home.

As to the "20,000 beds," it is indeed an immense work for you to do. However it is *something* that the War Office have arrived at *thinking* even of such a matter.

You were to speak today at the Volunteer Ambulance Association. And I hope you have won over Sir Algernon Borthwick.[233] All this will tend to the "educating of public opinion."

Thank you for the copy of Sir T. Longmore's letter to the *British Medical Journal*.[234]

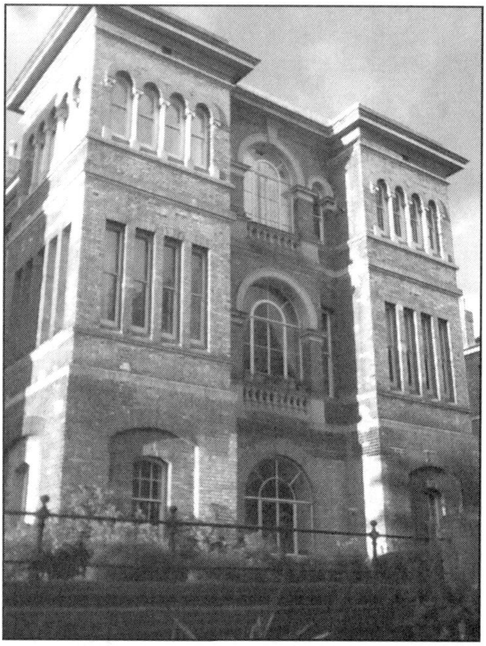

One pavilion of the "Royal Herbert Pavilions," now luxury residences, renovated from the Herbert Hospital, Woolwich (picture on p 232).

233 Algernon Borthwick (1830-1908), Conservative MP, later Lord Glenesk.
234 Thomas Longmore, "The Early Care of Wounded in War," *British Medical Journal* 2 December 1893:1248-49.

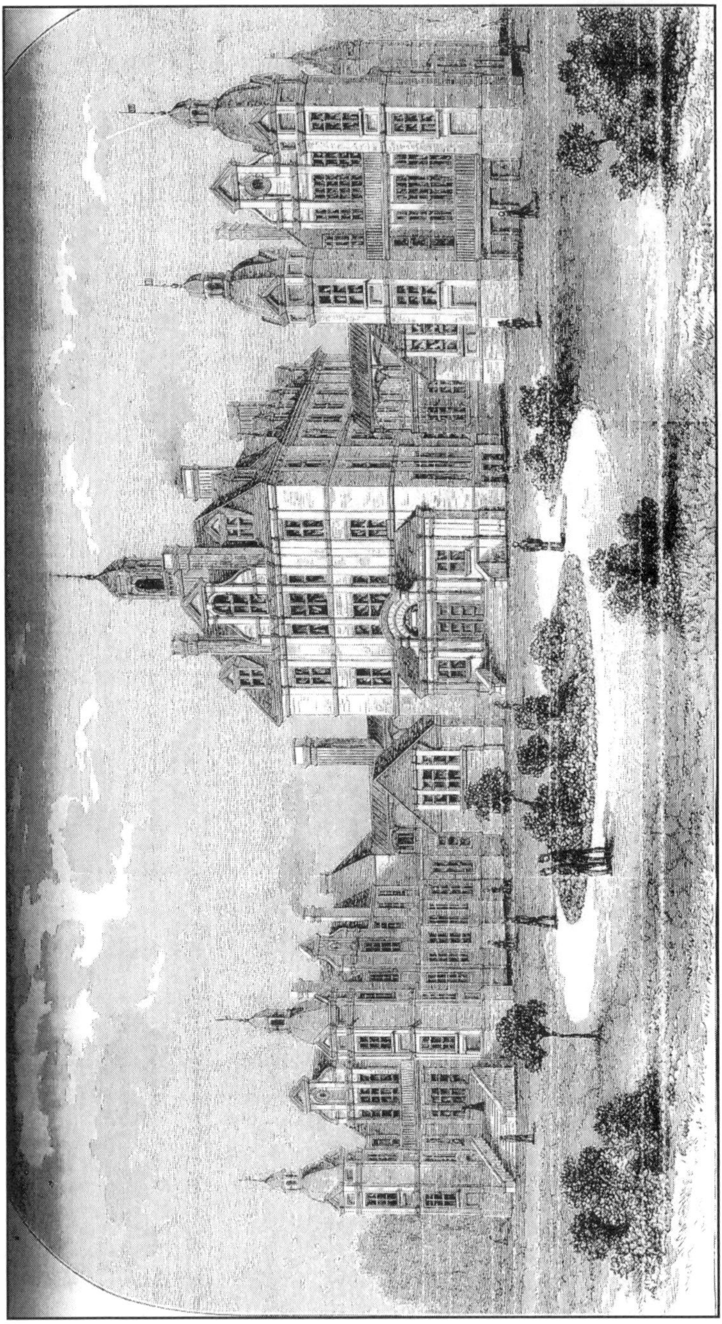

Lincoln New County Hospital. The hospital, however, was not of the preferred pavilion model. From *The Builder*, 5 July 1879, p 79.

CIVIL HOSPITALS: LETTERS AND NOTES

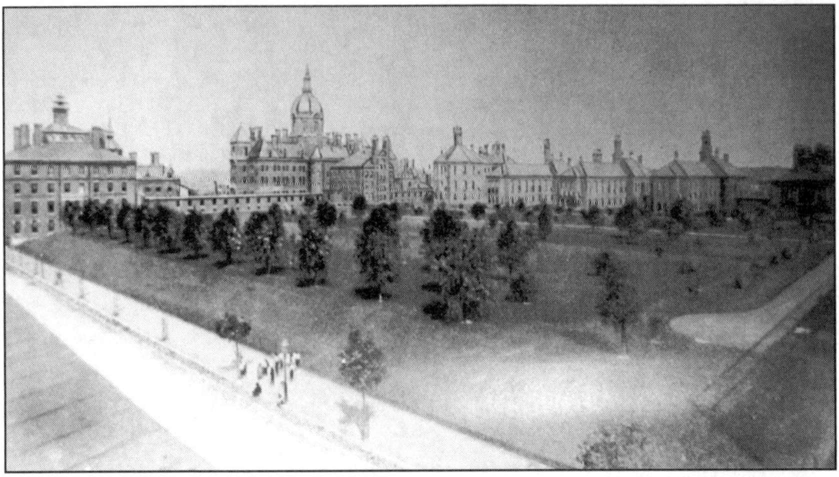

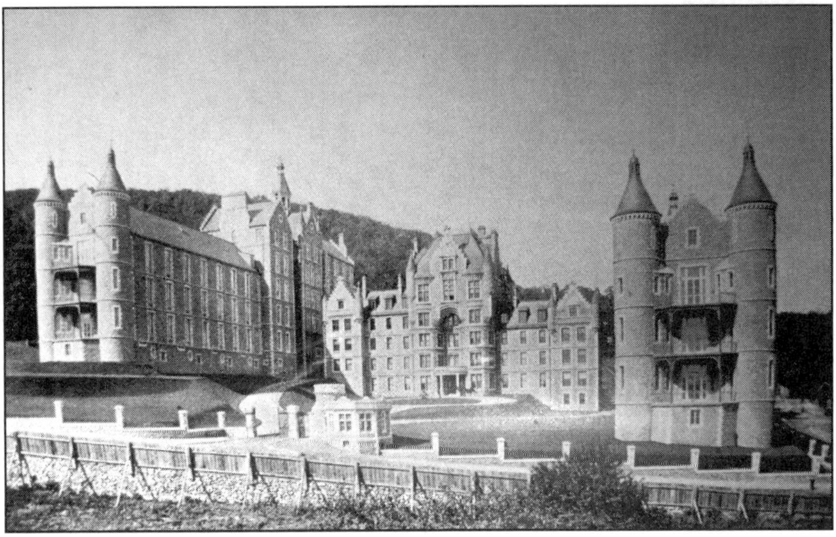

Top: Johns Hopkins University Hospital, Baltimore, Maryland, a model American pavilion hospital.

Bottom: Royal Victoria Hospital, Montreal, designed by Henry Saxon Snell, with input from Nightingale.

Civil Hospitals: Letters and Notes

Nightingale's need for data on civil hospitals is evident in her work on military hospitals, undertaken upon her return from the Crimean War. The same laws affecting health or disease held in both kinds of hospital; there were more civil hospitals than military; and peacetime conditions were the norm, war the exception. Part of the case she made on army hospitals in her Crimean War analyses relied on comparisons with civil hospital data. Then, soon after her return from that war she began to receive requests for assistance on civil hospital plans, which she continued to receive into old age.

Unlike military hospitals, there was a great diversity of types of civil hospital for Nightingale to consider, from general hospitals to convalescent and cottage hospitals, workhouse infirmaries and lying-in institutions. There was no system of hospitals in her day; the National Health Service was not even a thought; and the regular civil hospitals were independently managed by their particular boards. Decision makers ranged from reform-minded doctors to hospital committees, Poor Law guardians, architects and concerned citizens whereas, in the military, control largely lay with the Army Medical Department, sometimes the (civilian) War Office or (army command) Horse Guards.

Where there is sufficient material on a particular hospital, I have grouped it together and provided an introduction. In-between items are simply reported in chronological order. The last note available by Nightingale dates to 1901, the last action by her to 1908. Both of these, tellingly, concern her first hospital, the Establishment for Gentlewomen during Illness in Harley St.

Topics of the correspondence and publications range from the basic principles of the pavilion model, issues of site and materials to statistics to track results. Nightingale focused on design to facilitate patient care and efficient nursing from early on to late in her career. Concerns about specialized hospitals, especially children's hospitals and children's wards, again are present from early to late in the correspondence. There are sections on convalescent and cottage hospitals.

Gathering and maintaining statistics to enable effective decision making continue to be important in this section, and Nightingale sought advice from experts as to how to improve them. For example, she asked Dr Farr in 1861 to go over the statistics for St Thomas' Hospital. Both she and James Paget at St Bartholomew's wanted his assessment, obviously for the purpose of making them more useful (see p 574 below).

Broader health conditions in cities, towns and rural areas emerge periodically, although the main subject is general, acute care hospitals in major cities.

There are several short articles, first published in the reliable *Builder* (one on preventible disease and three on the site for St Thomas' Hospital), and a substantial paper, "Hospital Statistics and Hospital Plans," written for the National Association for the Promotion of Social Science.

Whistle blowing was another Nightingale activity, and since she held no paid position and needed none, she had nothing to lose. She was well aware that persons who complained could easily forfeit promotion or even lose their jobs. To put pressure on the Winchester Infirmary to build a new hospital at a healthier site she passed on the report of deaths there to the Registrar-General and to the "most eminent surgeons" of London. The plan was for the Registrar-General to call for a formal report, which would be public and damning.

Nightingale sometimes lost her battles on hospitals. She gave advice on plans and met with architects often to no avail. Thomas Bellamy, architect of King's College Hospital, went over his "execrable" plans with her (see p 588 below), but since every subsequent reference to those plans is negative, we can infer that her advice was not taken. She strongly urged that a new Manchester Royal Infirmary be built out of the city, but the hospital authorities instead chose to expand on the downtown site already occupied. She also at times gave advice on hospitals that were never built, for unrelated reasons: the Montreal General Hospital is a prime example.

Much of the correspondence is missing, a fact known from letters to her, to others she consulted, and notes she made about the hospital or architect in question. To attempt to give an overview of the whole range of the work she did on hospitals the following list is provided. It gives, in simple alphabetic order, the names of all the hospitals, with dates, on whose plans Nightingale is known to have advised (including the smaller number of military hospitals). Those hospitals for which significant correspondence or notes are available are indicated in bold. This list complements the chronology given in the Introduction. Architects are listed in Appendix A.

List of Hospitals on which Nightingale Advised

Birkenhead Borough Hospital 1862
Blackburn Infirmary c1858
Bucks Infirmary, Aylesbury 1859-62
Carlsruhe Clinique and Training School 1886
Children's Hospital, Heidelberg 1861
Coventry Infirmary 1862
Derby Infirmary 1865-69
Derbyshire Royal Infirmary Extension and Nurses' Home 1891-94
Devonport Women's Hospital 1861
Edinburgh Royal Infirmary 1879
Glamorganshire Home for Convalescents 1871-74
Glasgow Royal Infirmary 1859-61
Gordon Boys' Home 1885-89
Winchester Infirmary (Hampshire County Hospital) 1858-64
Haydock Cottage Hospital, Lancashire 1885
Herbert Hospital, Woolwich 1859-65
Herbert Memorial Convalescent Home 1865-67
Johns Hopkins Hospital, Baltimore 1876
King's College Hospital, London 1857-58
Leeds Infirmary 1861-62
Lincolnshire Convalescent Home 1869
Lisbon Children's Hospital 1859-61
Liverpool Royal Infirmary 1882-85
Malta Hospital of Incurables 1862-65
Malta General Hospital 1862
Malta Military Hospital 1858 (not built)
Manchester Convalescent Hospital 1860-61 (not built)
Montreal General Hospital 1874-76 (not built)
Moscow Children's Hospital 1874
Norfolk and Norwich Hospital 1875
North Staffordordshire Infirmary, Stoke-on-Trent 1861
Oldham Infirmary (no date)
Prince Alfred Hospital, Sydney, Nurses' Home 1882, 1891

Reading Hospital c1861
Regimental Hospitals (generic plans) 1858-59
Royal Hospital for Incurables, Putney 1861
Royal Victoria Hospital, Montreal 1888-89
Royal Victoria Hospital, Netley 1856-63
St Marylebone Infirmary (Supplementary) Nurses' Home 1882-83
St Pancras Workhouse Infirmary, Highgate 1868
St Thomas' Hospital 1859-71
St Thomas' Nurses' Home 1882-85
Städtisches Allgemeine Krankenhaus im Friedrichshain, Berlin (City General Hospital) 1868
Swansea Infirmary 1864-65
Sydney Infirmary and Nurses' Home 1866-69 and 1874
University College Hospital 1877 (not built)
Women's Hospital, Euston Road 1888
Woolwich Female Hospital 1862
Yoxall Cottage Hospital 1872

Source: From a letter to William Farr, Add Mss 43398 ff3-4

Combe Hurst
Kingston on Thames, S.W.
8 January 1857

I am not going to worry you. This is only to be a "retainer." I have received from the Registrar-General[1] the mortality statistics of the London hospitals, which are very much the same as what I had been led to expect from the private returns I have. You would, however, derive great joy and satisfaction from them (as I should say if I were writing a *Chadwickiad*) for the one fact they point out is that the mortality increases as the number of patients. There are some differences between the hospitals which, however, can only be explained by some taking in worse cases than others.

7.59 deaths on every 100 cases treated is the general rate in general hospitals, 9.38 in workhouses, 11.48 in "special" hospitals.

The rest of my agreeable information I defer till I have the pleasure of seeing you again. I shall go up to town early next week to stay, as I cannot be away longer. I am sure that you will be glad to hear that I have prospect of active employment, as this pen-and-ink employment drives

1 For Nightingale's visit to the General Register Office see p 239 above.

me mad, and I am sure, if the love of God and mankind entail much pen-and-ink work for a continuance I, for one, would not go on loving them. (I have a wretched slave from Vacher's working with me at 1/ per hour, which I consider cheap.)

I hope you are better and will remember to let me know when you come back.

Source: Notes, Add Mss 45825 ff12-14

[ca. late June 1857]

The arguments on the much-controverted point of large versus small wards may be shortly summed up. The French have decided in favour of wards of not less than twenty beds; the corners of wards always make a whirlpool of still air; it is as well to multiply these as little as possible, on account of greater facility of attendance and administration.

The London civil hospitals seem generally to adopt the same plan: Guy's, London, King's College, etc., give us double wards with from ten [to] twenty beds in each partition. The effect of this is to have four rows of beds with a partition down the middle, in order to impede the ventilation.

Military hospitals in England seem to decide the question in favour of small wards, of about ten beds each, on grounds of discipline. It is true that the discipline in military hospitals is very imperfect, but from other causes, it has been attempted to show, than that of number of beds. Again, the question of facility of attendance, important as it is, is not to be put into competition for a moment with that of the sanitary condition of the ward. (It is often urged, in civil hospitals, that a ward of forty beds is the most convenient for attendance.)

When clinical instruction is to be given, as at Netley, another question enters into the question. Dr Zdekauer, professor of the Academy of Medicine of St Petersburg, who has recently been sent by the emperor of Russia[2] to inquire in France and England as to hospital construction, appears to have solved the question with regard to all these matters, for his acquired knowledge and natural capacity.

He appears to have arrived at the following conclusions:

1. That the "block" plan, as shown in the Lariboisière Hospital, but with the blocks farther apart, with two storeys only and each ward to

2 Nicholas F. Zdekauer (1815-1901), professor of pathology; Tsar Alexander II (1818-81). Dr Sutherland wrote Nightingale about Zdekauer's visit, letter 26 June 1857, Add Mss 45751 f20.

contain twenty-five sick only, without artificial ventilation, but solely with doors, windows and open fireplaces and air shafts, with self-acting water closets, contain the elements of the best hospitals constructed.

It might not appear at first sight what is the connection with clinical instruction. The facts are these: there is more than twice the room proportionally for students in a ward for twenty patients than in a ward for ten; on the other hand, in a ward for forty patients, the twenty very bad cases are much disturbed while the students are examining the other twenty slight cases. Therefore, a medium ward for from twenty [to] twenty-five cases is considered the best.

This is the only humane and Christian view of the subject. Expense is another consideration, and, on account of economy, one roof for 100 patients is better than two roofs, one for each fifty, according to the Zdekauer's plan. But then let there be four wards for twenty-five patients each on two flats. But *all with opposite windows to each.* None, double wards. Vincennes illustrates the putting wards end-to-end, still preserving the "*block*" shape.

Editor: Before being recruited for the Crimean War, Nightingale had accepted an offer to head the nursing at King's College Hospital, London. Naturally, she was greatly interested when shown the plans for the new hospital building in 1857—architect Tite sent them—by his friend Thomas Bellamy. She wrote Dr Whitfield about the plans, but her letter only refers to "an idea about King's College Hospital," which information she asked to have returned "immediately, as I mean to do something about it." Whitfield evidently replied with substantive points, for her next letter to him stated that she agreed "with every word of your plan for King's College Hospital."[3] A letter to Dr Bowman (the next item below) fleshes out her concerns.

3 Letters 17 and 19 July 1858, Florence Nightingale Museum (LMA) H1/ST/NC1/58/4-5.

Source: From an incomplete letter to William Bowman,[4] Bowman Private Collection

[ca. July 1858]

The following have occurred to me as among the more obvious objections to the plan of extending King's College Hospital:

1. placing any part of the new buildings upon the old saturated graveyard of St Clement's, which was for so many years a nuisance to the metropolis;
2. the existence of so many close corners formed by high walls, which must necessarily obstruct the free circulation of air;
3. the small enclosed court between the theatre and chapel and the proposed mass of building in front;
4. the immense [line missing];
5. the proposed back-to-back wards.

It would be well to consider whether it is for the benefit of the sick to place so many of them upon so small an area of ground, on such a site and neighbourhood; (2) whether the proposed front buildings could not be dispensed with altogether—whether another wing, consisting not of double but of single wards, might not be constructed parallel to the new buildings on the chapel side—so that the whole building would consist of three sides, like the letter **E**, leaving nearly the whole of the old burial ground unoccupied; (3) whether the two-storey corridors might not be removed from their present position.

The corridor next the present wards cannot be otherwise than obstructive to light and ventilation of the lower wards. The object to be aimed at should be to make the building as simple as possible to avoid all unnecessary angles and corners and [illeg] all closed courts, so that the sun and air may have free access to all parts of the hospital building.

Editor: The next letter explains Nightingale's long-held negative view of Dr John Simon. Her concern here was with his promotion of the statistical analysis of death rates by Edward Headlam Greenhow, a pathologist and the first lecturer on public health at St Thomas' Hospital. Greenhow, on undertaking his work at St Thomas', discovered many flaws in the available data and also became unhappy with the conglomerate term "zymotic" being used as a synonym for preventible

4 William Bowman (1816-92), later Sir, ophthalmic surgeon, member of the original Nightingale Fund Council.

disease. Simon commissioned a report from him, which he incorporated into his (Simon's) annual report for 1858, along with a substantial, laudatory introduction.[5]

Source: From a letter to Edwin Chadwick, Add Mss 45770 ff30-33

Great Malvern
11 August 1858

Have you yet seen Dr Greenhow's report to the Board of Health, with an introduction by Mr Simon? We do trust that you will take this up without delay and criticize it in the *Examiner* and move the world about it before next year, when the Board of Health question will come on again.

In this publication a sixth only of the districts are taken; all occupations are dealt with collectively to show the effects of one, and the difference of age is neglected as an element of mortality. The consequence of this extraordinary sanitary method is that all sanitary precautions are undervalued, infantine epidemics declared inevitable. Dr Farr is coming out with an account of the effect of occupations, which is to have all the truth of which this report has all the error. And, as your draining and ventilation have become unpopular, so they are here deemed unnecessary. It is quite obvious what Mr Simon's intention in writing the report is, to succeed Pym[6] as quarantine officer at the Privy Council. For quarantine regulations are to be substituted, in this enlightened publication, for sanitary improvements, in order to prevent zymotics. They are extremely proud of this work, which has doubtless been sent to you. If not, may I send it you? We shall hope to see you cutting it up in your own manner and with your own thunder. But it is lamentable to see the falling off of the sanitary party.

---

5 John Simon, "An Introductory Report by the Medical Officer of the Board on the Preventability of Certain Kinds of Premature Death," in General Board of Health, *Papers Relating to the Sanitary State of the People of England* i-xlviii; Greenhow's report, in the same volume, is titled "The Results of an Inquiry into the Different Proportions of Death Produced by Certain Diseases in Different Districts in England."

6 Sir William Pym (1772-1861), superintendent general of quarantine.

Source: From a letter to Lord Stanley, Liverpool Record Office 920 Der 146/6

15 August 1858

PRIVATE. IN RE MR SIMON. There are few things more painful to have to do than to discredit a professional man, and one would only do it for the sake of numbers. Mr Simon's work has always been what may fairly be called "scampish," in the language of the trades; his writings must always be considered as the result of a "prospecting" expedition, as they call it in the gold countries.

The last report of the Board of Health, to which I have alluded, and the report on Netley Hospital, are indications of this. "All sanitary precautions are to be undervalued," because they have become unpopular, "epidemics to be declared inevitable," and "quarantine to be substituted for sanitary improvement," quarantine which it was well nigh hoped had become an extinct superstition.

Source: From two letters to Edwin Chadwick, ADD MSS 45770 ff38 and 39-42, both from Great Malvern

16 August 1858

Has it occurred to you that your article (written for the *Quarterly Review*) might be read with advantage at Liverpool at the approaching meeting of the Association for the Advancement of Social Science (?), Mr Holland, being the secretary for the Public Health Section? I do not know. I only ask whether it would do for your article.

19 August 1858

I am very glad to hear that you mean to press the India question at Liverpool. It cannot fail to do good. Would you, when you have read through Simon and Greenhow's Board of Health papers,[7] send us your opinions of them? Dr Farr has done so. And if we do anything, we should like to be at one with you. You are the only man who can answer them properly. But, if you do not mean to do so at once, you will perhaps give us your opinion to go on with.

It seems to me that they are based on a shallow and erroneous system of statistics, intentionally perverted to cry up contagion and quarantine and other (extinct) superstitions, and to discredit sanitary precautions, draining and ventilation, and all that you have devoted your life to promote. Simon is in a "prospecting" expedition for the Privy Council, that is evident. I rejoice to hear that you mean to put down

7 For Nightingale's critique see p 352 above.

this kind of thing yourself, at the Health Section, and I only ask for a cursory view of what your opinion is about it now.

Would you not think of stirring up Liverpool a little about itself at the same meeting? asking it how it comes still to have a mortality of 36 per 1000? whether it has done away with cesspits under its houses, etc.! I do not suggest, because you will know best what is to be done. I only ask.

Have you seen the letter of "A County Surgeon" in the *Times*? I think they should be answered. (It is very easily done) and the *Times* shown that the time is come for compulsory utilization of the sewage. I write these few words merely to save the post and get your opinion of Simon and Co., not to express (which I cannot do) our sense of our great obligation to you or how earnestly I hope you will not relax your exertions in our favour. (You can do for us what no other man can do) especially with the supreme importance of this juncture for India under our eyes.)

Source: From three letters to Robert Rawlinson, Boston University 1/1/10-11 and 1/1/14

9 September 1858

I think, for our IDEAL ward, which you are so good as to intend to draft, either of the enclosed sets of dimensions would do. The first is modified from Lariboisière—the second from the cubic space given in our best hospitals. More cubic space is required in London than in Paris for sick. Each ward is for thirty-two sick. Either I should think a very good ward. But less than No. 1 I would not accept.

Ward	No. 1	No. 2
	Ft.	*Ft.*
Lengths of ward	111.6	128
Width	30	30
Height	17	17.6
Wall space between end wall and window	5	6.4
Wall space between windows	9.2	11.4
Window space	4.8	4.8
Beds	32	32
Cubic space	1760	2100[8]

8 This list was used in the third *Builder* article (see p 302 above).

12 September 1858

I am always very slow (as a person with nothing but practical experience and no scientific knowledge generally is, I believe) in criticizing plans. Upon going over yours again, I think:

1. That it would be inadmissible to carry up the chimney breast through the ceiling of the ward. The fire must have its chimney carried under the floor and up the side wall, if possible. (I have been told this is now done with success.) If not, then we must have the fireplaces in the side walls. Are not the fireplaces too near each other?

2. I think that we have practical experience enough, as regards the appurtenances at the ends of the wards, to know that they will be perfectly safe, although they do *not* project in width beyond the width of the ward, and although there is no lobby, *except* down the middle.

3. The ventilated ceiling introduces a new element. We wish to ventilate solely by doors and windows. If we go farther, we must study farther what the effect of the ceiling would be with doors and windows. We have made ventilation a matter of regulation in the army hospitals. It should be so in civil hospitals. We assert that doors and windows, if properly constructed, are enough.

4. I am afraid of the ventilating shaft or area carried through the floors at the bath end, for the same reason as I am afraid of the ceiling. It is unnecessary and will interfere, which is worse, with the door and window ventilation.

5. I think we will keep, please, to showing the arrangements for a *single* ward, not a *duplicate* one. For a *duplicate* one, which however I don't want to consider just now, I think I can imagine a rearrangement which would be better than a repetition of the same parts, viz., nurse's room, scullery and staircase. Upon the whole, then, so far as my experience goes, I think a more economical construction, as shown in the first rough sketch, will answer all sanitary purposes.

P.S.S. 1. We have collected a great deal of information about hospital ventilation. We find *ceiling* ventilation often very unsuccessful. If you would like at some future time to put a paper in *The Builder* upon ventilating methods, all our experiments should be at your disposal, if you would put them into form.[9]

---

9 Rawlinson published two signed articles in *The Builder* in 1860, the second with much information on ventilation; see "Sanitary Progress," 18,900 (5 May 1860):275-77.

2. Also, I see in a note to the present number you offer a detail plan of the Lariboisière. I have plans drawn to scale of that hospital and notes (or I could write notes) if they would be of any service. But the plans, being rather dilapidated, I should not like them to go farther than your office.

3. The internal lobby, see plan, need not exceed 7 or 8 ft. wide, nor the door from the ward into it 4 ft. 6. A lobby 20 ft. by 24 ft between W.C. and lavatories is unnecessarily large. So is a door into it 6 ft wide.

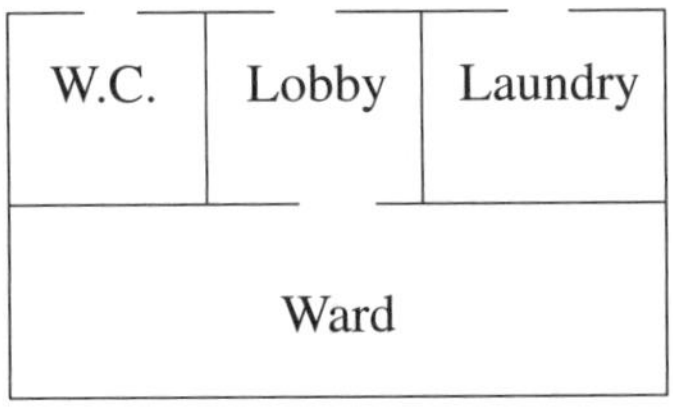

[rough attempt of sketch of a ward] ward (solid walls) except for opening from lobby into the ward, unable to enter to ward through W.C. or the laundry.

4. I have made a summary at the end of the paper, taken out my evidence, and made a few alterations. Upon measuring steps for sick, I doubt whether the rise should be more than 4½ inch. I need not say how unfeignedly I feel that I ought always to be cautious in differing from your better judgment and how much I feel your patience and kindness in doing all this.

7 October 1858

I am going to ask your most valuable advice and in doing so I must be allowed to ask it professionally or not at all.

A friend of mine has built a school for 120 boys and girls,[10] and is desirous, instead of the usual barbarous out offices, to introduce water closets or water latrines with lavatories. The water supply is from a well, 21 yards deep and between 4 and 5 ft. across, in which the water stands 4 ft. deep. It is proposed to raise it to the surface by the labour of the boys—the mouth of the well being 14 ft. above the ground, where it is proposed to place the water closets.

How many pans would be required? of whose construction? and about what would be the cost? And would the water supply (this is the

10 Probably a new building for Richard Dawes's innovative Hampshire school, King's Somborne, which began on a small scale in 1842.

main thing) be sufficient? What form of lavatory would also be the best? It is proposed to conduct the drainage to a field about 30 yds. from the school wall. The place is a hilly spot in Derbyshire. Please write me your advice on the subject—I know no other upon which I can depend.

I think what you were so good as to send me last night on hospital construction most important—so much so that I do not think it is *my place* to use it. My paper (as you will see, if you hear it at Liverpool[11]) is written without any more knowledge than any experienced nurse *might* have (I wish I could say *has*). What you ought to do with what you have sent me is to write a paper yourself, from the engineering point of view, and back mine with it at Liverpool.

Please remember that my report, which I sent you, is really and strictly PRIVATE and CONFIDENTIAL. Unless it is laid before the House of Commons (which I don't desire) I have no right to send a copy, even to you.[12] . . .

If you will not make any use of the enclosed, I should like to have it back very much, as I approve cordially of every sentence. But I think it would be of essential use if you were to draw up, were it but a few sheets, a paper on the subject for Liverpool. My paper refers exclusively to observed defects in hospitals and calls upon others for the remedies.

Source: From a letter to T. Graham Balfour, Add Mss 50134 ff47-50

Great Malvern
28 September 1858

I was not aware of the extent of Neison's iniquities,[13] although I had seen a report of his paper quite sufficient to infuriate me. That it must be answered there is no doubt, or it will do our cause much harm. It is (what my old nurse used to call me) "mischievous." If I were you, I should answer him from your point of view, I mean from the army sta-

11 Nightingale's original "Notes on Hospitals," read at the meetings of the National Association for the Promotion of Social Science at Liverpool (see p 47 above).

12 A reference to her *Notes on the Health of the British Army*. Rawlinson's copy in fact made its way into a university library, was microfilmed and was used for the *Collected Works*.

13 The same material has already been discussed relative to army hospitals (see p 314 above).

tistical point of view, in which, of course, you have the best right to meet him.

Not knowing that you were in town, I wrote yesterday to another gentleman to get him answered from another point of view. And in order that we may be all "in the same boat" about it, I will give you the substance of what I said. (The sudden death of Mr Herbert's eldest sister at a little wayside inn on Loch Etive has taken him down to Scotland, and I did not like to worry him on the subject just at this moment.)

Neison reproduced at the British Association at Leeds, in full, his fallacies about overcrowding having nothing to do with consumption. He adduces the Registrar-General statistics as to overcrowding, totally mistakes the question, and produces great mischief to our cause, on account of these population tables being quoted as authority. Thus, if (2) were Manchester and (1) were Liverpool, the dotted circles being the registration districts, of which the population is given by the Registrar-General, the black circles the actual densely inhabited parts, then Dr Greenhow compares the density within the dotted circles, and not within the black circles, and concludes that, inasmuch as (2) is much less densely peopled than (1) and yet has the same mortality from phthisis, therefore overcrowding is rather a healthy thing, and density does not influence phthisis.

Neison appears to have done the same thing. The real fact is that the density for Manchester and Liverpool is very nearly the same.

Again, surface density has in reality nothing to do with the subject. It is density in *rooms*. Our barracks have a smaller surface density generally than any town or perhaps village population in the kingdom, but they have generally a far higher *room density*. This is the substance of what I have said which I am, of course, not giving you as information, but merely in order that we may be all one about it.

I am exceedingly glad if Neison has laid himself open to your *tangible* correction. Because I think you ought on public grounds to correct this public error. What should you think of addressing a correction to Mr Herbert, as chairman of the royal commission, leaving us to reply to Neison and Greenhow on the other grounds?

Source: From five letters to Edwin Chadwick, ADD MSS 45770 ff50-51, 54-59, 60-62, 63-64 and 77-80

7 October 1858

I have just received your kind note. You will probably have heard at Leeds Neison's absurd paper to prove that overcrowding is rather a healthy thing. Could you not notice it and refute it in your papers at Liverpool? Saving this, I have no suggestion to make. So little is known and so much has to be done as to sanitary affairs in India that I think you must treat it from your own point of view. I know no one who can do it so well. You see no one has come up to yours in the *North British*.[14]

I read your paper on competitive examinations which was in the *Daily News*, in full. Someone was so good as to send it me. It would take up too much of your time to say what I thought of it. Like everything you do, it is masterly. I hope we shall hear that something is being done by the government about Indian sanitary matters soon.

I sent a copy to your house at Richmond of my Crimean reports to the War Office. There is no need of your either acknowledging or returning it. And I only mention it now to say that it is strictly PRIVATE and CONFIDENTIAL. I thought, however, I was in duty bound to send a copy to you who have always been our leader.

9 October 1858

It is in the highest degree important that your paper should be read at the Liverpool meeting. The Manchester Statistical Society would not answer the purpose at all. I should, if I were a known authority like you, select the main points and read them, then print at my own expense, if the council will not print in full. Afterwards they will print it out of shame. Or I would read to the end of their (absurd) twenty minutes and then say, "I have a great deal more to read, but the council says we are only to be interesting for twenty minutes."

I am quite aware of the inestimable mischief Simon and Co. are doing. I wrote a paper on hospitals for Liverpool. After I had written it, I made my uncle read it aloud to himself. It was longer than the *sacred* time so I remodelled it and cut it in two. *You* should cut yours into three. I dare say it would make into ten. It is utterly impossible to write anything worth writing to last twenty minutes. At all events,

14 Chadwick's critical analysis in "Our Army in India," which included a condemnation of the Netley site, in *North British Review* 29 (August-November 1858):211-43.

bring the paper before the meeting, were it only to make a protest against the course which would-be sanitarians are taking. . . .

The strength of the British troops in India may be safely assumed at 60,000. The loss of a British army in India from death and invaliding could hardly be brought down so low as 12 per 1000, could it? If you assume the possible *death rate* at 12 per 1000 and the customary death rate as 70 per 1000, and the permanent force at (say) 60,000, the annual loss at the *present* rate would be equal to a division of 4200 strong, and at 12 per 1000 to the loss of a battalion 720 strong. Suppose your divisions to consist of six battalions, each 700 strong, you might save about five out of the six by sanitary improvements.

11 October 1858

I still hope you will read your paper before the Liverpool meeting. From the information which I have received, I should say that it would be unsafe to recommend the system of cultivation and settlement to which you allude. For you might be met by a statement that cleaning and cultivation are uniformly attended by pestilence. One of the great points with regard to Indian inquiry is to ascertain how to cultivate (not only with safety but) with increase of salubrity. The statement almost amounts to a proverb in India, wherever you make a garden, you make a graveyard. The West India experience is too limited to establish a rule.

With regard to my papers, I am desirous that they should not be printed from the manuscript until I have an opportunity of revising them, which I had not time to do. (I was so driven by other business.) Of course I cannot help the newspapers reporting.

If Mr Whitly does so, perhaps he will be kind enough to send me a proof for correction. (I have no copy of the manuscript.)

I quite agree with what the newspaper you sent me says about the twenty minutes. If the whole of the first volume of *Transactions* had been burnt, the world would have been none the worse. The association has mistaken its object. If I were the council, I would devote each day to reading *two* (or at the most three) papers of the calibre of *yours*, and on subjects as large. And I would rather have no association at all than accept papers on specialities like mine, which ought to be read in quite a different place.

12 October 1858

Thank you very much for your note of this morning.[15] I do not anticipate that my papers will raise any storm. The subject is so little understood. And if they do not, I think it better to say nothing and leave the time of the association open to the more important paper which will follow.

If, however, any objections are raised to my paper, it will be on two scores: the attack on the doctrine of contagion [and] the sweeping away of all the principles at present adopted in London hospital construction. I think then a few words from you would be important, because (1) you have done more than any other man against the absurd contagionists, the lazy fellows; (2) you are thoroughly well acquainted with the *pavilion* principle of construction for hospitals [folio cut off]

6 November 1858

With regard to "contagion," it is a great advantage to me to hear what people say, for I see no one. Sanitary experience has so completely disproved the invisible "seminal" contagions that I can only see a mania for being wrong in such letters as Greenhow's and Simon's. With regard to the *material* "contagions," I have acknowledged them.

With regard to "infection," I believe in it just as much as I do in the emanations from sewage, and put them just on the same footing. But I say, where there is "infection," the fault is in those who have charge of the disease, not in the disease. Give cubic space, keep your patients clean, ventilate your wards and there is no infection. I never knew a case of "infection" but there was gross mismanagement and carelessness. I never heard an anecdote of "contagion" but it had *less* evidence than have witchcraft, magic, etc., to support them. . . .

In the well-constructed hospitals I could mention, I have never heard either doctors or patients complain of the bad effects of either light or ventilation being too strong. Please to look at the answer to Greenhow in today's *Builder*.[16] I honour the development of the pavilion system and the ventilation principle in Paris. But there is not a hospital in Paris where the latrines, the sewerage or the water supply are not things to be avoided, rather than to be imitated. They are quite behind hand there. . . .

---

15 Probably his letter of 8 October [1858], written from the Liverpool meetings, where Nightingale's first papers on "Notes on Hospitals" were read, Add Mss 45770 f52.

16 An anonymous article by Nightingale, the next item below.

I must just say, with regard to "cause and effect," I don't want to go into any metaphysical disquisition as to what they are. Just let Messrs Greenhow, Simon and Sir C. Hastings[17] try the ordinary rule (diminish, increase or remove the "cause" and the "effect" will be diminished, increased or removed also) upon "contagion" and "infection."

With regard to patients "catching cold" in bed, if they did so in fresh air, all the patients in the Crimea must have died, for they lay looking up at the open sky through the chinks and slits. Yet even in the worst time, the mortality was one half what it was at Scutari, and afterwards it became a mere trifle, and this with the thermometer near zero.

Source: "Preventible Disease: Scarlet Fever," *The Builder* 16,822 (6 November 1858):740

In our last number we inserted a communication from Dr Headlam Greenhow on the non-preventibility of scarlet fever, which appears to show a vagueness and uncertainty of view on sanitary subjects prevailing among many able and excellent members of the medical profession. Although in no wise connected with that profession, we are backed by much experience in all that concerns the sanitary improvement of towns and dwellings, and have directed our attention, amongst other things, to the question of children's diseases, and to their origin and spread.

The question as to the cause of these diseases is one of evidence, which any person with ordinary opportunities and powers of observation can decide, whether he be in or out of the medical profession, and from what we know, we could feel nothing but surprise when we read the following passage in the communication in question: "No one, so far as I know, has ever been able to trace scarlet fever to any other origin than intercourse, either direct or indirect, with persons already sick with that disease."

This is not sanitary doctrine, and would be sustained, we venture to say, by no careful sanitary observer.

But, if Dr Greenhow's view be correct then, considering the fatal nature of scarlet fever, and the many hopes it has blighted, the public can but arrive at one conclusion as to the method of preventing it,

---

17 Sir Charles Hastings (1794-1866), founder of the British Medical Association.

viz., a quarantine of the most unrelenting nature upon affected towns, houses, rooms and even persons. The quarantine ought to extend, above all, to members of the medical profession itself, who are the most constantly in communication between the sick and the healthy, between persons affected and unaffected with this disease.

If scarlet fever spreads in the way stated by Dr Greenhow, then the conclusion is inevitable that medical men are the great agents in propagating the disease, and should be dealt with as such for its prevention.

In regard to what is said as to the non-exemption of families of the rich from this fatal disease, it is too true. But has Dr Greenhow ever considered whether the way in which children, even of the rich, are in too many cases brought up, and the state of their sleeping rooms are such as to require no improvement? Has he ever estimated the probable effect upon health of the air in the dormitories of public schools, from which institutions so much of the scarlet fever among the children of the higher classes proceeds?

The fact is that children's epidemics have this peculiarity—that young people appear to become liable to them from sanitary defects which produce comparatively little evil to grown-up people.

It never appears to occur to the advocates of specific "contagions" that there must have been a *first* case in the world, which could not have received its "infection" or "contagion" from any other case, and hence, according to Dr Greenhow's doctrine, the Supreme Being must have directly inflicted it. In the absence of all proof of this, it is a far more rational thing to consider children's epidemics as belonging to the category of mitigable and preventible diseases, arising from the infringement of certain laws, either known or unknown. If they are known, and those influencing children's epidemics *are* to a great extent known, they ought to be obeyed. If they are unknown, we should endeavour to discover and obey them. It would show more common sense to do this than to put medical men in quarantine, and draw cordons round all infected houses, rooms and persons, which is the only logical result of the "contagion" doctrine.

"So far as we know," we are satisfied that children's epidemics of all classes are mitigable or preventible, and the lay public, with their present advance of sanitary knowledge, will support this view. The cure for "infection," if there be "infection," is cleanliness and fresh air. And this, notwithstanding Dr Greenhow's assumption to the contrary, and we say it with due respect for him, is the only remedy consistent with common sense.

Source: From a letter to R.G. Whitfield, Florence Nightingale Museum (LMA) H1/ST/NC1/58/6

8 November 1858

Thank you very much for your kind offer of doing anything for me at Edinburgh. Do you know the infirmary? I think, if you would go over the wards, especially the new surgical and the high school wards, with the particular view of comparing their *construction* with what *we* think ought to be the requirements (in sanitary respects) of the construction of wards, it would do much good. I went over them at the beginning of last year with this view,[18] and I shall be curious to know how far your views and mine agree. It would be very desirable, if they would let us have ground plans.

I think there are "R." Infirmary and "High School" and "Fever Hospital" to examine. But I have not a very distinct recollection of the local names, though of the wards I have much too distinct (and painful a one as regards some). If you could get from them any statistics of the mortality of nurses, such as you were kind enough to send me from St Thomas', nothing gives such a really good criterion of the sanitary (or non-sanitary) construction of hospitals as this.

I have got all the nurse statistics of all the London hospitals now. And into your ear I will privately whisper this fact, which I have deduced from them in figures, viz., that 54 percent of all the nurses' deaths are from preventible causes.

You take in *The Builder*. Did you notice Dr Greenhow's letter on contagion in last Saturday's but one—and my answer in last Saturday's?[19] (Please however to keep my secret.) I hope YOU agree with ME.

I hope you are better—I write from my bed and therefore not with much distinctness.

Editor: John Roberton, a Manchester surgeon and member of the Manchester Statistical Society, was the first doctor in Britain to take up the issue of safer hospital construction, doing so only a short time before Nightingale herself did. He gave his first paper to the Manchester Statistical Society on 21 March 1856, when Nightingale was still at work in Crimean War hospitals, which by then had been sub-

18 Nightingale was taken through the Edinburgh Royal Infirmary by Dr James Syme (1799-1870).

19 On which see p 514 above.

stantially improved. He later wrote a highly complimentary review of the royal commission report, with copious quotations from Nightingale on hospital issues. Nightingale naturally sent him a copy of her "confidential report," the lengthy analysis of the causes of the high mortality in war hospitals.

In the following covering letter, Nightingale not only introduced her confidential report, but remonstrated with him on his views of nursing, on which he had published comments she regarded as harmful. The two "pamphlets" she mentioned were papers Roberton had read to the Manchester Statistical Society in 1856 and 1858, which were published in its *Transactions* and then reprinted for wider circulation.[20] In the second paper, Roberton praised the nursing by nuns at Bordeaux and deaconesses at Bethanien, in Berlin, specifically stating that it was better to have "a lady of rank and pastor over them" than a physician (42). The possibility of a trained and experienced nurse as superintendent was not raised. In that paper also he extensively quoted Nightingale's evidence to the royal commission (39-41).

Source: Letter to John Roberton, in "An Unpublished Letter of Florence Nightingale," *St Thomas's Hospital Gazette* 27,8 (February 1920):247-48

22 November 1858

I have ventured to send you a copy of a "confidential" report of mine to the War Office, in spite of its being an old story now, and I will tell you why.

I know no one except yourself, Mr Whitfield of St Thomas' Hospital here, the officers of the Middlesex Hospital and the Army Sanitary Commission who have at all taken up the question of hospitals on the large sanitary ground. Your two pamphlets were read by us all with the greatest interest. (I differ with you upon the nursing system. But of that anon.)

It is only inasfar as the Crimean question bears upon the sanitary problem generally that I think my report will interest you. I must ask you to consider it as quite "confidential," i.e., it is not to be read by anyone else—for the war secretary has never laid it on the table of the

20 John Roberton, "On the Defects, with Reference to the Plan of Construction and Ventilation, of Most of our Hospitals for the Reception of the Sick and Wounded," *Transactions of the Manchester Statistical Society* (1855-56): 133-48; and "Additional Suggestions with a View to the Improvement of Hospitals for the Sick and Wounded" (1857-58):23-48.

House of Commons, and therefore it is in NO sense a public document.

As to the nursing question, my experience is this—and I ought perhaps to add that I have lived and served in almost every nursing system of Europe. I deprecate equally the system when nurses, whether male or female, are under the command of the authorities of the hospital solely—in which case the arrangements as to hours, proprieties, sanitary things, etc., generally strike me as all but crazy. And the system where the nurses, whether religious or secular, whether their head is male or female, whether they be Protestant or Roman Catholic, are in entire command of the hospital, the arrangements are generally equally crazy as in the first case.

In the first case, the nurses are destroyed bodily and morally. The patients are (generally, not always) well nursed. In the second case, it is the spiritual good of the nurses and not the care of the sick which is obtained (generally not always). But the care of the patients is the object of hospitals.

The collision (often disagreeable) between the secular administration and the nursing staff (whether nurses or nuns), as in the hospitals of London and Paris, is always salutary for the care of the patients. The mutual impertinences even between doctor and nurses (or nuns), equally observable in London and Paris, is far better for the interests of the sick than where authority is solely vested, as it generally is in Germany, either in the male authorities of the hospital, which is the case in their great general hospitals, or in the spiritual head of the nursing establishment, which is the case in both their Catholic and Protestant hospitals nursed (?) by orders. Take the nuns, brothers or deaconesses out of their parent institutions, and set them to work on a great secular hospital in daily contact with the exigencies of doctor and governor, and they will work admirably.

I do not like to print this, because I have lived on so intimate a footing with *all* these orders that it seems almost like treachery. But having seen the expression of a contrary opinion in your last pamphlet, and considering you as our greatest hospital authority, and being myself little likely ever to be able to work in hospital again, I have wished to trouble you with a record of my opinion.

Source: From an incomplete letter to an unidentified recipient, Boston University 1/12/151

[c1858]

I dare say you are aware that the results of some test cases, such as amputation, lithotomy,[21] etc., in London and in county hospitals have been published—showing a very large balance in favour of the county hospitals. But this tells us only a general fact we knew before, viz., that country constitutions are in a better state to endure operations than London ones, and that when even, as is often the case, the London operations are on countrymen, yet still in spite of inferior medical art and often inferior buildings in the country, still the country hospital, with its purer air, affords a better chance of recovery than the London—with all its magnificent professional excellence.

Source: Undated note, Add Mss 45751 f68

[c1858]

	Cubic feet of air per person per hour	Cubic feet of air per person per minute	
Chambre des Députés	635	10½	Amount not enough
Institut	1024	17	Can be increased
Conservatoire Arts et Métiers	469	7	Hall contains 494,000 cubic feet

In all these cases, there is a large balance of fresh air to begin with, from the great size of the salles [halls] in proportion to the audience. And the séances [meetings] last only one or two hours and are rarely full, except in the case of the Corps Législatif. (Perhaps the state of the air was the cause of the Revolution of 1848.)

Source: Questionnaire, Florence Nightingale Museum (LMA) H1/ST/NC1/58/3

[1858]

Particulars requested as to the "Enfant Jésus" at Paris

1. No. of beds and cubic space per child
2. Size of wards
3. Best number of beds per ward
4. Ages at which separate wards for different sexes are required

21 Surgery for the removal of kidney stones.

5. No. of operations and whether performed in ward or in a theatre
6. Approximate no. of surgical/medical cases
7. Best bath, W.C., kitchen arrangement
8. No. of children per "soeur"

Personnel under the "soeur" as to wardmaids, "frotteurs" [floor polishers], etc. Whether it is considered that any rearrangement of this would work better?

9. A slight sketch of what is considered necessary as to playgrounds and play halls, gymnastics, exercise, etc.

10. Generally, with regard to *frottage* [floor polishing] is a portion done before the "visite," and a portion after? or all at once? This last question refers to Paris hospitals in general.

Source: From two dictated letters to Sir John McNeill, Florence Nightingale Museum (LMA) H1/ST/NC3/SU108-09, both from Great Malvern

13 January 1859

Would you be so good as to send me the following information, viz., what the daily expenses of a patient at the Edinbro' Infirmary is supposed to be? You were once good enough to give me this information relative to pauper patients, and what was paid for them, but this was, I believe, *below* the actual expense, and I should be very much obliged to you, as it is for a county hospital in England, to let me know the *exact* expenses. I am very sorry to give you the trouble of procuring this information. . . .

If you could add the average number of days of a patient in hospital, it would make the information complete and I should be very grateful.

7 February 1859

I was so very glad to hear from you. I had looked in the paper every day for the arrival of your grandchild with much more interest than for that of the queen's grandchild, though I don't despise the little prince either.[22] I was so glad to hear that Lady McNeill and Mrs Stewart continue well.

I am sorry to have given the treasurer of the infirmary, and above all you, so much trouble. In many hospitals the information specified is made up at the end of every year as a matter of course. I don't think it will do the treasurer any harm to make it up for his own information.

22 References to the births of two first sons. One was born to McNeill's daughter, Margaret Ferooza Stewart (1834-71). The other, born to the crown princess of Prussia, became Wilhelm II, the "kaiser" of World War I.

Source: From two letters to William Farr, Wellcome Ms 5474/4-5, typed copies Add Mss 43398 ff115 and 117

21 February 1859

As you see, I am back in the land (not of figs but) of soots. And I beg to report myself to you by the same token and humbly to hope that you will come and see me. I am entirely enchanted by your summary of the *weeklies* for 1858, and especially by the paragraph about the "2000 medical men" and the "midnight rush."

Could you tell us whether you can give us the mortality returns of the schoolmasters and mistresses of the schools which receive the Privy Council grant, *separate* from the others? The census, I suppose, does not distinguish?

I enclose a paragraph from a newspaper, which please read. Is this done since [Charles] Trevelyan left the office? And if so, would it not be the time to press for more? to ask for a wider circulation of your reports?

Many thanks for all you have done for us in the way of newspaper articles. I had *not* sent a "green" "contribution" to the *Times.* If you would do it, our gratitude would be the greater. And I will send you some more copies, if you say yes. Otherwise I am ashamed to trouble you.

If you could look in upon me on your way home from the office this evening, you would find Dr Sutherland here between 5 and 6 o'clock.

25 February 1859

Have you done anything about the scheme of hospital statistics for the *universe*? In reading any medical book about nursing, I am always struck by the advance that *common* sense has made lately upon *medical* sense. If I were a mother I should dismiss a nurse (for doing what Dr West[23] recommends as very great lights) as being in very great darkness.

Source: From a letter to T. Graham Balfour, Add Mss 50134 ff71-72

9 March 1859

First let me return your valuable books, which I have kept only too long, and let me thank you very much for them.

Secondly, could you send me a list of the infirmaries, hospitals and lunatic asylums in Scotland (which I cannot find in the *Medical Directory*) without much trouble to yourself? Or could you tell me where to find one?

---

23 Charles West (1816-98), pioneering pediatrician at the Children's Hospital, Gt. Ormond St.; possibly a reference to his *How to Nurse Sick Children, Intended Especially as a Help to the Nurses at the Hospital for Sick Children*, 1854.

Thirdly, is *The Army in Its Medico-Sanitary Relations* (a copy of which has been sent me "by the author"), by Dr Combe of the Artillery?[24]

Finally, could you come and see me on Saturday at 12 o'clock? I have no business, only gossip.

Editor: An anonymous article in *The Builder* in June 1859 has a long quotation from Nightingale, with the advice that architects should obtain the volume with her papers on hospitals that were read at Liverpool. A footnote gives publishing details.[25] The article also promised more on the planned (pavilion-style) Blackburn Infirmary.

The second letter below shows how Nightingale used her status as life governor of St Mary's Hospital to press that hospital to use the new forms pioneered at St Bartholomew's. She sent a nearly identical letter to an unnamed official at the London Hospital, again using her connection as a life governor.[26] The correspondence to her from St Mary's officials is missing, but her follow-up letter of 1 October shows that they did offer to use the forms as requested.

Source: From a letter to William Aitken, Wellcome Ms 5471/4

Montagu Grove
Hampstead, N.W.
21 September 1859

I have to thank you very much for a copy of Dr Lyons's report on the yellow fever of Lisbon.[27] It seems to me very well done—but I had wished the government to send out an engineer to that unfortunate city. Now, all Dr Lyons has told us is (not how it can be prevented but) what it has done, which he has told very well. I should like, if you could send mè his direction, to thank him myself.

---

24 Matthew Combe, Royal Artillery, was indeed the author; Nightingale had a copy of the first edition of her *Notes on Nursing* sent him.

25 "Hospital Construction: The Hospital of Lariboisière," *The Builder* 17,855 (25 June 1859):417.

26 Letter 29 September 1859, Wellcome Ms 5482/34.

27 Robert D. Lyons, *Report on the Pathology, Therapeutics and General Aitiology of the Epidemic of Yellow Fever which Prevailed at Lisbon, During the Latter Half of the Year 1857.* Dr Lyons (1826-86) was head of the pathology commission sent out to the Crimean War; Aitken was the chief assistant on that commission.

Source: From two letters to L.G. Wilkinson, copied into the minutes of the Board of Governors, St Mary's Hospital, Paddington

28 September 1859

I have received so much kindness from the authorities of St Mary's Hospital that I venture now upon that plea to ask a favour.

I have had a set of new forms prepared for hospital statistics with the Registrar-General's sanction. I should be very glad if St Mary's Hospital would have the kindness to fill up for one part/year a copy of these. But before asking leave to send one for this purpose, I should like to ascertain to what extent the information could be obtained from the hospital books.

The following are the data required to fill up these forms. Of these will be required the remainings on the last day of any year/day/1857 and the remainings at the end of 1858, a full year.

1. Age
2. Sex
3. Disease

Also the Admissions
Discharges
Deaths
Discharges Incurable, with the Duration of the Cases.

N.B. The age, sex and disease must be shown for each of these headings.

St Mary's Hospital, having done me the honour to make me a governor, I have ventured to hope that it would not be at least presuming too much to ask whether this information is readily obtainable from the hospital books. Indeed the Registrar-General himself considers that St Mary's Hospital is a more likely institution to supply this information than any other.

1 October 1859

I beg to thank you very much for your most kind offer of filling in the set of forms, which I enclose.

Perhaps the readiest way of doing so will be to tick off in pencil case by case out of the hospital books according to their ages and disease on the blue line opposite the diseases, under the proper sex and age. And after the hospital books are gone through to fill up the sum of the ticks in figures, black for the men and red for the women, the duration of cases will be obtained by adding together the numbers of days intervening between the admission and death or cure of male and female cases at each age, and by dividing the sum by the number of cases for each sex and age. These figures entered in the line of the disease under their proper ages and sexes will give what is wanted. If any disease in your books does not appear on these forms, please write it in.

I fear that I am inflicting a great deal of trouble upon you. Perhaps you will be kind enough to let me have them back as soon as your convenience permits. If there are any points on which further explanation is required, perhaps you will be kind enough to let me know. . . .

P.S. I take the liberty of sending for your acceptance some pamphlets on similar subjects. At page 2 of the "Notes on Hospitals," in a footnote,[28] you will find the reasons for my desiring the favour which you have granted so kindly.

The Lisbon Children's Hospital, 1859-60

Editor: In 1859, Nightingale was asked, by Sidney Herbert, who had been approached by Prince Albert, to assist in the planning of a new hospital in Lisbon in memory of the recently deceased queen of Portugal (in the first letter below). Pedro V, king of Portugal, had married a German princess, Stephanie, in 1858. The two visited at Windsor Castle the same year, when he was made a knight of the garter. The couple had been married only five months when the queen died of diphtheria; the king himself died two years later. The hospital was named after her—in Portugese, Hopital Dona Estefania—but the name never appears in the letters. As this volume is printed, the hospital is still in use, and can be seen on the hospital's website.

The initial correspondence seems to be about a general hospital, and only later do references to a "child's hospital" begin to appear. The architect selected was Albert Jenkins Humbert, and while the full correspondence between him and Nightingale is not available, her advice to him is (the third item below). Two letters of Humbert to her are extant, the second of which includes a lengthy memorandum.[29] The plan is reproduced as No. 11 in *Notes on Hospitals.*

Portugal was not part of Nightingale's European travels. Consequently, all her observations about the city and site are from indirect sources.

---

28 In the separate publication of the papers; the footnote gives eight points on which Nightingale thought London and Paris hospitals should be providing information annually.

29 Letters 23 and 27 April 1861, Add Mss 45797 ff175-76 and 179-80, memorandum 181-87.

Source: From a letter to Douglas Galton, Wellcome (Claydon copy) Ms 5482/35

Hampstead, N.W.
22 November 1859

Mr Herbert told me on Sunday that you were to be applied to for a plan for a civil hospital at Lisbon. From what I know of that odious place, it will be very important, before you begin, to have

1. A plan and section of the ground and its elevation above the Tagus. There is scarcely level ground of the size of a sofa in Lisbon. And there are horrible gullies in which no hospital ought to be built.

2. The number of beds, of course, which Mr Herbert did not know.

3. The building materials to be used. Has there not been, since the great earthquake,[30] a kind of *wattly* stuff used? Do not however take any trouble about or make any use of this information till you are properly applied to.

The king of Portugal wishes to erect this hospital to the memory of the dead queen, and consulted Albert about it, who consulted Mr Herbert, who spoke to me. . . .

I think it is rather a triumph for Albert to consult Mr H. about a hospital, after having been thwarted by him about his Netley!

Source: From a letter to Sir Charles Phipps,[31] Royal Archives PP/Vic/1860/6403

24 December 1860

I have this morning forwarded to the architect, Mr Humbert, of the new *Lisbon* Hospital, his plans, with my suggestions, and with five questions, the reply to which will be necessary in order to be able to trust to one's own advice being correct.

I need hardly say that I shall be most happy always to give any result of my experience to help in the details (floors, walls, appurtenances) of this admirable hospital.

The proportions of the large wards are beautiful. They will certainly be the finest wards in Europe. Having had some experience of hospitals in southern as well as in northern climates, I can safely say this.

I am sorry that I have been compelled to delay so long in giving Mr Humbert his first instalment of advice. Perhaps he will not be so sorry.

30 The great Lisbon earthquake of 1855 killed up to 100,000 people.

31 Sir Charles Beaumont Phipps (1801-66), private secretary to Prince Albert.

Source: From a draft or copy probably to A.J. Humbert, Add Mss 45797 ff188-95 and 45825 ff92-99

24 December 1860

Lisbon Hospital information wanted.

1. *Site.*

(1) a description of the ground about the site, whether it be more or less built upon or open, or laid out in gardens or the ventilation obstructed by higher ground;

(2) whether there are extensive views from it, and in what directions;

(3) at what point or points there are easy means of entrance to the ground for sick;

(4) a common plan of Lisbon showing the streets and houses, with the proposed site marked on it, would be a great help.

2. *Nursing.* Will the ordinary system of Roman Catholic nursing, viz., Sisters of Charity (male attendants, female, etc., under the "sisters"), be adopted in this hospital? If so, "*communauté*" [community] accommodation must be provided for the "sisters" and dormitories for the men.

3. *Diseases.* Some general idea must be obtained from the books of any hospital in Lisbon what kinds and proportions of diseases and accidents there will be, e.g., among the women are there but a very small proportion of capital operations, or of accidents, and are fever cases admitted?

Is it intended to have a midwifery ward? Is it intended to admit venereal cases? If so, they *must* be separate. What is the average annual number of *noisy* cases (male, female)? Are there delirious fever cases, or is there any delirium tremens? What is the average annual number of *offensive* cases (male, female), requiring segregation, such as erysipelas, hospital gangrene, etc. What is the average annual number of operations (male female)? . . .

4. *Soft* pure water (and a plentiful supply) is so essential to a hospital that it would be well to have information about the water supply and especially whether there [are] any sulphates in it.

5. Is the hospital intended to be also a medical school?

Lisbon Hospital.

1. The wards should have a cubic capacity, about 1600 or 1700 feet per bed, the length and breadth remaining the same as in the plan. This determines the height.

2. There is no sufficient accommodation for nurses; one for eight sick is the number required in France. If there be Sisters of Charity, and if there be male attendants, as in France and Germany, this makes a difference in the kind of accommodation required.

For each ward of thirty-two sick (men): one sister, one nurse, two men attendants. For thirty-two sick women: one sister, two nurses, one man (attendant). The sisters, if they belong to a religious order, will always live in a "communauté" building by themselves, kitchen and sleeping room to be in this. The "matron" then becomes the supérieure, living in the same. The nurses' rooms at the end of the wards are occupied by the sisters in the daytime. *Dortoirs* [dormories] for the male and female attendants must also be provided. It would be desirable to have all these points known, before proceeding to criticize.

3. A north light is preferable, and from only one large window or skylight.

Lisbon Hospital.

(1) The wards are perfect. They will be among the (if not the very) finest wards in Europe. I only regret that adults are not to be intermingled with the children. But one thing I would strongly urge, let the age of admission be raised to fifteen years, especially on the female side. It is matter of universal hospital experience that this intermingling of ages is essential.

(2) There seems a confusion of the idea of a military hospital with that of a children's hospital (in the plan): the ideas ought to be the very reverse. (a) Not one *woman* more than is absolutely essential ought to be in a *military* hospital. Not one *man* more than is absolutely necessary ought to be in a *children's* hospital.

If the female quarters ought to be locked up in a military hospital, certainly the men's ought to be in a children's hospital. Undoubtedly the best plan is for the whole of the women attendants of each ward to sleep near their own ward, for the kitchen and bath, other attendants (all women) to sleep near the matron, and for the men's quarter to be quite separate.

But no information whatever has been afforded as to what the staff, (essentially) quite different in a child's from that of any other hospital), is to be. Where, for instance, are the "sisters" and nurses not attached to the wards to eat? Lifts must be provided. (b) In a children's hospital, the nursing staff, so far from requiring separate staircase and all that, had better be as near their wards as possible. (c) The W.C.s and baths fitted for a military [hospital] are quite unfit for a child's hospital.

The only men who ought to sleep in a child's hospital are (1) director, (2) resident medical officer (supposed to be men of weight and experience), (3) porter (who should be as far off the wards as possible), (4) chaplain (if this is conformable with the usages of the clergy).

Sweep away the steward in so small a hospital; the director can want nothing but a clerk, who should not sleep on the premises. The cook and her assistant or two assistants must be females. (This is not *may* but *must.*) It is in these little things that I see the confusion of idea between a military and a child's hospital.

In Continental hospitals, where men do far more of household work than in ours, the necessity of having as few men as possible is fully recognized as to *children's* hospitals. Women must be in undisputed charge of a child's hospital, saving, of course, the direction and medical service.

4. In all children's hospitals abroad, the classification is (1) medical, (2) surgical, (3) cutaneous [diseases of the skin]. And in all Continental hospitals, the proportion of the cutaneous is so large that I would fain know *what it is expected to be at Lisbon,* before going farther. It is a great pity that precise information and instructions were not afforded on all these points. In no experience that I have would the small wards here planned be in proportion for the cutaneous cases.

5. Day rooms are not necessary (see p 164 above).

In all hospitals (in children's hospitals *much* more than in others) the patient must not stay a day longer in hospital than is *absolutely* necessary.

Physical exercises, in and out of doors, are a part of its treatment, in all but acute cases. Bathing also. Teaching also. But secular as well as religious teaching should be conducted by the chaplain in the chapel, which should be contrived for this purpose. It must never be forgotten that children can never be left alone for a moment, and that you must provide a separate staff for every room. I had almost said a nurse for every child.

6. Every hospital is a bad moral atmosphere for a child. This must never be forgotten.

7. Boys and girls may sit on opposite sides of the chapel. This is the only place where they should meet.

8. Without knowing the proportion of cutaneous cases,[32] it is impossible for anyone to make a plan. If at all commensurate with what it is in other countries, the cutaneous wards should be separate, under a staff of their own, as to nursing, baths, playgrounds, etc.

9. The operating theatre seems MUCH too large. (Croupe operations, the most frequent, are always performed in ward.)

---

32 The memorandum was split here by mistake; it continues (mid-sentence) in ADD MSS 45825 f92.

10. The baths seem MUCH too small. Outdoor patients are always (to their own great advantage, and the in-patients' great disadvantage) admitted to baths and gymnastics in these institutions. This must be taken into account. But, in this as in some other things, it is very much to be regretted that the projectors of this hospital do not make known their intentions more precisely. Considering the above fact as to outdoor patients, there should be: one boys, one boys cutaneous, and neither sex should ever come on the side appropriate to the other; one girls, one girls cutaneous, separate bathing place. Each bathing place *must* be under the charge of a separate, competent, sister, with one or more attendants under her. Otherwise your lists of mortality by drowning and scaldings alone will be fearful.

Each bathing place *must* have a number of small baths, separable by a curtain or slight partition, with one or more large baths, in which several children may be bathed at once. The girls *must* bathe alone—the infants together, unless the disease is something special. The medical officer must decide when the age comes when boys should bathe alone. Girls should *always* be bathed in frocks, unless the special disease prevents it.

11. The bathroom at the end of each ward is only (here) calculated for men. It should consist of two small baths, being for acute cases or infants. There should be a portable bath besides.

12. I must make the same criticism about the W.C.s. They are not calculated for children. They are too intricate. As a general rule, there should be no possibility for a child to fasten itself in to communicate with another child, when in—they should be self-acting and well lighted by day and night. This is one of the great difficulties of a child's hospital that, whereas experienced authorities utterly repudiate the *separation* by several doors or turnings of the W.C.s from the ward, *without* this separation they can hardly be made healthy.

13. The kitchen seems good. I have nothing to add except that it requires more attendants than in an adult hospital and that they must be female. I have already said that all cleaning which must be done by men (and *frottage must* be) should be done by men not attached to the hospital. *No* male attendants *must ever* be attached to children's *wards.*

14. It is almost needless to say that the lavatories for children must not be lavatories for men, as to height, handiness or anything else. And that the children who will have to be washed in ward are much more numerous than adults in hospital—consequently, there must be a much greater provision of portable basins, etc. In this point, foreign

hospitals are woefully deficient. To prevent a child's skin from becoming chafed (in certain diseases) it has to be partially sponged many times a day.

15. A large garden ground, laid out in sward and green hillocks and such ways as children like (*not too pretty* for the children to be scolded for spoiling it) must be provided for

1. Boys
2. " Cutaneous
3. Girls
4. " Cutaneous

combined with gymnastic grounds and halls (*in* and *out-of*-doors). A professor (a man) *must* be attached to superintend these exercises. (The girls especially will otherwise injure themselves.) I have already said that out-patients are always admitted to these, which form a very important part of the treatment. Singing in chorus accompanies some exercises. A "sister" must superintend each of the playgrounds—besides the professor for all. The gymnastic covered place (for bad weather) is also used as a play room and day room.

16. To foreign children's hospitals, two schoolrooms, one for boys and one for girls, are generally attached. And these again are each under the charge of a sister, who teaches *besides* the teaching in the wards and the teaching by the chaplain.

Special care is taken to occupy the children only enough to conduce to their recovery. Prizes, etc., are given. The two schoolmistresses *need* not live in the hospital. (The day rooms might be retained as schoolrooms.) If the habits, feelings, of the country would not be outraged, the chapel (in so small a hospital) might be employed as schoolroom.

17. There must be some place to deposit the dirty linen in—which can hardly be carried to the laundry more than once a day. A chute into a light closet in the basement is the best. There must also be lifts.

18. I do not like the position of the deadhouse. In R. Catholic countries, this is a matter of importance. A separate building, in a quiet corner, beyond the possibility of being overlooked, with two *separate* entrances, one into the dissecting room, the other opening from the outer wall (for the relations to come in) into a small mortuary chapel, which opens into the dead room, where each little corpse lies on its own little bed, separated by white curtains all round, so that the friends see *only it*.

19. All experienced children's doctors lay immense stress upon this: *that every child's hospital ought to have a convalescent branch* at a dis-

tance, in the most healthy spot that can be found—best a watering place, and this, however munificently the hospital itself is furnished with air and exercise. Almost all the operations required on children, especially tracheotomy, need to be done in such a hurry that *the* hospital cannot be very far from the city.

20. My estimate of the nursing staff for a child's hospital is as follows: for every ward of thirty beds one head [nurse], two nurses, one night nurse. This is the minimùm and can only be, by having

for every bath place	= 1 head	= 4
for every exercise place	= 1 head	= 4
for every schoolroom	= 1 head schoolmistress	= 2
for kitchen	= 1 head/ 2 assistants	= 3
for clean linen store	= 1 head	= 1

21. These "heads" must all be women of the calibre of "sisters." There seems an inordinate quantity of (much too good) accommodation for servants. The matron must have one woman servant. The rest must be settled by custom. It will not, therefore, do to give them the accommodation of "director's servant," etc. (as in plan). Also, where are they to eat?

22. I don't much understand the distribution of storerooms, etc. It must be decided whether the kitchen and stores are to be under the same person. If they are, then the steward comes in rather oddly. If not, the cook's and steward's jurisdictions ought to be more separate.

23. The porter must sleep on the premises.

24. Even if the nurses all do sleep in the administration, there must be at least two head nurses' rooms on the nurses' dormitory flat (at each end) to keep order. Often the porter would do for director and medical officers. Or one woman would come in and do for both. Anyhow, two grand rooms are not required.

25. Even if the little wards are preserved, the corners must be arranged wide enough for beds.

26. The nurses of the wards *must* dine in the sculleries. These are hardly large enough.

Finally, I must repeat that the perfection of all these arrangements abroad and the obstinate mortality of the children are equally remarkable. Sometimes an epidemic disease will sweep a whole ward.

Source: From a letter to Douglas Galton, Add Mss 45759 f125

Upper Terrace
Hampstead, N.W.
Xmas Day 1860

Cry of fire! The *Lisbon* Hospital (the plans of which are now passing through our hands) and the Bucks Infirmary are both going wrong about their *end* appurtenances to the wards. Could you be so very good as to send me a tracing of the *ends* of the Woolwich Hospital wards for these misguided individuals?

Glasgow Royal Infirmary, 1859-61

Editor: While Nightingale was the major force bringing in professional nursing to the Edinburgh Royal Infirmary, in 1872, she had only peripheral dealings with the equivalent institution in Glasgow, the Glasgow Royal Infirmary. Trained nursing was started at Glasgow much later than at Edinburgh, with a superintendent, Rebecca Strong (1843-1944), who had trained at the Nightingale School. Nightingale is remembered at the Glasgow Royal Infirmary with a stained glass window in the chapel, and a fine marble statue (sculptor unknown) in the main lobby.

The dealings with the hospital reported here concern its physical defects, of which there were many—although probably no more than at Edinburgh at the same time. However, Edinburgh redeemed itself by building a new pavilion-type hospital and bringing in trained nursing (with a matron and staff) long before Glasgow.

The original building of the Glasgow Royal Infirmary, opened in 1794, was designed by the distinguished architect Robert Adam (with James Adam). Nightingale's involvement was on a new surgical block that had opened in 1861, the site, in fact, of Joseph Lister's pioneering use of antiseptics in surgery in 1865, work he then continued at the Edinburgh Royal Infirmary. From the correspondence on the state of the hospital, it would seem that he had plenty of germs to work on. Specific flaws Nightingale raised on the new building were its five storeys (counting the basement), when she held that there should be no more than two; the placing of nurses' rooms in the basement, and possibly putting patients there as well. Proximity to a burial ground was a fault of the original building—with the new building, Nightingale lamented, its mistakes had been tripled (see p 534 below).

Source: From a letter to William Aitken, Wellcome Ms 5471/3

8 June 1859

I was only able to open your kind note of 3 June yesterday. I think the system of arranging the beds (in the Glasgow plan you send me) far better than that of arranging them against the dead walls, but far worse than that of arranging them between the windows.

In the plan, the patients cannot read in bed without straining their eyes (and Scotch patients read much more than English ones). If the windows are along both sides the ward, as they ought to be, the light is then always just opposite the patient's eyes—which, however important light is to recovery, is by no means always desirable.

Again, the irritability peculiar to many diseases makes it distressing to the patient to have any noise behind him which he cannot SEE. A patient dying or coughing, or who required much fidgeting attendance, would make the bed back-to-back with him almost uninhabitable. Noise which a patient cannot *see* (!) always partakes with him of the character of *suddenness* and injures him. This is, believe me, the fruit of long experience with the sick.

Again, I think, in cold weather, when the doors are opened, or when the doors and windows, being shut, the fire is acting, it will be found that the cold air will come right down upon the heads of the patients under the ventilator in a way which is not at all anticipated.

The forms for the eight heads mentioned in the note to p 2 of my "Notes" are under process of preparation by Dr Farr, and we hope to try them quietly at our London hospitals and to propose them at the next European Statistical Congress, which will take place in London.

Will you allow me to enclose a copy of the "Notes" for your friend, Dr McGhie?[33] There is a misprint at p 30, which I have corrected in this copy. Please to look at it.

I enclose for your own private eyes a little pamphlet I wrote on nursing (which is really "confidential"). Perhaps the article *noise* will illustrate what I have said about patients.

33 James McGhie, medical superintendent at the Glasgow Royal Infirmary.

Source: From a letter to Douglas Galton, Add Mss 45759 f91

Hampstead, N.W.
30 October 1860

I have been referred to with regard to the new Glasgow Infirmary (detestable place) as to cements for walls. Keane's cement is the one they affect. I know you have been looking into these cements lately. Which do you recommend for inside hospital walls?

Source: From a letter to William Aitken, Wellcome Ms 5471/17

1 February 1861

The *Glasgow Medical Journal* was sent me. Dr McGhie's article betrays either willful misrepresentation or helpless, hopeless, ignorance of his own subject. It is impossible to answer. Many of his principal facts are wrong. I would instance those about the Lariboisière Hospital. It is nothing but a defence of an indefensible mistake, and not very ably pleaded.

The best thing that could happen to the Glasgow Infirmary (and what would save much human life) is that it should be burnt down. There will be no other safety for it. Almost all its air reaches it over burial ground. Now the mistake has been tripled.

But, depend upon it, Dr McGhie knows all this just as well as you or I.

Source: From a letter to James Paget, St Bartholomew's Hospital Archives X102/1

13 February 1861

I have kept your Topinard[34] a most unreasonable time. But the truth is I was so excessively interested in it—the more as I have been *out of* that kind of hospital observation for three years and I have also made the most unscrupulous use of it—specially in its condemnation of Glasgow Infirmary, against which I am waging war.

I shall only permit myself "old nurse's" remarks upon the book to you—except one: I have not the least doubt as to French surgery being inferior to English surgery, and the remark is less presumptuous than it seems. Because it is the hygienic side of English surgery that I so much admire.

1. But to my "old nurse's' " remarks: I entirely concur with M Topinard in all he says about the great inferiority of French hospitals to ours—as to diet, cleanliness, etc. The vile way they have of not removing

34 Paul Topinard, *Quelques aperçus sur la chirurgie anglaise.*

instantly the surgical dressings taken off—their hot, damp, saturated, smelling, greasy packages of dressings when on, like swaddling clothes, instead of our nice, light, clean, water dressings, with a nurse, if necessary, to mop up the discharge.

Then the French have not the least idea of our expenditure of water, hot and cold, in the ordinary ward work; then their system of artificial ventilation and warming the air is destructive of freshness; then their latrines are always offensive.

With regard to wound dressing, you may poison a patient through his wound just as well as you may poison him by foul air. And this the French are constantly doing. And all the fresh air in the world will not save him from being poisoned thus—in the finest pavilion palace in the world.

2. A person accustomed to the look of patients, even without professional knowledge, could instantly pronounce on what the fate of certain operations in the French hospitals will be. Pyemia is an indigenous disease among the French poor. It is constantly taken into hospital. With our poor, we of course sometimes see it. But it can hardly be called an indigenous disease.

Healing by the first intention is scarcely possible with the French constitution. The French surgeons whom I have seen at work rarely attempted it. They would cram two or three pounds of charpie into an operation wound, and say they could only heal by granulation.[35] And I have no doubt this was true.

But you yourself, I suppose, would say that if you had operations upon half a dozen sedentary, scrofulous, factory, ill-fed drudges, perhaps pyemic into the bargain, and upon six well-fed out-of-door Yorkshire labourers—ceteris paribus [other things being equal] and with the same first-rate surgical skill in both, the results would be very different. M Topinard never takes these things into account.

3. The *London* hospitals, adding up together *all* the conditions which constitute the health of hospitals, have undoubtedly a greater sum of these than the Paris hospitals. I should be very sorry if I had said anywhere that ventilation was more than cleanliness—or that either would stand in lieu of efficient drainage. But, in writing about construction, you cannot put in about diet or cleanliness, in both of which we are undoubtedly superior to the French. In fact, in all in

35 Formation of grain-like sores on a wound.

which we are as a nation superior to the French, our hospitals are superior. And the converse also is true.

M Topinard's conclusion that, because our mortality is less high than it is in Paris hospitals (which I have no doubt is true), therefore construction and site go for nothing, is not logical and certainly not according to experience. I might as well say that, because Scutari mortality was higher than Paris mortality, therefore surgery goes for nothing.

4. M Topinard's statistics, though true in themselves and excessively interesting, cannot bear out any general conclusion. He takes no account of age, sex, previous occupation and condition of life, etc. Now ceteris paribus [other things being equal] these things are well known to have influence upon the results of operations. The law of life after operations has not yet been ascertained. And no hospital statistics have yet been kept so as to ascertain it.

5. Taking into account the local position of St Bartholomew's, the results obtained are most creditable to all its scientific and administrative authorities. I have always been struck with the exquisite management of its wards. I should have no difficulty in believing that it is more healthy than any Paris hospital; e.g., Boudin,[36] tells us that Beaujon has lost pyemia out of its newly ventilated wards. But pyemia has not disappeared out of its other wards.

The magnificent Lariboisière, I do not believe, is healthy, because it won't open its windows and will artificially heat its air. The vast wards of some of the Paris hospitals, I am quite sure, are unhealthy and impossible anyhow to keep fresh.

I should have a great deal more to say. But my only apology for having said so much and so lengthily is that I have very great difficulty in writing at all, but I am so anxious that you should not throw your great weight into the scale against improved hospital construction.

Mine has always been an unrequited love for St Bartholomew. I have worshipped that saint. He has never taken any notice of me.[37]

I have got two kittens, the finest ever known (angoras) already as big as large Spitz dogs. One is called Thomas and the other Bartholo*mew*. It is a mercy *she*, the latter, does not answer to her name. Or it would be heard all over the housetops.

36 Dr Jean Christian Marc François Boudin (1806-67), who published much on French medical statistics.

37 Nightingale hoped that St Bartholomew's would start a nurse training school, but it did not until 1877.

Your late patient, my maid, of whom you made such a "good job," is come back to me full of health—and takes a particular pride in her *thumb.* As also does her husband, who would make a capital "infirmi*er*" [male nurse] himself. . . .

I wonder whether you would despise the fag end of this year's game.

Editor: David Smith, chair of the Glasgow Royal Infirmary, sent a defensive letter to Nightingale on their decision to proceed with building on the existing site:

> Had we ground and means, a close approximation to your own suggestions might have been made. We have done the best we could with the means at our disposal. It was the desire of the directors to retain the lofty and airy site, with the former portion of the hospital occupied, to combine unity of management with convenient proximity to the mass of the friends of patients, and also to retain their position near to the two great medical schools of Glasgow.

He explained that "a suitable" site was as difficult to find in Glasgow as in London. Dr McGhie's points were based on those considerations.[38] The correspondence is difficult to sort out as one letter of Nightingale's to him, of 29 July, is not extant, and only a copy of his to her of 7 August is available, the second letter below.

Source: From a letter to Samuel Smith, Add Mss 45792 ff213-16

[August 1861]

David Smith, chairman, house committee, Glasgow Royal Infirmary.

(He is a shoemaker.) Please write very respectfully "to thank him very much for the reports, to say that I do not know how to thank him for the kindness of his invitation, but which it is quite impossible for me to accept, because I am confined to bed, have not been out of these walls for six and one half months, nor for three and one half year have been out except to be moved in an invalid carriage." (It is necessary to say this because, you see, Isa Craig, who knows it perfectly well, does not.)

I have looked over the plan of the new part of the hospital and should have felt the greatest diffidence in criticizing it, had not reference been made to the 'central fireplace' in the wards as being a suggestion of mine. I have certainly suggested central fireplaces with the

38 Letter 31 July 1861, Add Mss 45797 f243.

view of saving heat and increasing window space and bed space. It certainly never occurred to me to carry the chimney up inside the wards.

In a large hospital about to be erected, every long ward will have two central fireplaces, but no chimneys. The flues will all be carried under the floors and up the outer walls. It is of the greatest importance in any system of good nursing and administration to have the ward clear from end-to-end.

The pavilion plan of structure I have also advocated on account of its great sanitary advantages for sick. This plan, you say, has been adopted in the present instance (of Glasgow). But it has been so adopted as to negative many of the results aimed at. For example, there are beds against the end walls, whereas the pavilion structure says a window between every two beds, at most, and no more than one bed therefore in any corner. Again, the wards, instead of being open from end-to-end, are shut up by water closets, scullery, nurses' rooms, day room and small wards.

It would have simplified the construction immensely to have had all your administrative offices at the end next [to] the stair. Besides, for really good hospital discipline, you *must* have your sculleries and nurses' rooms *not* at the far end of the ward, but at its entrance. For the patient's sake, certainly, no small wards should be there, viz., at the far end. The wards of each pavilion should open straight into the air at the far end by a large end window. The W.C.s, bath and ablution rooms should be at the far-off corners on each side of the large end window, with windows to the open air on *three* sides, and should not open *directly* into the ward.

Again you have no less than four flights [storeys] of wards, whereas one floor (and never more than two) of wards is the best, and now the actually adopted principle. Again your nurses are in the basement, whereas in dwellings even the use of basements is becoming (and always should be) discontinued altogether.

I can hardly understand the intention of putting "forty patients" into these basements "in case of pressure upon hospital space" (Report, page 6). Does it mean that, when the hospital is most crowded, and most care is required, it is contemplated to put the excess into cellars, where experience teaches that no serious case will recover?

Again, is it true of these basements, where the report proposes to put sick, that the back wall is near an old burial ground? If so, is not the exercising ground over the same burial ground (as shown in elevation), so that the living above will walk over the dead below? It puts me in mind of a London hospital lately extended by excavating and removing thousands of corpses.[39]

As it is intended to present the plans before the "Social Science meeting" at Dublin, I have (sadly and unwillingly) felt it the more necessary to do what I can to guard the principles of hospital construction from misapplication. Certainly, as applied at Glasgow, they are hardly to be recognized as the same principles. (I laid a short summary of these before the Liverpool "Social Science" meeting.) A number of new hospitals are now being built in which these principles are correctly applied. . . .

P.S. It would be quite essential to pull down the small houses on the fourth side of the square to secure a better external ventilation. . . .

The mortality, as indicated in the report, is exceedingly high. Paul Topinard, a well-known French medical writer, has lately published the fact that the ill success of surgical operations in Glasgow Infirmary is notorious among the hospitals in Great Britain (from no want of surgical skill but from circumstances connected with the hospital itself).

Source: From a copy of a letter probably to David Smith, Florence Nightingale Museum (LMA) H1/ST/NC5/3/9

Hampstead
7 August 1861

I ventured to send (by the post) as you expressed a wish for my *Notes on Nursing* for your nurses, five copies of the last edition [*Notes on Nursing for the Labouring Classes*],[40] which is also the cheapest, although it contains many additions, particularly in the first and second chapters, and the sixteenth chapter on "Minding Baby," which I added at the request of several "national schoolmasters, who found they could make their schoolgirls mind *me* by telling them it was for baby's sake."

I like your address about a building act. It is admirable, shows a complete mastery of the case as regards densely peopled towns. Your proposals would not altogether suit ours, because we build every man on his own ground, and flats are almost unknown. However the Paris experience shows it to be quite possible to have healthy houses in flats, and we too have "model buildings" in flats which yield the average

39 King's College Hospital, Strand, from St Clement Dane's churchyard.

40 David Smith wrote Nightingale 31 July 1861 from Glasgow, saying that he had her *Notes on Nursing* and would get more copies for their nurses, Add Mss 45797 f243.

mortality of the other parts of London. If you would like to send me a draft of a building act "suitable for Glasgow," directed against the most prominent existing evils! always those most likely to recur, I could obtain for you every assistance, conforming it to our principles of sanitary legislation and police. But perhaps you have already done this.

God's hand has been very heavy upon me, for besides increasing illness, incessant business, He has taken from me the powerful friend, with whom for five years, this very 7 August[41] I had daily co-operated for the welfare of the army and the loss is severe indeed. You must therefore excuse hurried letters.

Editor: The unnamed recipient of the following letter must be R.G. Whitfield, the resident medical officer at St Thomas'. Certainly he toured provincial hospitals in the north of England around this time and reported to Nightingale some months later on them.[42] The diversity of sizes and layouts he reported would be an ongoing problem for planning the introduction of trained nursing. Nightingale's cousin Joanna Hilary Bonham Carter at that time often stayed with her to help with correspondence.

Source: From a letter written on behalf of Nightingale by J. Hilary Bonham Carter, Add Mss 45797 ff79-81

9 January 1860

In answer to your letter (of the 4th inst. [January]), for which Miss Nightingale wishes first to thank you, she bids me say that she much values your offer of services during your approaching expedition, and would be particularly obliged to you if, in visiting those provincial hospitals which you mention, you would kindly bear in mind the following queries, in order to tell her the result of your observation and conviction in regard to them.

1. What is the present system of nursing, and what the construction of building for it?

2. What you think *should be* the system of nursing, and of construction for it in a provincial hospital? E.g., take *as a unit* a provincial hospital of fifty patients (it may be doubled—trebled),

(a) Should there be one head nurse to fifty cases?

41 The date of her return to England from the Crimean War; Sidney Herbert died 2 August 1861.

42 Whitfield letter 7 April 1860, Add Mss 47742 f71.

(b) Where should she sleep?

(c) Should there be one night nurse?

(d) Where should the assistant nurses sleep?

(e) Should there be *two* wards only for fifty patients, one for men and one for women? Or should there be *four* wards, two for medical and surgical cases (men), two for medical and surgical cases (women)?

(f) Would it be well to continue the London hospital system of the nurse sleeping in command of her ward, even in the provincial hospital where there is but *one* head nurse, and to construct any new hospital that might be erected so that there should be a nurse's room attached still to each ward, arranging that the head nurse should sleep in that adjoining the ward in which the worst cases happened to be (probably the men's surgical ward?), the assistant nurse (or nurses) of each ward sleeping in contiguity each with her respective ward?

Lastly, in a hospital (say) of four wards of only twelve patients each, what should be the nursing personnel of each ward? Could one head nurse, one night nurse, with assistant nurse to each ward, do it all?

Source: From a letter to John Sutherland, Add Mss 45751 ff149-50

14 February 1860

You would be puzzled to see Sir John Forbes's book *Nature and Art in the Cure of Disease*[43] arrive by the post. It was I [who] sent it. It just occurred to me that you might possibly like to put another book at the head of your article. If so, this is the only medical book I know in *our* sense at all. Sir John Forbes, who is slowly dying and *chair*-ridden, wrote to me when my little book came out, saying that he "went along" with it entirely, a great deal for a *medical man* to say. I was not able to write and tell you why I troubled you with the book yesterday.

Many many thanks for your letter.

Source: From a letter to William Farr, Wellcome Ms 5474/22, typed copy Add Mss 43398 f190

31 May 1860

Mr Herbert has sent me the enclosed, with the remark "in answer to your letter" "probably Dr Farr would be able to obviate the objection." Dr Sutherland is gone on inspections. He saw Dr Balfour yester-

43 John Forbes (1787-1861), also founder of the *British and Foreign Medical Review.*

day, who told him his grievance. And, as I understood Dr S., he, Dr S., agreed with him.

I asked Dr S. to write to you, but I have no doubt he did not make it intelligible what he wanted, viz., as I understood, that you should not pledge the War Office to adopt the congress's conclusions, when your own were likely to be so much more well founded.

Source: From a letter to T. Graham Balfour, Add Mss 50134 ff80-84, typed copy Add Mss 45772 f235

12 July 1860

Private. You are quite right in what you say. We are all of us in the same boat. And, if it were not that England *would not be* the mercantile nation she *is*, if she had not business habits somewhere, I should wonder, from my experience, where they are.

Certain of us, who were asked to do business for the Statistical Congress, had it all ready since December last, and were not able to get it out of the General Register Office till this week. Certain of us were asked to do business this morning, and to have it ready by tonight, which, if *not* done, would arrest the proceedings of the congress, and, *if* done, must be the fruit of only five hours' consideration, when five months might just as well have been granted for it.

I don't say that this is so bad as the treatment of you, who are secretary. But still it is provoking to see a great international business worked in this way. What I want now is to put a good face upon it before the foreigners—let *them* not see our shortcomings and disunions. Many countries far behind us in political business are far before us in organization power.

If anyone has ever been behind the scenes, living in the interior of the maison mère [motherhouse] of the "Sisters of Charity" at Paris, as I have, and seen their counting house and office, all worked by women, an office which has twelve thousand officials (all women) scattered all over the known world, an office to compare with which, in business habits, I have never seen any, either government or private, in England, they will think, like me, that it is this mere business power which keeps these enormous religious "orders" going. I hope that you will try to impress these foreign delegates, then, with a sense of *our* "enormous business power" (in which I don't believe one bit) and to keep the congress going.

Many thanks for all your papers. I trust you will settle some sectional business with the "delegates" here tomorrow morning. And I trust I shall be able to see you, if not tomorrow morning, soon. . . .

I send back your American big book with many thanks. But if you would like the delegates to see it here, pray send it back by bearer. Mind, I don't mean anything against your office by this tirade, on the contrary, I believe it is one of the few efficient ones now in existence.

Editor: The next letter is to Nightingale's great mentor on statistics, L.A.J. Quetelet (1796-1874), head of Belgian statistics.[44] Nightingale did not know it, but Quetelet had suffered a stroke in 1855 and was no longer undertaking new research.

Source: Letter to L.A.J. Quetelet, Edith Cavell Institute, Brussels, copy City University, London

13 July 1860

I would greatly desire to solicit your sympathy in favour of a project I must submit to the congress to obtain uniform hospital statistics. It was your books which awakened in me (to a much lesser degree) the idea of statistics for the sick.

My life, all my work have made me envisage only the practical side.

I dare to send you, Sir, several of my small works on hospitals and ask you to interest your confrère Dr Berg[45] in them who, I know, is particularly occupied in hospitals. I have sent him a similar package.

If you deign to read the note on page 2 of my "Notes on Hospitals,"[46] you will see the reform which I desire and to which I presume to request the loan of your great name.

Be assured, Sir, of my deep devotion,

Florence Nightingale

Source: From a letter to Sir James Clark, Add Mss 45772 ff162-63

26 July 1860

Private. Dr Engel,[47] the delegate from Berlin, has asked me to give him a letter to our princess royal.[48] I told him that I was not at all in a posi-

---

44 For other Quetelet material and a biographical sketch see *Society and Politics* (5:11-128 and 827-28).

45 F.T. Berg, Swedish delegate to the International Statistical Congress.

46 For reference see p 524 above.

47 Ernst Engel (1821-96), leading German statistician; Nightingale invited him, with others, to breakfast at her home to strategize on statistics.

48 Princess Victoria (1840-1901), daughter of Queen Victoria, crown princess of Prussia and later the Empress Frederick.

tion to do so. But he said that he was very little known at Berlin, where he has only recently been made director of the Statistical Bureau, having hitherto held that office in other German states, not Prussia, that the whole direction of the next meeting of the congress at Berlin would devolve upon him, and that every support he could have would be useful to him. Do you think there is any propriety in my writing to the princess? (Of course he would not present himself till after her recovery.[49]) And if so, *how* may I write? May I tell her how useful and effective these congresses are? As her own father [Prince Albert] has been president of ours, she may be induced to give her cordial influence in favour of the next, and of Engel. Do you know whether she is on good terms with the princess regent?[50]

Source: From a letter to William Farr, Wellcome Ms 5474/24

6 August 1860

I consider Engel and myself ill-used individuals. He asks me to write to the princess royal; Sutherland says nothing ought to be done till the Prussian Embassy here is requested to act. Dr Farr makes no answer, and poor Engel, an unbusinesslike *savant* [scholar], is quaking meanwhile in his shoes at Berlin, without any *renseignement* [instructions] whatever.

Source: From a letter to Douglas Galton, Add Mss 45759 ff49-50

29 August 1860

I should have sent you my calculation of water supply per day per patient yesterday, but that I wanted to have the experience of the hospital surveyors of some of our largest civil hospitals, which I now have and which confirms mine.

My calculation is 24 gallons per *individual* in hospital, of which 16 gallons must be soft, *at least.* My calculation is based upon this: that *all* the water which touches the inner and the outer man ought to be soft water—the water used for cleaning, washing up, etc., may be hard, if it likes it.

My calculation includes baths, and does not include washing, exception the wringing out of certain things, therefore used for severe cases,

49 The crown princess gave birth to her second child on 24 July.

50 Augusta of Saxe-Weimar-Eisenach (1811-90), spouse of the later King/Emperor Wilhelm I of Prussia.

which must be done before they are sent to the general washhouse, and the washing of bandages, etc. Therefore, patients 650, other persons (say) 150, [total] 800; 800 persons at 24 gallons per day each = 19,200 gallons per day. Of this 12,800 gallons should be soft water. One gallon of soft water per patient per day will be required for the pharmacy. (This is in civil hospitals condensed water from a steam boiler, collected in slate cisterns for the purpose.)

I have had both your letters about Dr Gibson's objections to the plans, and Mr Robertson's remarks. I have looked them all over. Some are futile—others imply a mistake in apprehension—some are good. I will return you all the plans, with answers, tomorrow.

(Certainly there is a singular want of managing appreciation in our Army Medical Department. Compare what the kitchen of a civil hospital, like St Bartholomew's, cooking for perhaps 900 persons, does, with what Dr G. thinks your kitchen cannot do, but must have a vast number of little *succursales* [branches] to help.)

Source: From two letters to William Aitken, Wellcome Ms 5471/14-15

3 September 1860

I shall be most glad to give my proxy for Mr Couper,[51] if you will tell me how. It is a matter upon which I can have no opinion. I can only choose my advisors. Perhaps you will tell me some governor voting for Mr Couper, who will take my proxy.

12 September 1860

I venture to trouble you with my proxy for Mr Couper. Perhaps you know some governor of the London Hospital voting for him who would take it.

Dr R.D. Thomson[52] sent me the enclosed card. Perhaps he is a governor—Mr Couper would probably be able to indicate one.

I am assured by Captain Galton that the fittings will positively be all ready by 1 October. I hope that you have had no farther hitch.

51 John Couper, assistant surgeon, London Hospital, fellow of the Royal Medical and Chirurgical Society of London.

52 Robert Dundas Thomson (1813-71), doctor and chemist.

Source: From a letter to William Farr, Wellcome Ms 5474/26, typed copy Add Mss 43398 f204

Hampstead,
16 September 1860

I hear that the Liverpool Town Council has taken deep offence at something you have said. Newlands,[53] McGowan and others are going to try their hands again at Glasgow[54] to prove, not only that your statistics are all wrong, but that Liverpool, with cesspits and middens, is the healthiest town in England. As I understand, this is not the old story raked up again, but something new; I hope you are to be at Glasgow to refute it. Therefore I have heard *nothing* from you about *anything.*

I wish that my letter about Engel to the princess royal could have been written before the prince consort went there, who, for his own credit, would have urged it. But I fear that is too late now. The queen starts this week.

I wish the hospital statistical forms could have been out before the Glasgow meeting. Already I think the objections in the *Medical Times* have told against them in the provincial mind.

Source: From two letters to Edwin Chadwick, Add Mss 45770 ff178-86 and 187-94

Upper Terrace
Hampstead, N.W.
16 September 1860

I hear that the Liverpool Town Council has taken offence at something in the Registrar-General's reports and that, at your meeting at Glasgow, Newlands, McGowan, etc., are going to prove that the Registrar-General's statistics are all wrong, and that Liverpool *with* cesspits and middens is healthier than any town *without.*

I wish you would set them right. Dr Farr is grown quite comatose. If you are coming up here to see your boy[55] before you start for Glasgow,

53 Probably James Newlands (1813-71), civil engineer at Liverpool, who went with the sanitary commission to the Crimean War hospitals in 1855.

54 At the fourth annual meeting of the National Association for the Promotion of Social Science, which opened on 24 September.

55 His son Osbert Chadwick (1844-1913), later Sir; he did important engineering work in India, in 1898 named the first Chadwick professor of municipal engineering at University College, London.

would you bring him to dine here? And I would get Dr Sutherland to meet you, if I knew beforehand. We could offer *you* a bed, but alas! our "spare room" is not one which would accommodate Mrs Chadwick. For we are just now a sanatorium for babies whose parents are away.

You and I do not mean the same thing by the "water cure." I am not at all prepared to dispute that Mr Roebuck[56] was "built up" at Malvern. But does he think that, if he had had Dr Gully[57] at Ashley Place, Westminster, he would have "built" him up, with any number of wet sheets? It is *because* Dr Gully is a brave and a sensible man and says, It is I *and Malvern* who must do it that he succeeds. But would it not be better to call this the "absence from Parliament cure" or the "quiet life and exercise cure" or the "Malvern Hill cure" rather than the "water cure"?

My objection is really only a practical one. The quack name has done mischief. It has (in a measure) prevented, as all quack idolatry (of *any* specific) does, the recognition of the hygiene treatment of disease. Admit fully the utility of water, hot and cold, as an adjunct in recovery. But it is not all.

How wicked it would be in me to disparage what is (unwisely) called the "hydropathic" treatment. But this treatment, so humane because so successful, includes much more than "water" (either hot or cold, or both). Take Mr Roebuck's case. There was absence from Parliament, absence from head excitement, absence from night hours, proper diet, quiet life, exercise, fresh mountain air and different kinds of bathing.

In my own case, which I only mention because it is that of thousands, I recognize, just as much as I recognize that 11 oz. of solid carboniferous food are necessary for a man in health, that I should not be here, were it not for Malvern. In August 1857, after my work at the royal sanitary commission, and after four years of anxiety and exertion, I was told that my life was not worth twenty-four hours' purchase, and I knew it too. I owe three years, at least, of (not useless) life to the

---

56 John Arthur Roebuck (1801-79), MP for Sheffield, whose resolution for an investigation of misconduct in the War Department brought about the defeat of the government and the sending of a committee of inquiry, which he chaired.

57 James Manby Gully (1808-83), water cure doctor at Malvern; treatments Nightingale took at Malvern and Umberslade are described in *European Travels* (7:677-80).

"water cure" at Malvern, although it could not "*cure*." Just as little does, however, water *per se*, as calomel succeed, e.g., in pulmonary phthisis, I *know* that water cannot arrest, it cannot even delay the diseased action. But gentle gymnastics with good air and water can. Dumbbells, if the patient's strength permits, horse exercise, if the patient can bear it, or other modifications which a wise and careful "hydropathic" doctor introduces. But these cannot be called *water* treatment exactly. Let us have "nature instead of drugs." But don't let us erect, or degrade, water into the *status* of a "drug."

Again, "I am not at all prepared to dispute" (as the doctors say) that the water cure *gets out* mercury and other deleterious drugs through the skin. But all sufficient perspiration, whether excited by friction or other means, does the same. And the true sanitary conclusion is, don't take the mercury, etc.

I don't disparage the wet-sheet packing; I know it has saved many lives in fever. I am sure it saved mine. I believe to a weary rheumatic labourer, before or after he has been at his day's work, it would be even more healthful than the Turkish bath. Russian, Turkish, Roman, *hot air* and vapour baths are all under the same category as hydropathy. None is a specific, none best for *universal* use, all good as part of a hygienic system. Praise them all in their places, all these forms of bath. This is all I contend for.

But, above all, I am anxious (and venture to suggest that it is *most* important) that the medical profession should not be indisposed to you, to the sanitary movement generally and to the Social Science Association in particular. Hitherto, to do them justice, I must say, I think they have behaved very well. And they have contributed their fair quota to the Social Science meetings. In particular forms of treatment and of disease, they can (or the public think they can) give *powers* to lay civilians "interfering in medicine."

I am most anxious that their opposition should not be roused. The sick are the most credulous of human beings. They will believe anything the "Doctor" (whether allopathic, homeopathic or hydropathic) says to them. For their sakes let us be most careful to carry the "doctors" with us.

18 September 1860

Mr Hutchison's Hospital Reports.

I am afraid I have kept Mr Hutchison's book a most unreasonable time. Were the answers fully and freely given, which is the case in remarkably few instances, and were an abstract and correct index made of the whole, I can fancy few "*recueils*" [collections] more important or more curious. As it is, one does not obtain much from it except a general idea of want of system and management.

Take the nursing. It appears that the generality of provincial hospitals (even those of the size of Birmingham) have no head nurse or nurses, that they have a number of women, all equal among themselves, under a matron, that these women are in many cases paid as low as 5/, or even 3/6 a week sometimes, that the night nurses are sometimes one to as many as 100 patients, in one case (to as many as seventy patients, even when these are all "accidents") as specified where all the nurses are paid £8 a year, without rations, but that, on the other hand, the night nurses have sometimes fewer patients than the day nurses; one cannot tell exactly why, and are sometimes better paid than these.

On the other hand, the answers are so careless and imperfect that, even in some provincial hospitals, there appears to be head nurses, although the answer to this (printed) question is "no." Sometimes, in the enumeration of how many patients to a nurse, the head nurses are counted and sometimes *not*, giving, in the latter case, a most erroneous idea of the disproportion of nurses to patients. Sometimes it is specified, and sometimes not, whether the nurses have rations, etc. But, in a few instances, it would *appear* that literally all they receive is 5/ a week. It is probably not so. But, of course, whether it is makes all the difference.

If a proper analysis were made of the book, all these imperfections would appear and could be reduced to certainty by fresh information. And a most valuable body of evidence would then exist. As it is, I think it almost misleading. The Liverpool hospital, where the information is most complete, appears to require a very ample reform as to nursing, as to adopting a plan of head nurses especially, etc.

One question entirely omitted is as to whether there is a "steward." I conclude, from the absence of the *question*, that there never *is* one in provincial hospitals. I have recently found, in several cases, when questions had been referred to me from these hospitals, that they usually have one matron, *no* steward and *no* head nurse. The matron performs the duties of the steward and *no one* performs the duties of the head nurse. (The nurses are all equal under the matron.)

I am certain that this system of no steward and no head nurse is extremely bad *economy* (in the large provincial hospitals, say, those which contain above 200 beds, these being actually larger than some of our London hospitals, such as King's College, University, etc.). Upon this question of stewardship, which is a very important one, Mr Hutchinson's book throws no light. In provincial hospitals, I don't at all dispute that a woman often makes the best steward. But then I would have a head matron who should be also superintendent of nurses (for, after all, the hospital is for the *patients* and not for the stores), and an under matron who should be steward. Even in prisons, the head matron is for the female prisoners, according to Sir J. Jebb's plan, and, under her, is, I believe, generally, an under matron. We take more care of our prisoners than our patients.

One thing which makes Mr Hutchison's book appear more defective than it really is (in its information) is that, in many cases, the answer is only "(See Rule --)," printed Rules and Reports having been apparently sent with it, which are not bound up in the book. And while I am all on the tiptoe of expectation, this is all I get. See Sheffield, Hereford, etc. As far as one can judge, the Scotch are, of all hospitals, the worst nursed. In one I find three nurses (serving in both capacities of night and day nurses) attending upon seventy beds, at a salary of £5.10 per annum each, apparently no rations. No head nurse. (The Glasgow Infirmary is quite a curiosity of mismanagement. See P.S.)

In some hospitals, there is a duplicate set of night nurses, sitting up *alternate* nights. But the answers never specify whether they do anything on the alternate days. I conclude, however, they are only night sitters-up, not nurses at all. It is curious that, in *very few* instances (my own town of Derby, I regret to say, among the number) is the blunder committed of having no *fixed* staff of nurses. Whereas, in military hospitals, there is *never* a fixed staff. As if there could be any *nursing* without one.

P.S. The Glasgow Infirmary has 540 beds, and might be as complete a sample of administration as any hospital in the world. It has *no* fixed staff of nurses, *no* head nurse. For every ward of twenty patients it has only one day nurse at 19/, and one night nurse at 17/ per *month*!! apparently *no* rations. (The supernumerary nurses appear to make up the whole number of nurses at present to forty-six, twenty-three day, twenty-three night.)

Source: From five letters to William Farr, Wellcome Ms 5474/27-30, typed copies Add Mss 43398 ff204, 207, 208 and 210, all from Hampstead

7 October 1860

I was exceedingly edified by your letter to the *Medical Times* upon hospital statistical forms.[58] I think it is the very best thing I have ever seen of yours *in that line*. And that is saying a great deal. They will answer it, if they have any pluck.

Thank you very much for the enclosed. Balfour is cross. Poor old Quetelet. His letters are very characteristic of himself.

I have had a perfect war of correspondence with Mühry.[59] Some day I hope to show it you. In the meanwhile, I keep to my opinion that they have to learn the very ABC of *practical* sanitary science. Mühry throws at me all the long-forgotten prejudices of thirty years ago in England by way of arguments.

I have received from Bongaels [?] (from Heuschling?[60]) several pamphlets about this and late congresses.

I see Lord Brougham[61] says that all politics must rest upon statistics.

11 October 1860

On looking over the book you have just sent me, I find the decision of the Vienna Congress[62] at p 235 (in capitals), which settles the principle upon which classification is to be carried out, viz., "in reference to the bearing on statistics, medicine and the public health." You have only to show that your classification fulfills these conditions and that the others do not.

I have applied at St Thomas' for Dr Stone's[63] papers, etc.

---

58 William Farr, "Hospital Registration," *Medical Times and Gazette* (29 September 1860):316-17, which also defended Nightingale's papers to the International Statistical Congress.

59 Dr Adolf Mühry (1810-88), advocate of environmental conditions as causes of disease, author of a map of diseases; the correspondence is missing.

60 Philippe François Xavier Heuschling (1802-83), head of the Office of Statistics, Belgium.

61 Henry Peter Brougham (1778-1868), 1st Baron Brougham, founder of the National Association for the Promotion of Social Science, and chair of the Glasgow meetings.

62 At the third meetings of the International Statistical Congress, 1857.

63 A published letter by William H. Stone attacked Dr Farr's classification scheme, while fully approving of Nightingale's paper to the Statistical Congress: "Hospital Registration—Letter from Dr Stone," *Medical Times and Gazette* 2,536 (6 October 1860):342.

20 October 1860

Dr Stone has not shown the slightest sign of life as to sending me his hospital paper, although he has promised it every day during the last week. My own idea is that we have seen the last of it we ever shall see.

I enclose a note of his, which apparently grants the whole case, viz., that he has attacked your scheme without having one to propose of his own. He will answer your letter of today though, depend upon it. And then I think you should bring out your whole serious rejoinder.

Mr Tripe's letter of today[64] grants all we want. And indeed there has never been any serious objection made excepting "this will take trouble and labour." And we answer, "yes, we want correctness, which certainly does imply labour. And it is because you have not given it that we have no hospital statistics worth having."

You see that the Paris hospitals are bestirring themselves to organize *their* statistics. And now is the time for M Legoyt[65] to bestir himself and see your classification adopted.

I return the two reports with many thanks. They are highly satisfactory in this sense, p 235, 1857. Some months ago, I got inserted into the leading medical journals of Paris an article on the proposed hospital registration. And you see they are at work. Look at p 383 of today's *Medical Times.*[66]

Dr Sutherland showed me your correspondence about Stark and Co. and he is going to send you an answer.

22 October 1860

If this is not a quack, what is? Should you be walking over Hampstead Heath some day, and would look in here, you might perhaps find the sacred trust lying on the table. It is certainly not the work of a "scientific nosologist." For all such purposes, it would do just as well if arranged according to the letters of the alphabet. As a practical nurse,

64 Dr John W. Tripe, medical officer of health at Hackney. His letter in the *Medical Times and Gazette* was a reply to Farr, arguing that doctors would be faced with an immense amount of unpaid labour to fill in the new forms (20 October 1860:388).

65 Arthur A. Legoyt (1815-85), French statistician.

66 This note reports an announcement by the director of the Assistance Publique in Paris acknowledging the lack of adequate medical statistics, which he said would be remedied the following year; fourteen leading physicians and surgeons had been appointed to advise on the preparation of new forms.

it stirs my strongest feelings of indignation, ignoring as it does all causation, and treating diseases as if they were accidents to organs.

I shall tell Dr Stone that, though I may (perhaps) keep his secret, yet the joke is much too good a one to be kept—the quack attacking and not choosing to be attacked in return.

23 October 1860

I was exceedingly amused with Dr Laycock's allusion (in his letter to you) to "a person of the name of Trevelyan," who had deprived him of your weekly statistics. You will perhaps remember that the last thing before Trevelyan went out of the Treasury, I had a correspondence with him on this very subject. And he said I had made out my case. But he could not rescind his resolution.

On Sunday I asked Mr Herbert whether he would lay the case before Mr Gladstone[67] (to this gentleman the undoing what "a person of the name of Trevelyan" has done will be a strong inducement).

To make an effective case, will you get for me the weekly circulation of the London weekly return at the time it was distributed gratuitously from your office? (2) the weekly numbers sold at present (3) the weekly numbers at present gratuitously distributed?

Mr Herbert says the *postage* is what the Treasury will object to!

Editor: In 1861, Louisa (1838-1923), grand duchess of Baden and daughter of the king and queen of Prussia, sent Nightingale a package of material about her "clinic," or hospital. The item below gives Nightingale's extracts from that material, to which she added her own comments. Her points included both better conveniences for nurses and the location of the mortuary or "deadhouse." Its position was not a safety issue—it was in a separate building—but Nightingale thought it too close for psychological comfort, as people had to pass it routinely going to the washhouse. There are cautions also about avoiding a "labyrinth" and superfluous exits in the hospital itself. Night supervision would pose a problem.

Nightingale's comments for the grand duchess on plans for a children's hospital in Heidelberg appear later in this volume. There also is correspondence with the grand duchess on nursing in *Extending Nursing* (13:466-69).

---

67 William Ewart Gladstone (1809-98), chancellor of the Exchequer, later four times prime minister.

Source: Extracts from a letter of the grand duchess of Baden, with Nightingale's comments, Add Mss 45750 ff111-14, and a note f109

[ca. late 1860 or early 1861]

[Grand duchess:] Our little clinique is intended to be as well a clinique for patients of *chirurgical* [surgical] kind, as for *eye* patients—two specialities. The surgical wards and department are on the left from the main entrance, the eye patients' wards on the right. On the upper floor there are, besides the nurses' rooms and some more wards, some rooms for the purpose of being occupied by sickly persons, invalids, etc., wishing for a quiet place to be taken care of and restored to health.

We intend to offer some rooms to several doctors in town if they wish to have them for their patients. But you see the whole is very small—not much more than sixty patients—the *home* for our *nurses* to be one of the chief objects of the new building. There we shall place, too, the stations for the nurses going into town to nurse the patients (in their own homes). There too is to be the training school for our nurses. So the objects are rather numerous. And I know well that their influence on the whole of the building has not been quite favourable.

In the souterrain [basement] there are rooms for disinfection of nurses' dresses. We have but four or six deaths in the year, therefore there seems no objection to put the mortuary room near the washhouse—a thing impossible in large hospitals with cases of inward illnesses and inward infectious diseases, of which we have none in our clinique.

Some changes will yet be made in our plans for providing, I hope, one more large room for the benefit of the nurses, and for cross-ventilation in the passages. The wards are intended to be provided with folding doors, so as to allow of using the passages as *day wards*, shutting them by folding doors likewise, and making them comfortable little rooms, obtaining, too, cross-ventilation. . . . Let me add for explanation that the kitchens are in a *half* souterrain under the chapel.

[FN:] The kitchen department appears good. But are all the nurses to have their meals in that Speisekammer [dining room]?

Mortuary? Though there are so few deaths, is not the effect on the imaginations and the gossip of the patients bad of having, if but one dead body a year, in such close proximity to washhouse and kitchen?

Is there a lift from kitchen to upper floor? Is there hot and cold water laid on all over house?

One sick room for nurses [is] very desirable. Above all, a little scullery with stove and dresser where late at night a poultice may be made or hot drink, which so often prevents an illness.

The night nursing will be difficult to arrange for in the number of small wards, especially on the surgical side. It is desirable, if possible, that the same nurse, especially by night, should not attend *men and women* patients. Indeed it is desirable, where only possible, that *women and children* should be on *one floor* or in *one wing*, and *men* on *another*. There would almost need to be three night nurses. But supposing there is one for the women and children, and one for the men and single-bedded rooms, they would require a small room or scullery, would not they?

Where are the night nurses to sleep *by day*? They should have sleeping rooms undisturbed by *day* noises.

The clinique seems difficult of supervision whether by night or day.

[FN note:] Generally speaking: rule without exception that there should be only one door and one entrance—*and that under supervision* for every unit in a hospital. Thus, a ward and its offices should have only one door, guarded by two sentinels. Sister's room on one side, duty kitchen on the other, so that at any moment of day or night, sister or nurse should see where every patient is or is not. No labyrinth. No superfluous exit or regress.

Ovariotomy[68] room should be isolated. . . . Night supervisor: what head night nurse? Probationers should be employed by day, while head nurses, matron and everybody about. What is assistant matron to do?

Source: From a letter to William Farr, Wellcome Ms 5474/34

9 January 1861

Would you be so good as to look at the enclosed (returning them to me) and tell me whether you think it is of any use asking for the imperfect information therein offered?

2. I had another inquiry from a London hospital last week asking if my scheme of hospital statistics were *not* OUT YET!!!

3. Mr Herbert's failing health (he has disease of the kidneys) and retirement from the House of Commons, which has cost him a severer struggle and greater pang than anybody knows of, of course makes a great difference to us—although at the earnest request of those who know him best, he retains office. Lord Stanley has been offered and accepted the Indian commission. We are making haste to do as much as we can before he comes on. But, anxiety has made me more unfit

68 The removal of an ovarian cyst.

than I was before. Mr Herbert (I cannot bear to call him by his new name [Lord Herbert of Lea], nor will I) is just as eager about things however as ever.

Source: From two letters to Robert Rawlinson, Boston University 1/2/23-24

15 February 1861

1. My ideas about the Reading Hospital are much too vague to help you. I have a general impression of inefficient drainage. The same description would do almost for every small provincial hospital in the kingdom: a private house, ill-fitted and worse, adapted for a hospital.

Light, air and cubic space about half what is requisite—all that has to do with sewerage imperfect. . . .

2. I enclose a fragment about Winchester. Would it not be desirable for you to send them the account of some town by you drained and sewered, *with the actual cost*—where you have been within or exact to your estimate? This would remove the distrust, expressed in my enclosure, as to expense. I shall be most happy to place my services at your disposal in all that concerns the Reading Hospital. It is quite possible that you may find it capable of improvement, and not necessarily to be removed or rebuilt. And I shall be very glad to help in any such plan.

3. I will send you the specification for the regimental hospital as soon as I get it. I am asked to tell you that the plans are private and for you alone, till they are lithographed and published.

20 February 1861

I have read your Reading papers, and Dr Sutherland has seen them too. There are a good many questions which I should wish to ask before I could have any confidence in the opinions I should like to give. But it would take you too long to answer them in writing. Dr Sutherland says the same thing. If, therefore, you would appoint an hour, when you have considered your report, to walk up here, I would get Dr Sutherland, and we would come to a conclusion.

The Reading plan is certainly a very bad one. It looks like a gibbet on which patients are to be hung, and the whole seems to depend from the cesspool, as from a peg. . . .

In general, for a provincial hospital in an open situation, I think 1500 cub. ft. enough, and 2000 cub. ft. a useless expense. King's College Hospital in London does right to give 2000 cub. ft. But perhaps you may say that, where 2000 cub. ft. are required, hospitals ought not to be at all.

I must say that the Reading people have given us "a Roland for our Oliver."[69] We say, give us the statistics of erysipelas and pyemia. And *they* say fresh air gives us erysipelas and tetanus.

Under the ground floor of the plan I sent you are at least two feet [of] space—with air brick back and front. In India we say feet where we here should say inches. Could you contrive for India my No. 2? They are singularly deficient there in such things.

Source: From two letters to Douglas Galton, Add Mss 45759 ff199-200 and 203

Wednesday [27 February or 6 March 1861]

I have done your work of art and written you a treatise on sinks. I will send you down your model and my treatise at once, if you like it. But if you could come up here today rather late, or tomorrow at any time in the afternoon, we might talk it over.

I have seen Lord H., and he says he will set about your committee as soon as ever you like. Make haste, for he is like the "son" who said "I go, and goeth not."

[Enclosed treatise]

Three sinks for a ward of thirty-two beds.

1. The scullery sink must be exclusively reserved for eating and drinking vessels and suchlike. It would be better if the model were two inches longer, broader and deeper. The border should be two inches broader on the side of the *washer.* On the side opposite, the water will be apt to splash up—it would be better if it could bulge outwards a little. I prefer the straighter end, and would make both ends the same. Great pains must be taken to have the earthenware thick enough to stand the wear and tear of hospital scullery washing.

In order to make unnecessary the nasty practice of putting a tub into the sink to "wash up," the sink ought to be made, if possible, so as to retain a few inches of water, at pleasure. The cock must be of the best kind. Some cocks turn on water too abruptly, and some too slowly.

2. The lavatory would be a great deal the better for a sink of exactly the same kind, with exactly the same improvements as No. 1. This must be exclusively reserved for emptying wash-hand basins and basins for dressing wounds, etc. But if the lavatory be not large enough, the lavatory sink need not absolutely be this size. Wall and floor to be, of course, protected.

69 Roland, a medieval French poet; Oliver, his companion.

3. Bedpan sink to be used only for emptying all secretions, all excreta, all expectoration, blood and vomit. This should be a circle, about 18 inch in diameter and 1 foot deep—with broad rim and a trap like a W.C. This should be placed high enough not to be used for any other purpose. The space underneath will do for hooks to hang up bedpans, etc., which should never be put in the W.C.

I should like to see the model of the bedpan sink. The walls round the sink must be protected with slabs of enamelled slate or tile. The cock over the bedpan sink should come right over its centre, so that the water may fall straight into any vessel to be cleansed.

All sinks must be lighted at night. A faint gaslight is enough—a pane of glass high up is sufficient to introduce light into the various compartments. This of course will be done in lighting the lavatory and W.C.

8 March 1861

The question might now be settled by an examination of each of the surfaces with a magnifying glass—dry and wet—to see how the surface takes water.

The colour also should be carefully examined. Otherwise one may look on the thing as decided.

Source: From three letters to William Farr, Wellcome Ms 5474/35-36 and 39, typed copies Add Mss 43399 ff2, 3 and 8

14 March 1861

Why my dear Dr Farr, are you not the greatest impostor that ever was? What did I wait for my paper from July till March for, except to have the names and opinions of all the wise men appended to it, which goes so far in this country? If it were not for the honour of the thing, I had a great deal liefer [more willingly] have printed it myself in July. The hospitals who wrote to me for it then, and have been waiting for it ever since, will think I am laughing at them if I send them this naked skeleton now.

But, as life has its natural term, even according to you, would you tell me how many years it will take to have printed the adoption by the pundits and their several additions to it? and don't you think I had better have it done at my own expense?

yours sincerely ever
although in extreme old age
Florence Nightingale

21 March 1861

Is it an "eternal law" that McCulloch should print my papers? Then I submit. But would you allow me (there are "perturbations" even in "eternal laws") to print the recommendations of the congress on my own account? To do this, I must have the page of the report which refers to them. I observe you have as little "expectation of life" to see the report done as I have. But it may turn out otherwise ("averages" you know I have denounced).

I eagerly snatch at your offer to send "copies to the principal hospitals, with a note signed by the secretaries of the congress," because, you see, that is all which makes the paper likely to be practically followed, viz., the adhesion of the congress. Otherwise I might just as well have printed the paper on my own account last December twelvemonth.

I meant, with your assistance and Dr Sutherland's, to have prepared and printed hospital books (for distribution) to *carry out* the system. But this is your busy year.[70] Dr Sutherland is capricious (in all his work). And I am *non compos.*

6 April 1861

I have drawn up the enclosed two varieties of a hospital book to get the particulars required by our forms and by the congress additions. I have not included numbers 8, 9, 10, 12 of the latter. I should propose to put these in another book. And these numbers should be published with the annual hospital report.

I have enclosed the articles for this summary, which might be extended, if you approve, into the form of a table, and put in type. Should not these forms of table be printed on the back of the flysheet and go out with the paper itself? What of your own letter? It has not come back to me.

Source: From a letter to Edwin Chadwick, Add Mss 45770 ff236-37

12 July 1861

Both your papers are admirable and complete. And I think your project will do a great deal of good, as you always do. Have you observed that Art. 6 in your shorter memoranda is wanting in your longer paper? Could you not include sanitary construction generally, such as healthy arrangement of rooms, number of windows, healthy

70 The decennial census, conducted in April of that year.

arrangement of streets and blocks, etc.? Could you not include in Art. 7, soldiers' tents? (There are one or two clerical errors in both papers.) . . .

When you come to details, don't forget cottage bedding, best and cheapest material for cottage mattresses, best cottage bedstead, etc. The ladies of a county recently asked my advice on this point, specifying particularly bedding for poor cottage penitentiaries, and I was obliged to answer that practically we knew nothing at all about bedding. The best was undoubtedly hair, but quite out of many cottagers' reach, after that *quilted*, not stuffed, straw. But straw is cold and hard.

Proportion in cottage furniture is another important subject. Cottagers often buy a bed at a brokers which fills up more than half this room, etc.

"Hospital Statistics and Hospital Plans"

Editor: The need for accurate, relevant statistics went to the heart of Nightingale's mission: the finding of "the laws of diseased action." Her paper "Hospital Statistics and Hospital Plans" is a continuation of her plea for what would later be called "evidence-based health care." She sent it to the National Association for the Promotion of Social Science, after some two years of preparation. The creation of a list of diseases, by class and order, and a list of operations and accidents, the latter of which Nightingale said was the first for England, was the cause of the length of the process. Of course she had not been trained medically, and so she had to rely entirely on the information sent her. Making up the lists required an enormous amount of correspondence with hospital officials and doctors. For some hospitals, she said, she had to send three times to obtain the needed information.

The forms provide for the collection of related data on age, sex, marital status and birthplace, to permit analysis of what people were most vulnerable to what diseases. These would become standard variables for data collection in the sociology of health. Data on hospital outcomes, by ward, and by disease, would permit crucial comparisons to be made.

The material on plans can be seen as an update of her original "Notes on Hospitals" of 1858. Now, in 1861, Nightingale explained that when she wrote those first papers on hospital construction, there was not a "really good plan" for a civil hospital in Britain. She had had to use French examples for good plans, and British only for the bad. Since then, several excellent English hospitals had been planned and were under construction, but they were military only.

The person Nightingale asked to read the paper was Robert D. Lyons, head of the pathology commission sent out to the Crimean War. She appreciated his work and strongly supported pathology research in the Army Medical School. Dr Lyons's letter to Nightingale agreeing to read the paper at Dublin recalled his own appreciation of Sidney Herbert: "one such man's work is worth more than the centuries of the pitiful efforts of our medical corporations."[71]

Source: From a letter to Isa Craig, Columbia University, Presbyterian Hospital School of Nursing C65

Hampstead, N.W.
10 August 1861

I send by rail (today) my paper with forms and plans, for the "Public Health" Section. My paper is very short. I have requested Dr Lyons to read it.

Source: Florence Nightingale, "Hospital Statistics and Hospital Plans," *Transactions of the National Association for the Promotion of Social Science* (August 1861): 554-60, reprinted London: Emily Faithfull 1862

In my paper on the sanitary condition of hospitals (read before the meeting of this association at Liverpool, in 1958[72]) the defective state of hospital statistics was pointed out, as well as the necessity for all hospitals coming to a common agreement on the number and nature of the data to be tabulated for future use. It then occurred to me that the best thing to do to forward the object would be to prepare a set of forms to give effect to these suggestions, and to bring them for discussion before the International Statistical Congress in London last year, the subject being one of interest for all hospitals, foreign and British. To do this, it was necessary to adopt a common nomenclature of diseases as the foundation. Such a nomenclature had been already adopted at a previous meeting of the congress at Paris, and was used in substance in the forms I laid before the London meeting.

It was most important to arrive at some common agreement as to classification of diseases, in order to give the requisite facilities for reducing the statistical data and obtaining the results. This matter is

71 Lyons letter 11 August 1861, Add Mss 45797 f252.

72 Her original "Notes on Hospitals" (see p 47 above).

confessedly beset with difficulties not likely to be soon solved. But, as it would never do to leave hospital statistics in the unsatisfactory state they were found in till everybody had agreed on a classification, that one in use by the Registrar-General of England (and by now by a large section of the United States) was adopted.

The paper and forms which I now lay before the association are those which, after a lengthened discussion, were adopted by the Statistical Congress. I thought it right to bring them before the Dublin meeting, because of an implied engagement to follow up improvements I had myself urged on the Liverpool meeting of the association, as above said, and also because I have been given to understand that several eminent hospital medical authorities in Dublin (in that spirit of improvement which distinguishes medical science there) had wished that the subject should be thus introduced.

It is proposed that one and the same form would be used for each statistical element. Seven such elements are required to enable us to tabulate the results of hospital experience; they are as follow:

1. *Remaining in hospital* on the first day of the year
2. *Admitted* during the year
3. *Recovered or relieved* during the year
4. *Discharged* incurable, unrelieved, for irregularities, or at their own request
5. *Died* during the year
6. *Remaining in hospital* on the last day of the year
7. *Mean duration of cases* in days and fractions of a day.

These seven elements printed as separate headings and attached to copies of the same form, or written in, would furnish us with the means of tabulating every fact we require. Provision can be made for different sexes in one or two ways: the column for each age may be subdivided for males and females, or it might be more convenient to have two sets of forms, one for each sex.

Again, surgical cases and injuries may be included in the same form with medical cases, or, in large hospitals, a separate set of forms might be devoted to surgical cases.

For small hospitals, one set of seven forms might easily be made to contain the annual statistics of ages, sexes and diseases (medical and surgical), but for very large hospitals, possibly four sets might be required.

The primary object of these tables is to obtain a uniform record of facts from which to educe statistical results, among which the following may be mentioned:

1. The total *sick population, i.e.*, the number of beds constantly occupied during the year by each disease for each age and sex.

2. The *number of cases* of each age, sex and disease submitted to (medical or surgical) treatment during the year.

3. The *average duration* in days and parts of a day of each disease for each sex and age.

4. The *mortality* from each disease for each sex and age.

5. The annual proportion of *recoveries* to beds occupied and to cases treated for each age, sex and disease.

In reducing the data to give the annual results, either percentages or per thousands may be used.

The number of beds constantly occupied may be obtained by taking the mean of the numbers remaining at the beginning and end of the year, if the hospital has been fully occupied, or the mean of the numbers remaining at the beginning and end of each quarter, or oftener if the hospital be irregularly occupied, or the total number of days spent in hospital by all the cases during the year might be obtained, and by dividing the sum by 365, the mean daily sick would be arrived at. (The total daily "*diets*" issued during the year divided by 365 would give the same result.) The "*sick treated*" during the year may be obtained by taking the mean of the admissions and of the discharges from all causes, including deaths.

With fixed data arrived at on these principles, we can readily obtain the proportionate mortality, not only of the whole hospital, but of every ward of, and also the proportionate mortality and duration of cases for each age, sex and disease.

The laws which regulate diseased action would thus become better known, the results of particular methods of treatment, as well as of special operations, would be better ascertained than they are at present. As regards their sanitary condition, hospitals might be compared with hospitals and wards with wards.

The whole question of hospital economics as influenced by diets, medicines, comforts, could be brought under examination and discussion.

The liability of particular ages, sexes, occupations and classes of the community to particular forms of disease might be ascertained; other data, such as "married" or "single," previous attacks of illness of the same or different kinds, birthplace, etc., might be added for comparison, and hospital experience might thus be made to subserve sanitary improvement. The data for these latter comparisons would have to be kept separately, as indeed they generally are in all well-regulated hospitals.

A. is a leaf of the hospital "Admission and Discharge" book, proposed by the secretaries to the Statistical Congress for entering those details required for filling up the annual forms proposed by me and adopted by the congress, and also for registering the additional particulars regarding the patients required by the congress.

B. is one of thc annual forms referred to.

Especially I wished to call attention to the additional points of hospital statistics agreed to by the Statistical Congress, and which will be found at the end of my paper. They did not come within the scope of my forms. But they are of great importance, particularly those referring to the sanitary condition of hospital wards and to the method of recording fresh attacks of disease *in* hospital in the "Admissions and Discharge" book. These data, if properly used, will enable a check to be kept over the sanitary condition of the hospital, at least as regards hospital diseases.

But it must not be forgotten that a hospital is in a bad sanitary state before such diseases can appear. They are evidence of bad constructive arrangements or of culpable sanitary neglect having produced their results, rather than indices of the actual sanitary state of the wards. All careful hospital physicians and surgeons, as well as nurses, can generally tell to what extent a ward is healthy, or otherwise, by the manner in which cases are progressing, before actual hospital disease appears. *This* is the time to prevent the occurrence of hospital diseases, not after they have occurred.

I refer to the point because, since my papers were read, some melancholy instances have occurred of fatal hospital diseases arising from distinctly preventible causes. In one such case, in a small provincial hospital in one of the healthiest counties in England, twenty-four poor creatures ran the gauntlet of their lives in nine months from erysipelas, of whom eight died. And this after very trifling accidents or operations, none of which ought to have produced erysipelas at all—much less to have ended fatally. In this case there were both local causes of disease about the hospital, and there was also defective structure.

Especially am I anxious to recur to this latter point. I have seen several misapplications of the principles of hospital construction (briefly laid down in my former paper) defended because, it was said, they were adaptations of those principles, also bad principles of construction defended because they had been "already adopted"! This is not the way to hasten human progress. Defects, the result of want of knowledge, must disappear; improvements, the result of experience, must advance.

I can do no more in the matter but reiterate the appeal (at the end of my former paper) that the real practical object and intention of these principles should be very carefully considered and embodied by those on whom it falls to design, to construct or to manage buildings for the care of the sick. Let us look forward to the time when the necessity of providing even for the record of *hospital* diseases, so much insisted upon by the Statistical Congress, will thus cease, and when the stigma of these diseases will be wiped out from hospital records.

Explanation of the Plans

At the date of my former paper (1858) there was no really good plan of hospital construction in this country to refer to. Since that date, however, several excellent hospitals have been planned, and are now in process of construction. These will, when completed, practically show forth the principles required to give pure air to the sick, and to ensure economical and efficient administration.

I beg to submit plans of two of these hospitals. They are both military—I am sorry I cannot give any civil ones as models, for they do not exist. Some, however, will soon exist, and it is fairly to be hoped that in all future hospitals generally, the same principles will be substantially adopted—yes, and improved upon. It need hardly be said that the details in civil must be somewhat different from those in military hospitals.

One of these plans is for an infantry regimental hospital for one hundred and twenty sick.[73] The other is the plan of a general hospital for the Royal Artillery Garrison, at Woolwich (six hundred and fifty beds [Herbert Hospital]).

The infantry hospital consists of one double pavilion containing four wards, each of twenty-eight beds, and four small wards of two beds each. The larger wards are open from end-to-end, so that the attendant in the nurse's room can see every bed in the ward. The small wards have windows on three sides, and are so arranged as to be under constant inspection from the same nurse's room. The water closets and baths are at angles of the wards, opposite the entrance, and are entirely cut off from the wards by a method of ventilation which ensures any foul air being blown away from the ward. The large end window allows of easy ventilation during the night.

73 This is the larger version for regimental hospitals, designed by Galton, with input from Nightingale.

In this hospital the fireplaces are in the walls, with a window over them. Each large ward has a separate scullery, a matter of necessity, not choice.

The two pavilions are cut off from each other by a large passage and staircase traversing the building. The kitchen and stores are under a separate roof. The hospital sergeant and orderlies are quartered in the centre of the building, and surgery and waiting room are in the same position, as also a day room for convalescents. Thus the whole administration is concentrated in the middle, and the hospital sergeant can always know at any moment where each of his orderlies is, and where he is not, and what he is doing, and the same of each of his patients. There are no dark corners nor spare rooms, and "skulking" is all but impossible. This plan, then, combines the greatest facilities for economy in administration with efficiency of discipline (which includes the utmost care for the sick and the utmost obedience from the convalescent), and pure air for all.

The Woolwich Hospital plan is simply an arrangement of a number of these pavilions—each having two floors of wards, connected by a corridor one floor in height—under one general central administration for the whole hospital. There is one kitchen in a half basement under the library and chapel. It is connected with all the pavilions by a basement corridor, along which all diets, etc., are transported on rails and raised by lifts to each pavilion. There are separate chutes for foul linen and dust; hot and cold water are laid over the whole building, and there is a central bathing establishment besides the ward baths.

There are separate wards for sick prisoners and for lunatics and others requiring segregation.

There is a large library, also a dining and day room for convalescents.

The axes of the pavilions are arranged north and south, so as to have both walls exposed to the sun. The nearest pavilions are sixty-four feet apart, or double their height. The others are much more. The eight wards in the end pavilions have a free look out to the open country.

The outer walls will be of white brick, to give the building a more cheerful appearance. The inner walls and ceilings are to be of polished Parian cement.

In this hospital there will be two fireplaces in the centre of each ward. They are to be of terra cotta, constructed so as to give the greatest warmth. The flues will be carried under the ward floors, and up the side walls of the pavilions. This leaves the view of the ward open from end-to-end, and enables the nurse to see every bed from her room window. (There are to be female head nurses in this hospital.)

The principles embodied in this plan are: subdivision of sick under a number of separate roofs; separation between the hospital proper and the administration; no more than two floors of wards; opposite windows in each large ward, with the beds ranged between them, one window for every two beds; sufficient isolation and free ventilation of the water closets and baths; one scullery and one nurse's room for each ward, and placed at the entrance end, so that the attendants, while overlooking the patients, can be themselves overlooked; large separate day room for convalescents; building to be placed on high ground in the open country; abundant external ventilation.

The wards of each of these hospitals are 14 feet high. Each bed has from 93 to 97 superficial feet, and from 1200 to 1400 cubic feet. The width of the wards between the opposite windows is from 26 feet 6 inches to 26 feet 9 inches. The cubic space of military hospitals is not so large as that required for civil hospitals, because the greater bulk of the patients in military hospitals are what we should call convalescents.

This building is to be called the "Herbert Hospital," after the great and good statesman whom we have lost, who was himself its founder.

Let Dublin, who knew him so well,[74] join with us, who loved him so well, to give him worthy tears—such a tribute as he would have liked—he, who suffering under a fatal disease—he, who with every possession which God could bestow to make him idly enjoy life—yet ran like a racehorse his noble course, till he fell—and up to the very day fortnight of his death, struggled on doing good, not for the love of power or place (he did not care for it), but for the love of mankind and of God. His glorious death would be almost too sacred to mention here, but for the sake of calling on those who loved him—and who did not? to carry out his purposes.

It is five years since he began to carry out his chief purpose to restore the health of the British Army, and how well he worked at it all know. But the soldier was not his only care. His cares were national, and one of his cherished principles was the reconstruction of all hospitals according to the latest improvement of the pavilion structure. It

74 Sidney Herbert was a landowner in Ireland, but unlike many absentee owners, provided relief during the potato famine.

is not often that we find a man, born to politics and high position, who would master, for the love of his kind alone, every dry detail of this almost technical subject. Yet he did. His loss is irreparable. Time will only show more and more what we have lost in him. But at least let his purposes and principles outlive him in us.

Forms:
B Proposed Hospital Statistical Form
This sheet will serve for the classification of cases in hospitals under the following headings: "Remaining, 1st January," "Admitted," "Cured (or relieved)," "Dead," "Discharged incurable, for irregularities, or at their own request," "Remaining, 31st December," "Duration of cases in days."
Write the Name of Hospital, the Sex, the required Heading, and Date with the Pen.

Class I, Order I (Zymotic Diseases): [a row each for each disease, separated by, / indicates on same line]
smallpox, measles, whooping cough, croup, scarlatina, quinsy, diphtheria, coryza/catarrh/influenza, ophthalmia (purulent), erysipelas, metria (puerperal fever), pyemia, hospital gangrene, carbuncle/boil, dysentery, diarrhea, cholera, typhoid fever (thyphinia), ague, remittent fever, rheumatism, others.
Order II: gonorrhea, primary syphilis, secondary syphilis, tertiary syphilis, others.
Order III: scurvy, purpura, alcohol/ (1) delirium tremens, b) intemperance, others.
Order IV: thrush, porrigo, scabies, worms, others.
Class II, Order I (constitutional diseases): gout, dropsy, cancer, canker (noma), mortification, others.
Order II: scrofula, tuberculosis mesenterica, phthisis, hemoptysis, pneumothorax [page torn here, not sure], hydrocephalus (tubercular deposit), others.

Class III, Order I (local diseases): A. Brain/spinal marrow and nerves, meningitis, cephalitis (including acute hydrocephalus), paralysis, chorea, mania, epilepsy, hysteria, tetanus (idiopathic), convulsions, others.
B. Sense organs: ophthalmitis (not purulent), cataract, amaurosis, glaucoma and other diseases of the eye, ottorhea, otitis, deafness and other diseases of the ear.
Order II: carditis, pericarditis, endocarditis, disease of heart valves, heart hypertrophy, heart atrophy, heart fatty degeneration, aneurism

of heart, aneurism of aorta, etc., angina pectoris, fainting, phlebitis, varix, others.
Order IV: gastritis, enteritis, peritonitis, constipation, colic, ileus (obstruction of bowels), intussuception, hernia, stricture of esophagus, stricture of intestinal tube, ulceration of intestinal tube, dyspepsia, pyrosis, gastralgia, hematemisis, apoplexy, melena, hemorrhoids, fistula, pancreatic disease, spleen disease, hepatitis, jaundice, gallstones, cirrhosis, ascites, others.
Order V: nephritis, ischuria, nephria (Bright's disease, albuminuria), diabetes, stone (uric acid, etc.), gravel (uric acid, etc.), hematuria, cystitis, disease of prostate gland, other.
Order VI: varicocele, hydrocele, ovarian dropsy, others.
Order VII: synovitis, ostitis (including periostitis and endostitis), exostosis, curvature of spine, curies, necrosis, muscular atrophy, others.
Order VIII: phlegmon, whitlow, abscess (external), ulcer (external), other skin diseases.

Class IV: Order I (developmental disease): spina bifida, other malformations, teething, others.
Order II: chlorosis, childbirth (miscarriage, abortion, etc.), paramenia (including amenorrhea, leucorrhea, turn of life, climacteria).

Class IV (violent deaths or disease):
Order I (accident): burn, scald, fracture, contusion, concussion, gunshot wound, cut/stab, poisoning, others.
Order III (homicide).
Order IV (suicide): gunshot wound, cut/stab, poisoning, others, sudden deaths (cause not ascertained), causes not specified or ill-defined.
Total
[to the right of the form, explanations]
Most of the diseases in the following marginal list are of less frequent occurrence in hospitals, and all, with some exceptions, are classed as "others" in their respective orders in the left-hand column. They will be distinguished in abstracting the diseases by writing the *ages* of the persons attacked, cured or dead, etc., against the particular diseases in the margin below. Thus, a person aged sixteen would, if admitted for "*mumps,*" be indicated in the body of this sheet by a *tick* against "others" of Class I, Order I, and his age (16) would be written against "mumps" in the margin. And so of other diseases. The diseases not found printed in the margin must be written in their proper compartments. A summary of the facts in the margin should be given in an appendix to the general table.

Class I, Order I: varioloid, varicella, miliaria, mumps, erythema, dysentery with abscess of liver (placed to *dysentery*), yellow fever.
Order II: leprosy (Greek elephantiasis), yaws, glanders, hydrophobia, malignant pustule, necusia (infection by puncture in dissection or by handling the parts of dead animals).
Order III: rickets, bronchocele, cretinism, ergotism.
Order IV: phthiriasis: *hydatids, tapeworm and other entozoa should be distinguished here. In the capital table they will be added to the head "worms."*

Class II, Order I: anemia, lupus, dry gangrene, bedsore, melanosis. *The several forms of cancer comprised in the capital table under the heading "Cancer" should be distinguished as under the ages, and parts affected should also be distinguished:* soft, colloid, osteoid, schirrus, epithelial.
Order II: psoas abscess, scrofulous abscess of joints (placed to *scrofula*), tubercular peritonitis.

Class III, Order I: myeletis, shaking palsy (placed to *paralysis*). *The parts affected in all cases referred to "paralysis" in the capital table should be distinguished here and the ages stated:*
neuralgia (tic douleureux), neuroma.
Order II: arteritis, atheroma (of arteries).
Order III: hydrothorax, empyema, pleuripneumonia (placed to *pneumonia),* congestion of lungs, spurious melanosis.
Order IV: glossitis, stomatitis, pharyngitis, esophagitis. *Distinguish here the following varieties of hernia, all of which are classed in the capital table under hernia:* congenital, femoral or crural, inguinal, scrotal, umbilical, ventral.
Order V: diuresis, stricture of urethra (not a consequence of gonorrhea). *In cases of stone and gravel, the composition of substances should be specified here.*
Order VI: orchiteritis, hysteritis, ovarian tumour, uterine tumour, polypus of uterus.
Order VII: fragilitas ossium, mollities ossium.
Order VIII: roseola, urticaria, eczema, herpes, pemphigus, ecthyma, impetigo, acne, mentagra, lichen, prurigo, psoriasis, pityriasis, ichthyosis. *In abscess and ulcer the parts affected should be distinguished here.*

Class IV, Order: explosion of powder, gas, etc. (placed to *burn*), chilblain, frostbite, lightning (where struck and how?), sunstroke (state circumstances). *The circumstances attending deaths by violence should be shown in detail, as, for example, how many persons, at their several ages, were burnt by their clothes taking fire, how many died by falling from scaffolds or heights, how many were poisoned by arsenic, opium, quack medicine, overdose, etc. Gunshot wounds should be distinguished as regards the species of weapon—rifle, pistol, cannon, etc., other wounds as whether inflicted by knife, dagger, etc. When cases of privation, drowning, hanging, suffocation, fall within observation, they should be placed to "others" in the general table, and the particulars should be stated here. All violent deaths should fall under one or other of the three orders: accident, homicide, suicide.*

Columns for: No. of case, Date of admission, Name, Age, Sex, M or F, Residence, and place where ill or injured, Trade or occupation, Disease or accident; Date (sub-columns) of attack, of recovery, of death, of discharge (relieved) or (unrelieved) or otherwise, Of transfer to other division of hospital; Duration of case in hospital, in days and quarters, Remarks (previous diseases of patients and of parents).

Source: From a letter to Samuel Smith, Add Mss 45792 ff233-36

Hampstead, N.W.
2 September 1861

I enclose you a second letter of Mr Whitfield's about his son and beg you to be so kind as to answer it. I have made every inquiry at the fountainheads (magnify to him the extent of my exertions as much as you can) and find:

1. as to government dockyards, they do employ some, but "very few," civil engineers; it would be most "difficult" to introduce one there now;
2. as to the War Office, they employ "*none*," of course;
3. as to contractors, they choose their own "and generally NOT" (with a great *not* underlined a great many times) "gentlemen."

My authority concluded his answer to me with a very strong caution "that a man is always spoiled and lost who goes into government employment." My authorities also said: "his best chance of employment is from the leading men of his own profession, who are always wanting assistance of some sort, perhaps he is too grand for that." However correct or incorrect this information may be, it is quite obvious that my authorities do not intend to do anything. Therefore it is useless my going on.

I trouble YOU to write this to Mr W. because he is quite capable, from my five years' experience of him, of writing to me next, if I write to him, to ask me to apply to the sultan at Constantinople for his son, "in consequence of my known influence in that quarter" (that is his favourite formula).

A.H. Clough says "there is nothing people think too selfish, exacting, mean or false to do for their own families." He does not often give us a sentiment. I re-echo this.

Source: From a letter to Parthenope Verney, Wellcome (Claydon copy) Ms 8999/56

[ca. December 1861]

But I cannot see Mr Simms without knowing more about him than this. And I entirely deprecate special hospitals. The only reason which militates against the immense evils of having hospitals at all is to have them *general*.

But if Mr Simms chooses to write me questions, I will answer them in writing. And I shall then see whether he is worth seeing and telling general principles to. Even now, were I to answer all the letters and see all the people (who apply), it would take my whole TIME and that of one clerk. I think your house beautiful.

Source: From an incomplete letter to James Paget, Clendening History of Medicine Library, Kansas University Medical Center

[late 1861-62]

Several of our hospitals have been good enough to send me their statistics this year. Among these, St Bartholomew has unquestionably the best. (Though I think he might do still more in improving his statistical forms.) And Guy, who used to be the best, is now unquestionably the worst.

I wish I could say that I had done anything yet in utilizing your invaluable materials for the record of "Causes of Death after Operations." But I have not. I do not, however, despair of doing something this year. We are overwhelmed with business at the War O., business almost hopeless, now that we have lost our head [Sidney Herbert].

I am like Professor Tyndall, if he had broken both his wrists at the top of the Weisshorn.[75] Our chief is dead. Also, since Albert is dead, too, the commander-in-chief[76] has gone to the dogs entirely.

---

75 John Tyndall (1820-93), physicist and the first person to ascend Weisshorn. He is referred to in Dr Croft's lectures to probationers for a lecture on disease and dust. Tyndall wrote also on greenhouse gases and global warming.

76 Prince Albert died on 14 December 1861; the commander-in-chief was George, 2nd duke of Cambridge (1819-1904), cousin of Queen Victoria.

Source: From a letter to Douglas Galton, Add Mss 45760 f55

22 January 1862

If we could get an adaptation of our principles to a thirty-two-bed hospital by such a man as Mr [T.H.] Wyatt, we should gain much. You know we have never done a thirty-two-bed hospital. What would do most good would be to get Mr Wyatt to apply his genius to the principles, and for us to go on objecting to details till we get the best possible.

Source: From a letter to Robert Rawlinson, Boston University 1/2/31

24 February 1862

I have not yet thanked you for your report on West Ham sewerage—one of the most interesting things, I think, you have done. I am very glad that you found the drainage of Windsor in so good a state. But one of the great evils of the present time is to ally typhoid fever exclusively with bad drainage or nuisance. And hence the real cause, which no doubt exists, is overlooked.[77]

Editor: The next letter refers to Nightingale's efforts to get two questions, one each on housing and illness, added to the decennial census.[78] The "illogical" letter of Major Graham referred to in it is not extant.

Source: From a letter to William Farr, Wellcome Ms 5474/41, typed copy Add Mss 43398 f205

20 April 1861

It has been "sung and said" in various places that women's letters are illogical. Now Major Graham's letter says:

1. That I generalize from one instance, and then proceeds to do the self-same thing;

2. Lays down a principle in human nature in which I think all the world will be against him, viz., that family people are *less* likely to give accurate information about themselves than a landlord is to do it for them;

3. Ignores the only point in our communications, viz., that it is *not* of travellers we are speaking (those who sleep one night in an inn) and that a superintending registrar might decide to what class the inn

77 The bacillus that causes typhoid fever was not identified until 1880.

78 For other correspondence on this, see *Society and Politics* (5:95-103).

belongs. It would be a curious thing to know. I take it (in hotels of this character) the proportion of passers-through, beds let by the night, would be *nil*.

You have not criticized my apostle's [St Thomas'] statistics for me, and Paget and I are waiting breathless upon your voice. You have not even returned me the copy to comfort myself with.

Source: From a letter to an unnamed recipient, Columbia University, Presbyterian Hospital School of Nursing C66

26 April 1862

My reason for not answering sooner your kind note of 2 April is that I have been and continue to be very ill.

It is most desirable both for private houses and for hospitals that every effort should be made to improve (and to improve *cheaply*) porcelain sinks and baths.

If you would like to send a specimen of each kind to this house, and allow it to remain for twenty-four hours so that I may be able to look at it when least unwell, I should be very much obliged.

Source: From a letter to William Farr, Wellcome (Claydon copy) Ms 5474/47, typed copy Add Mss 43399 f58

Hampstead
8 October 1861

Your friend, Dr Mühry of Göttingen, has written to me to know the fate of a certain paper of his upon "sea currents," which, if you remember you were kind enough to send (about December last) to the secretary of the Geographical Society (?) for him. He does not ask for it back, as he has a copy of it. He only wants to know "what has become of it." If the Geographical secretary did not approve of it, it would be very easy to make some excuse, as that it does not fall in with the rules of the society to, etc. . . .

I enclose you a review by Dr Mühry out of the *Göttingen Critical Journal*, merely for you to look at (if you do not care to read the rest) the passage marked p 1588. Please return it to me.

Source: From a letter to James Paget, Add Mss 45798 ff60-61

10 May 1862

I dare say you will have entirely forgotten what the enclosed refers to. Some time ago, you were so kind as to lend me Topinard on hospitals, a book which stirred up all the old dog's hospital enthusiasm, both by its truths and its errors, errors, i.e., to the old dog's hospital experience.

You then wished for Paris medical authority to an assertion of mine that pyemia was indigenous in Paris. The man in whose wards I had seen it, M Roux of La Charité,[79] was dead. I asked others and got no answer. Lately Dr Shrimpton (whose name may be known to you as having been many years in the French Army Medical Service, and all his life a practising physician at Paris), and Baron Larrey[80] began a correspondence with me about the artificial ventilation of Paris hospitals.

I am entirely unacquainted with Dr Shrimpton, but in the course of our correspondence I asked him my question "promiscuous." I enclose a copy of an extract containing his answer, *telle quelle* [such as it is], in order that I may not give the trouble to you of returning me his letter. I also enclose a "discours" [speech] of Baron Larrey, which I am afraid I must trouble you to return. I think it shows them to be about thirty years behind us in the "hygiène des hôpitaux" [health of hospitals]. Also the *Gazette médicale*, in which is the conclusion of the hospital controversy (no conclusion at all, as usual) I am afraid.

Source: From a copy of letter to Lady Easthope,[81] Florence Nightingale Museum 0522

25 June 1862

My dear Lady Easthope, First of all, let me thank you for your beautiful roses, and for all the trouble you have taken about the Paris hospital questions so interesting to me.

Secondly, about Mr McIlroy's bedstead. If you wish to make him an answer, will you tell him merely that my health entirely prevents me from entering into discussions and inquiries of this kind?

But, that I might not seem to neglect any request of yours, I sent a person on whom I could depend to the exhibition to look at the bedstead. I am told that it is an invention (and its parts were described to me) which does not improve upon the thousand and one bedsteads invented of this kind, and the execution of the one exhibited is considerably inferior to what we already make in London. Mr McIlroy

79 Joseph Roux (1780-1854), French surgeon, from Nightingale's visits to Paris hospitals in 1853.

80 Charles Shrimpton (1815?-?), surgeon general in the French Army; Félix Hippolyte Larrey (1808-95), son of Dominique-Jean Larrey, the famous surgeon of the Napoleonic Wars. The letters are missing in both cases.

81 Lady Easthope (1803-65), née Elizabeth Skyring, an artist and family friend who had lived in Paris, and who was also a French translator.

appears to have gone to the expense of a patent, which he wishes to sell in England.

Generally, I must confess, from my own experience, that it is quite impossible to judge from inspection (much more impossible from inspection of a model) of these things. Use only in a hospital can *determine* what really adds to comfort (for the patient). I have seen, I believe, almost all the inventions that ever have been made of this kind, have invented some myself, and I could not judge even of my own, except by use among my patients.

Source: From a letter to Samuel Smith, Add Mss 45793 ff20-21

21 February 1863

I am afraid you are almost as little able to attend to these things as I am. But I am told that the Craven Charity, now worth about £700 a year, to provide the London poor (of certain parishes) with hospital accommodation for *plague*, is now before you,[82] to all which information I attach as much importance as I do to all the other information I receive (now that Sidney Herbert and Clough, each the most accurate of men, are both gone).

It seems to me I never hear a word of truth. But if there should chance to be 1 gr. of truth in this, may I say that £700 a year is quite useless to afford hospital accommodation, of which there is enough and too much, but of *convalescent* (country) accommodation, of which there is hardly any for the London poor, it might afford enough to be signally useful.

E.g., St John's House (King's College Hospital) has long been trying to establish such at Hampstead. A china merchant has guaranteed £500 a year for the first two years *and a house.* Some besides myself have given all we could afford, viz., £100 each. But a part of the Craven Charity, even *yearly*, would enable it to be set up, which it is not yet. It would not be confined to the patients of King's College.

St John's House has a large number of out-patients, nursed at home. Do not trouble yourself to answer this, if there is no truth in it.

82 Nightingale's uncle Samuel Smith was clerk to committees at the House of Commons.

Source: From a letter to James Paget, Add Mss 45798 ff93-95

21 February 1863

I sent you copies of the operation tables, completed in the flower of their perfection (from the printers) the other day by my sister. I had no time to write and thank you for these tables, which I must call yours. I trust that their utility will spread to other hospitals, and thus recompense you for the invaluable labour you have bestowed on them.

I am sending copies to our principal London hospitals. I am not so young as to expect now that they will be accepted on the face of their obvious usefulness at once. But the hospitals will carp and alter this and amend that. And in the end a great deal of good will be done, if only by directing attention to the subject, and awakening them to make their own criticisms.

I intend, if I live so long, to bring the whole subject before the next Social Science meeting.[83] And it is then I hope to make use of the information you have given by filling up those tables. I mean also to propose a form for registration since the first step in the way of improvement is to obtain a terse and accurate registration of the elements of the problem.

Every well-kept hospital record ought to contain these as:

1. age
2. sex
3. occupation
4. accident or disease leading to operation
5. date of accident and of operation, or date of operation, if from disease
6. nature of operation
7. constitution of patient
8. complications occurring after operation
9. date of recovery or of death
10. fatal complication (a) resulting directly from accident, (b) resulting from operation.

I imagine that the agricultural county hospitals, who have perhaps but one or two operations a year, will not go farther than keeping such an operation book as this. But all London, Liverpool, Leeds, Manchester, Glasgow and large town hospitals should tabulate these elements for use on your operation forms.

83 Nightingale sent a seven-page "Proposal for Improved Statistics of Surgical Operations" to the International Statistical Congress, Berlin, December 1863, published in *Notes on Hospitals*, 3rd ed. (see p 205 above).

Source: From a letter to Lord Stanley, Liverpool Record Office 15/11

22 April 1863

A remarkably stupid advertisement has been appearing in the *Times*, asking everybody to send in plans for a civil hospital at Bombay, without giving any information, such as would enable any living being to make a plan, and "topping up" with stating that the local authorities and the railway authorities were to be judges of excellence. The whole thing was so absurd, and it was besides such a re-enacting in India of what we have given up here, that I made an effort to prevent mischief, as far as I could.

I am told that Sir Charles Wood will consult you about it, which I was very glad to hear.

Some time ago, we recommended Mr T.W. [T.H.] Wyatt as architect for a civil hospital at Malta. And he produced, with our aid, one of the very best plans in existence. Would you think well to put the matter into his hands? He has shown great ability. Any help we could give him would be willingly given, for the good of helping.

Source: From a letter to Hilary Bonham Carter, Add Mss 45794 ff209-10

20 May 1863

Dearie, You could not have given *me* a greater pleasure than by *your* going to Paris (!) I only hope you will stay longer than a fortnight.

Do you know Dr Shrimpton? If not, would you merely take this parcel and letter and send it to him—if yes, give it him—you can roll up the parcel, if more convenient, though it is better to carry it flat.

It has taken my odds and ends of time for two years to prepare these forms, simple as they look. For (at least in England) this is the first complete list of operations and of complications (curious as this sounds) that has been made. I had to appeal to every large hospital in London to send me its own list of *complications*, all imperfect. And the forms had to be sent back to people and revised three times (after they had been looked over each time by our most eminent surgeon), to add in the names of important operations which had been left out—so laborious is it, when you come to *do* a thing of this sort, to include everything.

Perhaps you will tell Dr Shrimpton this, as a proof that the forms have received the fullest consideration, not only by me but by our great surgeons. I should ask you to take the copies to your friend M Legoyt, to M Husson and to M Larrey. But I am sure you will have no time.

My best love to dear Monsieur et Madame Mohl[84] and thank *him* for his letter.

ever your F.

Source: From an incomplete letter to an unnamed recipient, Radcliffe Infirmary Archives RI/1/39

10 July 1863

As the conviction of my hospital life has been that no curtain should be allowed to come near any hospital bedstead, to obstruct its fresh air, I cannot advise on how to hang curtains.

If the patient requires privacy, low moveable screens should be used, just high enough to prevent him seeing into other beds or other beds seeing into him, i.e., not higher than the patient's head when sitting up in bed.

This is the best way not to obstruct ventilation and not to obstruct the head nurse's view when walking about her ward—very serious accidents with sudden hemorrhage, etc., having happened owing to the patients not being all and always under the sight of the head nurse at the same time.

Source: From a letter to W.J. Little, Wellcome Ms 5482/55

31 July 1863

I am extremely obliged to you for sending me the statistical tables of the London Hospital. They are the best I have hitherto seen of any of the great London hospitals. But I think, without altering the form, they might be drawn up so as to lessen the expense.

Would it be too much to ask you to send me two or three copies? I would return one to you, with the suggestions which occur to me.

Source: From a letter to William Farr, Wellcome Ms 5474/61

Hampstead, N.W.
7 August 1863

I am extremely sorry for the Berlin Congress. I believe there is a dead set of Louis-Napoléon[85] and the Austrians to put it down. Engel per-

84 Julius Mohl (1800-76), professor of Persian at the Collège de France, and Mary Clarke Mohl (1793-1883), English-born and a family friend. Nightingale stayed with the Mohls when in Paris.

85 The fifth meetings of the International Statistical Congress; Louis-Napoléon (1808-73), Emperor Napoléon III.

haps does not look upon it quite seriously enough. What a curious Germanizing brain process his letter shows. Also why Germans cannot succeed at liberal institutions as we do.

He is thinking (and writing to you) of the *subjective* good effect upon his own character of political vexations. We in England should just lay our heads together as we did in James II's time and say *this shall not be.*[86] And the *objective* action would follow directly. However, one thing he says is perfectly certain, viz., that all this vexatious opposition has the effect of advertising the thing much more than our own utmost effort could do.

So it will be with the attacks upon our India report at Newcastle[87] and elsewhere. But why are you not there to answer them? There will be no one else to do so. Why did not Berlin time its meeting better?

I don't think I could get anything ready for Berlin. I have no time or strength, unless you thought the surgical operations tables would do, with a paper of which the enclosed is an uncorrected proof, in which case I must ask you to get somebody to translate it into French. I have no time. You will see that your own proposition recurs on the second page and extended.

Source: From two letters to Douglas Galton, Add Mss 45761 ff130-32 and 135-36, both from Hampstead, N.W.

28 September 1863

You differ from Mr Mennie as to the quality of the Parian cement. At least, the meaning of part of his memo was that by mistake the second quality had been used.

Miss Jones says that at King's College the best quality was *not* used. Any quality is very much superior for hospital purposes to plaster. An impervious surface is the first necessity. Glass or enamelled slate or glazed tile would be best, except for the cost. Next best would be an impervious cement of a good colour (imperviousness in any case).

If you cannot get this together with colour in the material and polish, then you must paint, varnish and polish the surface of some impervious material. The surface should require renewal only at distant periods. And the usual renewal of paint should not be required, i.e., as it is applied to plaster.

86 James II (1633-1701), upholder of the divine right of kings; he was defeated at the Battle of Boyne in 1690 and forced into exile.

87 The meetings of the British Association for the Advancement of Science were held in Newcastle in August that year.

The Lariboisière surface has been in use ever since it was born and will continue so for the next twenty years. All paint work that requires renewal frequently is imperfect and hardly suitable for hospitals.

Plaster for hospital wards has been distinctly relinquished. And it won't do for us to go back upon that again, in such a building. The only question has been about the ceiling. Again I say we *must* have an impervious, polished, good-coloured substance and surface.

Miss Jones says that she has seen the workmen mixing (like mortar) the cement, and she is quite sure that the not being able to get "large surfaces" with an "even colour" is owing to their doing this, without regular quantities, in a rough careless rule-of-thumb way.

1 October 1863

I have heard from Dr Sutherland the disastrous intelligence about the Parian. But I am not at all prepared to surrender to paint. Can no better substitute be? Scagliola [stone-like plaster]? Pray inquire about it more.

I am not at all convinced that the "very best" Parian *was* used at the Herbert H. It was "ordered," I know, but your own officers differ as to whether another quality was not used by mistake. A certain good specimen of the cement was shown to the foreman, but was not adopted in practice—vide [see] Mr Mennie's minute.

Miss Jones says that the best was *not* used at K.C.H., and says, moreover, that the way the workmen mix it is quite enough to account for any failure. If we were to mix our medicines and our poultices in that way, we should not be surprised at the result, I assure you.

Source: From a letter to T. Graham Balfour, Add Mss 50134 ff116-17

Hampstead, N.W.
30 September 1863

I will gladly wait till you can send me those tables (which you are so kind as to promise) at your own convenience. I will write more fully about your admirable report another time.

The International Statistical meeting has been sadly plundered. But it was doubtful till the last moment whether Prussia would have it at all—whether Austria would join—whether the crown prince[88] would be allowed to preside, etc. And poor Engel, a thorough German (and

88 Friedrich (1831-88), the (liberal) crown prince of Prussia and husband of Princess Victoria, later, briefly, emperor.

not a native of Berlin) thought less, as we should do, of the businesslike manner of bringing things straight than of the subjective effect of these trials to his own idiosyncrasy *sic!!!*

Source: From a letter to William Farr, Wellcome Ms 5474/65

22 December 1863

With regard to your question, there is no civil hospital of a large size in England which can be called "a model." The Herbert Hospital is a model for a military hospital, i.e., having respect to the character of the ground, the pavilion system is there applied in a model manner. But I am not sure that, did the ground allow of it, it would not be better to arrange similar double pavilions in the shape of a square, with open corners, as in the form of Yarmouth Naval Hospital.

For a civil hospital, I think the entire separation between the sexes, and the *single* pavilion far preferable, as in the Lariboisière. The defects of the Lariboisière are its three floors, its pavilions too near each other, and its abominable artificial ventilation, which neutralizes half its good. In a civil hospital, each ward (and each floor consequently) should be as separate and complete in itself as a family living on a flat in Paris. This is why I prefer the Lariboisière plan. The Bucks Infirmary is a good adaptation for a *small* civil hospital of the pavilion.

You don't want a cat! do you, for your young people, a Persian, NOT thoroughbred, 4½ months old?

I ought to send a copy of my *Notes on Hospitals* to *Varrentrapp*. Can you tell me his address and how to send it? Did you see him at Berlin?

Royal Hospital for Incurables, 1861

Editor: Nightingale was consulted in 1861 about a new building for the Royal Hospital for Incurables. The hospital had been founded in 1854, and was then in temporary quarters near Croydon, adjacent to a related charity. It is not clear what role she played as there was great dissension on the board about moving or staying at the original site. Some leading members left and formed a new society, and built on the Croydon site. The (remaining) board had a new building put up in Putney, later expanded. Nightingale wrote two detailed letters to the person who had requested her advice, but it is not clear if her advice was used for either building.

After a major extension was made to the Putney building, finished in 1881, Nightingale assisted the hospital in finding a new superintendent of nursing, St Thomas'-trained Ulrike N. Linicke.[89] In 1995 the hospital was renamed the Royal Hospital for Neuro-Disability.

Source: From two letters to Frederick Andrew,[90] Royal Hospital for Incurables, both from Hampstead, N.W.

4 September 1861

I have only this morning received your note of the 26 August. To answer your questions first, i.e., as well as I can without knowing your selected site, upon the character of which, of course, every requirement of cubic space, etc., must depend.

1. "A single room for *one* patient" cannot have less than 2500 cub. ft., or about 150 sq. ft.

2.3. For every patient where the number exceeds two, I should give 1500 cub. ft., or about 100 sq. ft. It matters not whether they have a "day room" or not.

4. For "day rooms" 600 cub. ft. for each patient, or about 50 sq. ft.

I regret to see the word "corridor" used. A "corridor," if it means a long room with windows on one side, can rarely be kept healthy. As you do not "enclose" the "list of maladies under which the patients suffer," nor any indication of the proposed site (which, however, I take for granted is in the country, as it ought to be), I can but add a few general hints.

1. *Superficial area signifies a great deal more than cubic space.* Indeed a height of about 17 ft. is actually, in my opinion, prejudicial. But a height under 14 ft. is certainly so.

2. In a *very* airy site, the "1500 cc. ft." I prescribed might be lowered to 1200 cc. ft. But *only in large wards.*

3. All the wards and day rooms should be ventilated and warmed on the new principles of the "Barrack and Hospital Improvement" Commission.

4. Of course it is not intended that *anyone* at all should sleep in the day rooms.

5. I have given my reasons (in all my published books) for objecting to "wards of from three [to] eight beds," and for preferring "wards of from twenty [to] thirty-two beds." Privacy does not extend beyond the bed on each side the patient. And if he has one bed on each side

---

89 In *Extending Nursing* (13:167-73).

90 Letters also published in G.C. Cook, *Victorian Incurables: A History of the Royal Hospital for Neuro-Disability, Putney.*

of him, he may as well have ten, whereas nursing, in any sense of the word, is impossible in the smaller wards.

Women fit to be head nurses are not, alas, so common. And one such can easily overlook thirty-two beds in the same ward, cannot possibly overlook them in "wards of from three [to] eight beds." In like manner, I would only assign single rooms to "noisy" or "offensive" patients, or such as require absolute quiet and a *constant* watcher.

I do not presume to say more. Because I do not know the character of your requirements, I will only add:

1. I have had large experience among both patients who go into hospital and those who ordinarily do not.

2. Among the "incurables" whom I have nursed, there has always been a large proportion who required that kind of nursing which, in my opinion, can only be given in large wards, and who would certainly have been neglected in the smaller wards, each of which *can*not be put under one head nurse.

I shall be most happy to render any assistance in looking over plans, or in answering any questions. But it must be before the 12th of this month, or after 1st November. And in my state of health, which may terminate my power of work at any moment, you are much more certain of having me this month than in November. I shall be very happy to contribute towards your building if it is on principles conducive, in my opinion, to the welfare of the sick.

3. In some *new* convalescent institutions abroad, wards of three or four have been found to answer, with day and exercise rooms. But as soon as the convalescents became PATIENTS they had to be transferred to the infirmary wards. I imagine that some of your "incurables" are like the "convalescents," in the sense that they don't require the nursing of *patients*. For such I should not object to the three-bed wards and should think three or four better than eight-bed wards. For such I should not object to single rooms, except on account of expense. But, for those who require Nursing, whether "incurables," operations, accidents or "sick," every year only confirms my experience that from twenty- to thirty-two-bed wards are the best.

4. The material of your walls and ceiling and of your floors is of immense importance.

5. As a *general* rule, hospitals cut up into small wards require more cubic space than hospitals with large wards. In a certain sense, a patient profits by all the space (the air) in his ward, e.g., an "offen-

sive" case does more mischief in one eight-bed ward than in a thirty-two-bed ward. Popularly, it is supposed to be just the reverse.

10 September 1861

The list of patients you have enclosed rather confirms me in what I have stated, but is too small in numbers for me to come to any definite conclusion. I should require to know the numbers for whom you intend to build, whether equal for men and women, etc. One curious fact comes out of your list of "candidates" "as home patients" that there are two men to thirty women.

I should classify such cases as those in the list into one large and seven small wards. But, as I say, the numbers are too few to judge. It is certainly impossible to put an aneurism of the aorta into the same ward with an epilepsy case.

I am not aware whether your "out-patients" tally with what we call "out-patients" at general hospitals, or whether they are cases waiting to come in. I think the list bears out the remarks I have made, on the whole, and shows that more than ordinary care is requisite in arranging the details of the plans. If you desire me to look at them, I should prefer seeing the rough draft plans first, in order to avoid expensive alterations afterwards.

Your site is well chosen. The gravelly soil about Croydon is good. But it requires to be very carefully drained and for your hospital to be well raised [breaks off]

"Winchester Infirmary," Hampshire County Hospital, 1858-64

Editor: Nightingale's involvement in the lengthy and complicated process of planning a new hospital at Winchester[91] was considerable and ultimately successful. The Nightingale family home was at nearby Embley Park, so that she (and her family) knew the main actors. When she found out how bad the existing hospital was, she was incensed that such death rates should occur in a hospital "in my own county town" (see p 589 below). After some years of manoeuvring, the decision was made to build a completely new building on a healthier site.

The correspondence reveals family strains. Her father was a governor of the hospital and supported the old guard, who merely wanted

91 For background on the hospital see Barbara Carpenter Turner, *A History of the Royal Hampshire County Hospital.*

expansion (see p 620 below). By 1860, however, Nightingale herself had become adamant that both a new building and a different site were essential for good health. Cubic space at the existing hospital was inadequate—less than that required for a workhouse infirmary—and the sub-soil was contaminated as the town was unsewered. No amount of cubic space would make the wards healthy, Nightingale repeatedly said.

The correspondence begins in 1858, with information from family members about rebuilding the infirmary. Nightingale was keen to advise on the planning, but had not been formally invited to do so. She had let it be known that she would be willing to go over the plans, but she was not sent any at this point. The next stage starts in 1860, with the publication of data about the hospital's inordinately high death rate from erysipelas. No less than twenty-four patients had fallen ill of the disease, of whom eight died and another sixteen barely escaped death (see p 589 below), out of a total patient load of only 100. Nightingale was so disturbed by the data that she showed them to "most of the eminent surgeons in London," and to the Registrar-General (see p 594 below).

A major breakthrough occurred early in 1861 when Robert Rawlinson, in his capacity as chief engineering inspector for the Local Government Board, was asked to inspect the hospital along with the local sewerage and drainage. A friend of Nightingale's from his time on the sanitary commission during the Crimean War, Rawlinson naturally consulted her before going and shared his findings with her later. The hospital was situated within the town, the sub-soil was wet, and such sewers as there were ended in cesspools. The hospital rooms were not large, but were said to be clean. "Erysipelas prevails at times," he had been told, but his informant had added that "erysipelas is common to all hospitals." Rawlinson rhetorically wondered why he was needed if the ventilation was as "good" as he had been told it was. He would decline a fee, he told Nightingale, as he did not expect his findings to be liked. She replied promptly, with advice. Rawlinson in turn promised to report back to her as he was to meet the chair of the building committee, Sir William Heathcote, and the county gentlemen.[92] He duly produced a strong and unambiguous report, which Nightingale would cite in making her case for a new building and site.

---

92 Rawlinson letters 11 and [12-14] January [1861], Add Mss 45769 ff3-8 and 9-10.

By January 1861 Nightingale was able to state that she and Rawlinson would fight to the bitter end for removing the existing building and constructing a new infirmary. She used numerous connections to get through to decision makers. For example, she asked Douglas Galton, who was both a close collaborator and husband of a cousin, for help in persuading another cousin, the local MP: "would you please devote the first day of every week—till further notice—in driving nails into Jack Bonham Carter, MP, about the Winchester Infirmary? (see p 592 below).

The husband of an old friend, Louisa Ashburton (1827-1903) was Lord Ashburton (1799-1864), a major local landowner and prospective donor. Nightingale requested that her friend urge her husband, when asked for his contribution, to insist on first seeing the expert report condemning the old hospital and its site. In fact, Lord Ashburton made his £1000 donation conditional on a new building and site (see p 592 below).

It took a long time to persuade the head of the leading local family, Sir William Heathcote (1801-81), fifth baronet of Hursley, of the merits of a new start. One complication was that his family had owned the old building. When he did accede, Nightingale was magnanimous in crediting him with bringing the committee around. She was clearly hurt that her father did not respect her expertise, but was instead complacent about conditions that killed large numbers of people, conditions that Nightingale called "willful murder" to two other correspondents (see pp 589 and 594 below). The charge was reduced in another letter to mere "manslaughter," for repeating "experiments on the sick poor" (see p 595 below).

In 1862 Nightingale declared "victory" with the decision to move the hospital to a new site (see p 608 below). Her £100 contribution to the building fund was promptly publicized in the hospital appeal. Her father, though much wealthier, also gave £100.[93] The queen made a personal contribution, perhaps because her private home, Osborne, was nearby. Lord Ashburton's £1000 contribution led the list.

Generally referred to as the Winchester Infirmary, although sometimes abbreviated to "Winton," the proper name for the hospital was the Hampshire County Hospital, Winchester, with the "Royal" designation added when the queen gave it this honour in 1868. Further

93 Hampshire County Hospital, Winchester Building Committee 3 February 1862, Florence Nightingale Museum (LMA) H1/ST/NC2/V3/62.

background is given later on the selection of the architect, as the person mentioned as the architect in the letter immediately below was not in fact chosen (see p 620 below). The letter, however, is of interest also for its condemnation of the plans of King's College Hospital, perhaps Nightingale's star example of bad design.

Source: From two letters to Parthenope Verney, Wellcome (Claydon copy) Ms 8997/71-72, both from Great Malvern

Sunday 1 August 1858

I saw the architect, Bellamy, before I left town, à propos to the new plans of King's College Hospital, which are his, which are execrable and which he brought me. (Farr and Bellamy are my darlings.) I was so good as to hold forth upon sanitary architecture, which he received as from the mouth of an oracle. (Of course he ought.) But the gist of this is that he told me he was to build the new Winchester Hospital for Sir W. Heathcote and would be glad of my advice (sic). Nothing is to be done directly but, as you gave me some message from Sir W. Heathcote about it once, I should be very glad, as Bellamy is the architect, to help and to make it the model of its set, an example for all time.

14 August 1858

My dear, I never answered your note about Sir W. Heathcote. I would never undertake to give advice about the administration of any hospital, unless I were able to go and look into it personally. Cela va sans dire [that goes without saying] it seems to me. And this was what I understood from you, a long time ago, Sir W.H. wanted of me.

Plans are quite a different thing. I could give a judgment about plans, both as to sanitary and administrative points, by simply looking at them. And this was what Mr Bellamy told me was what was wanted, with regard to Winchester. But he also said the plans were not even planned yet. If, when they are, Sir W.H. would like to put me in communication with Mr Bellamy on the subject, I am very much at his service, and have no hesitation in offering mine, because it is very evident, from recent showing, that the subject of the health of hospitals is a totally unknown and unstudied one, and chiefly so to and by doctors and architects.

Source: From a letter to James Paget, Add Mss 45797 ff198-99

29 April 1860

I enclose you some papers with regard to the Winchester Infirmary. Please return them to me as soon as possible.

Here is an indictment to which the verdict must be "willful murder." Here are, in nine months, in a country hospital (of only 100 patients) and by no means the worst of its class, twenty-four poor creatures brought together to run the gauntlet of their lives, through erysipelas, contracted *in* the hospital, of whom eight perish and sixteen just escape with life from this fatal building. Depend upon it, other hospitals, if as well inquired into, would give as disastrous or *more* disastrous results.

It is not the cubic space but the ward construction (other causes which make foul the ward air) which produces the result in *this* case. We are trying to get this hospital removed and rebuilt, and I think I have a fine handle in my hands with this table.

Source: From a letter to Robert Rawlinson, Boston University 1/2/21

13 January 1861

I am very sorry to be able to give you so little assistance in my own county town in such a good work. With regard to the sewerage your only hope is to convert the farmers and to show them the advantage of the sewage in agriculture. They will not let you turn the sewage into the Itchin [River]. And Winchester is without an outlet. We had all this up, *à propos* to the Winchester Barracks, two years ago. With regard to the hospital, it is many years since I was there. But my impression is that nothing but rebuilding and removing it would be of any use. That this impression was shared by others, with recent local knowledge, you may infer from this—that two years ago I was consulted about the rebuilding of this hospital, and I offered my assistance in plans, etc., *but the plans never came.*

I am quite sick of the old excuse heard by me some thousand of times, "gratuitous medical advice must not make the doctors go too far," etc. Then all I can say is, *let the doctors stay at home*, and *let the patients stay at home.* Or do you wish the alternative to be ten lives out of every hundred sacrificed to a bad hospital?

I am happy to say I know at least one surgeon in a city of the North who, to his own great personal inconvenience, rather chooses to attend his own poor patients (accidents) at their own homes, than to send them to the infirmary in the town—and this, although he has vast distances to traverse. Gangrene and erysipelas, he says, are what they will find *there.* And these Winchester people dare to say that, in what *ought* to be as healthy a little county town as any in England, these hospital diseases are "inevitable"!! They *don't have a hospital at all.*

You have so little notice—else I could have helped your good work by writing to my cousin, Mr Bonham Carter, MP, Sir William Heathcote, Lord Ashburton, Lord Eversley,[94] all of whom I believe might be enlightened and stirred up. My father has little or no influence in the northern division of the county. But I hope, if you are going to sleep out, you would do so at Embley (Romsey Station) and I will write to him and say so.

Would you give me an answer as to these gentlemen?

Source: From a letter to Harry Verney, Wellcome (Claydon copy) Ms 8999/3

18 January [1861]

Mr Rawlinson, C.E., and I are going to fight the battle *à outrance* [to the bitter end] for removing and rebuilding the Winchester Infirmary. I think I have got the perfection of a plan now, which I invented for one of our regimental hospitals. It is on the same principle as your Bucks Infirmary, and as a pencil sketch I sent you, and which you have returned, but is, I think, an improvement. It consists of two wings of two floors of wards, each with small wards in front, but open space between, up to the door—kitchen and offices pushed out behind.

Would you be so good as to tell me the rough general estimate of your plan, without the ground, and the number of beds? This would help us much. . . .

Would you be so good as to tell Parthe that I have received a request from a celebrated man, Dr Ross of Altona, through a Dr Lappenberg of Hamburg,[95] to translate my *Notes on Nursing* into German. I cannot help thinking that poor Frances Bunsen[96] would be very glad to be relieved

94 Charles Shaw-Lefevre (1794-1881) made Viscount Eversley, on his retirement as speaker of the House of Commons, a Hampshire family friend.

95 Dr Ludwig Ross, a much-published classicist and archeologist; Johann Martin Lappenberg (1794-1864), a medically trained historian. Altona is a district of Hamburg.

96 Frances von Bunsen (c1791-1876), an Englishwoman married to Christian von Bunsen, former Prussian ambassador in England.

of it. This is the fifth I have had from *good* German doctors. I have forwarded the letter to Mr Clough and asked him to write to Parthe.

Source: From a letter to Douglas Galton, Add Mss 45759 ff145-46

19 January 1861

Mr Rawlinson, c.e., has been called in to examine the town and hospital of Winchester, *qua* drainage. Winchester is not sewered and he wants to know whether the government would bear its share of the expense for the barracks, instead of shirking it, as it always does—whether it would pay £1000, which would be about its proportion for the barracks to the population, on condition that it were satisfied as to the plan of sewerage proposed—which is, as I understand, to find the barracks with an outlet, which now have none. If I am indistinct, please talk to Dr Sutherland, who will be with you today.

2. The removal and rebuilding of the hospital comes into the plan. I am going to send Mr Rawlinson your pencil plan for the Bucks Infirmary, which they have copied and returned. Also, could you give me a tracing or lithograph of the last duplicate regimental hospital, with wards (little) sticking out in front and space between up to front door? Also, a rough general estimate of expense, with number of beds—Mr Mennie said, I think, that this one, which has two floors of wards, would be £80 or £90 per bed.

The Winchester Infirmary would require 112 beds, and I think, with a few civil modifications, this last regimental plan would do. I have written for the Bucks estimate to Mr Brandon in like manner.

Source: From a typed copy of a letter and a letter to Robert Rawlinson, Florence Nightingale Museum (LMA) H1/ST/NC5/3/16 and Boston University 1/2/22

19 January 1861

1. I have written to the W.O. to ask it what it will do to help in sewering Winchester.

2. I am getting estimates of the cost of sundry hospitals for you per bed.

I send a pencil sketch which was made to revise sundry defects in a plan for a new Bucks Infirmary which is building. If the lower floor, instead of being offices, were wards, and the offices pushed out behind, it would about meet your requirements.

I have written to the W.O. for a tracing of a new regimental hospital on this plan, which will cost about £80 or £90 per bed. Civil building might probably reach £100 per bed.

20 January 1861

The W.O., with unusual promptitude, which shows it thinks itself getting off very cheaply, "will certainly be prepared to support the proposal of paying £1000 towards sewerage for Winchester Barracks." x x We "have never been able to get any outlet."

I could not ascertain whether you thought I had better write to Sir William Heathcote and others about the removal of the hospital. When you saw them, what was their temper about it? Sometimes one only complicates matters by putting one's foot in the dish.

I asked Dr Sutherland to find out from you what you thought best. My sister is going down to Embley on Wednesday and would drive over to Sir William Heathcote's and say anything we wished. I certainly never would advise any of the old hospitals to spend money on alterations.

Source: From a letter to Douglas Galton, Add Mss 45759 f180

10 February 1861

Also, would you please devote the first day of every week—till further notice—in driving nails into Jack Bonham Carter, MP, about the Winchester Infirmary?

Rawlinson, C.E., who has been down to look at it (as well as at the drainage), told me that the sub-soil was tainted past the power of cure—that there were wards so bad they could not let the committee into them (only the patients), that erysipelas was confessed to, that the cubic space is scanty, the site overcrowded—that they allow they must add to the hospital to the sum of £6000—for £12,000, he says, they might (selling the old hospital and site perhaps for £3500) have a new hospital on virgin soil, with light and air. . . .

I have been pegging into Sir William Heathcote. Do tell J.B.C. that they are quite behind the times—Rawlinson has sent in his report—a very good one.

Editor: At this point Nightingale appealed to Louisa Ashburton to get her husband to use his influence as a major (prospective) donor:

> They must rebuild on a better site. I hope that, if Lord Ashburton is applied to, which he is sure to be, he will require a copy to be sent him of the report of Mr Rawlinson, a civil engineer (who was sent for to examine it) and which is admirable. And I trust you will persuade him to give his influence to *rebuild and remove.* Patients had much better stay at home than go into the present hospital. So much for the ancient city of Winchester.[97]

97 Letter 11 March 1861, in *Women* (8:720).

Source: From a letter to Robert Rawlinson, Boston University 1/2/26

29 April 1861

I don't know whether you have seen the enclosed papers with regard to the Winton Infirmary. Please return them to me.

Here is an indictment to which the verdict must be "willful murder." Here are, in nine months, in a county hospital (of only 100 patients), by no means the worst of its class, twenty-four poor creatures brought together to run the gauntlet of their lives—of disease contracted in the hospital. . . .

It is not the deficient cubic space so much as the ward construction and other causes making foul the ward air which produces this result. Depend upon it, other hospitals, if as well inquired into, will give as disastrous results or more so. I mean to threaten the hospital authorities with publishing this, in order to make them do what we like.

Sir W. Heathcote is quite come round to our side. I send you a report which Colonel Kennedy has made for me in Paris on the new Male Convalescent Civil Hospital there—near Vincennes. I think it more nearly approaches to your idea of the separate cottages for convalescents than anything that could have been planned. There are obvious defects in it, on which we could improve. But I am afraid we might have waited long before an English architect's ingenuity would have produced such a plan. It strikes me as so very good. . . .

Please return this report to me as soon as possible.

Source: From three letters to Harry Verney, Wellcome (Claydon copy) Ms 8999/18-19 and 34, typed copy of the first Add Mss 45791 f12

25 May 1861

As my name has been dragged into a discussion before the committee of Winchester Infirmary, with reference to a request that the facts (almost unparallelled in a civil hospital) of the enormous mortality from erysipelas in that infirmary might be used as a proof of the absolute necessity of shutting up the present building as soon as possible, and as the committee have declined to grant such permission, I feel bound at least to enter my protest against the continuance of such a state of things for one moment longer than necessary to provide new buildings.

The table, viewed in any way, is a sentence of condemnation of the existing building. What can you call it but a pest house, when a number of people are exposed to the risk of fatal illness from a special hospital disease, while several have been literally killed offhand?

The question for the county is whether this is to be allowed to go on? Are we Hampshire people to go on tolerating an institution which sends a number to their graves by a disease which I, with my hospital experience, know need never appear at all in a well-constructed [breaks off]

26 May 1861

I am most happy to be able to say that, before I received the resolution of the Winchester Infirmary in favour of having erysipelas within their walls, I had already shown their table to most of the eminent surgeons in London, and given it to the Registrar-General.

I have arranged with him that he should only use it thus. He is to call for the Winchester Infirmary deaths, which are just coming in. He will see that they are too many. And you will then be all struck with astonishment at the *unfailing sagacity* and at the *unerring law* with which he will make out the excess of deaths from erysipelas, and all upon your paper, which he is not to see.

I send you a note, which you can forward or not as you think best, to the Winchester people who prefer erysipelas. I have had the statistics of St Thomas' Hospital ransacked by the resident medical officer, who was also always in the wards besides. And I find that in this, one of the largest hospitals and one of the worst situations in London, the comparison with a small infirmary [Winchester] in one of the healthiest counties in England [Hampshire] stands thus: St Thomas' 1860, twelve months, 500 beds (upwards of 450 constantly filled), erysipelas *occurred in hospital* thirteen cases, *no* death, *admitted* seventy-two cases phlegmonous [inflammation] and simple erysipelas, of which (phlegmonous erysipelas) *three* died. Winchester, 1860, nine months, 120 beds, erysipelas occurred in hospital twenty-four cases, eight deaths, and possibly they did not *admit* any, while St Thomas' admits seventy-two cases of this (said to be) most infectious disease. It is, you know, willful murder. . . .

I am going to show the Winchester resolution in favour of erysipelas to the Registrar-General. It is quite as strong a case against them as the facts themselves. Or rather it completes the case against them.

Hampstead, N.W.
12 September 1861

I will answer Sir William Heathcote's note first:

1. Mr Rawlinson's *report* entirely settled the question of the Winchester Hospital. The sub-soil is tainted beyond the power of cure. The construction and internal arrangements are bad. In nine months in a hospital of only 100-120 beds, they cause twenty-four unfortunate

creatures to run the gauntlet of their lives with erysipelas—of whom eight die—a circumstance wholly unprecedented in my experience of hospital massacres—excepting at Scutari during a short period. So that Winchester aspires to rival the most colossal calamity of history in its small way.

In a London hospital of 500 beds, badly situated by the river, in the twelve months of 1860, only thirteen cases of erysipelas occurred *in* the hospital and without a single death—whereas seventy-two cases of erysipelas, simple and phlegmonous, were admitted in the same period, of which three only died (all of the latter severe form when admitted).

To the tainted sub-soil alone the Winchester deaths cannot be referred, but to the other errors of its construction also. The Winchester Hospital committee is therefore going to meet to discuss whether they shall try to do a thing which is impossible—or whether they shall not rather do what is in accordance with common sense. They are going to consider whether they can make a hospital which killed eight people by erysipelas alone kill fewer in future—or whether they should not build a hospital where erysipelas will not show its face.

Judging by what I know about the present building, I have no hesitation in saying that, if they try their hands at "adaptation," they will fail, and not only throw away their money, but kill more patients before they finally make up their minds to give up a site and building where sick ought never to be placed. Hampshire should have as good a hospital as any county in England. And why in these days men should even raise the question of preserving the present building passes my comprehension.

I understand that Lord Ashburton will give £1000 towards a new hospital if built upon a new site. If not, nothing. I would gladly give what I can out of my own earnings,[98] which would be £50 and might be £100, and I believe my father would give as much more. And I would gladly revise and consider the plans for a new building, if desired to do so. But I should be guilty of that crassa ignorantia which lawyers tell me is a ground of verdict of manslaughter if I helped the committee in any way to repeat experiments on the sick poor.

Captain Galton is now building a pavilion hospital (sixty beds) for a regiment at £70 per bed—with every modern appliance—the more

98 A reference to her royalties, as Nightingale did not ever receive income for her work as a nurse or administrator.

extraordinary in cheapness as the number of beds is so few. The pavilions are end-to-end as in your new Bucks Infirmary—two wards of twenty-eight beds and two of two. It will become cheaper to build good hospitals than bad.

With regard to Sir W. Heathcote's other questions:

2. I send him by post today (to save time) a copy of my *Notes on Hospitals*, second edition. But will you tell him that I am at this moment employed by Parker to write a third edition, leaving out all the Crimean part—and adding to all the construction and arrangement parts which refer to all hospitals. And I shall be undone if he does not return me my copy (at his convenience) as this edition is entirely out of print. And, strange to say, the War Office continually refer to me for information out of it.

The report of the Barrack Commission, in speaking of *military* hospitals, really refers to *all*, as far as construction goes. But I shall be most happy, when it comes to building, to say in what internal arrangements consists the difference between civil and military hospitals, hospitals where both sexes are, and all nurses are female, and hospitals where adult men only are patients, and all or most of the nurses are men. Otherwise, that report is a capital guide.

3. I know of no better "authority" than Mr Rawlinson on the points on which he has already reported. And he "examined the hospital on the spot." When it comes to construction, I am sure that Dr Sutherland, either with Mr Rawlinson or alone, will gladly "examine any sites which may be suggested and advise." I wish that Sir W. Heathcote's letter had come one day earlier, as Dr Sutherland and Captain Galton have just sailed for the Mediterranean inspection.

But I regret this the less as, having fully discussed the subject of the Winchester Infirmary with Dr Sutherland and Mr Rawlinson, I am able to say that Dr Sutherland declared that "nothing would induce him to have any hand in recommending any alterations in the present building on the present site." And if he "were to examine the hospital 'on the spot' twenty times" (he has inspected it) "he could not say otherwise."

I know no authority in Europe to compare with that of Dr Sutherland in the sanitary construction of buildings and the inspection of sites. He will be home early in November or before, and I will let you or Sir W. Heathcote know. Finally, I repeat, I shall be too glad to advise, criticize and consider any draft plans which may be sent me, but only for a *new building on a new site.*

Source: From an incomplete letter probably to Parthenope Verney, Wellcome (Claydon copy) Ms 8999/60

[ca. September 1861]

Winchester Infirmary existing site and buildings worth to sell, say, £3500; alterations as estimated 6000; £9500 for an old building—patched up—on a FOUL SUB-SOIL in a crowded situation and with only two thirds the requisite cubic space ("a sub-soil so tainted as to be beyond the power of cure." This is the report on this infirmary). For a new hospital, on a VIRGIN *sub-soil*, with air and prospect, sun and cubic space and offices complete, *as now made*, for 112 beds, say, £12,000.

Suppose you ask Sir William Heathcote to send me a copy of Mr Rawlinson's report—this is a way to "entrer en matière [get into the substance]," although nothing can make me think the place worse than I do.

I will return Mr Brandon's letter to Sir Harry: £7250 for fifty beds [Bucks Infirmary]. I do not think by a rule of three that £12,000 for 112 beds is an unlikely proportion. Of course the smaller a hospital, the dearer it is.

A regimental hospital for 112 beds would cost us from £80 to £90 per bed. Civil building is dearer—say £100 per bed. That is, for the two pavilions-*in-line* plan.

Source: From a typed copy of a letter and a letter to Harry Verney, Add Mss 45791 ff17-20 and Wellcome (Claydon copy) Ms 8999/36, both from Hampstead, N.W.

14 September 1861

It occurred to me to send you again the heads of our indictment against Winchester Infirmary (for Sir William Heathcote), as Mr Rawlinson, Dr Sutherland and I considered them after consultation last January, in consequence of Mr Rawlinson's inspection.

1. The present building stands in the midst of houses on an undrained sub-soil. There are sewers and drains ending in a cesspool and forming part of the cesspool, with an overflow outlet in the hospital grounds. The surrounding sub-soil is saturated with its contents, and for many years past. The site could not be drained unless Winchester is sewered, and even then would be improper for a hospital, which ought to be on a proper site outside the town.

2. There are twenty-eight patients in five wards on the ground floor, with an average of under 1000 cub. ft. per bed; forty-three patients in four wards on the first floor with an average of under 1000 cub. ft. per

bed; forty-one patients in three wards on the second floor with an average of 900 cub. ft. per bed.

The proportion of surgical patients is sixty-eight out of 112 beds. *Half the beds ought to be removed at once.* Mr Rawlinson says 2000 cub. ft. per bed would not be enough. I have no hesitation in saying that a hospital which requires 2000 cub. ft. per bed ought not to be there at all. And this fact is in itself *prima facie* evidence against any hospital. If you want 2000 to make your beds healthy, your beds won't be healthy with 20,000. 1500 cub. ft. per bed is the proper allowance in any hospital which ought to be a hospital, excepting, of course, in a single or double-bed wards, which ought to have 2500 cub. ft.

The Barrack Commission gives only 1200 cub. ft. per bed, but this is in military hospitals, where half the patients are not patients, but only not fit to be on duty. This is one of the great differences between civil and military hospitals.

The small wards in the Winton Infirmary are altogether objectionable. What an idea to distribute twenty-eight patients in five wards. There is not one good ward in the place. I understand the average patients are as follow:

	Male	Female
(1) Accidents	7	--
(2) Venereal	6	6
(3) Surgical	36	25
(4) Medical	16	16
	65	47

I would follow this distribution and have six or seven wards accordingly, instead of twelve, which there are. But, excluding the (2) [venereal], which ought to be quite separate, you might have a very nice double pavilion, for men and for women, with one large medical and one large surgical ward on each floor or each side. It is useless, however, to show how this might be done when the question of removal is not yet decided.

3. I think I mentioned to you that, upon my application to the War Office—alas! during my dear master's reign—government consented to bear their fair share of expense for the barracks, if Winchester were sewered.

4. I understand that the committee (hospital) had estimated proposed alterations to give 1500 cub. ft. per bed at £6000. Existing site and buildings might sell at (say) 3500 [total] £9500. Therefore you have an old building, patched up, on the foulest of sub-soils, in a

crowded situation, and with only three fourths the requisite cubic space (for in that situation certainly 2000 cub. ft. will be necessary—and then it will not be healthy) to cost £9500. Whereas you might have a new hospital, with air and light and view and virgin sub-soil, to cost £12,000 *or less*. . . .

Mr Rawlinson, who is quite the first authority in England on drainage and sewerage, says that he can sewer Winchester for £12,000, and that the annual rate to extinguish the debt in thirty years will not exceed sixpence in the pound. As he has great works to show of this kind, in which the cost of main sewers in each city or town he has done never exceeded sixpence in the pound of the local rateable value, he deserves to be believed. And this is to make a sinking fund as well as to pay interest on the money borrowed and pay for local management.

25 September 1861

I don't know that I have any more to say about these terrible trees. It is obvious that one ward will *not* be affected by them, but that the others will. But as they do not appear to grow in a thick line or screen, and as they are to the north, it seems to me that, if necessary, to cut down any, the cutting down of one or two at most would do. And I can only say again what I did before that I could not take upon myself, *from what I know*, to advise the cutting of these fine trees.

But that, in the course of the winter, I could send somebody to look at them. And the committee could then decide which, if any, need be sacrificed. As I understand, the situation is an airy one, and rather exposed than the contrary. This makes all the difference.

Pray do not suppose that I said I had "rather Sir W. Heathcote should write to me." On the contrary, I had rather he wrote to you, but for the trouble to you. As it is, I am quite agreeable, if he likes to write direct. That is to say, I shall be very *dis*agreeable if he does not carry the removal of the hospital.

Source: From a letter to Robert Rawlinson, Boston University 1/2/29

Hampstead, N.W.
7 October 1861

Private. I have been engaged during your absence in furthering the removal of the Winchester Infirmary. A sub-committee has met for the purpose, but had adjourned decision till 5 November. Strange how little the best men will take the trouble to master the subject! I have had to write out the substance of your report all over again for

Sir William Heathcote. Lord Ashburton has however promised £1000, if the hospital is removed. If not, nothing.

You know that I have lost my dear master. Seven years this very month I have fought the good fight[99] for the army, in and out of the War Office, without the intermission of one single waking hour, and have lost it! Have you had an invitation from Malvern to give them a water supply?

Source: From typed copies of three letters to Sir William Heathcote, Add Mss 45798 ff5, 7-11 and 19-21, all from Hampstead

8 October 1861

I am glad that my hospital remarks were of any use to you. Of course what you call my "strictures" were meant only for the private consideration of yourself and Sir H. Verney. But Winchester is not sinning in ignorance so much as you think. Winchester sent for Mr Rawlinson in January and his January report did all that could be done in the way of information and advice.

I am glad you are going to see Aylesbury Infirmary. But I venture to remind you that their estimate was for £7377 for fifty-four beds, including cost of oak floors and polished Parian cement walls and ceilings in the wards—that their architect himself estimated the cost of *doubling* the accommodation for sick at only £1500 more, i.e., two wards under the original two—offices put out behind, operating room over offices. For, as you will see in the Aylesbury Infirmary, only 4508 square feet (out of more than 9000 square feet) are occupied by sick, the administrative offices actually occupying more room than the sick whom they are for.

The elevation also, though simple, is handsome and expensive. So that I should not fairly put the estimate of a hospital of *over* 100 beds at more than £90 to £95 per bed—*excluding* in each case the outpatients' offices, which cannot fairly be charged to the "per bed" expense.

I will most gladly put the whole of my hospital plans at your disposal, when you are farther advanced—as also consider and revise your draft plans, if you are so disposed—if you ever come to any. At this moment, I am being consulted by the Staffordshire Infirmary upon exactly the same premises. They want to do as you do.

99 Nightingale left for the Crimean War in October 1854; the biblical allusion is to 2 Tim 4:7.

In the War Office, we are now building regimental hospitals (with all the modern appliances) at only £70 per bed. But local institutions must make their own plans and their own estimates. Others can only revise them. Our Barrack and Hospital Commission will be home before 5 November and could be consulted by you (Captain Galton and Dr Sutherland). But we are so overwhelmed with business during the month of November that we hope this will not be done without necessity. . . .

Let me also remind you that it is not only cheaper but far more healthy to run all administrative offices out behind—instead of putting them under the wards, as at Aylesbury, and to have the sick and their attendants in the main building apart—which, after all, is built for sick.

12 October 1861

In answer to your note, I feel almost inclined to ask you (if, as I hear, you are passing through London this month) to drive down here and look over such plans as I have by me of hospitals. It would best answer Winchester questions. Should you have time and opportunity to do this, I would ask for a day's notice, that I may not be too much occupied to see you—also, that I may send you my address so as to find the house.

The points I would press by means of plans are:

1. That it is quite possible to "put the offices out behind" (connected with a covered way) at such a distance as neither "to form two corners," nor to be inconveniently far. The trouble to attendants is often objected. All that I answer is that it is actually done—in hospitals too of vast size—that the meals, etc., are conveyed upon a truck (and tramway, if desirable) and then up to the wards on lifts, and that the meals arrive hotter and with less trouble to attendants than with the ordinary rush and bustle and tray-carrying upstairs and sending nurses (or, what is worse, patients) to wait at the kitchen. All that is wanted is a little system, and you actually save one attendant to every thirty sick by this.

Whether the offices are one or two storeys high depends upon the nature of the site. In some confined sites, two storeys would be too high, but as they are behind the administrative and not the sick part rarely so. If too much, then have one.

The operating room may either be placed elsewhere (in a county hospital operations are comparatively few and the room may be comparatively small). Or even if it is put on the top of the offices (for the sake of wheeling the patient without difficulty into a ward on the same plane) it does not constitute a screen to free external ventilation or a whole second storey.

The main want in an operating room is to have *one* large high *north* window—no cross lights—easy access to a ward and not to be overlooked. All this may well be obtained over the offices.

2. I quite agree with you as to some points in the Bucks Infirmary. I am not its godmother. Indeed, I contended with Mr Carrington[100] about every single point you mention. Some I carried, because they had used my name in print without my authority, points left in (which I had expressly condemned). Lord Panmure once called me a "turbulent fellow" because I contended with him when in authority. I hope you will not do so.

I can readily understand that those who have not seen, with their own experience, the sick recover with direct fresh air, who would not otherwise have recovered, and the sick die (who would not otherwise have died) with foul air or air passing over other beds and not direct from the fresh air to them do call me a very "turbulent fellow." I am sure Mr Carrington does.

With regard to your prints, then, I do not know which were the Bucks Infirmary plans sent to you. (Nor can I send you mine for the North Staffordshire Infirmary have got them.) But there were considerable alterations made in the working plans from the lithographed set—unless indeed they have gone back to their old errors again. Among these were: kitchen removed to central building, laundry put out behind, three beds at *end* of each ward (which were quite inadmissible) abolished altogether, ward end window opened, ward end conveniences very much improved, fireplaces put on *opposite* sides of ward and not on the same side, etc. (My calculation of comparative sick area and administration area was made on the first plan. I throw all the *ward* offices, which are perfectly necessary—including nurse's room—into the sick area sum and call all offices *not* belonging directly to wards into the administration area sum. Probably this is our difference.)

The cubic space was, I believe, from the first plan enlarged. All civil hospitals should have 1500 c. ft. per bed in my opinion; 2000 may be necessary in London. But if necessary they show that the hospital ought not to be in that position at all. In other words, where a hospi-

100 George Carrington, chair of the Bucks Infirmary.

tal is unhealthy without 2000 c. ft. per bed, it will not be healthy *with* 2000 or 2500.

A wall space of 16 feet in width for *two* beds is certainly not too much. But it would be impossible in construction to put each bed exactly in the middle of its own territory. Let us not sacrifice the window space, whatever we do. Still it is better, if possible, to have an interval of *three* ft. between any two beds.

It is generally found that the more apart the out-patients' entrance is the better. It is particularly undesirable that there should be any possibility of communication, by signs or otherwise, between the out-patients and ward windows. And none of the attendants on the in-patients ought to be able to communicate with the out-patients. In well-regulated, large hospitals, even where the out-patients enjoy the advantage of the hospital baths, they are allowed no communication whatever. And the out-patients and in-patients bathe at different times. So with all dispensary work.

It would be impossible otherwise to preserve discipline. It is difficult enough to prevent spirits, etc., from being smuggled into the hospital, as it is. And all honest hospitals will tell you so. And alas! it is too difficult to prevent fresh appointments for vice [prostitution] being made for the women already in (from vice). This is again an experience of hard hospital life—not to be controverted by the inexperienced.

I enclose two tracings of a regimental hospital plan to illustrate my proposition of putting the offices out behind, and the possibility of having four little airy wards in front, if the doctors insist upon such small wards—I send it not for imitation but for illustration. Of course a civil hospital must be widely different. Would you kindly return these to me at once? I also send the foul copy, which turned up quite accidentally, of my criticisms on the first Bucks Infirmary plan, which suggested alterations that were, I understand, adopted. I only send this in case it should have been the *first* plan they sent you.

Please return me this memo, as these memoranda, which I had myself forgotten, are sometimes useful to me.

My cousin Bonham Carter, MP of Winton, has applied to me for information about the Winton Infirmary when he returns from abroad. Would you be so kind as to direct his attention to Mr Rawlinson's report? And would you kindly let him see all my letters to yourself and Sir Harry Verney forwarded to you—as I am unable to write any more than is absolutely necessary? I will desire him to apply to your kindness. . . .

P.S. The covered way to the kitchen should be a mere light, iron-pillared arcade (with glass to fill up the arches in winter, if you are inclined to be extravagant). If there is no operating room above, this covered way is only one storey high. Thus there can be no possibility of any "stagnation of air" thereby.

28 October [1861]

It is almost impossible to get the opinions of the practising physicians and surgeons of a hospital as to its healthiness: so many interests prevent them from even investigating the circumstances which would lead to any opinion worth giving, e.g., in London, one always hears that the hospital must be in the heart of the great thoroughfares, "because of the accidents." But ask to look over the hospital books, and you will find that, with the single exception of the London Hospital, which is near the docks, the majority of the accidents, in some cases a vast majority, come from a distance. St Thomas', the second most important of the London hospitals, showed upon examination of his books a complete refutation of the argument universally used against removing him, and that he would be positively nearer the majority of his cases at Blackheath than in London. I do not believe that, if this fact were really recognized, physicians and surgeons, who more than any other profession give knowledge in charity, would ever again bring forward the plea that it is too far for themselves and their schools to go to a healthy hospital a little out of town, instead of to an unhealthy one *in town*.

You often hear the argument used—oh but any hospital is more healthy than the poor people's homes. In the first place it is not true, and in the second, would it be an argument for not making the hospital as healthy as possible?

I would bring as authorities Mr Whitfield, the able resident medical officer for fifty years of St Thomas' Hospital, [and] Mr Roberton, the well-known Manchester surgeon and perhaps the first medical authority in England on hospital construction, whose letter on the Manchester Infirmary I enclose, begging that it may be returned to me. These are two men who have nothing to gain or to lose, and who speak their experience—the experience of half a century—freely, which is, that patients, doctors, schools, would all alike gain by being removed out of town, and that another century will consider it the most barbarous proof of a nation's want of civilization that any hospital should be found within the precincts of a town. . . .

Of course in crowded cities the Paris plan must be adopted, which is to have an accident ward or two near any place where accidents *are* continually happening (which are after all, very few) as a succursale [branch] to the great hospital on the outskirts. Or, you must frankly calculate the percentage of life you will sacrifice to a neighbouring and a crowded site for your hospital.

I also add the letter of a Dr Pincoffs[101] about the Manchester Infirmary, also begging that it may be returned to me. (He is half German, half Manchester, was employed at Scutari, afterwards in Syria during the massacres—and is well known to me as an able man who has thoroughly studied the hospital question.)

Mr Paget, the great surgeon of St Bartholomew, has given it as his opinion that healthy accidents, strong men coming in from the country, suffer materially from their hospital sojourn in towns. And the opinion is so well recognized in Paris that it is as little questioned there as the reverse is questioned here.

Source: From a letter to Robert Rawlinson, Boston University 1/2/30

Hampstead, N.W.
30 October 1861

I must congratulate you on having taken the Home Office position[102] and congratulate you all the more because I am afraid it involves a considerable money sacrifice on your part. I don't know any man (or hardly any man) but yourself who would have done it.

I hope and believe that the good you will do will be equal to your motive in thus accepting. For you are our only sanitary engineer. Does the appointment exclude you from private practice? entirely?

[continued]

Since I wrote this, I have your note about Winton Infirmary. Sir W. Heathcote, my cousin [John] Bonham Carter and my father, and Lord Ashburton have all expected me to write them information separately, which information was of course only a résumé of your report and of my book (on hospitals). Still, I have done it, although these gentlemen might have read the originals. I do not think that I have anything to add to you.

---

101 Peter Pincoffs (1816-72), a civilian doctor who served during the Crimean War, and later settled in Manchester. Thousands were massacred in 1860 in Christian-Muslim conflicts in what is now Lebanon and Syria.

102 Rawlinson became chief engineering inspector for the Local Government Board.

The Bucks Infirmary was contracted for at £7377, including polished Parian cement for walls and ceilings of wards, and oak floors for wards (beds fifty-four). But Mr Brandon (the architect) himself estimated that the beds might be doubled, at a farther cost of only £1500, i.e., two wards under the two present ones, where the administrative offices now are (much too good) these put out behind. (This does not include the cost of out-patients' offices, which it is not fair to put down to cost of beds).

The plans (which you saw) are, as you will perhaps remember, two pavilions end-to-end. And the elevation is by no means an *in*expensive one. Captain Galton, R.E., of the War Office, is now building a regimental hospital of only sixty beds at £70 per bed (exclusive of cost of site), with all the modern appliances (two pavilions, also end-to-end). But this is a wonder of cheapness. Also the cubic space is only 1200 feet per bed. On the whole, I think a civil hospital of ABOVE 100 beds may be built at a cost of £90 to £95 per bed (exclusive of cost of site). And if you say £100 per bed, you will be quite safe—cost of materials, labour, etc., varying so much in different counties. I put 1500 cubic feet per bed to this estimate.

Blackburn Infirmary was, as you know, of a monstrous and useless cost (eight eight-bed pavilions). I speak of pavilions exclusive of cost of site and also of out-patients' offices of reasonable size, i.e., wards of twenty-eight to thirty-two beds at 1500 cubic feet per bed. And two floors of wards.

If you will look at the Barrack Report of this year, p 185, Fig. 87, you will see the regimental hospital now building at £70 per bed.

The N. Staffordshire Infirmary is also going to build, and they have all my plans and estimates now to look at.

Source: From a letter to W.E. Nightingale, dictated to Hilary Bonham Carter, Add Mss 45790 ff231-34

Saturday 9 November 1861

Dear Uncle, Flo bids me write for her. "The reason why a hospital should always be" kept at above 100 beds, if possible, is a vital one, for by the medical acts the graduation of a medical man depends upon it. In this graduation no attendance at a hospital of *under* a hundred beds counts. For London hospitals the number has even been raised recently. You will see at once that it is fatal to a provincial hospital, even pecuniarily, if it cannot rank as a medical school for medical educational purposes, and this is the reason why Winchester does quite right to struggle if possible to keep itself up above 100 beds, and if Winchester is going to build a new and healthy hospital on the best type, it seems to me a most extraordinary discouragement to the good side if you withdraw your subscription from good and energetic Winchester to give it to Southampton or Salisbury or Reading or Portsmouth, all of which are worse one than the other, all of which are sunk in the blackest depths of sanitary ignorance, and not one of which has made the slightest effort to better itself, Reading excepted, which got itself reported upon by Rawlinson last winter, but has satisfied itself with getting itself reported upon and has done nothing since.

It seems to me that the logically good act is for you to subscribe to the *best* and not to the *nearest*, hospital and to send the patients where they will get well, though it may be a little farther off. I even told Sir William Heathcote, some time ago when I communicated to him Lord Ashburton's message, namely, that if the hospital were removed he would give £1000, if *not* nothing, that I thought you would give from £50 to £100 on the same condition. I fancied I had understood this from you. It was the condition I made for myself, viz., that I would give £50 to £100 from my own private earnings, if they removed, and I am sure I understood from you that you meant to encourage them by money.

The hospital movement is becoming general throughout the country, and you Hampshire people will be left quite in the dark ages if you don't take care. You ought to force Salisbury, Southampton, Reading and Portsmouth to go and do likewise[103] by your example at Winton. I am doing the very same thing just now for the North Stafford Infirmary, to which I have furnished plans, and for the Royal Hospital,[104] which I am striving to do for the Winton Beotians,[105] so let them draw back and stay in the last rank if they like it. But surely there will be enough in the advanced guard to prevent that!

---

103 Luke 10:37.

104 Possibly the Royal Hospital for Incurables, but only scant information is available on the point (see p 583 above).

105 In the Persian Wars, fifth century B.C.E., the Beotians sided with the invaders against Athens; they were treacherous again during the Peloponnesian Wars of the next century, siding first with Sparta, then Athens. Nightingale's father had studied classics at university and would have appreciated the classical allusion.

Source: From typed copies of two letters to Sir William Heathcote, Add Mss 45798 ff43 and 50

23 December 1861

I admire your resolutions, *qua* Winchester Hospital, which are very thorough. As to sites, the shortest way would be to look out for them. And when a few have been fixed upon, to have down Dr Sutherland (or better still Dr Sutherland and Mr Rawlinson together) to choose you the best out of those available.

Dr Sutherland is in the employ of government and you could not offer him money remuneration. But I have already communicated your note to him, and he will be very glad to go down and advise for the day. But we are so excessively busy just now, as you may suppose, that it could only be for the day. And even that is difficult to spare now.

23 January 1862

It is a great victory to have persuaded Winchester to remove her hospital and mainly, if not entirely, due to you.

In answer to your question, it would be unadvisable to build a hospital near a railway. If the four acres were nearly square, the distance would not be more than 150 yards. The hospital would look on the rail much as the north wing of St Thomas' Hospital, London (which hospital is now about to be removed), looks on the road leading up to the railway at London Bridge. The noise is found to be intolerable to the patients, and they are actually obliged to keep the windows shut. It is true that, in the country, trains pass only occasionally, but they pass day and night. And there is the inevitable whistle too. I should much prefer a quieter site.

I am astonished at the cost (as now stated) of Bucks Infirmary. The estimates I saw amounted to under £7500. There must be some mistake, £200 per bed is most extravagant. A hospital for 100 beds may be built for £10,000, unless there are local disadvantages.

Source: From a letter to W.E. Nightingale, dictated to Hilary Bonham Carter, Add Mss 45790 ff245-46

23 January 1862

The Winchester is a great victory. I will not ask you to put my subscription down under yours, because mine is entirely contingent upon whether I approve the plans at sight. I have made this condition with every hospital I have assisted. I promised the Winton from £50 to £100 if they made the hospital what I consider "conducive to the welfare of the sick." N.B. I hope you know that I pay all my charities out of my own earnings, including the £50 to the Herbert Memorial and £300 for the printing of the "stuff."[106]

You have been so exceedingly liberal to me that I should be sorry you thought that I gave these things out of your pocket. I have taken enough out of it without that, or more truly *you have given* me enough! I have managed my donation to several county hospitals, i.e., to the building of new ones, in the same way as I propose to do with the Winton. I have no doubt it will have to be made £100.

Will you tell Parthe that I will answer Sir William Heathcote's question about "site" to him direct tomorrow?

Source: From a letter to Harry Verney, Wellcome (Claydon copy) Ms 9000/6

5 February 1862

My father asked me "for the last edition of my *Notes on Nursing*" for Sir W. Heathcote. *I* think he meant the "last edition" of my *Notes on Hospitals*. It is not done—not even begun—though promised to Parker above a year ago. And now my first strength must be given to the Indian report, for which there is not a bit of my "evidence" yet written.

But if Sir W.H. would like my old copy, or rather yours, of *Notes on Hospitals* for immediate Winchester purposes, and will return it to me (he has had it before), I will send it him.

Editor: Rawlinson wrote Nightingale that he had met with Heathcote and would be inspecting the proposed sites with Dr Sutherland. An architect had been settled on, and Dr Sutherland and Captain Galton were "to approve the plans—this of course means your approval."[107]

Source: From a letter to Harry Verney, Wellcome (Claydon copy) Ms 9000/56

27 June 1862

I am beyond measure astonished and grieved that these people should have printed, without my knowledge, garbled extracts out of my private letters.

Had they selected only my facts, there would have been some excuse. But to print an *opinion*, without asking leave and without giving the context, such as that I "think the British Army hospitals the

---

106 For her three-volume *Suggestions for Thought*.

107 Letter to Nightingale 4 March 1862, Florence Nightingale Museum (LMA) H1/ST/NC2/V5/62.

worst in the world" is quite unjustifiable. These are the things which do mischief.

And I must insist, if not too late, that this paragraph be omitted. It is irrelevant, useless, mischievous. When I gave the details of expense of [horse] hair in our army hospital mattresses, it was because I thought such detail might do good. But *this* is pure and simple mischief. And, besides, it relates to a state of things which has passed away, as they presently show in the very next clause of the same paragraph, quoted from me, which I have no objection to let stand. . . .

I think that, after the trouble I have taken about their hospital, the least thing they could have done would have been to have sent me this paper for my remarks, before adoption.

Source: From two letters to W.E. Nightingale, Wellcome (Claydon copy) Ms 9000/68 and Add Mss 45790 ff295-96

Hampstead, N.W.
18 October 1862

I hear that six acres have been bought for the new Winchester Infirmary "on the road to Hursely and Romsey." If so, it must be the *best* site which they have taken. But how could they get "six acres" there? Do you know anything about it?

27 October 1862

I forgot to say, about the Winchester Dispensary, that the very best thing that can be done is to leave it, with the six doctors (and their ridiculous requirement of "six rooms") inside Winchester. Dispensaries never did any good—do do great harm. And let the two evils stop together.

Editor: In 1863 Nightingale asked her colleague Mary Jones, then superintendent at King's College Hospital, to review the plans for the Winchester Infirmary (letter not extant). Jones sent back the plans with three recommendations, on windows, fireplaces and dirty linen chutes. In a subsequent letter, Jones commented on the adequacy of space for nurses, especially for sleeping accommodation for night nurses.[108]

108 Jones letters 28 and 29 June 1863, Add Mss 47743 ff215-16 and 217-18.

Source: From typed copies of three letters to Sir William Heathcote, Add Mss 45798 ff160, 183-84 and 185-88, the first two from Hampstead

11 September 1863

I feel bound to send you my opinion as soon as possible, as you ask for it. My experience is very conclusive and my feeling very strong on all three points. I had written what I enclose before I read the sheet of "opinions adverse," as one does not want to read what is similar to one's own view.

But now I have read it, I must say, Miss Russell's is a good practical opinion, which all who are *really* conversant with hospital patients will echo, particularly. . . . This applies to day rooms and small wards too. I often smile to think how little people really know of the feelings of hospital patients, who have not nursed them. These actually prefer a full large ward and think it "so cheerful."

Mr Davis and Mr Yeo have also given excellent practical knowledge, showing that they know their work. If you would like me to get you Dr Sutherland's opinion, he will be in London (41 Finchley New Road) on Tuesday. I would have kept the papers for the purpose, had you not wished for an immediate answer. Should you like to send him the two sheets of your own, and the two of mine?

19 October 1863

1. The Lariboisière Hospital at Paris is the one which I remembered as having had day and dining rooms, and having discontinued them on account of the men patients making themselves rather worse than better in them. Both in St George's and the fever hospitals in London you may see day rooms in all the perfection of their discreditableness. But then I don't know that these hospitals wish to leave them off.

In the fever, they look much like the parlour of a discreditable public house. In St George's, a nurse is told off, who can do nothing else, to attend to them. And you see the patients gossiping and lolling out of window.

The lady superintendent of King's College Hospital [Mary Jones] is totally against them. She says, as we do, to put a nurse to sit there and expect her to check the gossip and tricks! of course she gossips too! She also conceives it totally impossible for a ward nurse to have a day room (to each ward) under her care. And I can't conceive it architecturally, or rather constructively. But, after all, nothing can be added to the evidence you have already. People who do not object to badly managed and badly constructed hospitals will not object to day rooms. But those who think that hospital administration has a very serious effect on the results of cases will see that the cost involved by having a whole separate staff, which is necessary for convalescent day rooms, had much better be spent, because more efficiently, on a separate convalescent establishment or "home" or country branch.

2. I send a separate memo on the subject of lock wards[109]—I had rather not be quoted on this subject. It is strictly private.

28 October 1863

1. "Convalescent wards" are, properly speaking, merely dormitories, which the "convalescents" leave in the morning and go back to at night. They must therefore have "day and dining rooms." This does not entail a double staff, because the sleeping rooms are left in the daytime (in some establishments locked up expressly in order to prevent the "convalescents" lounging on their beds. But this is unnecessary).

In all convalescent establishments, small or large, there must always be separate sick wards, in which relapses—or even "convalescents" (?) unable to leave their [ward]—are nursed with a staff of their own.

The difference between your wards (or those of any provincial hospital) and "convalescent wards," strictly speaking, is that yours will *always* have some cases confined to bed, and therefore can *never* be shut up in the daytime. Farther than this, in convalescent establishments every means is (or ought to be) taken to employ the patients, both in and out of doors, in the daytime.

Now the question manifestly is: is it not better to transport this "convalescent" establishment quite away, requiring, as it does, a different staff, and different, I had almost said opposite, rules, from the hospital? and to make a sick ward an apanage of the "convalescents," instead of "convalescent wards" an apanage of the sick?

2. Sir John McNeill told me that he had never succeeded in all his life in making the most intelligent (civilian) medical man understand the difference between military and civil hospitals. If he can't, I can't. I can only repeat, all military "hospitals, especially during war and in warm climates, must have convalescent wards *and* day and dining rooms," because you can't send "convalescents" from diarrhea, dysentery, fever, cholera, back to barracks. To leave them in the sick

109 Nightingale's eight-page printed "Note on the Supposed Protection Afforded Against Venereal Disease, by Recognizing Prostitution and Putting It under Police Regulation," 1862, in *Women* (8:428-35).

wards is simply to consign them to relapse. To make them sleep at night in the sick wards is as bad. And what *are* you to do with them?

I have looked all through my *Notes on Hospitals* to find the sentence attributed to me that "*all* hospitals should have convalescent wards and day and dining rooms," and I can't.[110] But the question is now not what I have said, but what is right?

If Dr Crawford will send me the quotation, chapter and verse, I am quite ready to cry "peccavi" [I have sinned]. I never aspired to be infallible. But I cannot remember to have ever had a different opinion from what I have now, though my present opinion has been strengthened by experience. (The first and second editions of my *Notes on Hospitals* were composed mainly of my evidence before the royal commissioners, in answer to certain definite written questions, which referred exclusively to military hospitals. And the first edition was reprinted without my even correcting it. It is very possible therefore I may have said, "*all* hospitals," meaning all *military* hospitals.)

In the third edition, which is entirely rewritten and has long been in the printers' hands, I am quite sure there is no such sentence with regard to *civil* hospitals. It must be remembered, too, that all that has been published of mine hitherto on the hospital subject has been the *odd times* and not the substance of my life—carelessly written, and sometimes not even corrected by myself. I have often been overruled by medical men. And I would rather appeal to my practical arrangements than to my writings. But, as I say, the question is not this, but what is the best?

So far upon the general principle. But everything depends upon the case in point. If you were building a large hospital in the heart of an unhealthy city, or even if you had determined to continue your old unhealthy hospital of Winchester, in either case you must, if you will not have a convalescent branch by the sea or in an open country, have convalescent wards *in* the hospital. And you will find that the very medical men who most advocated day rooms in the old hospital will, when they come to have their patients in the new, be the first to say that neither day rooms nor "convalescent wards" separate from your fine large wards are wanted.

110 *Notes on Hospitals* says that day and dining rooms are essential for convalescent hospitals but "objectionable in a civil hospital," for if patients are well enough to use them, they would be better out of hospital, in a convalescent institution (see p 171 above).

The proposal of the glass screen amounts to having a day room or convalescent ward as a vestibule to the W.C.s, with all the sick passing through it. It has been found that the large end window is the most popular part of the hospital for all patients able to leave their beds. But a screen is not necessary. It obstructs the ventilation.

There is danger of your sacrificing simplicity while you seek for so many classes of accommodation in so small a hospital. And again I say, have a convalescent "cottage home" at a distance—if at all.

Source: From two letters to Samuel Smith, Add Mss 45793 ff35-38 and 42

15 January 1864

Private. Very many thanks for sending me Mr John Bullar's[111] friendly letter. But we read it twice over before we made out that it was anything but a bad joke, such complete ignorance does it show of the subject. I mean it is as if I were to write to Mr Mohl (and date my letter "11:30 p.m.") pointing out to him a "serious error" in his version of the *Schah Nameh*,[112] without knowing my Persian letters. Mr John Bullar obviously does not know his letters in statistical methods and, though we thought it better to answer him as Dr Sutherland has done, certainly a man who could write such an exposure of his own ignorance as *this* is incapable of being convinced by being told what the methods *are* in such a letter as that, Dr Sutherland's. (It is as if Mr Mohl were to try to teach me the Persian grammar in a note sheet of paper.)

For (1) had Mr John Bullar had the smallest acquaintance with the existence of the General Register Office as by law established, in his own country, since (I believe) 1827, its Weekly Tables, Quarterly Reports, Annual Reports, Census Reports, he would never have set up his own authority against that of the national statistics, or fallen foul of poor me, who have simply quoted the only statistics which *are* "national" and authorized.

And (2) if he had read the last section (on statistics) in my own book, he would have seen that I have myself suggested a better method of

111 John Bullar (1778-1864) established the Royal South Hampshire Hospital in Southampton, where his son, Dr Joseph Bullar (1808-69), was a physician. Nightingale considered the hospital not good enough to train probationers; see *Extending Nursing* (13:199). His letter is not extant, although several others by him on nursing are.

112 Julius Mohl was a distinguished Persian scholar, who published a multivolume translation of the classic *Schah Nameh.*

noting hospital statistics, which has been adopted by two International Statistical Congresses, and which is (not against Dr Farr, but) an improvement on the present methods, and which Dr Farr himself has sanctioned by sending copies to all hospitals from the General Register Office, three years ago (and again this year, as to the Sub-Section "Surgical Operations"). And (3) Mr John Bullar's own method is no method at all. It is obviously impossible to get any hospital statistics at all by his method.

ever yours
in great haste of business
F.N.

What I am afraid of is that Dr Bullar, who is attending at Embley now, will be open-mouthed to tell (and they to believe, open-eared) my dreadful "mistakes" and "serious errors." And that my own people will be the first to say, "poor Flo!" And that I shall have letter upon letter to write, in the thick of my business! just as I had about the Indian statistics, to people, *not* my own people, who ought to have known better. But even this is far better for me than to let me be in ignorance of these attacks. Pray believe I feel this.

2 February 1864

Thanks for the note about the Dr Bullars. An attack in the *Medical Times* came out on Saturday on my book,[113] as intemperate as Mr J. Bullar's was courteous, but in the same sense. It was a covert attack on the Registrar-General. Dr Farr is going to answer it; *he* calls the writer "the savage," but says his (own) anger must cool down first (at the "stupidity") before he can answer.

The article is so inconceivably ignorant, beginning its onslaught upon me by stating that "it has been clearly proved that hospital death rates are almost *wholly independent* of sanitary conditions," and then warning me of my "serious and elementary errors," that the sting of it is taken out for me.

If you like to send us Mr John Bullar's *second* letter, my party are rather curious to see it. (I cannot say I am. I am too weak for curiosity.) It was as I anticipated. Dr Bullar ran straight to Embley. And Parthe fell foul of me.

113 Discussed (see p 225 above).

Source: From a letter to Edwin Chadwick, Add Mss 45771 ff42-45

5 June 1864

General Morin's report is by far the most satisfactory that has yet appeared on the Paris ventilating systems. But there are evidently questions still needing solution, with which the report does not deal. Duvoir's system of "aspiration" is without doubt better and more reliable than the system of "insufflation." But the report shows that all such systems are liable to irregularities, not admitting of immediate remedy, liable to accidents affecting patients injuriously and that, after all, none of them up to the present time has succeeded in keeping the air of wards fresh. The report itself is the best witness to the causes of Lariboisière high mortality. It shows that the ward air is never *fresh* and that patients, irrespective of conditions, are all *cooked* at the same temperature.

I accede to the desirableness of churches, theatres and other public places, where there are no open fires, being warmed and ventilated by such means (and, of existing mechanical methods, Duvoir's is the best). I demur *in toto* as to what constitutes ventilation in a hospital. If the wards are ever so free of "smell," the simple absence of *freshness* in the air and of variation in temperature shows the system of ventilation to be wrong. Nature has given variety of temperature as a condition no less favourable to health than to recovery from sickness. Let them remove all their ventilating machines, put in open fireplaces, and open their windows so as to keep the wards both fresh and free from odour *at all times*; let them give more blankets in cold weather; and the Lariboisière Hospital will become as admirable as its construction, instead of furnishing a very high death rate, as now, which I hold to be solely due to its artificial ventilation. I should feel it a great honour, if you would read my last (Longman's) edition of my *Notes on Hospitals.*

M Husson sent me last year his quarto on Paris hospitals, which I have quoted largely in this. When I return you your *washing* books, I shall write farther, I hope.

Editor: It was not until some time in 1864 that serious decisions were made concerning the plans for the Winchester Infirmary. The architect finally selected was the eminent William Butterfield (1814-1900), who was well known for his church restorations but had not previously designed a hospital. He sent Nightingale his working drawings on 20 September 1864, to which her answer was obviously negative, for Sir William Heathcote told her that he was "distressed" by the "severity" of her comments. He asked if the site should be sold and the scheme abandoned.[114] A further letter from Heathcote to Nightingale stated that the tender for the hospital had been accepted, that Douglas Galton had persuaded the governors that the cost was moderate.[115]

Butterfield wanted and got a spectacular chapel built as part of the Winchester Infirmary, contributing substantially to the additional expense himself. Correspondence on the chapel is lacking, but it seems that Nightingale wanted it to be in a separate building, as it was large, but it stayed in the hospital, up three flights of stairs. A book on the history of chaplaincy at the hospital concluded: "Had her wishes prevailed, the difficulties which caused the Butterfield Chapel to be closed a century later would not have arisen, and we should still doubtless have the chapel in use."[116]

As with the chapel, Nightingale did not get her way on everything. A sarcastic letter to the editor of the *Medical Times and Gazette* was critical of her, and even more so of Butterfield:

> The plans for the new building have been concocted by the following personages: 1. Miss Nightingale, 2. an architect named Butterfield, only known to me as a defacer of fine old churches and a builder of ugly new ones, 3. a domineering baronet of the neighbourhood, who has put a ring in the nose of the Hampshire hog, and leads him about as he will.

The author signed himself "Epicuri de Grege Porcus," a hog from the sty of Epicurus, a learned joke from Horace, who had so described himself. "Porcus" noted that the building had five storeys, including the basement, and that its axis was east-west, so that every ward had a row of large windows facing north, pointing out "how far these peculiarities agree with Miss Nightingale's published opinions."[117]

In the end, and with some misgivings, Nightingale gave her approbation and money, even a higher contribution to the hospital than she had planned. She told her mother that she had been "deluded into

---

114 Butterfield letter 20 September 1864, Florence Nightingale Museum (LMA) H1/ST/NC2/V5/64; Heathcote letter 28 September 1864, H1/ST/NC2/V7/64.

115 Heathcote letter 16 November 1864, Florence Nightingale Museum (LMA) H1/ST/NC2/V18/64.

116 Cyril Moxley, *Cathedral College and Hospital: An Account of the Chaplaincy of the Royal Hampshire County Hospital 1736-1986* 39.

117 "The New County Hospital at Winchester," *Medical Times and Gazette* 20 February 1864:211, and reprinted 27 February 1864:243.

giving another £100 to Winchester Hospital."[118] The next year she remarked to her mother that "hospitals and convalescent homes bear so very hardly upon me," mentioning the £200 she had given to Winchester, the £50 to the Herbert Memorial, and a promised £25 to Swansea.[119]

Source: From a typed copy of a letter to Sir William Heathcote, Add Mss 45799 f34

18 November 1864

I thank you for your note about the new Winchester Infirmary. I am very glad to hear that your way is so far clear out of your difficulty. I wish an attempt could be made at once to raise the additional funds. Otherwise, when the building is up, people may be less disposed to give. But I hope, from what you say, you have promises to a considerable amount.

I beg you to be so kind as to take charge of my (£100) contribution (which I enclose) now, not because I am afraid, if I live, of being unwilling to pay it, but because I am fidgety lest, if I die, there should be some stupidity, as I think generally happens in this kind of thing.

But more than all other feeling, I feel regret at your state of health, and can only hope in the winter abroad being a safe restorer.

Source: From a letter to W.E. Nightingale, Add Mss 45790 ff324-27

23 November 1864

The second proposition (second in order of importance), in your letter, about which you cannot be serious—it is impossible that you can be serious—at least not in making such a proposition to me—is about the new Winchester Infirmary. "Your model at Winton," you say, "helps *us* not." If you were thoroughly convinced that you were sending a person to a place where he would have nine chances to one of being killed, instead of to a place where he would only have three chances against him to seven for him, or to a place where he would have nine chances of life for him against one of death, which would you choose?

But then you have no convictions; I have—and so strong that I have just paid my second hundred out of my hard-earned store (which I

118 Letter to Frances Nightingale 25 October 1864, Wellcome (Claydon copy) Ms 9001/72.

119 Letter 29 September 1865, in *Life and Family* (1:180).

shall never be strong enough to earn again) to Sir W. Heathcote for the new Winton Infirmary. I think you would have been perfectly right, if you had stoutly refused to subscribe to the *old* Winton Infirmary and said I *won't* send people there to be killed. I think you would have been perfectly right, if Southampton or Salisbury were going to build a new *and healthy* infirmary, to refuse to contribute to the new Winton Infirmary, *however healthy*, on this ground: that your people prefer going to Salisbury or Southampton.

But, as for your being "constrained to give a ticket to Salisbury" WHEN the new Winton Infirmary *is built*, I'd be hanged if I would send these poor, ignorant people to their deaths, when you know better. It is just what Cavour's physician (who bled him) said: "he was constrained," *and he killed him.*[120] But then, as I say, you have no convictions about these things. You have repeatedly referred to them to me in these terms—repeating the third-class apothecary's (of last century's) arguments, used by Dr Crawford and Jack's constituents, who ought to be ashamed of them, explaining away the awful loss of life from erysipelas at the old Winton Infirmary, asking me again and again "*how*" our inspectors "could tell that the ground was saturated"—"did they dig holes?"

Why these are mere schoolboy's lessons to us (and let me say that the saturation of the ground was only *one* of the awful evils of the old Winton Infirmary). You say "North Hants ought to have been ashamed to *solicit us*," *only* "ashamed" if you South Hants people had been going to build an infirmary for yourselves. (*I* should be ashamed if *any* "constraint" made me send a patient to any but the new Winton Infirmary from the county of Hants or Wilts, *until* South Hants and Wilts have built infirmaries for themselves.)

Then you say to me: "So and so has got well at such and such an infirmary." We don't deny it. But do you think we don't know (at the General Register Office here) *exactly* the proportion that has got well and that has died which ought not to have died (which is very like saying that has been killed?)

I began my book [*Notes*] *on Hospitals* with saying, "The first requisite of a hospital is to do the patient *no harm.*" This has been quoted in every review since as if it had never struck anybody before.

---

120 Count Camillo Cavour (1810-61), Italian independence leader and prime minister. On his bad medical treatment, but glorious death, see *European Travels* (7:330).

Poor Dundas Thompson, who is dead, said (quietly) in his evidence before our royal commission, "I conclude therefore that the Vauxhall Water Company killed 1600 persons in that year." I tell you that we know exactly the proportion that your Winton, your Southton, your Salisbury Infirmary has, each of them, killed, over and above the proportion which *ought to* have died from such and such diseases.

That people who have not made these things a study don't know them does not surprise me, any more than it surprises me that they don't know Persian. But for people, especially those Dr Bullars of Southampton, to write to me these worn-out and exploded arguments (which are exactly like the arguments for a belief in witchcraft) does surprise me, just as much as if I were to write to *M Mohl*! a theory of *mine*!! upon *Persian*!!!

Yes, I feel so strongly upon a subject (on which I am said to be the first authority in Europe) that I have just promised a contribution to Swansea, much larger than I can afford, who is just building a new hospital on the condition that I shall revise the plans, which I have just done, and that I shall withdraw my contribution if they job[121] the plans. I have done the same, and shall do the same, for every healthily constructed hospital, *wherever* it is, and shall steadfastly refuse *any* subscription to any unhealthy one.

(You know I gave £30 to poor Sidney Herbert's memorial convalescent cottages, of which I made the plans myself. I did the same with Aylesbury, i.e., I revised the plans and gave £25.) I do not expect you, though you are my father, to Quixotize about the country in this way. But neither must you expect me to reply anything farther to your arguments for your *triad* of *wretched county hospitals)* but "you cannot be serious, it is impossible that you can be serious."

Editor: In 1868 Heathcote wrote Nightingale several letters, the first announcing that the hospital was "nearly completed."[122] Her replies are not extant, but a draft note in Dr Sutherland's hand commends him, with a proviso about costs:

> Your first year has been a great success, for apparently your death rate has been 23 per 1000 treated in the hospital, which is just the death rate of the whole metropolis. Would it not be admirable to

121 To get a kickback for a contract.

122 Letters 11, 16 and 22 April 1868, Add Mss 45801 ff8, 21 and 35.

> get out the death rate of the whole infirmary for a series of years? It will be your best justification for the outlay. Still I must say that the hospital has cost too much. The beautiful new Swansea infirmary has, I am told, cost £110 or £f120 per bed.[123]

When I visited the hospital in the course of research for this volume, the old building, except for the chapel, was still in use, but surrounded by larger, later, buildings.

Midlands Hospitals, 1860-67

Editor: Nightingale knew the Midlands well, not only from her time spent at the family home at Lea Hurst, Derbyshire, but from visits to her grandmother Shore, who lived in the outskirts of Sheffield. There were other family travels when she was young and she held fond reminiscences of visits to Manchester and Birmingham.[124] Post-Crimea, when she could not travel for pleasure, Nightingale continued to visit Lea Hurst. Her considerable work on the Derby Infirmary was doubtless fueled by ongoing local contacts. It is reported in a section of its own (see p 705 below). There is also material on Leeds, site of the first civil hospital built on the pavilion principle, and on Liverpool, with its many hospitals and also the city of Nightingale's close collaborator William Rathbone.

The work in Manchester was particularly important as it was the location of the first English doctor to call for hospital reform, John Roberton. A Nightingale letter called him "our greatest hospital authority" (see p 518 above), and she referred to him in another as "the well-known Manchester surgeon and perhaps the first medical authority in England on hospital construction" (see p 604 above).

It seems that Nightingale was informed in 1861 of the intention of Manchester city authorities to enlarge their—in her opinion—highly defective hospital, the Manchester Royal Infirmary. It had been located in the downtown core from the time of its foundation in the mid-eighteenth century, and Nightingale evidently tried to dissuade the officials from renovating in favour of building a whole new hospital on a new site. She appealed to Dr Roberton, with whom she had been in correspondence earlier on general principles—each approved

123 Undated note, Add Mss 45801 f12.
124 In *European Travels* (7:675-98).

of and quoted the other. Her letter to him (see p 627 below) apparently sparked serious reconsideration, and both William Rathbone, who had initially apprised her of the situation, and Harry Verney were brought to use their influence.

Correspondence is lacking on Nightingale's involvement with the Blackburn Infirmary, one whose plans "passed through" her hands and Galton's, as she recalled it years later (see p 730 below). It was to have been Britain's first pavilion hospital of the nineteenth century. A competition was held for the plans, which was won by Manchester architect James Turnbull. The foundation stone was laid in 1857 and construction begun in 1858, but it was interrupted by the massive layoffs in the Lancashire cotton mills.[125]

Rawlinson, in 1861, reported to Nightingale of having seen the new Blackburn building, but only at a distance. It was "painfully fine and costly," he said.[126] She told him that the cost was monstrous, on account of the use of eight-bed wards (see p 606 above). She always disapproved of wards that size, for each would require its own nurse as much as a twenty-eight bed-ward (or larger) would, resulting in a much higher operating cost per patient. A Blackburn matron who met with Nightingale in 1876, however, told her that the infirmary had more patients on average than Preston, Halifax, York or Hull, and got them out sooner, in "a less average of *days*," a point Nightingale made note of.[127]

In 1861 Nightingale worked on plans for the North Staffordshire Infirmary[128] at Stoke-on-Trent. There are passing comments about those plans, but no surviving letters. A secondary source explains that the planning committee, after consulting Nightingale, had decided on a pavilion plan, the actual construction to be supervised by the medical board. The two architects selected, G.B. Nicholls and Charles Lynam, visited the new hospitals in England and Paris (George Gilbert Scott's new Leeds Infirmary was then under construction). The result was a "French type," with a glazed cloister, resembling the Lariboisière on a more modest scale.[129]

---

125 Nightingale worked with others, unsuccessfully, on a scheme to find alternative employment for the workers, reported in *Society and Politics* (5:163-65).

126 Rawlinson letter 30 May 1861, Add Mss 45769 f81.

127 Note of meeting with Miss Whitton 14 December 1876, Add Mss 47762 f226.

128 On which see R.A. Hordley, *A Concise History of the North Staffordshire Infirmary and Eye Hospital*.

129 Jeremy Taylor, *The Architect and the Pavilion Hospital: Dialogue and Design Creativity in England 1850-1914* 77.

When the hospital later sought a matron from Mrs Wardroper, the matron at St Thomas', the claim could be made that North Staffordshire was "a new infirmary, in an excellent situation, on a hill with a country aspect. . . . built on the pavilion plan, for 200 beds."[130] It later became the "Royal North Staffordshire," and still later was merged with other hospitals to become the University Hospital of North Staffordshire.

In 1865, Nightingale was involved in providing trained nurses for the Manchester Royal Infirmary, although there is little surviving correspondence on the subject by her.[131] A letter to Nightingale from Dr George Greaves (d. 1869), who was also vice-president of the Manchester Statistical Association, thanked her for her encouraging letter regarding the hospital.[132] In 1866 Sir Harry Verney asked Nightingale to give her opinion for "friends in Manchester" regarding founding a children's hospital there. Her lengthy reply covers both recommended principles and existing defects.[133]

The correspondence reported here begins in 1860 with a reference to Joseph Adshead (1810-61), a successful Manchester businessman who took up the cause of hospital reform in a large way after reading Nightingale's *Notes on Hospitals*. She called him her "best pupil" (in the second letter below). Whether or not Adshead gave the paper at Glasgow referred to in the first letter below is not apparent. However he did give one to the Manchester Statistical Society.[134] Unhappily, he died the following year and his projected new convalescent hospital was never built.

---

130 Godfrey Wedgwood letter to Henry Bonham Carter 21 July 1872, Florence Nightingale Museum (LMA) H1/ST/NC18/11/30.

131 See *Extending Nursing* (13:271-73).

132 Letter 27 November 1865, Add Mss 45799 f172.

133 Her reply has already appeared, in *Public Health Care* (6:530-32). A further letter she wrote on the subject is in *The Nightingale School* (12:163-64).

134 "A Plea for the Establishment of a Convalescent Hospital for Manchester and Its Surrounding District," 10 December 1860, published in the *Transactions of the Manchester Statistical Society* (session 1860-61) 1861:38-43.

Source: From a letter to Edwin Chadwick, Add Mss 45770 ff168-70

Upper Terrace
Hampstead
14 September 1860

Mr Adshead of Manchester is to moot the question of convalescent institutions at the Glasgow meeting.

None such are as yet projected, excepting the one for which the late A. Morley bequeathed some £100,000 odd, in connection with St George's Hospital.[135] The Manchester one is not yet brought before public notice, although I have seen and revised their plans. It will be brought forward at Glasgow. I had rather not give any general sanction to plans, but only to principles. Plans must vary according to ground and local circumstances and exposure. And people are so stupid they will not see this, so that I am always afraid of laying down anything like a universal plan. Since my "Evidence" was out, plans for some dozen hospitals have been sent to me, purporting to be constructed on my "principles." And in all I have had to make the most essential alterations.

Source: From a letter to Samuel Smith, Add Mss 45792 ff136-43

25 February 1861

Adshead of Manchester is dead, my best pupil. I wrote to condole with a friend of his, intending my letter to be sent to his widow, whom I do not know, saying how great the loss was and how I hoped that Manchester would pay his memory the tribute which, of all others, he would have liked—the carrying out his plans (all finished) for a country hospital. The friend writes me back the answer (enclosed) asking me to let my letter be published.

This is what I want to consult you about. I am afraid you do not know who Adshead is, so I must explain. How often I have called him my "dear old Addle-head," and now he is dead. I had a letter from him about his plans—perhaps the last he ever wrote—saying he was "better." Then the next thing was a pair of black gloves and a fine white mausoleum printed on a black card from the undertaker—dear old custom of my north country, which I have so carefully fulfilled for my own old people, and cannot laugh at, minus the mausoleum.

Adshead was a man who could hardly write or speak the queen's English (I believe he raised himself) and was now a kind of manufac-

135 Discussed further (see p 626 below).

turer's agent in Manchester. He was a man of very ordinary abilities, commonplace appearance, vulgar but *never* unbusinesslike, which is, I think, the worst kind of vulgarity. Having made "a competency," he did not give up business but devoted himself to good works for Manchester. There is scarcely a good thing in Manchester of which he has not been the mainstay or the source: the schools, infirmary, paving and draining, water supply, etc.

At sixty he takes up an entirely new subject, hospital construction, fired by my book, and determines to master it. This is what I think is peculiar to the Anglo-Saxon. He writes to me whether I will teach him (this is about eighteen months ago) and composes some plans for a convalescent hospital *out of* Manchester, to become the main hospital, if the wind is favourable. He comes up to London to see me about these.

The working plans passed eight times through my hands and gave me more trouble than anything I ever did, *because* Adshead *would not* employ a proper builder, but *would* do them himself, which is part of the *same character* I believe. The plans are now quite ready, but nothing more. He meant to *beg in person* all over Lancashire, and had already some promises of large sums. Now all this is cut short.

He had been ailing for about a year, but never intermitted anything. I don't know whether you remember that I had a three months' correspondence with him (and oh! the immense trouble he took) about the transplantation of the Spitalfields and Coventry weavers to Manchester and its districts, Preston, Burnley, etc., And how ill Miss Sellon[136] behaved. It never came to anything about *her* people. I hate Miss Sellon now for it, because I think it hastened his death, though *he* would not have minded it, if it had come to good. He was sixty-one when he died.

This is the character, which I believe is quite peculiar to our race, a man, a common tradesman, who instead of "retiring from the world" to "make his salvation," or giving himself up to science or to his family in his old age, or founding an order, or building a house, will patiently (at sixty) learn new dodges and new-fangled ideas in order to benefit his native city.

Oh how superior I do feel this sort of character to the Sutherlands who pursue the same things for the love of science and capriciously—

---

136 Priscilla Lydia Sellon (1821-76), founder of the Anglican order Society of Sisters of Mercy of the Holy Trinity, Devonport.

to the Sellons who cut themselves off from the world and from all progress in ideas to found "orders," to the statesmen, like Lord Spencer,[137] and to the Roman Catholics like Pascal,[138] who retire from their life's business for their own "individual salvation."

How I do feel that it is the strength of our country and worth all the Roman Catholic "orders" put together. I hate an "order" and am so glad I was never "let in" to form one.

Do you know that St George's Hospital have embezzled A. Morley's legacy for a convalescent branch?[139] and that Adshead was actually employed, when he died, upon my information, in trying whether it were legally possible to institute Chancery proceedings against them? For it was *not only* Manchester that he cared about. However, that is all over now, and his plan for Manchester is the only one which will fulfill my ideal of a country hospital. Now what is to be done? For that is the question.

I don't want to be dragged into holding subscription lists, neither into an opposition to all the Manchester doctors. There is a hot controversy in the Manchester papers now. EVERY day one side or the other sends me an article. Please return the enclosed.

Source: From a letter probably to William Rathbone, Florence Nightingale Museum (LMA) H1/ST/NC1/61/8

Hampstead, N.W.
5 October 1861

I was grieved to hear from your letter that Manchester was adding to and enlarging the already overgrown Manchester Infirmary. It is built on the worst of hospital plans: gangrene is never out of its wards. One of the most eminent surgeons, who is also surgeon to the railway, never sends his accidents to the infirmary, but prefers, at immense personal

---

137 John Charles Spencer (1782-1845), 3rd Earl Spencer, who explained his decision to retire from politics, at age forty-nine: "Only one object which is worthy of the ambition of a man of sense, and that is to obtain the favour of God. Political pursuits and political rivalships are not the means to conduce to this end" ("The Life of Earl Spencer, Written by himself," in Denis Le Marchant, *Memoir of John Charles Viscount Althorp, Third Earl Spencer* xv).

138 Scientist Blaise Pascal (1623-62) experienced a "second conversion" in 1654, which prompted him to abandon his scientific work for contemplation; his *Pensées* were published posthumously from his reflections.

139 A convalescent hospital, however, was opened in 1869. See "The Atkinson Morley Convalescent Hospital, Wimbledon," *The Lancet* 17 July 1869:104.

labour and loss of time, to attend them at their own homes, because they are sure to incur erysipelas or other hospital disease at the ill-placed, ill-constructed, ill-ventilated infirmary. This is the evidence of a brave man, and what few even brave men would venture to give.

Two years ago, I was employed by some rich and benevolent Manchester men to give a verdict upon the plans of the present Manchester Infirmary, which were sent me, and to construct plans for an infirmary out of Manchester, where first convalescents and, it was hoped, subsequently cases which could not recover in Manchester, would be sent.

I was then convinced—and others too were convinced (men important in Manchester)—that no improvement in the present infirmary could make it a place where patients would have a good chance—that to *enlarge* it would be fatal. And the plans for the *convalescent* hospital out of town were entirely finished and in the hands of the principal mover of the whole (a Manchester man) when he died almost suddenly. Nothing has since been done. And the peccant [sinning] hospital is actually being enlarged.

The reason why I tell you this long story is that, as you may possibly become connected with the Manchester Infirmary (by training a superintendent for it) you might be able to avert a great evil and spread a sounder knowledge there. I am actually engaged at this moment on the plans of four provincial hospitals or branches of London hospitals—where the principle of sound construction in country air is to be observed. It would be hard, if Manchester with her high civilization and generous public spirit, should not recognize this principle.

Source: From a letter to John Roberton, Wellcome (Claydon copy) Ms 8999/37

Hampstead
London, N.W.
7 October 1861

I have heard with great regret that the Manchester Infirmary is being added to and enlarged. I hope you will be able to tell me that I have been misinformed.

I thought it was agreed among you that the ill-placed, ill-constructed, ill-ventilated Manchester Infirmary was not a place to give the sick a fair chance, however improved, and that, if added to, it would be fatal. Sold, it would make an admirable warehouse, being indeed fit for nothing else. And the price would be available for a new building out of the town. But, if all this is out of the question, would you not renew poor Mr Adshead's proposal for a convalescent hospital (to receive also those sick who cannot recover *in* the Manchester Infirmary) a little out of Manchester?

It is hard indeed if Manchester, with her high civilization, with her magnificent public spirit, never failing in the utmost generosity towards her public institutions, and with her advanced principles of progress, should fail in doing what the pettiest county town in England, as well as London, is now planning on proceeding with.

I am at this moment engaged upon propositions made to me, and plans laid before me for revisal, from no less than five of these institutions, all to be built upon your pavilion principle in county sites, where alone the sick can be expected to recover.

My health and time will ill afford my writing a single extra letter, yet I could not but appeal to you, upon this bad news, concerning a city I respect so much, reaching me.

Source: From a copy of an incomplete letter probably to Peter Pincoffs,[140] Woodward Biomedical Library, uncatalogued

Hampstead, N.W.
8 October 1861

I wish you could do something at Manchester about the infirmary, which I grieve to hear they are enlarging. That ill-placed, ill-constructed, ill-ventilated infirmary will be fatal to the sick, if its already overgrown bulk is added to. How much better to sell it for a warehouse. They have also abandoned the admirable project of having a convalescent branch hospital *out of* the town.

Source: From a letter to William Rathbone, Florence Nightingale Museum (LMA) H1/ST/NC1/61/9

Hampstead, N.W.
19 October 1861

I return Mr [Murray] Gladstone's letter with many thanks. But you will see that his opinion as to the infirmary at Manchester being very much improved (or improvable) is not shared by the best Manchester medical authorities. Please return to me Mr Roberton's letter [missing]. I have also another *nearly similar* from another Manchester man, with which I do not trouble you. But as you may have some future

140 He is referred to later (see p 605 above), as having written a letter on the Manchester Infirmary, which was what Nightingale asked him to do in this letter.

influence in this line, I should be glad if you would glance at Mr Roberton, who has written two of the best tracts on hospital construction extant.[141]

I must add that there is yet a third authority (a Manchester surgeon) who told me that he *never* sent his accidents into the infirmary, although at the greatest loss of time and money to himself, if it were possible to help it—as they were almost sure to do badly.

I understand that an old Mr Harker (query is that the name?) is the main hindrance to removing the infirmary. 100 years hence I expect it will be considered as impossible to put sick down in the middle of a crowded city as it is now to leave jails in the state these were in 100 years ago, or to chain lunatics to rings in the wall.

Editor: Early in 1861, people from the Leeds Infirmary began to approach Nightingale regarding plans to enlarge the hospital[142] and in 1862 she was asked explicitly for assistance. A letter from William Beckett Denison (1826-90), a banker and MP, explained that the planning had been entrusted to George Gilbert Scott (1811-78), a leading architect and director of the largest British architectural firm. Her *Notes on Nursing* and evidence to the royal commission had both been consulted and Denison had questions about the recommended north-south axis for wards, window sizes, etc.

Joseph Adshead, who was already involved in hospital reform at Manchester (see p 623 above), actively promoted Nightingale's ideas at Leeds. His letter to the editor of the *Leeds Mercury* quoted Nightingale extensively, drawing comparisons between Leeds and Manchester.[143]

Nightingale's advice of the following year (immediately below) is the only surviving writing by her on the project. Denison sent her a cordial reply the next day, describing their intention of making the new Leeds hospital "the great hospital of the North of England, and which we desire to be as perfect as possible."[144] He asked for a meet-

---

141 Referred to (see p 517 above).

142 Letter from the treasurer 21 January 1861, with a copy of a letter 19 January 1861 by George Wilson, physician, Add Mss 45797 ff160 and 163, with newspaper clipping f164. For background see Stephen Towers Anning, *The General Infirmary at Leeds* and Jeremy Taylor, *Hospital and Asylum Architecture in England* 130.

143 Clipping 17 January 1861, Add Mss 45797 f164.

144 Denison letter 18 April 1862, Florence Nightingale Museum (LMA) H1/ST/NC2/V8/62.

ing with her, while another letter from him a short time later asked about ward size and the placement of fireplaces.[145]

A letter Nightingale wrote Douglas Galton suggests that there was further correspondence or a meeting with the hospital promoters (see p 636 below). The infirmary, when built, was an early civil hospital example of the pavilion principle. The foundation stone was laid in March 1864, and the structure completed towards the end of 1867.

Nightingale was involved further with Leeds in 1868-69 on providing trained nurses for the new infirmary.[146] The newspaper story covering the formal opening in 1869 compresses a great deal: "For a few years, the question of enlargement or entire rebuilding remained before the public, and after much discussion, many public meetings and very anxious thought, the latter alternative was finally adopted." The story related the European visits made by the architect, George Gilbert Scott, along with a senior physician. The pavilion style adopted had Gothic touches, with coloured brick and stone, embellished by polished granite shafts.

The newspaper account delicately explained the nursing arrangements, notably the selection of "five of the most skilled nurses" from the old hospital, and nine new trained nurses from the Nightingale School in London. The lady superintendent was inaccurately described as "a pupil of Florence Nightingale," for Nightingale did not herself teach any nurses.[147] Moreover, the superintendent in question, Clara Rebecca Jones, had been poorly rated at the school and Nightingale herself would never have recommended her.[148]

Source: From a letter to William Beckett Denison,[149] Royal Institute of British Architects ScGGS/4/3/4

17 April 1862

1. One great reason for N. and S. wards, instead of E. and W., is that the whole wall surface should be exposed to the sun every day of sunshine. North walls are always more or less damp and cold.

---

145 Letters 15 and 21 April 1862, Florence Nightingale Museum (LMA) H1/ST/NC2/V6/62, with a draft reply in Dr Sutherland's hand, and H1/ST/NC2/V7/62.

146 In *Extending Nursing* (13:275-78).

147 "The Leeds New Infirmary," *Leeds Mercury* 11 May 1869.

148 For more on Jones see *Extending Nursing* (13:276).

149 This letter is the reply to Denison's letter to her of 15 April, noted above (see p 630 here). It largely follows Dr Sutherland's draft reply, but omitted a point he made about the defects of the Woolwich Marine Hospital.

2. The morning sun is always advantageous, the south sun not so much so.

3. The exact number of degrees of inlet for sunlight is of less importance than the E. and W. sun. Every ward should, besides, have an end window, and the sun would thus shine into the end of the ward when in the south, and give a nice sweeping light. In this way the ward loses no ray of sun.

4. Whatever the size of your ward, you must have one head nurse to overlook each, be it for four or for forty beds. A good head nurse can overlook forty just as well as thirty-two beds. (The French say just as well fifty or sixty as thirty-two, and I agree.) But we consider twenty-four, twenty-eight or thirty-two, *not more*, the best number for *sanitary* well-being.

If you go into the open airy suburb of the town, you will find 1500 cubic feet per bed enough. A hospital in a situation requiring 2000 ft. had better not be there at all.

5. The French and Belgian hospitals are not workhouses. They only receive the class of cases sent to our workhouse infirmaries. The medical cases are usually *worse* than in our hospitals, because they receive our hopeless workhouse cases. But *no* hospitals in the world (in time of peace) receive so many *accidents* as large English hospitals, our dockyards, railroads, manufactories, etc., supplying so many.

6. At the Cavalry Barrack, York, you will see the latest military hospital which, with some small defects in detail, is the best hospital in Europe at present existing. Its cost was £4160 for sixty beds.[150] It is plain and of course wants many things required for a civil hospital. But even with all these requirements, a *large* civil hospital ought not to cost more than £80 or £90 per bed. I send you a pamphlet by this day's post. The York is half the "Plan for a Regimental Hospital" therein contained, i.e., it has the ground floor wards, centre two floors.

Woolwich Marine Hospital is bad. Woolwich Military Hospital, now being built, you will find a plan of (the "Herbert" Hospital) in the pamphlet sent. It will be the most complete *large* hospital in existence, much better than any abroad.

7. Pray see the Vincennes Military Hospital at Paris and the Lariboisière. St Jean, at Brussels, is good in some, very bad in more points. Have you seen the general report (a Blue Book) of the "Barrack and

---

150 Dr Sutherland's draft says £75 a bed.

Hospital Improvement" Commission? It is full of good principles, requiring, of course, to be varied for civil establishments. If you have any difficulty in getting it, I will obtain it and send it you.

8. Ashton Infirmary[151] wards are too narrow (24 ft.). York and the "Herbert" Hospital will be 26 ft. wide.

You are fortunate in securing such a man as Mr Scott as architect. I will gladly look over and criticize any plans you choose to send me. I would gladly also see you or any of your committee, as you propose. But it is now four months since I have been able to leave my bed. And the chances are so few that I ever shall be able to do so again that I am afraid of troubling you to call upon so poor a chance.

Any questions I would gladly answer in writing. But I must crave indulgence, both in answering these and in examining plans, for any delay. I am overwhelmed with business. And many days I am not able to write at all or to do anything.

Editor: Nightingale knew the Warwickshire area through family friends Charles and Selina Bracebridge, with whom she had travelled in Egypt and Europe and who accompanied her to the Crimean War. Charles Bracebridge is probably the link to the following letter on planning for what became the Coventry and Warwickshire Hospital, when a new hospital was built amalgamating the old hospital, then in a private house, and the Coventry Dispensary, of which he was chair. He was also a local magistrate.

Nightingale was evidently asked to criticize the plans for Coventry. She duly proposed alterations, which were not agreed on, but the fund-raisers were nevertheless poised to use her name to publicize their campaign. Only by threatening to expose them for doing so without taking her recommendations, did she succeed in getting "some more of them" adopted (in the letter immediately below, the only surviving documentation). A site was acquired in 1863 and the new hospital completed in 1866. The hospital was destroyed in the massive bombing of Coventry in World War II.

151 In Ashton-under-Lyne, near Manchester. See "The Ashton Infirmary Designs," *The Builder* 17,855 (25 June 1859).

Source: From a letter to an unnamed recipient, Florence Nightingale Museum 0868, typed copy Add Mss 45820 f62

[23 June 1862]

Coventry Infirmary.

1. No plan can be recommended without knowing the (proposed) number of beds.

2. If the Aylesbury one is adopted as a basis, there are some grievous defects in it to be avoided: (1) the wasting the whole ground floor upon administration, which nearly doubles the cost and extent of building, (2) the having the operation room on the highest floor, (3) the having the kitchen *in* the building at all, etc. But it is impossible for me to write a book upon the defects of every hospital plan.

3. If they have sent you the lithographed plans, they have sent you the plans made *before* we introduced some essential improvements: (1) removing the laundry altogether out of the building; (2) removing the kitchen from under a ward and placing it in the basement under the centre part; (3) improving small wards, ward offices at end of large wards, access to operation room, distribution of ground floor, etc. But, as I say, it is impossible for me to write criticisms of plans which are *not* the accepted plans. (4) I would have nothing to do, either, in criticizing or in praising, with fever wards or fever hospitals. Both are simple murder for fever cases.

4. Without knowing the average number of accidents, it is impossible to know whether to recommend an accident ward or not.

4. [5] Dr Sutherland will gladly inspect sites, *if invited*, and *if* the number of beds and other particulars, such as he wrote to Mr Bracebridge about, are determined beforehand.

6. The *draft* plans must be sent me for criticism, which will save them much expense. Send me a mere sketch.

P.S. The commendation by me in the letter press was put in without my leave. And it was only by threatening that I would expose them for having put in the paragraph, *without* having adopted all my alterations, that I got some more of them adopted in the building, as now exists.

Birkenhead Borough Hospital.

Editor: John Laird (1804-74), a Scottish-born shipbuilder, settled in Birkenhead, across the Mersey River from Liverpool, where he founded a major shipbuilding concern and became a local benefactor. He was mayor of the town and, later, MP. The correspondence here concerns his offer to fund, entirely at his own expense, the building of a new hospital. There is no correspondence with the architect, Thomas Layland. Nightingale was evidently sent the plans, for she sent her advice to Sir Harry Verney, who acted as intermediary. In this case the site selected was not unhealthy, but simply too small. The administrative offices took up as much space as the wards, while the same space would do for a much larger hospital, she wrote. She saw the potential for a "beautiful hospital" on the site, if it was extended.

The description and plan show that Nightingale's requirements were all fully met, except for ward size: fresh air, light and ample space, superficial area of 110 sq. ft per bed, 1430 cubic ft.; nurse's rooms to overlook each ward; a matron's "parlour"; complete separation of sick wards and administration; separate entrance for dispensary; garden and ground to south overlooking a park; oak floors, stone stairs and walls of polished and non-absorbent surface. The foundation stone was laid on 20 November 1862.[152]

A bust of Laird, paid for by subscription by the workingmen of Liverpool, was later placed in the vestibule of the hospital in recognition of his gift. In 1926 the hospital became the Birkenhead General Hospital; it was closed in 1982.

Source: From a note and two letters to Harry Verney, Wellcome (Claydon copy) Ms 9000/19-20 and 24

[ca. March 1862]

Yes, I would gladly look over the plans, if Mr Laird will understand that I can't see *him*, and that I can't be hurried. I must have the plans for two or three days, so that I may take advantage of my better moments to look at them. I was obliged to keep the Devonport plans (the last I had from the War Office) since I have been in this house a fortnight.

5 April 1862

Mr Laird is doing a most generous thing in building this hospital. But, in doing so, his object is to obtain the very best building for the sick that his money will supply. The area is too small to allow of this being done. For although two acres per 100 beds is enough, this rule applies to large, not to small hospitals. Because, however small, the hospital wants administrative offices, and these offices will do for a large as well as a small number of beds.

152 "The New Birkenhead Borough Hospital," *The Builder* 21,1055 (25 April 1863):296-97, with plan.

In this case the offices cover almost as much ground as the wards. At the new "Herbert" Hospital they occupy about a fifth or sixth of the ward area.

This plan is very crowded. And there are things about the building much better away. While the plan (forced by the ground upon the architect) is very much the reverse of realizing my principles. I would enter more into criticism—but that my first advice would be that sufficient space be given over to the architect to enable him, in sketching new plans, to apply the principles more fully. I would then most gladly help. At present I cannot.

Birkenhead has magnificent capacities for a hospital of the very best construction. If the present site is kept, four plots, instead of two, will be necessary. Of course a hospital of this size costs very much more per bed than one of four or eight times its size.

If you ask me what are the main things I think injurious to patients in this plan, I would instance, among others:

1. The plan is in fact a closed court, open only to the north.

2. The accident ward (accidents requiring, to give them a good chance, the very best of all conditions for recovery) has the very worst place in the building.

3. There is a closed corridor from end-to-end, on one side of which these unfortunate accidents lie.

4. In a new building the nurses' rooms and sculleries should be put in convenient places, i.e., the scullery on one side the entrance to the ward, the nurse's room on the other, so that, day and night, she commands her whole ward by a window looking into its whole *length*. (In this case she might as well get up and look through the door.)

I hardly think the architect has understood some of the applications of his principles. . . . I don't know where I have said that a ward should be "23 ft. wide." I said "*not more* than 30 ft wide." We have however built wards of "24 ft. wide." They are rather narrow for convenience, i.e., for placing moveable dressers down the middle of the ward. Besides, I have said that the bed's territory should be 12 ft. (12 × 2 = 24) [which] gives breadth of ward.

15 April 1862

Inside Parthe's portfolio is a pamphlet of mine for Mr Laird, if you will kindly send it him. The hospital of which I sent you the details of cost (£4160 for sixty beds) is the same as "Plan of a Regimental Hospital" in said pamphlet, but without the first floor of *wards*, with the central first floor. The staircase is fit only for a nobleman's house. But you can carry a patient at full length up it, without the slightest danger of shaking or alarming him, in case we should ever build our first floor of wards.

The small ward, 1, is turned into an operating room when required, and is quite good enough. The nurse's room, 2, would be too small for a woman, but could easily be increased by projecting the side. The day room is most cheerful and pleasant. Some of the other dimensions would be too small for a civil hospital. Hot water is laid over the whole hospital and arrives boiling at the lavatories at the end of the long wards, so *that* question is solved.

By the end of this year we shall have five hospitals as good as or better than this in the army.

Source: From a letter to Douglas Galton, Add Mss 45760 f76

22 April 1862

Leeds has subscribed £60,000 for a new hospital, Beckett Denison and Mr Scott, the architect, at the head. I have sent them to look at your new York Cavalry one. Birkenhead is going to build too. And I have sent Mr Laird and his architect, too, to look at it.

Source: From two letters to Parthenope Nightingale, Wellcome (Claydon copy) Ms 9000/36 and 63

2 May 1862

My dear, I send back Mr Laird's plans, with criticism. I assure you it grieves me much more than him to criticize, when the good man has taken so much pains (and understands nothing at all about it). And yet, as it often happens to me to be obliged to say, you had better put the patients under the hedges than in such a building as that.

However in this case the present ground will really admit of a beautiful hospital.

4 September 1862

My dear, Mr Laird's letter (which I forgot to return) gives no "information" whatever. Unless he were to send me all the plans, it would be of no use at all. And I confess I feel but small heart for them. . . .

I will worry about the Portsmouth Female Hospital, which is well worth it.

Editor: In 1867 Nightingale was invited to the laying of the foundation stone (by Lord Stanley) of the new, 200-bed Southern Hospital in Liverpool. The building committee, she was told, had "endeavoured in the plans to carry out the suggestions that you have made on the construction of hospitals," presumably from her *Notes on Hospitals* rather than from any direct comments. "It is probable that, upon your seeing the site as well as the plans, some valuable suggestions may occur to you," the letter went on. Dr Sutherland's draft reply makes the obvious points:

> I regret that years of confinement to a sick room render my presence in Liverpool impossible at the laying of the foundation stone of your new Southern Hospital. All I can do is to send you my very best wishes for the success of your undertaking and to offer any little assistance in my power in looking over the details of your plans should you desire it.[153]

Also in 1867, a Manchester writer, Frederick Milnes Edge, wrote Nightingale requesting that she read a pamphlet on a proposed children's hospital and dispensary for Manchester, and address a few words to the committee. He had published a book on her, *A Woman's Example and a Nation's Work: A Tribute to Florence Nightingale*, in 1864. Evidently Nightingale did write an encouraging letter, for Milnes Edge wrote her with "heartfelt" thanks, and said he would read her letter (privately) to the committee. He stated that the committee were paying increased attention to sanitary matters and were striving to bring about the appointment of a health officer and a board of health composed of the leading medical and scientific men.[154] Nightingale's (missing) letter was probably more diplomatic than the draft Sutherland prepared for her:

> Your appeal is the second I have received from Manchester within the last few days. You appear to be trying to stem the torrent of [illeg] mortality by medical attendance, for you have two special establishments for children. It is right to get your hospitals out of Manchester, because Manchester is no place for sick people, especially for sick children, but the causes of the high death rate among children in Manchester are those which neither hospitals nor medical attendance can reach. Children are made to live—not to die—and if they die it is because the society in which they are born contains some element which directly contravenes the laws of God.

---

153 Hamilton letter 17 September 1867, with a draft reply in Dr Sutherland's hand, Florence Nightingale Museum (LMA) H1/ST/NC2/V39/67.

154 Milnes Edge's letters 23 and 28 July 1867, Florence Nightingale Museum (LMA) H1/ST/NC2/V30/67 and 31/67.

This element you have in your social system and in your town. Until mothers are left to do mothers' work, and until mothers and children have places to live in where the health of both has a fair chance of being preserved, you may do what you like in the way of children's hospitals, but you will leave matters just where they are.

We in this country like to do exactly what suits us. We even claim the privilege of dying [illeg] and children. It is an unfortunate offshoot of liberty, and one is compelled to ask sometimes whether some hand strong enough to pull down and cart away much of our cities and to rebuild them all, as is now being done by the French authorities.[155] In this would it not be in the end more economical than all our Christian "support of voluntary contributions." It is an abysmal subject, which the practical Lancashire mind ought to take up and deal with.[156]

Buckinghamshire Infirmary, Aylesbury, 1859-69

Editor: Work on the Buckinghamshire Infirmary at Aylesbury,[157] as for that at Winchester Infirmary above, involved personal connections, for Nightingale's brother-in-law, Sir Harry Verney, was a major landowner in the area, as well as being an MP and chair of the building committee. Sir Harry, however, fully deferred to Nightingale's expertise, in contrast with her father, who sided with the people she considered misguided.

As was so often the case with hospital rebuilding plans, Nightingale soon came to believe that it would be "most economical in the end to build a new hospital" (see p 643 below). Rebuilding the original Aylesbury building would require such costly work as raising the flooring, for example. A new building was, in time, agreed on, with a design based on the pavilion principle and with exemplary attention to the choice of materials to facilitate keeping it clean.

In 1860 Nightingale had Galton and his clerk work on the plans, with her criticisms. Their architect should have taken care of the problems, she noted, "but he can't" (see p 647 below). Work proceeded and Parthenope Verney laid the foundation stone on 30 April

155 A reference to the massive rebuilding of Paris, with spacious avenues, under Napoléon III.

156 Draft reply in Dr Sutherland's hand, Florence Nightingale Museum (LMA) H1/ST/NC2/V29/67.

157 For background see Robert Gibbs, *A History of Aylesbury*. The plan is reproduced in *Notes on Hospitals*, Plan 2.

(or 1 May) 1861. By 1862 correspondence had moved on to the subject of furnishings (beds and mattresses) and cleaning procedures for the walls and floors. In 1866, on viewing the architect's elevation, Nightingale said that Aylesbury would be "the most beautiful hospital in England" (see p 648 below). It indeed became a model, not only for its pavilion plan, but the excellence of its materials. For example, in responding to a query in 1868, Nightingale referred to it as "specially planned for a small number of beds and . . . an excellent model to follow." She urged her brother-in-law to "let them see the plans" to give a "true answer" on the problem[158] (see p 655 below).

The hospital is commonly referred to in correspondence as the "Aylesbury Infirmary" for its location in the town, and also as the Bucks Infirmary. Officially, it was the Buckinghamshire (later Royal Buckinghamshire) Infirmary. In 1948 it became a maternity hospital when a new NHS hospital was built nearby. When this editor visited it in 2012, it had been renovated and reopened as a private hospital for the treatment of spinal injuries.

Source: Memorandum, Buckinghamshire Record Office, typed copy Wellcome Ms 9029

30 September 1859

In building or extending a hospital, it is to be taken for granted that the object in view is to benefit and not injure the sick. To have wards with only windows on one side is to injure the sick. They had better be left at home.

Every sick ward must have windows on opposite sides. Whatever plan of extension is adopted, this must be a sine qua non [without which there is nothing]. The plans you have sent me to look at fulfill this essential condition tolerably well insofar as regards the two sixteen-bed wards and the eight-bed ward. But there are three smaller wards with windows on one side only, and one of these happens to be the operating ward. There appears to be plenty of space for these three wards in a position where they could have windows on two sides. And this change could be effected by a little rearrangement.

2. The position of the water closets is not very good. But if they are in a portion of the building not yet erected they might easily be so arranged as to have a lobby separately ventilated between them and the sick wards.

158 Letter to Harry Verney 7 November 1868, Wellcome (Claydon copy) Ms 9003/52.

3. I am afraid you will find the central corridor rather dark.

4. There appears to be no window to the scullery.

5. By the plan, the large wards are 73 ft long and 17½ ft. wide. This is very narrow. To give even 1200 cubic ft. per bed, they will require to be 15 ft. high. If the wards could be made 1 or 2 ft. wider, it would be a great advantage, even at the cost of a little of their length.

6. Would it not be cheaper to devote the whole of your "villa," as it is now, to the officer and officers, and to put all your sick into the new wings? I should put my matron into the two small wards on the first floor. And put the six beds thereby done away with where the matron is now, or better still at the other end of the accident ward pavilion, where the surgeon's room is, bringing the nurse's room a little lower down the accident ward, which would not [be] too short, even if shortened, but leaving it (the nurse's room) with 2400 cubic ft. space *between* the two wards.

If, however, there is some reason why a four-bed and a two-bed ward are preferable to a six-bed ward, it might still be managed; the servants' bedroom is almost the best room in the house and has room for eight or ten.

Why not take that end for sick? They ought always to have the best. Bear in mind however (1) that the less small wards are multiplied the better. All foreign and English experience confirms this. Noisy, offensive or operation cases ought alone to be put into small wards. Even the last is now considered doubtful; (2) that it is absolutely necessary that every ward should be commanded by its nurse's room, with a window looking into her ward. This alone is a sufficient reason against multiplying small wards. And the plan of attaching a small ward to a larger one is not found to answer, as at Lariboisière. The small wards ought to have a separate nurse or nurses.

7. The staircases are not necessary for a hospital. I presume they are already there.

Note to 2. Could not the water closets be put out at the ends of the large wards, if there are no patients in the central building?

Note to 1. The operation ward, if it must be left where it is, viz., next the operating theatre, should have a window broken out on a second side, which I see could be done. At the same time, it is not a good place to have the operation case and his nurse so far out of the reach of all surveillance, but possibly this cannot be helped.

Note. I don't think that either management or health can be secured if the large wards are without a lavatory each and a scullery each. I should even prefer taking it off the length of the long wards, as they are now, and putting water closet and lavatory in the end (scullery should not be absolutely contiguous to these because it must have a fireplace). It should properly be opposite the nurse's room. I suppose the kitchens are in the basement.

Source: Memorandum, Buckinghamshire Record Office

Hampstead, N.W.
2 October 1859

After the reply received from Lady Verney, we would strongly advise as follows:

1. Find all the accommodation you require *for sick* in the proposed pavilions;

2. Place nothing in the centre building except the administration; there is no room in it for sick.

3. The wards should be at least 20 feet wide and 15 feet high, three *with 1200 cubic feet per bed* AT LEAST.

4. Each large ward should have three water closets (in one), built out from it at the end. There should be a small separately lighted and ventilated lobby between the water closet and the ward. The same out-building should contain a fixed bath, with hot and cold water laid on, and an ablution table with a few small basins, with hot and cold laid on.

5. Room might be found for the operating theatre and operating ward in one of the pavilions—perhaps at the other end of the accident ward pavilion.

In the country, direct light can quite well be obtained enough for an operating theatre without having it lighted from the roof. It is very important that the accident nurse's room should be so situated as to look in (through windows) into both accident and operating ward. It should, if possible, be between. But I would fain do away with operating wards altogether, and let the patient be taken straight back into the large ward, which ought, however, certainly to be on the same flat as the operating theatre. There should be as few small wards as possible.

6. The accident ward should have water closet and lavatory, which might be built out like those of the other wards.

7. The pavilion should be ventilated with shafts and inlets (and warmed [with] Captain Galton's stoves, if these are to be had). The

centre building should be ventilated with Arnott's valves.[159] But, when the plan is decided upon, we will give our best advice upon the manner of ventilating.

8. All that is said in my previous memo stands.

9. The pavilion plan requires only widening of its pavilions, rearrangement of some of its distribution and building out of water closets to be very good—nearly perfect in fact.

10. I need hardly say that, in mentioning the desirableness of putting all the three small wards into the pavilions, it is necessary that all the female wards should be in one pavilion and all the male wards in the other. . . .

The post-mortem room and deadhouse should be altogether out of the building and no post-mortems should ever be made in the operating theatre.

Source: From two letters to Harry Verney, Wellcome (Claydon copy) Ms 8998/7 and Buckinghamshire Record Office, both from Hampstead, N.W.

5 October 1859

I should be very glad to write in *The Builder* (a discreet little paper which always puts me in!) for your hospital, and am only afraid of setting the Buckinghamshire backs up. If, however, things should go wrong, and before they have finally gone wrong, if you will tell me and tell me also exactly what you wish to have said, I could at any time give Buckinghamshire a "blowing up" in *The Builder*, which might make some difference.

As to the width of the wards, you might make only the two ends of the pavilions two feet wider than the middle part. Or, as you have plenty of length, make the wards only as wide as they are now and put the beds not opposite but alternate

I I I I I
 I I I I   to each other

—neither plan is sightly, but in either would the sick recover.

I should have gratefully accepted your kind offer to read a paper for me at Bradford, as there is a subject I wished very much to start there: hospital statistics.[160] They are, as well as workhouse statistics, at

159 Dr Neil Arnott (1788-1874), inventor of a smokeless stove and ventilator.

160 The third meetings of the National Association for the Promotion of Social Science were held at Bradford in October 1859, but Nightingale did not send a paper.

present an unworked mine, both in France and England, and these institutions, created for the relief of human distress, positively do not know whether they relieve it or not. But my facts are not all ready, so that I have not finished my paper, as I do not like to read up or get up a thing, but must have personal observation and experience to go upon.

5 November 1859

I will first answer your questions:

1. Should the *amended* plan be adopted, it will be quite necessary to raise the flooring of the two existing (first floor) ends, so that the ground floor wards should be *at least* 13 ft. high—the first floor wards ascending by two steps from the central passage and preserving also their height of 13 ft. This will necessitate some contrivance about the nurses' rooms and sculleries.

2. I think it very probable that it will be most economical in the end to build a new hospital. It is true estimates are almost always exceeded. But, in repeating this, which everybody knows, I think people don't sufficiently remember that you *never know when* you will have done in adding to, altering or repairing an old house. The excess is even more frequent and greater, and the result less satisfactory, than in building new.

3. I should like to look over the plans you mention very much. (I sent to Burlington St. last night for them, but they were not come. I shall send again.) I should like to see these plans before I try, if I do try, an entirely new one. And also I should like, when I have seen them, if they are *approveable*, to have some kind of estimate from Mr Brandon as to what your plan (of the amendments) will cost, and what the new plan will cost. It must be, also, Mr Brandon or a builder, after all, who will make the estimate for my plan, if I make one, because so much depends on the value of labour and materials on the spot.

It would also be necessary, if I make a plan, that I should have the contour of the ground you speak of.

Source: From four letters to Harry Verney, Wellcome (Claydon copy) Ms 8998/21, and Buckinghamshire Record Office, typed copies Wellcome Ms 9029

5 March 1860

I am very much obliged to my "half nephew" for his noble offer and, as I am often employed in drawing plans for hospitals, I may very likely avail myself of it with great gratitude. I am just now about some noble plans for a great "pavilion" Manchester Infirmary *out of* the town. This is the more promising, as I hear from a man who has just been making a tour of the provincial hospitals that they are only fit to make the sick into incurables, to put poor men on the rates [welfare] and that the new are on worse principles than the old. . . .

The information I have received about provincial hospitals makes me the more feel that, without some knowledge of the proportion of surgical and medical cases, and of *what* cases, I cannot give reliable advice about the "Bucks" Infirmary. I have a *folio* volume of information about all the provincial hospitals in the U.K., which has been lent to me (Aylesbury is included). But, oddly enough, this most important information as to the average proportions of medical and surgical cases, and their character, is nowhere given.

25 April 1860

1. As to the method of warming your Bucks Infirmary, I have made inquiries and I find: if two common grates would warm the ward you mention, viz., 75 × 25 × 15 ft., *which I doubt,* one of our improved military hospital grates would do so. But the ward contains 28,125 cub. ft. I should put in *two* of our improved hospital grates, *medium size,* 1 ft. 5 inch opening. They would *enormously* economize coal. Of the grates, Captain Galton, R.E., deserves all the credit.[161]

2. I find, upon calculation, that in your plan you allot little more than 1200 cub. ft. per patient. I have laid it down that there should nowhere be less than 1500 cub. ft. per bed. In the country it signifies so much less than in town (and with country than with town-worn constitutions) that I only mention the circumstance for your consideration. . . .

To allow 1500 cub. ft. per bed would make the ward 93 ft. 6 inch long instead of 75 ft.

28 April 1860

1. The ceiling of the wards might be coved to give the height required, and a plain moulding carried round the upper edge of the coving all the way. It must be an astragal not to harbour dust. In case the coving be adopted, the windows should come as high up the ward as possible. Three of McKinnell's ventilators should be placed, as you propose, along the centre line of the building thus. These should each have an outlet (not into the roof but) through the roof.

---

161 These became known as "Galton grates," and were widely used.

2. If Captain Galton's grates be decided upon, he must be applied to as soon as possible, for the flues must be built into the wall. They are easily done enough, but they must be done while the wall is being built. There is a cold air flue, etc.

3. Our criticism was simply on the *block* plan of the hospital. When this is decided upon by the committee, we shall have plenty to say as to *detail*.

4. I cannot conceive end windows being objected to. They may be seen at Guy's and many other hospitals, and are never complained of on account of the cold. They give a nice long sweeping light to the ward. I would not put a glazed door across them, any more than I would put a glazed door across the side windows, which are close to the patients' heads.

The doors of the lobbies should be placed diagonally, and every opening A, B, and C. C.C. should be *door*ed. The lavatory will probably have a fireplace of its own.

With Captain Galton's grates, there will not be three weeks in the year when there will be the least danger of cold. There will not be many months in the year when *both* need to be lighted.

A. Jackson's
Upper Terrace
Hampstead, N.W.
21 September 1860

Thank you very much for the prospectus of the infirmary. I rejoice to see that you are so far advanced in the matter of money. But I protest against "my authority" being used for a plan, against several features of which I have entered an objection, e.g., the three beds at the end of each of the two large wards have no windows and no direct ventilation whatever, except from the W.C. lobby. If you tell me that there is any time yet for sending you a criticism of the plan, I will do so with pleasure. But my last paper to you included all my objections.

To make the plan a perfectly healthy one would involve very little, if any, more expenditure. It would also involve no deception of those to whom the prospectus may have been sent, as people are much too ignorant on the subject to know the difference. . . .

We have to thank you for a beautiful basket of game, etc.

Source: From notes, Buckinghamshire Record Office

[October 1860]

The questions are:

1. What is the average proportion of men to women patients? It is supposed by the plan that they will be equal. If so, it is against all county hospital experience.

2. Do the medical officers agree to having medical and surgical cases *together*? i.e., only one large female and one large men's ward? What kind of proportion do medical bear to surgical cases, on an average? What is the actual number of female surgical cases *ever*?

3. What is the annual number of operations? And what the proportion of male to female? Are there *ever* any female capital operations?

4. I cannot help working away at the Bucks Infirmary plans—in spite of Sir Harry's prohibition. I could suggest some important alterations, which I believe would actually *lessen* the cost. But three questions I have asked have never been answered. And without these answers, you are working in the dark.

The printed paper Sir Harry sent me (*annual sheets*) gave no answers. Perhaps they *have* no statistics. But they *must* make out these things or they may be planning without knowing their own wants.

E.g., a common case in county hospitals is this: that the men patients are *always* two thirds of the whole number, that half of the men patients are *surgical* cases and that there is never (or hardly ever) a capital operation on a woman. So that the accommodation wanted would be:

1 male surgical ward
1 " medical "
1 female general ward

and one or two single wards.

Also, a hospital would never work if the medical men decidedly objected to mixing the surgical and medical cases, e.g., it would never be right to put amputation and Fever cases together should these form the average cases of the hospital.

Please preserve these questions, all of which I have written before, and don't build your hospital without having them answered.

Source: From three letters to Douglas Galton, Add Mss 45759 ff73, 87 and 92, all from Hampstead

6 October 1860

I send you the Bucks Infirmary plan, with criticisms, as you were so good as to say that you and Mr Graham[162] would do it. At the same time you know, if you are much pressed just now, I think their own architect *ought to* do it. *But he can't.*

24 October 1860

I send you *my* "minute" about St George's Hospital kitchen. I am no admirer of the civil hospitals, as you know. But what I send you about their kitchens is literally true.

I send back the Bucks Infirmary plan, with many thanks and one suggestion. But again I say, if you are pressed, this is obviously the business of the Bucks people to do themselves.

I should like to send some affecting attention to Mr Graham—a man for whom I have conceived the highest admiration.

Many thanks for your cottage grates. Could the oven be ventilated?

31 October 1860

If you would be so good as to come up here and dine *Friday,* we shall be all ready for you, I mean as to plans, not as to mutton chops. I am very sorry to write so late.

Thank you very much for the Bucks plans—I think them excellent. Much better than *their own,* and I should think less costly.

Source: From undated notes, probably for the architect, Add Mss 45791 ff8-9

[c1860]

Bucks Infirmary Plans. The following points require consideration:

1. The cost in proportion to the accommodation, on account of the great extent of the administration. The sick wards occupy an area of 4508 sq. ft., out of a total area of above 9000 sq ft.

2. Much of the accommodation for administrative offices is far too good.

3. All the kitchen offices must be removed from where they are. They spoil the ward above. Should they not go into the central basement, if not wholly detached?

4. The washhouse (now in the basement) *must* be detached.

162 Alex Graham (1847-1922), architect of Lincoln Hospital and the Swansea Infirmary.

5. The five corner beds at the end of each ward are out of the question. There must be only two, one in each corner, with 18 inches between wall and bed, and then a window. Take out the bed in the middle altogether.

6. Why no end window and why not ablution and bathroom in a projection at end? Is it on account of the ground?

7. Why both grates on the same side the ward?

8. I cannot conceive how the patient is to be got up those stairs and through that door to the operating theatre, still less how he is to be got down again. If the operating theatre is to be upstairs, for which there seems no reason, as it does not *appear* to be lighted through the roof, there *must*, in this case, be a contiguous ward.

Source: From four letters to Harry Verney, Buckinghamshire Record Office and Wellcome (Claydon copy) Ms 8998/40-41, typed copies of the second and third Wellcome Ms 9029, all from Hampstead, N.W.

24 November 1860

1. As to medical and surgical wards, this is purely a doctors' point. If they are satisfied, so am I. I will venture to say that I could keep a properly constructed ward so *safe* as to put medical and surgical cases *safely* together in it. But doctors are generally very strong against this. And I received one letter of remonstrance from an eminent London doctor who had accidentally seen your plans. But London cases are *very* different from provincial ones, and I had much rather mix surgical and medical cases in two good wards (male and female) than have them unmixed in four bad ones.

I have done:

2. Your male and female cases are nearly equal. That is well.

3. You have scarcely one female capital operation case in fourteen months. Therefore it is absurd to provide a surgical ward for her.

4. I was not a little (certainly) surprised to find Mr Carrington asserting that the plans were constructed upon my printed opinions, when the six beds at the two ends of the wards are placed there in defiance of every opinion I have ever printed or written.

5. I adhere to my opinion of a window at the end of the ward.

6. I think Mr Brandon's elevation by far the best I have ever seen. It will be the most beautiful hospital in England.

7. I was (again) not a little surprised to find Mr Carrington advocating the present arrangement of beds upon the difficulty of arranging the windows. All one can say is, if there is difficulty in arranging the windows, then arrange the windows. We *have* done it in all the new

military hospitals and it is curious indeed to see them taking the start of the civil ones.

8. I send you a plan arranged for a hospital of similar proportions and numbers, male and female, to yours. Please return it to me. I am assured that it will be cheaper than yours. The elevation may nearly be the same—the details are not all properly worked out. Its principal merit is the doing away with the upper storey of the centre—the pushing out the kitchen from the basement to the back of the hospital—the putting the operation theatre (so seldom used) over the kitchen, from which the cases may be safely carried to the wards.

I am sure that Mr Ceely[163] will agree with me in the propriety of this. An operating theatre ought always to be on the same floor as the wards.

The same architect who does our new military hospitals did this plan for me, which is for a civil one, and which is going to be worked out, detail by detail. . . .

9. It is certainly a great improvement (in the silver paper plan) not having the washhouse in the basement, nor the kitchen under the wards. But you had much better have neither kitchen nor washhouse in the building at all. *We* don't in the new military hospitals, which leave you completely behind.

10. To add another storey to this hospital, in order to double the accommodation, would be to be guilty of the grossest extravagance (this is Mr Carrington's plan) because for £500 more you could probably double the accommodation in the present proposed plan, minus two beds, for the receiving offices are much too large and expens[ive] for the size of the hospital. If you required two storeys of wards, [they] might be built *outside* at a very cheap rate.

11. An impression seems to run through Mr C.'s letter that it is necessary, in order to secure the greatest sanitary and administrative advantages, to incur great cost. Whereas the truth is that it is always cheaper to build a good hospital than a bad one.

15 December 1860

I am glad indeed to hear that you have carried the end windows of the Bucks wards and removed the beds. I hope that in removing these, you have left room for only one in each corner. Else they will be put back again. Also, that you have widened the staircase.

---

163 Robert Ceely (d. 1880), surgeon at the Bucks Infirmary.

We could give you a plan for the ventilation of the kitchen which would make it nearly innocuous where it is. (No plan could have made the washhouse harmless there.)

I should like very much to see the plans, when thus revised, and I will then write you as "handsome" a letter as I can, enclosing my £25.

We have carried polished Parian cement, plate glass windows and oak floors for our new Woolwich Hospital (650 beds) as being the *cheapest* in the end, and is done by women and girls.

Xmas Day 1860

With regard to your hospital kitchen:

1. Carry a tube or flue, one square foot in area, from the ceiling of the kitchen in the chimney stack up above the roof, to act as a ventilator to remove fumes and heated air.

2. Put a glass louvred ventilator ("Moore's ventilator") into the upper row of the kitchen window. It is of course better to put the kitchen where it *can't* do any harm. And upon this principle we act in all our new hospitals. But in old constructions we find this plan answer[s].

We have tried the plan for the end appurtenances of wards indicated in your tracing and have not found it answer. Also the end bed is much disturbed by the passing to and fro into the lavatory, etc.

Something like the enclosed we are now doing. And I am going to send you a tracing of what we have decided upon for the new Woolwich Hospital upon the plan of the enclosed, which I think will prove perfect. You have done so much in this new Bucks Infirmary that it would be a thousand pities not to have it quite perfect.

28 December 1860

I send you a tracing of the *ends* of our wards at the new Woolwich Hospital, which, after many alterations, we have adopted as the best that could be contrived.

Many thanks for your hamper.

I sent the letters to Mr Carrington and to Mr Brandon, as desired.

I am now doing a new hospital at Lisbon for the king of Portugal to the memory of his queen, by Prince Albert's desire. (The tracing I send you will be adopted there.)

Source: From a letter to Douglas Galton, Add Mss 45759 ff126-29

Hampstead, N.W.
29 December 1860

Thank you very much for the tracing, of which I have made two. I sent your Bucks Infirmary plan long ago to Sir Harry Verney and now I have sent this.

Although we have not got all we want (they *won't* build their kitchen out behind, and they *will* build their operating theatre in the roof where the cats go), they have certainly improved their wards very much. After your suggestions—which I did not give them the chance of refusing—for I told them you had made that plan for me and they think we are going to build it elsewhere. It is the only way—they were quite eager to have the plan then. And, by the same line of tactics, they have been got to adopt polished cement, oak floors, etc.

Source: From two letters to Harry Verney, Wellcome (Claydon copy) Ms 8999/3 and 6

2 January 1861

Please to consider the tracing I sent you (of the ends of the wards) as a bill for £25, which, if not accepted by the committee, will be dishonoured.

That blessed committee is still haggling about the "polished Parian." They want to have oil paint. Now paint requires renewing, which costs more. Paint is good, varnished paint is better, polished Parian is best. I have written to Mr Brandon about it and asked him to send on my note to you, for he, poor man, I suppose, has no power.

What you want to get into people's heads is this—walls, floors and ceilings may all be equally dangerous or equally safe—I know of no distinction. People say, oh yes, the floors are walked upon. Not *everywhere*, not under the beds and tables. Yet there is no matron but would have these washed. I would wash my walls just as often.

And the question is, how to make your walls and floors so that they can be washed with safety. Now paint is certainly *saturable* and *dampable*, though very much better than plaster. But to be safe it ought to be varnished, and varnish is very destructible. And in England deleterious substances are often put into varnishes and paints.

15 March 1861

I have only had a very good note from Mr Brandon about the cost of the Bucks Infirmary, no estimate. His note proves that a good county hospital could be built for £80 to £100 per bed for 100 patients.

Because your lower floor might be converted into wards and your offices pushed out behind, at a cost, *my* advisors tell me, of £1000 more, I should like to see the estimate.

Source: Notes, Buckinghamshire Record Office

25 November 1861

Bucks Infirmary. It is a *very* good scheme, with the exception of certain small faults of detail. The block plan is good for the size of the hospital. The following points appear to require reconsideration:

1. Have the medical staff consented to put surgical and medical cases together? There are only two (one male and one female) wards, besides the two small ones. Do they not desire at least an accident ward for men? Do they not desire it on the ground floor? Or are there too few accident cases to make this necessary? Do they not want an operating room? Or is this provided for in the centre upper flat, of which we have not the plan?

Two very minute criticisms I have to make. There appears to be no window into the closet off the scullery (men's side) nor over the W.C.

2. A window would be better than a door from the nurse's room into the small ward. A dark place in a hospital is always a dirty place, a skulking place and a receptacle of foul air. I do not much like a closet at all in a scullery. A press is a much better thing, coal box, etc. But, however this is settled, all these places must have windows, or not be there at all.

3. There should only be a foot between the top of the windows and the top of the wards.

4. The lavatories, etc., should not be placed at the centre of the length, but at the end. But, in the present "*end*" arrangement, the patients in five beds would be disturbed by the passing in and out of the lavatories, etc. The two *corner* beds are inadmissible for other reasons. There never should be more than one bed in each corner, and then a window between it and the next bed. How is the "store" off the staircase (men's side) intended to be lighted at all?

If a large end window is desired, it might be done thus: with a lavatory and lobby on one side, and a W.C. with lobby on the other. It is of great importance not to disturb the end patients with the passing in and out.

It is decidedly objectionable to have kitchen and scullery under sick wards (in the army hospitals we are trying to get rid of kitchens in such situations).

I will make inquiries whether a ward 75 × 25 and 15 ft. high cannot be warmed by one of our improved hospital grates, instead of there being two, as in the plan.

2. Is the accommodation for the rest of the nurses in the top centre flat, of which we have not the plan? Is it not an useless expense to have two lifts and two linen shafts? For so small a hospital, one lift and one linen shaft would do.

3. *Aylesbury Infirmary.* It is always desirable, where practicable, to put men and women patients on different floors. As both sexes are on the same floor, the women's pavilion should be cut off from the staircase by a swing door, with lock and key—always to be locked at night. One such door is better than two. The best place for it is at the head of the stair at + on the women's side. This gives all the isolation both obtainable and practicable.

Certainly not longitudinal but cross-ventilation is the intention of all good hospital plans. The staircase up to the roof is intended to cut off the atmosphere of one pavilion from the other, and by an up current to prevent as far as practicable the air of one ward from passing into the other. The partition between the large wards (one men's and one women's apparently) should be thick enough to prevent any sound from passing.

Provincial hospitals are very commonly nursed by one night nurse. It is a very objectionable practice, if only because the men's and women's side ought to be (especially at night) entirely separate. (But there are other grave reasons against that practice.) One night nurse there should be for the women's side and one for the men's. And "occasional" night nurses (women "had in" by the night) ought thus to be entirely unnecessary, which does away with a great evil.

Having answered the questions asked, may I once more enter my protest (1) against the *double* corner beds—*one* ought certainly to be removed from each end corner. And certainly there ought to be a screen, even if there be only one bed, to screen it from the ward offices and the patients going in and out. (2) One lift and one linen shaft is enough for so small a hospital, IF it saves expense not to have two of each. With proper discipline, there can be no difficulty, by day, when alone they are used. The remaining space might be made into a store closet, though rather too dark for it.

Source: From a letter to Harry Verney, and undated notes, Buckinghamshire Record Office, typed copy Wellcome Ms 9029

14 February 1862

When I was an Irish boy, I should have replied to this question about chaff, is it *chaffing* you are? that I would supply an unlimited quantity of it, without contract.

Hair is the only material yet discovered fit for the sick to lie upon. And it can be washed and cleansed without limit. Coconut fibre is good. But, like all vegetable substances, when it becomes damp it tends to decompose. Now hair is free from all these objections. It is now everywhere being introduced, even in the worst hospitals in the world, those of the British Army. And I never rested till I made this matter of secretary of state's regulation (in 1859).

There should be one or two fracture beds, according to the average number of fractures at Aylesbury. There are cases, but which I never saw in provincial hospitals, cases of inveterate infirmity, chiefly among old men and women, as at Greenwich, Chelsea and in workhouse wards, where the funds of the institution will not admit of hair being supplied. For these I prefer straw, not stuffed but *quilted* in. But as the Aylesbury Infirmary are accustomed to chaff, let them have chaff. It is more elastic *but* it allows the patient to slip down uncomfortably. But, I repeat, it is only for these cases that chaff is admissible, and I never saw these cases in hospitals. A little ingenuity and great care on the part of the nurse is all that is necessary to save the mattress of hair in cases of casual infirmity. . . .

Let me add that I *never* use a blanket under any of my own patients—that I never saw one used *under* a patient without great injury to the same—that it is one of the main causes of bedsores—that I never knew a good hospital nurse who did not lift up her hands in horror at the use of one *under* a hospital patient. It may be necessary where you use chaff or straw. But I would use neither. Lay your sheet on the hair mattress and your patient on the sheet. And with the most ordinary care, you will never have bedsores, even with the most prolonged cases of compound fracture.

[ca. March 1862]

Surgeons in ordinary on the most ordinary hospital furniture: what is bad is dear; what is good is cheap in the end. All hospitals, even the French military, who are actually going to have rheocline beds, have found out that good beds are the cheapest.

I have written to our purveyor-in-chief at the War Office to know the annual cost per bed of [horse]hair. I believe it is about 12/. If you like to wait for the answer, I will send it directly it comes, but I repeat, there is *no* question that what is bad is always dear.

Bucks Infirmary. Walls. I have no hesitation in saying that common plaster and limewashing is better than unpolished cement. Polished cement is very expensive, but it saves its cost in limewash (or ought to do so) in a few years. People never think of this.

Plaster hospital walls ought to be limewashed twice a year *at least*, and *are* so now in military hospitals (by a queen's regulation of 1859). The unpolished Parian cement of Netley Hospital retains dirt and completes the failure of that luckless concern. It costs 2/6 a yard, and will require limewashing (or ought to do so). Polished cement requires only simple washing. It costs 10d a foot. A *very* pale pink is "warmer" than pure white. The colouring is inexpensive. (At Guy's and King's College Hospitals may be seen the unpolished cement. Its only impression on the eye is that of dirt.)

Floors. Oak is preferable for the *white* floor. If the hospital provided the crutches, as it ought, and these are properly tipped with cloth, they will not slip. French hospitals which *frotter* [polish] make, however, no complaint of slipping. And we shall never get the amount of polish which their *frottage* obtains—consequently not the same amount of slipperiness.

I recommend the mode of cleaning at p 217 of the book which I send.[164] It is no experiment or crotchet of mine. It actually exists.

Editor: The new hospital was opened in June 1862. The following year Nightingale wrote Sir Harry Verney about putting in "a small plan and elevation of your Aylesbury Infirmary, as it now is." She asked for a lithographical plan, or the loan of the architect's plans if they were not available.[165]

Source: From a letter to Harry Verney, Wellcome (Claydon copy) Ms 9003/52

7 November 1868

I see your name on the enclosed (which however I can scarcely decipher). The true answer to it is let them see the plans of Aylesbury Infirmary, which was specially planned for a small number of beds

---

164 "Method of Polishing Floors," in the revised *Notes on Nursing*, 1861, in *The Nightingale School* (12:701-02).

165 Letter 22 June 1863, Wellcome (Claydon copy) Ms 9000/108.

and will be an excellent model to follow. But, if you have already answered, or are not going to answer, just return me the enclosed, please.

Pray tell Parthe that "I've been quite cheered and nourished in my heart for to read "Avonhoe."[166] . . .

I followed your advice about Mr Chadwick. Many thanks.

Editor: By (roughly) 1869, a note Nightingale wrote gave firm evidence of the infirmary's success with shorter hospital stays: "The effect (of the new infirmary) has been that we cure in two months patients who used to be three months in the old, bad, ill-arranged, ill-ventilated building."[167] The question of an extension came up in 1882 (see p 833 below).

The infirmary, in time the Royal Buckinghamshire Hospital, remained in operation until the formation of the National Health Service in 1948, when a neighbouring hospital, Stoke-Mandeville, was expanded to take on its functions. It then became a maternity hospital, and later still a private hospital for the treatment of spinal injuries.

Source: From a letter and an incomplete letter to William Farr, Wellcome Ms 5474/70-71, typed copies Add Mss 43399 ff192 and 193-94

16 February 1864

I have first to thank you for your "jolly" little inkstand, on the truly practical principle. Second, to thank you for your truly witty letter in the *Medical Times.*[168] But I also greatly enjoyed the two adverse articles—it is the only comfort and amusement I have to see men showing themselves up in that way.

I send a copy of *Notes on Hospitals* for *The Lancet,* as you desire. And I hope to see it distinguish itself. . . .

I have to thank you, and most particularly, for your census report, which is really grand. And, also for the copy of your letter to Mr W. Cowper about the honour due to the Registrar-General,[169] in which you

---

166 A book by her sister, first serialized in *Cornhill Magazine.*

167 Note c1869, Add Mss 47716 f67.

168 W. Farr, "Miss Nightingale's 'Notes on Hospitals,'" *Medical Times and Gazette* 13 February 1864:186-87.

169 William Francis Cowper (1811-88), later Baron Mount-Temple, commissioner of works in Cabinet; however no honour seems to have been given to the Registrar-General, Major Gordon.

may be sure I fully concur. If I have an opportunity, I will say so. But I am not much in that line now.

23 February 1864

Private. Your informant was well informed about the Privy Council hospital inquiry. Mr Simon, for the Privy Council, selected Dr Bristowe of St Thomas' and Mr T. Holmes of St George's[170] to make an investigation and report of all the hospitals in England and Wales, the principal hospitals of Scotland and Ireland, and some of the Continental hospitals.

It has been already going on for some months. And a great part of their report is in proof. It is voluminous and goes into foundation, construction, administration, general plan and minor details, with general statistics. Bristowe and Holmes divided England between them; Ireland, Scotland and the Continent they took as suited the convenience of each.

A man in whose opinion I have great confidence has glanced at the report and says that, "though it will have all the prestige of the Privy Council to back it," he does "not fear the result," that it contains gross blunders and that both Bristowe and Holmes are thoroughly inexperienced.

I take it their conclusions are at variance with your statistics. You will now understand Bristowe's letter in the *Medical Times.*[171] *I* say, *too,* let us have the whole matter out, the more discussion the better. Let us know whether they are killing or curing the people in hospitals. But I am not so sure that the Privy Council report will not damage us for the moment.

Source: From a letter to A.J. Humbert,[172] Florence Nightingale Museum 0549

1 March 1864

I have not yet received any reply from Sir James Clark. As it is left to us to be doctor and director as well as architect, I unhesitatingly pronounce in favour of keeping the thirty-two-bed wards. It would be a

---

170 Respectively, John Syer Bristowe (1827-95) and Timothy Holmes (1825-1907).

171 J.S. Bristowe, "Miss Nightingale on Hospitals," *Medical Times and Gazette* 20 February 1864:211; in it he took up Farr's defence of Nightingale, which he took to be a "grave charge" against hospitals, and demanded that Farr make public the facts on which his case was based.

172 Architect of the Lisbon Children's Hospital, but it is not clear to what plans this letter pertains.

pity to make imperfect wards out of wards which are perfect, without any instructions so to do. They must exclude certain cases, that is all.

The French, who are the only nation, except their cousin-Belgians, who have *at all* considered the question of hospital construction, have come, for very sufficient reasons, to the conclusions I have stated to you.

But I would fully equip the small wards with sister's room, scullery, etc., and every appurtenance, as these will probably contain the very worst cases, according as they are set apart, whether lithotomy cases, or the most severe cutaneous forms.

Editor: An article in the *Medical Times and Gazette* in 1864 credited the Norfolk and Norwich Hospital with low mortality rates post-surgery, not because of the Norwich air, but because of the hospital's adequate cubic space, natural ventilation and lack of crowding; further, surgeons and dressers did not come in with hands and clothes dirty from the dissecting room.[173] More on this hospital appears later (see p 808 below).

Source: From a letter to Charles Williams,[174] Florence Nightingale Museum (LMA) H1/ST/NC1/64/6

21 May 1864

Sir, I have to thank you for annually sending me your Norwich Hospital statistics.

Although affording a number of points of comparison, they are not sufficient for many practical purposes. I venture to send you a copy of St Bartholomew's Hospital statistics for last year, just out. They are the most complete I know. It is a pity that yours should not be perfect—especially now when the comparative mortality of different hospitals and of the hospitals of different countries is daily becoming a more pressing question. And Norwich has already done so much towards its solution.

I need not point out to your experience the different headings of interest in the accompanying report. . . .

I see great stress made (in the Norwich Hospital manifesto) on the night nurses having one or two nights in bed "during the week." I

173 B.W.R. [B.W. Richardson], "Commentary on Hospital Mortality," *Medical Times and Gazette* 5 March 1864:262-63.

174 Charles Williams, surgeon, Norfolk and Norwich Hospital.

should lay great stress on their having *eight hours* "in bed" *every day* "during the week," which allows for dressing and undressing. Many strong women cannot sleep at all by day—consequently never can be night nurses—*all* require an apprenticeship to begin with, a week's night nursing at first or so. But, the apprenticeship once accomplished, it is my experience that it is better to make night nurses altogether night nurses (at least for six months at a time) and not to endeavour to piece out insufficient day sleep with *occasional* nights in bed.

Editor: The following letter concerns an infirmary for Bradfield College, Berkshire, a school which had been modelled on the more prestigious Winchester School.[175] Nightingale was evidently approached by Sir William Heathcote when she was working with him about Winchester Infirmary plans. His letter outlining the problem is missing. Nightingale's reply follows immediately.

Source: From a typed copy of a letter to Sir William Heathcote, Florence Nightingale Museum (LMA) H1/ST/NC5/3/22

5 July 1864

I only received your note of 1 July yesterday afternoon. And I happened to be particularly busy that day. This must be my excuse for delay in answering.

If we were asked to provide an infirmary for twenty-five beds upon a population of 150, we should begin by asking (Hibernicé [Irish]) what horrible sanitary wrong is there at home to be put right that you should require accommodation for such a sick population?

If they really ever have such an amount of scarlet fever, or of any sick, as twenty-five to 150, there should be most serious inquiry into the sanitary state of the school. And we would indicate the points to be inquired into: drains, sinks, W.C.s, stuffy dormitories, bedding, etc. (In any building for 150 with which we have to do, we should consider seven beds an ample allowance and be very indignant if they were all filled.)

Position. If the school is in the open country, the hospital may be placed wherever it will get plenty of light and air. And if it is a long building, the end may be brought within 20 or 30 feet of the school—always bearing in mind that it must be out of reach of the noise of the

175 Arthur Francis Leach, *A History of Bradfield College* 4.

playground and that, if the diets are cooked in the school kitchen, the hospital part must be connected with the school by a covered way.

Accommodation. Assuming the sick at fifteen and the convalescents at ten, one sick ward for twelve, one for three, would be convenient. They should be on the upper floor with a nurse's room and scullery between them. The convalescents might be on the lower floor. And the matron should have her bedroom and sitting room on the same floor. Also clothes room and clean linen room. Also a surgery for medicines, etc. Two nurses would be quite necessary for the two sick wards, where there is certain to be much night work, besides a cleaning woman, who will have enough to do, and must sleep in the house and belong to the establishment. The convalescents must have a nurse, besides the matron, a bedroom and sitting room, a separate door and a separate playground.

Cubic space. The sick beds must have (in the twelve-bed ward) not less than 1200 cubic ft.—better 1500—and (in the three-bed ward) at least 2000 ft. each. The convalescents should have 1000 to 1200 cubic ft. each in the bedroom. Unquestionably they should have a day room too.

I have not had much experience among young sick of the educated class of men. But I once directed myself an establishment for the sick of the young lady class—chiefly governesses—and was both matron and head nurse. Now an establishment for twenty-five sick and convalescents (of the educated class) *is* in fact a hospital. And I should consider it better that it should have its own kitchen. For scarlet fever, especially, there must be numberless messes prepared, which *must* be done in the hospital fire range. If you do these, you may as well do all the diets in the hospital. At least I should think so.

I would give as a warning this: all ward offices, now as a rule admirable in public hospitals, are execrable in every *educated* infirmary I have ever seen—execrable as to position, construction, everything (I would point out the Rugby School Infirmary), whereas they ought to be better for the educated than for the uneducated.

Source: From a letter to Douglas Galton, Add Mss 45762 f75

10 March 1864

Parian Cement: obviously useless for corridors and open passages exposed to damp. There appears to be no complaint of the Netley ward walls. Does not this indicate damp as the cause of cracking in the corridor? The material is certainly very imperfect. Would it not be advisable to have a special report from Major Ravenhill on the condition of cement in wards which have been occupied?

Malta Civil Hospitals, 1862-65

Editor: In 1862 Nightingale was approached by Ferdinand V. Inglott, comptroller of Charitable Institutions for Malta, then on a visit in London. He asked Nightingale for advice on plans for a proposed house for the aged and infirm for 1000 inmates, and a hospital for incurables for 300. On the advice of Dr Sutherland, T.H. Wyatt had been appointed as architect. Before proceeding, Inglott wanted her advice on the general arrangements.[176]

Inglott's letter of August 1862 asked Nightingale for her "final approval" of the plans for the Incurables Hospital, "in their complete and finished state." He noted that "almost all your suggestions have been attended to and embodied in the several buildings, and the rest is *now* as perfect as the most perfect charity could have made it." He thanked her for her "invaluable assistance" and asked for her permission to quote her opinion of the hospital.[177] Plans for the Poorhouse and Incurables Hospital are in *Notes on Hospitals* (Nos. 8 and 9).

Source: From a typed copy of a letter to and notes for T.H. Wyatt, Royal Malta Library 396 1-4 and 7-16, copies Wellcome Ms 9084/15

23 May 1862

Sir, I sent your Malta Hospital plans, with my observations, to Dr Sutherland, at 41 Finchley New Road, yesterday. He has not returned them to me. I therefore suppose he intends to communicate with you.

The plans are so good (far better than those of any hospital for men and women I have ever seen) that the difficulty was how to find a fault. I could not discover a single sanitary lapse. And my criticisms are simply administrative, and probably some of them will not be admitted by you.

I assure that it was a pleasure to me (and no "trouble") to look at such admirable plans. And I am only sorry that my illness prevents me from going over them personally with you.

---

176 Inglott letter 21 May 1862, Florence Nightingale Museum (LMA) H1/ST/NC2/V15/62. For background, see Malcolm Borg, *British Colonial Architecture: Malta (1800-1900)* 74-81.

177 Inglott letter 15 August 1862, Florence Nightingale Museum (LMA) H1/ST/NC/V19/62.

Privately, might I be allowed to give Mr Wyatt a hint that the Royal Hospital for Incurables here is about to build, and that it would be a very great joy to me to learn that Mr Wyatt was the architect? They consulted me many months ago about plans. Since then, quarrels amongst the governors have put off everything. Were I sure that the planning was in Mr Wyatt's hands, I should be sure it would be well done.

Malta Hospital for Incurables. . . .

Special Wards.

1. If the two one-bed wards are necessary, they are certainly in the best place for being nursed. The objection is that they will be noisy and that things can be taken in to the patients without the head nurse's knowledge. An essential to them is that there should be a sink, W.C. and hot and cold water, lavatory basin, attainable without the "slops" being carried through the larger ward. (It is presumed that the patients in the small wards are bedridden and therefore they do not require conveniences for themselves. But it is all the more necessary that the nurse should be able to "wash up" for them apart from the other patients, since these beds are there for the purpose of segregation.) (2) Also W.C.s for the nurses are necessary in the building and apart from those of the patients.

2. The arrangement of the end offices is not better in the flyleaf than on the place [plan], provided the end window be left open in plan.

It is always found better, where practicable, to quarter the nurses of each ward together and apart from the staff of any other ward, so as to be completely under the surveillance of the head nurses.

A ward of thirty-two beds requires:

1 head nurse
2 day nurses
1 night nurse

or if, as is presumed, the majority of these cases are not acute, one head nurse could easily overlook both wards as [on] the same floor, and one night nurse sit up with them—the head nurse sleeping next, the night nurse sitting up in the ward where are the worst cases. In this case, where there are usually very many patients (among incurable), another day nurse (between both wards) would probably be wanted.

But this is a matter for the matron, not me, to settle. My point is that, if the wards on the same floor are considered as under one head nurse, the empty head nurse's room would accommodate one or two nurses, perhaps, by a little arrangement, all except the night nurse, who must have a quiet room to sleep in by day by herself.

Should this be not thought desirable, the matron's proximity to the nurse's quarters certainly makes that the best place for them. But the night nurse could still less (than in the other places) sleep there since she would be constantly disturbed by the nurses' day room. I am not generally for nurses' day rooms. Each staff of nurses ought to dine in their own scullery and make that their day room. And for this purpose the scullery ought to be comfortable and large enough.

3. Is it necessary for matron and wardmasters to have kitchens of their own? Would not their dinners be better cooked in the large kitchen? A small scullery where tea, etc., could be made is generally found all that is necessary, and more comfortable, where the great kitchen is well managed.

4. It is necessary to have some surveillance over patients' day rooms. Otherwise they are found to do themselves more harm than good in there. The bow window rooms seem to have no supervision.

5. Is the men's side entirely served by men? Or are there female head nurses? It is always desirable to have a female head nurse to each floor, besides the wardmaster, and men nurses under the female head nurse.

6. I do not know why the men's clothing is separated from the women's. In the strictest R. Catholic orders, the same "sister" has generally charge of both. There need not be two mending rooms, two mattress rooms, etc. It is optional whether to have a separate vestiary for men and for women. But both may be under the same charge. There is too much room for mending, too little for clean linen store. One mending room, one clean linen store, one mattress room and two vestiaries, if desired, I should prefer.

7. Also, there should be in each ward (not in sister's room or scullery) a movable dresser for clean linen and another (both to lock up) for such stores as are kept in ward.

8. There is no necessity for the storeroom opposite scullery at entrance of dining room. The dividing, if it does not take place in kitchen, should take place in scullery.

9. But the dining and day room seem without any kind of supervision. This "storeroom" might be an officer's room.

10. To every floor must be a lift.

11. And to every floor a foul linen shaft communicating with a well-aired, well-lighted, closet below.

12. To return to the clothing store range. If there are two grills, the one to give out clothing, etc., to the men's side, the other to the

women's, so that the attendants need not enter inside that range at all, this is the utmost division wanted.

13. It is found a great blessing where patients from first floor can be wheeled into gallery in chapel on same plane.

14. There must be not less than two nurses to each of the wards, even those as small as eight-bed wards. There hardly seems to be nurse accommodation enough.

15. Of course the men's quarters over the store clothing range cannot be too separate from each other.

16. Do not pinch up the head nurses' rooms too much. These women, whose room is their only home, ought to have space and comfort.

17. If the nurses are to sleep apart from their wards, the W.C. accommodation is very nice. But women must be allowed to have each her washstand in their own compartment. And there must be a sink at hand.

18. The matron must have a female servant and a linen nurse, the latter rather a responsible person. These two must each have a bedroom. There is ample room in the matron's quarters.

19. The wardmaster's quarters seem too large.

20. The linen nurse will certainly want women assistants. Probably these only come in by the day.

21. Is there sufficient accommodation for servants, cooks, kitchen servant, etc.? Are these men or women?

Source: From notes, Add Mss 45825 ff151-64

[c1862]

Outline Specification of Buildings Required for Proposed General Hospital at Malta.

The site proposed for the new hospital is St Michael's Bastion, together with some ground at present covered with private houses. The bastion is on the S.W. side of Valetta and overlooks the quarantine harbour. It will be sufficiently convenient for the troops and garrison at Valetta and in the forts to the west. Sick from the forts on the east side of Malta harbour would have to be brought by boats to the Valetta side as at present, and they would have to be conveyed up the steep ascent rising immediately from the water side and along a single line of street, about ¼ mile in length. The means of access to St Michael's Bastion are very nearly as good as those to the present hospital.

It is proposed to take about 10,000 sq. yds. of ground for the hospital and its appurtenances. The area is an irregular polygon, 500 ft. in its greatest length and 250 ft. in its greatest breadth. It adjoins the houses of the town on three fourths of one side. On all the other sides it is freely exposed to the sea and land breezes. The highest surface level is 164 feet above the sea level.

And so far as we can judge from the maps and plans, the site is a very good one for its intended purpose. The surface is somewhat irregular: 2400 sq. ft. outside the flanking battery are 24 ft. below the general level of the bastion, 14,000 sq. ft. of what is called the lower level are 7 ft. 3 in. below the surface. And 17,000 sq. ft. of Spencer's Bastion are nearly 12 ft. below the level. These differences of level could easily be removed where necessary; part of the difference indeed might be converted into an advantage. Thus the hospital kitchen, fuel stores and provision stores might be placed in the first-named hollow. And a space might be found there for a small hospital washhouse for washing the hospital bandages and dressings. Pavilions to be erected on Spencer's Bastion might have an additional storey under the level which, besides bringing the wards to the general level, would afford a large amount of accommodation for stores.

In this, as in other instances, the ground plan of the hospital must be determined by the form and extent of the ground.

We find that there is superficial area enough on which to erect a pavilion hospital for 300 sick, allowing ample space sheltered from the sun for convalescents to take exercise in the open air. The longest axis the ground lies from N.E. to S.W., and we propose that the lengthway of the building should be in this line. By adopting this principle, it will be easy to shelter the pavilions to a considerable extent from sun heat.

We propose that there should be six pavilions—that each pavilion should have two flats of wards, with an arched basement to allow the air to pass below the wards, that the pavilions should be arranged parallel to each other, with their axes running from N.W. to S.E., that there should be an interval of 50 ft. between the pavilions, and that the whole should be connected together by a corridor 12 or 13 ft. wide and 430 ft. long, running from N.E. to S.W. From the conformation of the ground, it will not be possible to make the pavilions all of the same length. The two to be placed on Spencer's Bastion will have to be shorter than the others. But we do not consider this a disadvantage, as it will enable the casualty and operation cases to be accommodated in smaller wards. Each pavilion should contain two wards, and each ward should have the following offices attached to it:

1. A nurse's room with a window to the open air and another to the ward.

2. A scullery for washing up and keeping the ward eating and drinking utensils, for making poultices, preparing ward drinks, etc. The scullery and nurse's room should each be the same size, viz., about 12 ft. square.

3. At the end of the ward opposite the door, a portion of the pavilion should be cut off to contain the lavatories, bathrooms, water closets, etc. These should be reached through a half glass double swing door 4 ft. wide, opening into a passage of similar width, which passage should be thoroughly ventilated. From one side of this passage should enter the ablution and bathroom and from the other the water closets. These rooms should be about 12 ft. wide by 10 ft. long. They should have plenty of windows and the freshest means of ventilation. In each water closet should be placed a white earthenware pan sink, properly trapped, with a water tap over it, for washing out bed slops, etc.

Each patient is to have 1625 cubic feet of (sixteen hundred and twenty-five) space. Each ward should hold thirty-two beds: sixteen on each side, except the wards in the two shorter pavilions, of which one will hold twenty beds in each of its two wards, and the other ten beds in each ward. The wards for thirty-two patients should be 110 (a hundred and ten) ft. long, 30 ft. wide and 16 ft. high, with eight windows on each opposite side, reaching from within 3 ft. of the floor to 1 ft. of the ceiling.

The twenty-bed wards should have five windows on each side, and the ten-bed wards three windows on each side. Six or seven small wards of one and two beds each could easily be built out of the space occupied by the small N.E. pavilion and the corridor leading to it. In any case, these small wards should have windows on two opposite sides. In connection with them should be built the operating theatre with a separate entrance from the corridor. These wards must be provided with separate nurse's room, scullery, water closet, sink and lavatory.

The corridor should be the same height as the wards and should consist of narrow piers supporting arches with glass folding windows capable of being opened or removed, to permit a free circulation of air between the pavilions. It would be advisable to consider whether the S.W. side of each pavilion, being the side most exposed to the sun, should not be built with hollow walls, with openings both above and below into the interspace to allow of a free circulation of air—in order to carry off the sun heat.

The roof should also be double and should have a similar circulation of air through it. The ward window space, which in temperate climates ought to be fixed at not less than one third of the entire wall surface, should be less in the Maltese climate.

The entrance front of the hospital would be about the middle of the Strada Genio. And the buildings to be devoted to the administration might be erected so as to form one entire side of the street. If they were two storeys high, they would be about two thirds of the hospital façade in elevation.

The administrative buildings should be connected with the centre of both flats of corridors. And at the point of connection there should be a wide, roomy, staircase giving access to the building. A courtyard would be left between the back of the administrative offices and the front of the hospital. And across the courtyard the communication would be carried. If, for the sake of obtaining more space for the administrative offices, it were necessary to connect these with the corridor at two points, it might be done. But the first method would be the better.

The following is the accommodation which we would propose should be placed in this part of the building:

1. a small guard room and porter's lodge with an entrance gate under an archway
2. a writing room
3. a recovery room
4. a surgery and drug store
5. governor, 2 rooms
6. principal medical officer, 1 room
7. superintendent of nurses, 2 rooms and store closet
8. orderly medical officer, 1 room
9. medical officers' day and consulting room
10. steward's room
11. paymaster's room
12. apothecary's room
13. captain of orderlies, 2 rooms
14. chapel
15. chaplain, 2 rooms
16. pack store
17. clean linen store near the superintendent's room
18. rooms for dispensers, storekeepers, cooks and servants
19. a room for sick nurses should be provided near the superintendent's quarters
20. sleeping accommodation for 30 orderlies
21. a general bathroom for medicated and other baths.

The space in front of the hospital and facing the Strado Genio, which could be used for erecting this accommodation, appears to be 230 feet long, by about 70 feet in depth. But it would be necessary to leave as wide a courtyard as possible between the back of the buildings and the front of the hospital.

The chapel might be erected in the south corner of the bastion. It might be the whole height of the pavilion and might be entered from the corridor. The bedding store, foul linen store, etc., might be placed in the arched basement of the N.E. pavilions.

The provision store and fuel store should be placed near the kitchen. All hot water required should, if possible, be warmed by a furnace near the kitchen and hence conducted over the whole building. If this be impracticable, a *chauffoir* for the purpose would have to be placed under the corridor at the centre of the building.

The cooking apparatus should be placed in the middle of the kitchen floor. And if the kitchen be placed under the flanking battery, it should have a lift to take up the dinners to each flat of the corridor. The lift should not open directly from the kitchen but from the outside.

The ward windows should be so placed that the beds can be ranged two and two between them, with one in each corner. The corner spaces should permit the bed to be 18 inches from the wall.

The walls and ceilings of the wards should be of white Parian cement, the floors of oak or olive or some equally close-grained wood—oiled and varnished or beeswaxed. The corridor might be done with tile. The ordinary Maltese stone should be avoided for flooring, on account of its absorbent nature and the dust it creates.

The whole hospital drainage should be conveyed away in glazed watertight, earthen pipes, none of which should pass under any part of the hospital. The water from lavatories, baths, urinals and scullery sinks should be discharged by an open pipe over the trap grating of the drain which is to convey the water away. The water closet drainage and that from the water closet sink is to be conveyed away in carefully trapped drains, which are to be ventilated, at a sufficient distance from the hospital to prevent the effluvia reaching the wards. Or the ventilating pipe might be carried up from the water closet pipe to 3 or 4 feet above the roof of the pavilion.

The only question in regard to the proposed pavilion arrangement is whether the distance of 50 feet between the proposed pavilions be enough. It would *not* [be] enough in this country, on account of the dull climate. Here the distance should be at least twice the height of the pavilions. Information on this point should be obtained from one conversant with the climate of Malta. Should this be an objection, the pavilions might possibly be arranged in line.

Required (for a general military hospital of 300 beds at Malta)

Medical case	200 to 150
Surgical "	100 to 150
including venereal	40 to 60
Convalescents	75 to 100

It is very desirable for all reasons that these two classes should form, as it were, a separate hospital. Either the whole ground floor should be set apart for them, or a certain number of pavilions. They may always be reckoned at half the whole number in hospital. They never require any female nursing. But the little nurses' rooms are yet more essential than in bad cases, as wardmasters should always be within hearing, *especially* at night, when discipline is too little observed among these cases.

Offensive cases	3
Noisy cases	2
Operation case	1

One small ward of three beds, two of one bed and one of one bed, are wanted for the above respectively. But the two one-bedded cases (noisy) should be as far as they conveniently can from the others. They should be dark and cool.

The operating theatre is so little used that no great expense should [be] bestowed on it. But it should be near the one-bedded ward. And *all* these cases must never be on the same floor or up the same staircase with convalescent or venereal cases.

Winter	6 to 15 fever cases
Summer	60 to 90
Winter	15 to 30 severe cases
Summer	30 to 45

Whatever plan is adopted, one or two pavilions with not more than twelve to twenty beds in each of their wards will be loudly desired by the surgeons for the severe cases and the fever cases.

One nurse may very well see to the twelve or twenty-bed ward *and* to the three- and one-bedded wards, if near to one another. (It is not at all necessary to have one nurse for every one of the tiny wards.) The three-bedded ward should have a sink, etc., of its own and means of washing up of its own.

Query, whether, in the oblong plan, the magnificent double pavilion is not too good for the convalescent cases, and too far off from the administration and too hot for the bad cases? I only ask the question.

Malta. 1. To adjoin each other, to have a separate entrance from the street:

(1) deadhouse and dissecting room, to be kept clear of the wards and hospital;

(2) hospital washhouse; day and night orderlies to have separate sleeping rooms, N.C. officers' room adjoining;

(3) orderlies' lavatory;

(4) casements to be built suitable for sick in case of siege. Offensive ward must have water closet, sink, bath and lavatory separate. Ward for four requires some rearrangement. Nurse's room would be dark.

Side corridor not good contrivance. End scullery not in a good place. Scullery next nurse's room is probably intended for the noisy cases. It is better, where possible, to cut off the offensive cases more entirely, with all their appurtenances. Beds for 3 (three) only were asked in the specification. Noisy wards should have inspection holes in doors. Little ward halfway downstairs very inconvenient—if avoidable, unless it has every appurtenance to itself.

5. Three one-bed wards were asked for (for noisy, delirious cases); one lavatory, water closet, a sink and one scullery will do for all the little wards, but must be exclusive of the offensive ward. No bathroom need be—a portable bath will do.

6. W.C.s of large wards not numerous enough.

7. To each pavilion, or at least to each pavilion for *sick*, two separate W.C.s, one above and one below, are necessary, one for orderlies and one for nurses.

8. Is the hospital to be lighted with gas or with oil? How are the ward offices to be lighted?

9. Three sinks per ward desirable (in the large wards) to make the service perfect, one in the scullery for "washing up," one for hot and cold water for the ward, one in the W.C. like a W.C. pan on Jennings' principle, with a cold water tap over.

10. What is to be done with the dirty linen? Are there to be chutes? or closets?

11. A general bathroom will no doubt be provided.

12. Should not the corridor windows have blinds?

13. Half-glazed ward doors are always desirable.

Would it not be better to have end windows to the wards? The whole disposition of the end offices of the wards might be very much improved by throwing them out in projections and leaving the end wall free for a window and balcony? above with shade to window below.

The superintendent's sitting room is in reality her *office* and should be accessible as an office, instead of being hid behind all the bedrooms. (Better give those two rooms to captain of orderlies.)

1. South end wall of administrative offices to be double.
2. Roof all the way along to admit of ventilation.
3. Kitchen and day room require shelter from sun.
4. Will not kitchen, being under day room, make it very hot? Day room must have superintendence from N.C. officer.
5. Inner corridor of mezzanine will be very dark. As much light as possible must be introduced from staircase.
6. Inner corridor (first floor) must be lighted from the roof.
7. Administrative offices all require very good ventilation.
8. Principal staircase should be lighted and ventilated from the roof. Two open arches should be put into it from mezzanine, instead of dead wall at present there. Nothing of all this has been done.
9. Call the "nurses' day room" clean linen store and the opposite little room "mending room" and put a door across, so as to isolate them from the women's rooms.
10. The superintendent must have a storeroom, linen nurse's and servants' room and a sink and a sick nurse's room. There is ample space for all this in the quarters indicated.
11. Must dispenser have two rooms? Should he not sleep near his store?
12. Better not call the "servants" in a military hospital by that name.
13. Does the room marked "Apothecary" (ground floor) mean apothecary's *store*? or where is this?
14. Storerooms should be near the kitchen, not distributed about.
15. Must there not be a steward's receiving provision room?
16. Does not Mrs. S. Stewart now ask for a small nurse's kitchen in the nurses' quarters? N.B. All will want kitchens, though I do not see that they need them.

Editor: The following notes appear to be from a meeting Nightingale held with Alessandro Borgia, grand master of the Knights Hospitaller of Malta 1865-71, but there is no correspondence with him.

Source: Notes, with comments by Dr Sutherland, Add Mss 45752 ff45-46

[1865]

Malta *1865. F.N.*

1. Overhauling the towns, with reference to reconstruction and opening up of worst parts.

2. Improved model dwellings outside lines, to provide for increase of population, and keep down crowding within lines.

3. Sewers to be relaid, outlets to be improved. (It would be a great benefit if all sewage were applied to land for manure, where practicable.)

4. W.C.s and water latrines properly constructed, instead of present Maltese stone troughs.

5. Improved house drainage by drainpipes.

6. Extended supply of water and better means of distribution, so as to have it always laid on to houses and barracks.

7. New cemetery and abolishing interments in churches.

8. New incurable hospital, [new] poorhouse, prison.

9. General improvements in education.

10. Oversight of progress of barrack improvements.

11. New military hospitals required for Valetta and Cotonera.

12. Day and reading rooms, game rooms for soldiers, soldiers' gardens, gymnasia.

The grand master is the keenest man I have seen for three years. *We are to write a memo today for him* and he is to come back here, after considering it, to discuss it. He wants to know whether he had not better begin on the Vittoriosa side, instead of at Valetta. He says they will spend £12,000 or £14,000 a year on sanitary works. He wants to write to us, to be written to, two or three times a day. He wants to know whether Sir John Lawrence's municipalities are elected? **JS:** Yes, so far as appears, are paid? **JS:** No.

He says he fears they will be corrupt, if they are. He had a *paid elected* municipality at Zante.[178] That was only by the way. He says there has just been an epidemic at Malta and three officers have died. He asked particularly about outlets, about laying manure on land, etc. He is quite willing to be guided by us, almost too willing. . . .

He says Floriana Barracks are improved, but no others. He would have succeeded if he had not been recalled, if Ionia had not been given up, *he says,* so he was very popular.

178 An island off the Peloponnesus, then administered as part of the Ionian Islands by Britain.

Source: From a letter to F.V. Inglott, Royal Malta Library Manuscript 396 pp 45-47, typed copy Wellcome Ms 9085/16

16 May 1865

I have to thank you for the photograph of Sanese's Works of Mercy, which, I understand, is coming by my niece, Emily Verney, who has not yet arrived in England.

Could you send me (it is for the Colonial Office) copies of plans of your prison—the very best plan for a tropical prison I have ever seen? It was among the plans for workhouse and incurables which you brought to England. It would be doing us a great favour.

I have recently sent you by book post one or two books on sanitary subjects, which I understood Dr Sutherland [say] that you wished for. I should be too glad to send you anything of this kind which you would tell me of.

I have also to thank you for some beautiful oranges through Mrs Sutherland.

Swansea General Hospital, 1864-65

Editor: Nightingale advised on the construction of a new 100-bed hospital at Swansea from the initial idea through finding an architect, considering costs, reviewing the plans and proposing revisions. She also, as she often did when both plans and site met her requirements, contributed to the building fund.

She was initially approached by a physician, Dr Thomas Williams (c1819-65), who had published a report on sanitary conditions at Swansea. He wrote her "as one ardently interested in the good cause," asking her to allow him "without flattery or nonsensical circumlocution, to crave a few words of advice and assistance?" He sought advice "for building with a view to economy," inquiring if there was a "particular architect especially informed in hospital architecture?"[179] She consulted Douglas Galton about a suitable architect, asking if Alex Graham "would do" (the first item below). Galton replied with his address.[180] Dr Williams asked her to see Graham,[181] which she probably did, for a

179 Williams letters 12, 16 and 28 September 1864, Florence Nightingale Museum (LMA) H1/ST/NC2/V3/64, V4/64 and V6/64.

180 Galton letter 2 October 1864, Add Mss 45762 f219.

181 Williams letter 30 September 1864, Florence Nightingale Museum (LMA) H1/ST/NC2/V8/64. The general committee sent her a formal letter with a printed vote of thanks on the same date H1/ST/NC2/V9/64.

serious correspondence with him ensued.[182] A note Nightingale made on the back of Williams's letter of 30 September to her states: "

> He means that I should look over with Mr Graham those site plans when it tells for himself. You think the "pigheaded" way has carried the day. It is the £25 subscription I had already. Well? then they have not got a drainage outlet yet.

Williams and the hospital committee took Nightingale's advice on the plans (on which much detail appears shortly), notably on her recommendation for small wards for women. He told Nightingale that Graham had been appointed "*because he was recommended by you,*" although they had gone through "the farce of an open public competition." His letter also recounted his visit to Paris and other hospitals, when he caught typhoid fever, but he recovered. A further letter explained that, while they had engaged Graham and adopted his plan, they wanted her advice "*again.*"[183]

There is also correspondence with Emily Markham (c1839-?), a nurse who had been trained in the second class at the Nightingale School in 1861-62, and then began nursing at Cardiff in 1863. Four letters survive by her to Nightingale, written between 1864 and 1866, but not Nightingale's replies. Markham visited the Swansea Infirmary and then acted as spokesperson for it. She described the motivation for the hospital by a Dr Lewis as benefiting his own patients in the ironworks district. He had studied Nightingale's *Notes on Hospitals,* Markham explained, and intended to carry out its principles.[184]

The material below is typical in giving detail about practical requirements for adequate ventilation and carefully relating the needs of nurses, including decent living quarters and privacy. The letters are unusual both for their quantity (so many survived, from several angles) and their positive quality—the plans were (relatively) good from the beginning. The hospital opened in 1869.[185]

---

182 Graham letters 5 and 10 October and 3 November 1864, Florence Nightingale (LMA) H1/ST/NC2/V11/64, V12/64 and V15/64.

183 Williams letters 21 November 1864 and 8 April 1865, Florence Nightingale Museum (LMA) H1/ST/NC2/V28/64 and V4/65.

184 Markham letter October 1864, Add Mss 45799 f23.

185 See T.G. Davies, *Deeds not Words: A History of the Swansea General and Eye Hospital 1817-1948.*

Source: From a letter to Douglas Galton, Add Mss 45762 f207

Hampstead, N.W.
17 September 1864

I have been asked by the Swansea people to recommend an architect to build them a new hospital. Would your Mr Graham do? And, if so, what is his address?

Source: From notes presumably for Alex Graham, Florence Nightingale Museum (LMA) H1/ST/NC1/64/22

7 November 1864

Swansea Hospital. These plans, taken as a whole, are admirable. I have never yet seen first drafts which require so little alteration. The main points of criticism arise partly out of the form, and lay and area of the ground, partly out of the requirements which the committee has asked you to fulfill.

The area and cubic space per bed are ample. And the height and width of the wards are well proportioned. The windows are so large that you may quite well leave more space between the top of the upper windows and the eaves, so as to give a better architectural effect outside, i.e., if you think it desirable.

Considering that the prevailing winds are from the S.W., the block plan No. 3 would bring these winds most favourably upon the building. This block plan would also keep the interior of the wards most out of sight of house windows. If you adopt this plan, you will have to alter the operating room and place it on the N. side of the central block, where the staircase is at present.

If the road were diverted, this plan would enable the hospital to be extended northwards, to give rather more than an additional third of accommodation at some future time.

Block plans Nos. 1 and 4 are, either of them, as good as No. 3, so far as the disposition of parts is concerned. They would enable the line of the wards to be brought into the line of the streets. This might, however, be a disadvantage from rendering the wards liable to be overlooked from neighbouring houses. But the chief disadvantage would be that the sea breeze would be partially interrupted by the central block, and that it could not fall so favourably against the sides of the wards as in plan No. 3. These questions, however, can be best settled on the spot. And if for any local reason Plan 1 or 4 be preferred, either will make a good block plan.

I would strongly recommend, however, that the proposed Turkish bath be not placed on the S.W. point of the ground. The place where it should be is at the northern angle. *As it is*, the site will in time become much more confined than might be desirable, and as much open space should be kept within the hospital enclosure as possible.

The wards on the men's side will do, with the slight alteration suggested in the position of one of the nurse's two inspection windows—see plan. The same remark applies to the first-floor female ward. But there is a serious administrative objection to the small (women's) ward on the ground floor—on account of increased difficulty of supervision and increased cost of nursing. That ward will require a day nurse and a night nurse to itself, and even then, being out of the way of the head nurse, would not be well nursed. Would it not be possible, by lengthening the women's pavilion, to have a twenty-eight-bed ward and a six-bed ward, which would give all the accommodation required and with infinitely greater advantage to the patients, being on the same floor? Women's surgical cases in the country are generally few. (No proportion between medical and surgical cases is given in the specification, but judging from experience, a twenty-eight-bed medical and a six-bed surgical female ward would be all that is required.)

If this were done, the abandoned six-bed ward might be turned to better purpose, such, e.g., as physician's and surgeon's rooms, hospital admission and waiting room, etc. For this purpose, a different arrangement of doors would be required. The committee must be consulted on this point of the small lower ward. But, if they judge fit to retain it, they must decide upon incurring the additional cost of nursing.

The whole of the lower floor of the women's pavilion, intended to be used as a dispensary for out-patients, must be completely cut off from the hospital. It is generally considered that it is impossible (too) to cut off inexorably enough all communication between men and women out-patients.

They should come in by separate doors—they should have entirely separate W.C.s should be cut off, in fact, from any possible overlooking of one another either in entering, waiting or departing. (See plan for rearrangement.) I would strongly suggest that the one-storeyed building, containing operating room and small wards, shown in block Plans 1 and 4, be removed, or at all events so reduced in length as to contain no more than the operating room, a one-bed ward, space for a W.C. and sink and one wash-hand basin.

What can be wanted more (for men patients' accommodation) than what is found in the pavilion, one large and one small surgical, one large and one small medical ward? An eye case (who has to be shut up by himself in the dark, poor fellow) may be put into this one-bed ward, if such is judged necessary. For he wants no more nursing than can be given him.

N.B. The operating room should have not only a skylight, but a large north window. . . . (The small wards of one or two beds for special cases, and the one or two small wards for surgical cases, would be found quite unnecessary in practice, while they would add greatly to the cost of the hospital and to the cost of nursing.)

I am very glad that you have missed out the convalescent wards. If, in such a place as Swansea, such wards are ever necessary, they should consist in cottages at the seaside.

The deadhouse and post-mortem room (and laundry, if there is to be one), should be placed at a sufficient distance from and on the north side of the hospital.

Central Block. Kitchen floor very good. Area to be sufficiently wide for plenty of light. Cook must not sleep there, but among the female servants.

Ground floor will answer with the slight alterations (vide [see] plan) suggested, unless part of the accommodation is to be transferred into the lower-floor women's ward.

(I presume the porter must *sleep* on the premises. He ought to sleep and take his meals as near the principal door as possible.) The room allotted to him seems scarcely large enough for him to sleep and take his meals, which he ought to do there.

First-floor matron's accommodation, linen store, etc., will answer. But, if by any rearrangement you can obtain access from the matron's floor by the terrace to the upper-floor wards, it should be done.

Upper floor. I presume there will be a cook, housemaid and one or two other female servants. These should have a room apart from the nurses, but divided by compartments. It would be preferable, however, if the cook could have a small room to herself. Also, if one female servant, who will, I presume, assist the matron with the linen, should sleep near the matron.

To nurse the three large and three small wards efficiently would require three head nurses, nine day nurses (two to each large ward, one to each small ward, three night nurses, and I am afraid an extra nurse, in case of extra night nursing in any of the three small wards). Or it might be *possible* to nurse the three floors with three head nurses, six day nurses, three night nurses and one extra nurse, one scrubber. (I dislike this latter plan. It is infinitely preferable that the nursing staff of each floor should be distinctly separate from the nursing staff of each other floor, and that no scrubber or nurse should go from one floor to another.)

The three head nurses' accommodation is provided for (in the ward nurses' rooms). The three (if not four) night nurses must have a separate room to themselves, divided by compartments. There remains nine (or at least seven) day nurses to provide for. These *may* be in the same room, with separate compartments. But it is preferable that the nurses of each floor should have a separate room, with compartments. It ensures better discipline—particularly that the nurses on the men's side and on the women's side should have separate rooms. (Day and night nurses *must* be separate, in order to allow the night nurses undisturbed sleep in the day.)

I have said elsewhere that, if the small wards are retained, which I have proposed to abolish, accommodation must be found for at least two more day nurses, two more night nurses. The sculleries should be roomy and comfortable enough for the day nurses to take their meals in (also the night nurse, but at a separate time, of course). The head nurses' rooms should also be large enough for each head nurse to have her meals in her own room.

The disposing of this accommodation cannot, however, be finally arranged until the committee has decided on the block plan to be adopted.

N.B. On looking at the plan of the ground, I see that all the houses have back premises. It should be ascertained whether the houses have proper W.C.s, drained, or merely open privies over cesspits. If the latter, they would be a fatal objection to the site. When these matters are satisfactorily arranged, Swansea will have one of the finest hospitals in the kingdom. I only wish the site had been as good as the plan.

Source: From a letter to Robert Eaton, West Glamorgan Archive Service, Swansea D/D HIS 129

18 November 1865

My dear Sir, The account of your meeting about the new Swansea Infirmary, which you were kind enough to send me, has afforded me very great pleasure. Your enlightened committee has rendered a real service to the cause of humanity in adopting Mr Graham's beautiful plans. When completed, you will have perhaps the finest and most perfect small hospital in the kingdom.

I was deeply grieved to hear of the death of Dr Williams, who is indeed a loss. I shall be very much obliged to you to add my name to your list of subscribers and to summon me to pay the £25, when you are ready for it.

I think it is an extremely good idea to interest the *men* (in the great iron and other works) in your hospital—as it takes away from the idea of a *charity*, and gives them a personal care and anxiety for a measure which ought to concern their feelings.

Editor: Nightingale wrote Alex Graham in December 1865 asking for his estimate of the cost of a 200-bed hospital (in response to a request for this information from William Rathbone). Her letter is not extant, but Dr Sutherland's draft for it is. Graham answered promptly that it was £30,000, based on a safe, rough estimate of £150 per bed.[186] Correspondence on other hospital matters resumes.

Source: From two letters to William Farr, Wellcome Ms 5474/79 and 83, typed copies Add Mss 43400 ff6 and 19

23 January 1865

Private. I have received a proxy paper from St Mary's Hospital and shall of course vote for Dr Edward Smith.[187] Can you tell me a governor who is going to vote for him whose name I may put in? Are you a governor, and may I use your name? And send the paper to you? The election is on 31 January.

You ask me what I think of his diet theories.[188] You must please take what I say with several grains of salt, for I have not yet had time to finish his book. It appears to me, if it is intended to be physiological, not to be physiological, and if intended to be practical, not to be practical. Take it and compare it with Lyon Playfair's article on diet in *Good Words* for January (?)[189] and Playfair strikes you at once as master of his subject—the other not.

As an illustration of what I mean, I send you Dr E. Smith's Indian diet, which doubtless you have seen, and the note which accompanied

186 Sutherland draft on Rathbone letter of 8 December 1865, Add Mss 47753 f183; Graham letter 12 December 1865, Add Mss 45799 f193.

187 Edward Smith (1819-74), who lost the election for the assistant physician's position, by a large majority (*Medical Times and Gazette* 4 February 1865:132). Dr Smith was appointed inspector, then medical officer, to the Poor Law Board.

188 Edward Smith, *Practical Dietaries for Families, Schools and the Working Classes,* 1864. Nightingale later objected strenuously to his views on cubic space in workhouses.

189 Lyon Playfair, "On the Nature and Composition of Food," *Good Words* January 1865:24-31; Pt. 2 156-63.

it. I pointed out to him that the statements in his own pamphlet did not at all bear out the conclusions in his note. And, if the *second* note means anything but that he wants a vote, it means that he retracts all he said in the first.

He appears to me to be continually generalizing thus on insufficient or ill-digested premises, and drawing unfounded principles for conclusions. Then he always ignores that, after chemistry has done her very best to compound for us exactly the best diet, nature often says she will have none of it. And she will have something else. And that it is experience only, not chemistry, which is the ultimate appeal.

But for all this, Dr Edward Smith is so immeasurably superior to those brutes who go on without observing or concluding or generalizing at all, vide [see] (1) the wretched medical evidence at the Holborn Union inquiry;[190] (2) about St Thomas' removal, etc. that I should always vote for Dr E. Smith's success.

25 February 1865

I have heard from Paris about your "weekly," the gist of what I have heard being that, if you agitate for it, you will get it: "The weekly list is not made out but Haussmann *could* get it made. He is an intelligent scoundrel, and if the Registrar-General can explain to him the utility and importance of the thing, and if Lord Cowley[191] will interest himself in it, and poke his ribs, it will be made." Haussmann has published lately "A Report of the Inspectors of Mortality on the Mortality of the Last Ten Years in Paris." No doubt you have this. He is going to send it to me.

2. About your affairs: "Dr Farr's affairs are going on tolerably. It was from the beginning hopeless to propose him for a foreign member.[192] They have now made their list: Gladstone, Stuart Mill, Whewell.[193]

---

190 "The Poor-Law Official's Report on Timothy Daly," *British Medical Journal* 11 February 1865:143-44.

191 Henry Richard Wellesley (1804-84), 1st Earl Cowley, ambassador to France 1852-67.

192 Of the prestigious Institut de France, on which further appears (see p 683 below).

193 W.E. Gladstone, then chancellor of the Exchequer and soon to be prime minister; John Stuart Mill (1806-73), MP, political philosopher; William Whewell (1794-1866), moral philosopher.

They will name Gladstone because they adore ministers, having mostly been so themselves, and are in general a superficial crew of political. But Dr Farr ought and I hope will be named correspondent. I think it will be done; only in elections one is never sure before the end." This is what I hear, I don't know what they call "tolerably." I am disappointed.

Source: Memorandum, Wellcome (Claydon copy) Ms 9001/116

[13 March 1865]

The "Surgical Society" of Paris, in a discussion 6 October/14 December 1864, attended by all the leading physicians and surgeons, civil and military, adopted the following principles:

1. Never to bring together more than 200 to 250 sick;
2. Never to have more than two floors of patients;
3. Free external ventilation—natural (as opposed to artificial) ventilation;
4. To construct the hospital in separate buildings, completely isolated, freely exposed to sun, wind and rains;
5. Wards to have ward conveniences, properly situated;
6. All cleansing to be amply and immediately provided for;
7. All hospitals to be placed under a committee of persons acquainted with hygiene, architecture, medicine, etc., to see that they are kept in a proper state.

All this is merely restating the pavilion question, as it was stated by the royal commission, 1857. (Generally) people no longer consider that the old makeshift system of hospitals will answer; the question at issue really is that of improving up to our present knowledge, or of going back. Nobody now thinks it humane merely to bring sick together. They should be brought together to recover, not to die. Besides, in none of our pavilion hospitals have we at all come up in architectural cost to what the French have done in new hospitals, civil and military. We have spent a small part of the sum in making our hospitals healthy which they have spent in making theirs fine.

People not conversant with the subject are apt to be led away by the idea that we have been extravagant, when they see our wards so much better than the wards of more costly buildings.

Source: From a draft memorandum for William Farr, Wellcome Ms 5474/77, typed copy Add Mss 43400 ff63-64

[1865]

1. The Post Office Savings Bank allows of the accumulation of capital of working men.

2. Mr Gladstone's Insurance and Annuity Act enables this accumulated capital to be vested periodically in two ways: (a) as annuity, (b) as insurance.

3. It would apparently be very advisable to add to this facilities for purchasing small freeholds.

4. The first step to enable this to be done is to remove every legal obstacle at present existing to title purchase, registration, transfer of land, within the specified limits, so that land could be as freely dealt in and as easily identified as any other commodity.

5. A limit must however be fixed, so that the existing law of primogeniture and entail should exist as at present, subject only to the exceptions to be mentioned.

6. In these exceptional cases, women must inherit freehold, even without will.

7. It would be unadvisable to apply the enabling law to the whole surface of the country. It should be limited to cities, towns, populous places, villages, indeed to all groups of population and to a certain distance beyond the outskirts or defined legal boundaries of these groups, in order to provide for increase of population.

8. Within the limits, the law should declare that the leaseholds of all lands and of houses built on them shall, in future, go together, i.e., that the lease of the land and the lease of the house must never be held by two different people, an existing abuse which has had a fatal influence on the interests of working classes in towns, as well as on town and house architecture, so that English houses are about the worst built in the world.

9. Having then abolished by law separate leaseholds, and introduced perfect freedom of trade in land within the prescribed limits, leave the price of freeholds to settle itself on the principle of supply and demand, granting every legal facility as already stated.

10. You will thus have land where it is wanted, as an investment by the workingman for house or cottage building brought into immediate relation with his savings in the P.O. Savings Bank and an investment offered which of all others the workingman most covets.

11. In all places where there are constituted authorities, the existing law provides that houses must be built after the plans are approved by the authority. In villages this would hardly be necessary.

12. The objects gained would be: (a) a new outlet for savings; (b) improved social position and independence (by giving the man an object in life); (c) all such men would have votes. N.B. Rest assured that *none* of them would vote for a "Radical" to take their property from them, and no man of this class would believe he was a "slave," because he was told so from the hustings.

Editor: As is evident in several letters, beginning with the one immediately below, Nightingale went to some trouble to promote Dr Farr's candidacy to the French Institut. She contacted members she knew, ascertained the correct section for him (of its five academies) and relayed comments back to Farr from her correspondents. The news was discouraging—political notables were preferred. Farr was not elected.

Source: From three letters to William Farr, Wellcome Ms 5474/80, 85 and 87, typed copies Add Mss 43400 ff14-15, 30 and 32

9 February 1865

I reproach myself with not having told you what I have done about you and the Institut.

The members I have written to say: "To be sure Dr Farr ought and must be of the Institut." (Unfortunately I know no members of your academy. And I can only work at it indirectly.)

"Barthélemi St-Hilaire"[194] has been "instantly lectured" (by one of the men I wrote to) "about Dr Farr, and what" he (my man) "knows of" him, and he will work zealously. There is one danger. McCulloch[195] was associé étranger [foreign associate], of whom there are only six, and for whom they choose flashy people, of the Broughamite class, mostly hollow drums who in their time have made a noise, such as "frivolous and superficial great men, like Guizot, Thiers[196] et id genus" [and that species], can hear. "Dr Farr is a much superior man but works officially." "But it must be tried, and if it cannot be, we must try to make him correspondent of the Academy; the correspondents are proposed by the different sections. In Dr Farr's case it would be

194 Jules Barthélemy-Saint Hilaire (1805-95), French philosopher.

195 John Ramsay McCulloch (1789-1864), in the Académie des Sciences Morales et Politiques.

196 François Pierre Guillaume Guizot (1787-1874), author and chief minister to Louis-Philippe of France; Louis Adolphe Thiers (1797-1877), historian, later president of the Third Republic.

the Section d'économie politique et statistique. It is composed of six members, with three of whom" he (my man) is "on a good and with three others on a bad footing. We shall see what can be done, but at first try the succession of McCulloch. There is much of a lottery in every election—the frivolity, ignorance and indifference of the electors being an unknown but enormous element." "I have preached today some members of the Académie Morale about Dr Farr, and it seems to me that his prospects are good."

4 April 1865

Thank you 1000 times for "Government Insurances and Annuities." Depend upon it, *you* are the great "bill," not the Union Chargeability Bill. *You* are the great president of the Poor Laws, not Mr Villiers.[197]

8 April 1865

I send you St Bartholomew's [statistics], though no doubt you have received a copy. Please to return it to me, with your remarks. I think the saint deserves the greatest credit, but, before I praise the saint and worship at his shrine, I should like to have your judgment, whether there is anything more he ought to do, before he is canonized by *us* (which, you know, is a much more critical thing than his being canonized by Rome). . . .

I want a great many more of your "Plain Rules" for government insurances and annuities. Are they to be bought? I cannot find that they are.

Editor: In October 1866 Nightingale received a letter from Julius Unger (1837-1909), of Erfurt, Prussia, about a "crystal hospital pavilion" he intended to build. His letter is no longer extant, nor is her five-page reply. That she sent him such a lengthy response on glass in hospital construction shows some serious interest. Only a (very short) précis of the reply is available.[198]

---

197 Charles Pelham Villiers (1802-98), Liberal MP, president of the Poor Law Board, a Cabinet position. Nightingale pressed Villiers to bring in legislation for radical reform of the workhouses, which he did not. The Union Chargeability Act referred to was a technical measure on the financing of workhouses.

198 Unger letter 13 October; precis of Nightingale reply 20 November 1866, in Sue Goldie, comp., *A Calendar of the Letters of Florence Nightingale.*

Source: From a letter to William Farr, Wellcome Ms 5474/100, typed copy Add Mss 43400 f104

13 March 1866

These people worry me past my patience. But I have looked now through all my stores, and cannot find one copy left of the forms which you were so good as to send out and which *they* have "mislaid"?

Have *you* any copies of the forms which you were kind enough to send round for us to all the hospitals? If so, would you be so good as to send me one copy? returning me the enclosed (which makes me so impatient).

Elizabeth Garrett on Hospital Nursing

Editor: In 1866 Dr Farr sent Nightingale a paper on hospital nursing[199] by woman medical pioneer Elizabeth Garrett (1836-1919), later Garrett-Anderson. Garrett, of course, was not a nurse, and Nightingale considered her views on nursing badly mistaken, as her lengthy replies to Farr show. She objected particularly to Garrett's treatment of social class issues and nursing.[200] Later, Nightingale gave advice on the design of a women's hospital Garrett was instrumental in founding, and herself contributed financially to it (see p 884 below).

Source: From three letters to William Farr, Wellcome Ms 5474/105-07, typed copies Add Mss 43400 ff127-38 and 143-46

17 October 1866

I am so puzzled by "first, second and third class" (as if Miss Garrett and Mr Stewart were dividing the human race into railroad carriages) that I don't know whether she considers governesses as "Ladies." But, if she does, she can't be ignorant (at least, *I* am not for I once kept a governesses' hospital) that there are unaccomplished "ladies" toiling away as governesses their miserable, useless lives at £20 or £30 a year, who as head nurses ("sisters"), but for her invidious definition of classes, might lead useful happy lives at £50 or £60 a year. But then hospital life is not for the "upper class" and governess life is. And this unnatural prejudice Miss Garrett appears to support. . . .

I am very sorry your cholera is still so bad.

---

199 Elizabeth Garrett, "Hospital Nursing," read at the 10th annual meeting of the National Association for the Promotion of Social Science at Manchester, April 1866, published in the *Transactions of the National Association for the Promotion of Social Science* 10 (1866):472-88, and reprinted as "Volunteer Hospital Nursing," *Macmillan's Magazine* 15 (April 1867):494-99.

200 For further on this see *The Nightingale School* (12:165-74) and *Women* (8:30-40).

Embley
Romsey
20 October 1866

Thank you for sending me Miss Garrett's paper. The looking it through has considerably mollified me, though I am afraid you will think the reason why a very impertinent reason. It is because the paper is so superficial and there are so many inaccuracies staring in the face of anyone in the least conversant with hospital life, that I don't think it will do our cause any harm. And I think it clears up the ideas very much of any person who is conversant with hospital life to read such a paper as this. (I will return to the subject of the inaccuracies.)

In the meantime, I think your own note the best commentary. You say, for which I thank you a thousand times, "it" (the Nightingale Fund) "aims at making nursing an *art*." This puts the whole question in six words. And I don't know that I want to add a word more. You never yet made an artist by paying him well. *But* an artist *ought to be well paid.* Agreed, agreed, a thousand times.

But Miss Garrett puts the cart before the horse. We get a better price for our article because it is a better article. We did not have a better article because we gave a higher price. (The article did not exist when we began, or exceptionally only. I will return to this.) You say truly, "the payment of the artist was a part of your plan" and we *have* secured good, and *shall* secure better pay for our artists. (Indeed, as I have mentioned, it is not the offer of good pay that is ever wanting. It is the capacity of the artist.)

It is, of course, impossible for me to go into Miss Garrett's paper at length. For it would be, in fact, rewriting the whole paper. I will mention only a few of the most palpable inaccuracies, e.g., I think the harm done is *incalculable* by striking the gap, page 2, between the "commercial" and "religious" "spirit." . . . I know none but the *most* fanatical of Roman Catholic archbishops who would write as she does on this? Certainly no Roman Catholic religious order.

Inaccuracies:

1. P 3, the "matron." In no hospital up to the last ten years had the "matron" anything to do with "overlooking" the nursing, scarcely even with "controlling the nursing department." Even at the present time, very few have. This is one of the most essential reforms we have introduced. P 5 (describing the "lady" system): "The main difference is that the control no longer rests with the matron." What *can* she mean by this? Is it because we have changed the word to *superintendent*

because a "*matron*" does *not* properly "control" or "superintend" the "nursing department" that she makes this blunder? She mentions "King's College Hospital" immediately afterwards as being under this régime, p 6. Now the only civil hospitals I know (though of course I must not be quoted on this) where the "nursing department" is *really* "under the control of the matron" are: King's College, St Thomas', though Mrs Wardroper[201] is called matron and Miss Jones lady superintendent. (Indeed, by the *enemy*, I have frequently been told that the latter "controls" too much.)

2. The question of "economy" is inaccurately introduced, not only by Miss Garrett but by *The Lancet* and Middlesex Hospital (pp 6, 7, 8 and passim). It is generally very little known that King's College Hospital pays as much for the services of St John's House as the usual price. Also, that a "sister" (lady) is never refused because she cannot serve gratuitously or pay for her board, and that many, including the very best superior I have ever known [Mary Jones], receive a salary. But, you see, Miss G. can assert this. And I can't answer her.

Of course I am not at liberty to publish these particulars. But I have repeatedly and positively refused to be a party in assisting any hospital to make a treaty with any sisterhood for the sake of "economy." Even in R.C. countries, where hospitals are, as a rule, nursed by sisterhoods, the civil administration always pays for them. Where the order has no foundation, this payment constitutes their only support, and that of their other works. They are earning their own livelihood in exactly the same sense as our paid nurses are, only that the payment is made to the "sisterhood" and not to the "sister." But, at King's College Hospital, the payment is made to the "sisters." Is it not a pity that Miss G. should not have informed herself on these subjects?

3. P 9. Where does Miss Garrett find that "a lady, with very little training, does hospital nursing (or any other art) in a first-rate way"? She must have very little idea of what "first-rate" hospital nursing is. The "idea" of even the French sisterhoods is so different from Miss Garrett's that they, who fall under her ban, consider from three to five years the time of training, and I consider two years the minimum.

Three fourths of the whole mischief in women's lives in England is that they suppose themselves exceptions from the laws of training to which men bow. And here is Miss Garrett encouraging this fatal idea.

---

201 Sarah E. Wardroper (1813-92), matron of St Thomas' Hospital and superintendent of the Nightingale School there. See the biographical sketch (12:885-87).

However, as Dr Stewart represents me as "giving up" "ladies" (as nurses) because they *can't* undergo the training necessary," he rather neutralizes Miss G.

4. P 9. Miss G. likens "nursing" to "cooking and dusting." I think the poor patient would find a very great difference if the "mistress of the household" were to send the "cook" or the "housemaid" instead of going herself and procuring a qualified nurse to attend upon her sick husband or child. The fruit of my whole life is indeed lost if people have not got farther than this, if they still confuse nursing with cleaning.

The head nurse has nothing to do with these farther than to superintend them, exactly as the "mistress of a household." But many a life has been lost because the head nurse did not know how (or did not choose) to do the operations of "la petite chirurgie" [minor surgery] especially for men patients. And the fact is that no "cook" or "duster" *can* perform these properly, and that the more "cultivated" the woman, if trained, the less she shirks them. But I would say the same, in an inferior degree, for the under nurse. Her work is not at all the same as that of an under servant, least of all is the night nurse's.

5. P 12. The two "reforms" which Miss G. suggests are what? (1) good wages, (2) supervision by night. I think I might perpetrate a very bad joke on this, but I refrain. I resume your immortal phrase about "an art." And I would ask Miss G. to apply her panacea, her Morison's pills,[202] to the "reform" of any other "art" and see how it will do.

Take the "art" of sculpture. (Michelangelo[203] is said to have worked very much at night at his sculpture, with a candle stuck in a ball of clay on his head, during the Siege of Florence.) Let us ask Michelangelo whether (1) good pay (2) night supervision would "reform" sculpture. But let us take what Miss G. gives as her reasons: (1) good pay. She quotes, p 12, a "report" which has received more blame than its utter incompetency was worth, for appointing the "reporters" of which the master was called over the coals. The offices of the hospitals (to which they belonged) laughing at the transparent job, the very passage which she quotes was known to be a covert assault on the two most valuable officers of the hospital, in order to insinuate that the "improvement" in the nursing was due, not to their training, but to

---

202 A purgative medicine, good for everything, invented by James Morison.
203 Michelangelo (1475-1564), Renaissance sculptor, painter and architect.

the higher pay which the "N. Fund" enabled them to give. And this very passage Miss G. endorses with her authority. . . .

(1) P 14, "Night supervision." The night is the only time when no real "*supervision*" or training *can* be given. And therefore the night nurses ought to be such and so trained as to require no "supervision." For (i) it is a fiction. Is there to be one night superintendent? How can she give assistance or "supervision" in an alarming case? in ten or twenty wards? How can she even see in ten or twenty wards whether the nurse is awake? (ii) or is there to be [a] night superintendent in each ward? Then she had much better be the night nurse herself. In ordinary wards there had much better be but one sitter-up, and that an experienced one.

To be giving directions or "supervision" at night is intolerable, other than what every competent head nurse gives (from her little room adjoining the ward, where she ought always to sleep) when she has bad cases.

I exclude wars and cholera epidemics from the above. In cholera epidemics such is the stress and pressure that the staff ought often to be exactly the same by night as it is by day, i.e., there should be two staffs, one for night, one for day. I exclude war hospitals because the orderlies are often new to their work—the cases are urgent. I, for one, found it necessary to be about nearly the whole of the night, "superintending the night nursing."

6. P 14. "Je suis de l'avis de monsieur pour la raison contraire" [I am of the view of monsieur for the contrary reason]. Je suis de l'avis [I am of the view] entirely "de" [of] Miss G. in what she says here about "remunerated work among women of the educated class." But she does not appear to be aware that it is done already. P 17, she does not appear aware that exactly what she recommends (paragraphs 1 and 2) is done already. The salary is taken and returned indirectly. It is done by my superintendent of the Liverpool Workhouse Infirmary[204] and by many others who are "ladies," with "private incomes." But Miss G. has so mixed up "religious," "volunteers," "educated," "ladies" and other words that not only I but others had not the least idea that she meant this. And this is done already.

I will only repeat here that she is not aware of the immense harm she does in the minds of what she calls the "commercial" class by separating, nay by setting in opposition, the "religious" and the "commer-

204 The independently wealthy Agnes Elizabeth Jones (1832-68) gave her salary back to the workhouse. Nightingale herself never took a salary.

cial" motive (or "spirit"?). She may explain it as she will. No explanation will remove it. The good ones say, what! won't she credit us with a "religious" motive? The bad ones say, ay, our betters allow that this can only be done for money. "The labourer is worthy of his hire."[205] The clergy work for pay, and yet are *supposed* to be "religious." Would Miss G. apply her "commercial" and her "religious" line of demarcation to the clergy?

7. P 19. I have already said what I thought about Miss G.'s view of "volunteer help" in emergencies. She really seems to think that "stimulus" is the main duty of a nurse, "novelty" the main importance of her presence. I can hardly say how curiously that passage reads to me who have had, really, charge of crowded war hospitals, including "cholera" and all other "emergencies." I am afraid I should indulge in a most indecorous laugh at her expense, but that the subject is really too fatally serious.

With regard to her conclusions, pp 19, 20, 21, they are incorrect or unproved. Conclusion 1, why should she limit it to a class? 2. is absolutely defeating her own principle of "supply and demand." The idea of limiting the maximum!! It is besides incorrect. A good *training* head nurse is worth more than £50 and gets more.

3. Incorrect. 4. Contradictory. A lady superintendent need *not* be unpaid and must be trained. In no case does the "volunteer," untrained system have such fatal effects as in that of a superintendent. 5. *Entirely agree.* But is it not contradictory to "4"? 6. Miss G. is ignorant of the conditions of her question. She omits altogether India, Australia and village nursing in England. If I could show her my correspondence for one year she would see how wholly incorrect her premises are. (In a requisition I had from India, *one* item was "193"!!!)

I will only just add (1) with regard to separating the "religious" from the "commercial" element, I never do so. E.g., I take up the first letters lying under my hand from this morning's post. It is from a Delhi missionary. It concerns a "*lady*" now training at our school. He entreats me to get her to wait till they can raise the salary so as to make the Delhi appointment worth her acceptance. We are now training "ladies," salaried "ladies," for New South Wales. This "lady" was to have had the appointment. She will now have to choose between Delhi and Sydney. She is not only "religious" but a missionary. (What

205 Luke 10:7.

can Miss G. be dreaming about?) And I am not at all above making the best bargain for my "ladies."

2. *Ceteris paribus* [other things being equal] it is not true, Miss G.'s principle (only that I scarcely know what her principle is). Good nurses are much the same all over the world, whether Augustinian nuns or paid nurses. But, ten years ago, the *average* nursing of the Paris hospitals (nursed by Augustinian and other nuns) was *far higher* than the *average* nursing of the London hospitals. This is a *fact*, and not a theory. The former were trained, the latter not. God speed the good nurse, I say again, wherever, whatever and whoever she is. But don't suppose that I advocate "UNpaid nurses," because I think "*paid* nurses" a ridiculous criterion of excellence of nursing.

Embley
Romsey
31 October 1866

Private. A thousand thanks for your wise, kind and suggestive note. In reply to your query, they have not yet sent us the information about Romsey, viz., what *is* the death rate of Romsey? What *ought to* be the death rate of Romsey?

In reply to Miss Garrett, I do not at all doubt as to "matrons" that she can cite "two hospitals" where she knows the matron to have no control over the nursing. I can cite all the hospitals in London, *except* "two," where the matron has no real control over the nursing. Those two are St Thomas'[and] King's College, and the latter of these is nursed by a sisterhood.

The fact is that a matron having real control over the nursing is a modern invention. Ten years ago it did not exist. Even now, in most English hospitals, a matron only walks through the wards once a day (at 10 A.M.) to see that it is clean under the beds, has little real control over the nurses, and none at all over the head nurses, who defy her, even in cases of drunkenness, by appeal.

I think one of the hospitals to which Miss Garrett alludes is University College. Now I should "refer" to University College as a hospital which *is* nursed by ladies, where the ladies are *un*trained, where the nursing is *not* improved, where the matron has no authority, nor the superintendent either. (She, the superintendent, signs herself "Mother of all the Saints"!!![206] She does not reside in the hospital.) I should

206 Harriet Brownlow Byron, mother superior and foundress of the (Anglican) All Saints Community.

appeal to St George's Hospital to show the utter failure of "night superintendence" (of nursing). I should appear to Guy's, etc., where wages *are* high and nursing is *not* improved.

Many other instances could I give her out of my perpetual correspondence with county hospitals. But you are quite right in saying that I could not enter into any controversy. We have years to work before we ought to begin to talk.

Though, of all people I am the one who most recommends publicity, who am always urging the utmost possible publicity in hospitals, yet such a discussion as Mr Hastings recommends would do nothing but harm at present. Miss Garrett and her discussion has done nothing but harm so far as it is known.

E.g., how could I put in the papers the facts I have given you in my letters? Besides, I have no time. I must work. Ten years hence, we will discuss. No discussion ever made an artist yet. . . .

N.B. I re-echo entirely and with my whole heart your wise sentence: "so I look to the ordinary organization of work on sound principles for the main supply of nurses as of doctors." So do I. But as I and others have understood Miss Garrett, she would exclude Rosa Bonheur[207] (unless indeed R. Bonheur was untrained and acted for an "emergency") from art. And, did you know a most remarkable woman aged twenty-three, a Duchess Colonna,[208] who exhibited sculpture at the Royal Academy this year—she works harder than a journeyman mason—works for money—and asserts that all she has done is: "J'ai bien travaillé" [I have worked well].

The test of fitness for volunteer, for "*religious*" work has been made by some—by no means all—R. Catholics, and Miss Garrett has been understood (perhaps misunderstood) to support this view—to be: the "*religious motive*" which trains itself so well as to be able to *command the highest pay*! Amen says F.N.

207 Rosa Bonheur (1822-99), a French realist painter; Nightingale gave an engraving of her "Horse Fair" to the Working Men's Reading Room in Derbyshire. Letter to Messrs Graves 10 January 1879, Duke University Medical Center.

208 Duchess Colonna di Castiliogne (1837-79), who used the name "Marcello" for her work.

Source: From two letters to William Farr, Wellcome Ms 5474/108 and 110, typed copies Add Mss 43400 ff149-50 and 152

Embley
Romsey
16 November 1866

Very many thanks for your Romsey statistics. You say, "something must be wrong. What is it?" Everything is wrong, particularly the drainage. Your mortality note has produced a "*sensation prolongée*" in the hands of the very energetic and enlightened doctor who is much interested about drainage. He says "I am *glad* that Romsey has so high a death rate in the tables; it certainly deserves it; the sanitary arrangements are detestable." This unusual sentiment I re-echo.

But you know, "la reconnaissance n'est qu'un vif sentiment des bienfaits futurs" [recognition is but a lively sentiment of future favours]. My doctor of Romsey now asks you the same questions for Winchester. What is the mortality of Winchester? What ought it to be? You know, I dare say, that the drainage arrangements of Winchester *are* "detestable," and that my cousin [John, "Jack," Bonham Carter], MP for Winchester and I are on terms of a "mortal and undying hatred"[209] because he won't do anything and I will.

I am sorry to give you this trouble, if you are so very kind as to take it for us, about Winchester, but I think it does good. You see a communication from the Registrar-General's Office to us provincials is a moving event.

23 November 1866

Do you remember sending me the card enclosed? I am exceedingly glad that you are going to "statisticate the convicts." This is one result of your work about the India prisons. I have been asked to ask you to send me a draft for us to see, if you will kindly allow it.

Very many thanks for the Romsey and Winchester statistics. I hope it will bear fruit.

Source: From a letter to Henry Dyke Acland, Florence Nightingale Museum (LMA) H1/ST/NC1/66/23

7 December 1866

I received a verbal message from the War Office today that you had telegraphed some days ago to the W.O. for a copy of my paper and forms for hospital statistics.

209 In Charles Dickens, *Old Curiosity Shop*, chap 38.

Although a telegram, plus a verbal message, is quite sure to involve a double mistake, I beg to enclose the paper, as finally adopted by the International Statistical Congress, and a filled-up report of St Bartholomew's Hospital, in which the method is substantially adopted. The whole is, however, given in the last chapter of my *Notes on Hospitals*, third edition, Longmans. If this is not what you wanted, but something else, perhaps I might still be able to serve you—if I knew in what.

Source: From a letter to W.E. Nightingale, Add Mss 45790 ff344-45

17 December 1866

I referred Messrs Berthon[210] and Lorhan's paper, enclosed, to the General Register Office, and you will see what Dr Farr says (enclosed). To which I will add: we should not admit the Burial Board returns as evidence of death rate. You may depend upon the Registrar-General's figures. Why? Because everything is taken into account, and with a labour and trouble little known outside that office.

For example, Roman Catholics often, and dissenters sometimes, take their dead to be buried at a distance. Such a vague statement as that of Mr Berthon's, p 2, would never be received. I have known every death scrutinized at a radius of ten miles round to ascertain the true death rate of a sub-district. Again, the sub-district of the Registrar-General may not be the same as that of a corporate town. This will make a difference both in population and number of deaths.

I do not say that any of these things is the case with Romsey. I only give them as instances of the excessive care with which the Registrar-General's returns are made. Again, inhabitants die in hospitals and in workhouses. All this is allowed for in Registrar-General's returns. Otherwise, all the deaths of Romsey people in Winchester Hospital would be put down to Winchester. This, too, I would only give as an instance. You see what care has been taken about Romsey Workhouse in the return.

Please return me Dr Farr's letter and the Romsey return (Registrar-General's) of which Mr Taylor has already a copy.

---

210 Probably Rev Edward Lyon Berthon, vicar of Romsey.

Source: From two letters to William Farr, Wellcome Ms 5474/111 and 113, typed copies Add Mss 43400 ff155 and 157

19 December 1866

Private. Middlesex Hospital Secretary. I have already had a request from Lady Herbert, very difficult to me to refuse because it was urged on the ground of Sidney Herbert, to whom Mr *Watson's* recommender, Mr Wyatt, was devoted. But I did refuse it and I am glad of it, because I should think your recommendation a much higher one than Mr Wyatt's.

(I have also had an application from a third person, a Mr Seymour, whom I don't think much about.) But I am obliged to refuse you, however unwillingly, for this reason: it is not only as secretary (to the Middlesex Hospital) for which your word for your protégé would be quite enough and more than enough for me, that the appointment is to be made—but as "secretary" *and* "resident superintendent." Now this may be an office quite as special (in a hospital) and requiring quite as special qualifications as that of a superintendent of nurses. I am quite unable, overworked as I am, to make such inquiries either as to the duties of the office or as to the competency of the officer for fulfilling them, as would alone justify me in voting.

I have told Lady Herbert that, when she remembers, in Sidney Herbert's days, the excessive care in inquiry taken to select officers—out of the whole army—for similar posts in military hospitals, she cannot but see that the superintendent (of a hospital) must not only be a competent man, but must have had training, and that I cannot give the time and strength to investigate these things. I would take your word for a statistical man sooner than that of any man in Europe or America—if that were all.

I fear poor "Middlesex" is in a bad way on many accounts.

4 January 1867

I have kept the enclosed P. Stat. too long. But I have looked them carefully over. And so has Dr Sutherland. (I had not the opportunity of showing them to him before today.)

The tables we think very good. But ought they not to have put in column for state of health (and disease, if any) at time of discharge from prison after expiry of term of imprisonment, or at time of transfer to another prison? At pp 6, 7 and seqq. such a column might perhaps come in best.

Editor: The following "Remarks" were Nightingale's comments, presumably solicited, printed as the last two pages of a pamphlet issued by Sir J. Clarke Jervoise (d. 1889), a retired MP for South Hampshire, and an opponent of compulsory vaccination. They reflect her views against the "germ hypothesis" at the time they were written (1867), and even repeat her extreme "witchcraft" charge. However, her position had mellowed considerably by the pamphlet's reissue in 1882. As it happened, bacteriologist Robert Koch published his definitive paper on the cholera bacillus in 1884, which discovery led Sutherland, and through him Nightingale, to accept germ theory. Her opposition to quarantine, however, remained strong.

Source: "Remarks by Miss Nightingale," in J. Clarke Jervoise, *Infection," with Remarks by Miss Nightingale*, 2nd ed. (London: Vacher & Sons 1882 [1867]):62-63

This pamphlet is ably written. It reminds one very much of the arguments which, in the Middle Ages, might have been brought by an enlightened man against witchcraft as a cause of disease.

The disease germ fetish and the witchcraft fetish are the produce of the same mental condition, both of them considered simply as superstitions or harmless theories; both of them spring from the same source, a desire to group together a number of detached phenomena, so as to make a kind of raft on which weak minds can float. This view can easily be confirmed by reading any of the trials for witchcraft and comparing the facts and inductions in the Cattle Plague Report, and in other medical treatises on so-called contagious diseases. But when either the witchcraft hypothesis or the disease-germ hypothesis is made the basis of legislation, on the assumption that any public good can follow from any acts of Parliament, then the matter becomes very serious indeed, and the fact of such legislation being possible can only be considered as a striking proof how rapidly the (so-called) scientific mind of England is sinking into a condition of abject superstition.

This is not the only evil; commerce will inevitably suffer to a greater extent than heretofore from these absurdities, unless a check is put on them. It cannot be otherwise, because the germ hypothesis, if logically followed out, must stop all human intercourse whatever, on pain or [of] risk of disease or death. The germ hypothesis, moreover, is directly at variance in its results with ascertained sanitary experience, and to adopt it as a basis of legislation is, in strict logic, to declare that the Public Health Act, the Local Government Act and all other local acts for improving the public health have been founded on error.

This pamphlet is the first protest made publicly against this downward course. The author deserves great credit for his audacity, and one can only hope that it will open the eyes of other members of the House of Commons to the course on which they have entered.

Editor: In 1867 Nightingale was approached by Duncan M. Forbes, a physician to a Nottinghamshire colliery, whose proprietor was willing to co-operate with the workmen to build a hospital for accident victims. Forbes had her *Notes on Hospitals*, but could not see anything in it pertinent to the size of hospital they needed, from eight to twelve beds. Nightingale's reply is not available, but a draft by Dr Sutherland gives much practical advice for a small hospital. Forbes wrote again after several months with appreciation, but it is not known what, if anything, came of this.[211]

Source: From a letter to an unnamed recipient, Wellcome (Claydon copy) Ms 9001/173

Tuesday 12 November [1867?]

With regard to the Salisbury and Southton [Southampton] Hospitals—you ask me to tell you what is bad about them—hic—the big prigs don't like to do what the little prigs do, namely, give an opinion without recent data. I had all the plans and Rawlinson's reports about Winchester and Reading before me when I gave those opinions. All that I can say generally about Salisbury and Southton Hospitals is that they are founded upon the prevailing mistake—that the construction of a private house will do as the pattern for a place where there is to be a congregation of sickness—whereas we know that the construction of a barn would be better and more fit for the purpose.

But I would suggest to you as a work worthy of you, and of your genius for construction, to look at my book (first and last parts) and particularly at the figures, and then to ride over to Salisbury and Southton and compare principles with practice. I hear from Malta that they have no disease in the huts—although the heat in them is much complained of, whereas in the building, although very much preferred for coolness, fever and epidemics are never absent—the same at Gibraltar.

211 Forbes letter 20 April 1867, with Sutherland draft reply, and Forbes letter 4 July 1867, Florence Nightingale Museum (LMA) H1/ST/NC2/V16/67 and V24/67.

Source: From two letters to Harry Verney, Wellcome (Claydon copy) Ms 9003/15 and 9021/15

17 March 1868

I have been asked to obtain your help about this. This quarantine inquiry, if granted, will either do much good or much harm. The *commission* should consist of merchants, sanitarians and a lawyer or two. The *instructions* should state clearly that the object is to obtain facts and evidence as to the practice of quarantine, its grounds and results, and finally the measures which (in the commissioners' opinion) would mitigate or prevent the outbreak of epidemic diseases at seaports and on board ship.

You will see that some of the best names in the medical profession are among the signatures, and the MPs for Liverpool, Manchester, Edinburgh, London, etc. The point is now to get good men for this *commission,* and good *instructions.*

The duke of Marlborough[212] has appointed *today* at *one o'clock* to receive the deputation at the Privy Council Office. The appointment of so early a day is considered a favourable symptom as to the probability of the duke's granting the prayer of the memorial.

I should be glad to do anything, as I moved for both the army sanitary and Indian army royal commissions, if I could be of any use—I mean as to writing "instructions" or looking out for men.

[1868-69?]

I do not know whether anything has been done about that letter for the *Alexandria Hospital* (to be written by H. Bonham Carter and signed by Mmes Bernstorff and Schwabe[213] and me), which you were so good as to propose to send about to a few people. Should I write to *Miss Coutts*?[214]

---

212 John Winston Spencer Churchill (1822-83), 7th duke of Marlborough, lord president of the council.

213 Née Cynthia Victoria Ames, Countess Bernstorff, the American-born wife of the Prussian ambassador; Julie Salis Schwabe (1818-96), voluntary aid worker during the Franco-Prussian War; see the biographical sketch in *Wars and the War Office* (15:1036). The Alexandria Hospital was probably Kaiserswerth's.

214 Angela Georgina Burdett-Coutts (1814-1906), philanthropist, later Baroness Burdett-Coutts.

Source: From a letter to Douglas Galton, ADD MSS 45764 f140

19 April 1869

Most Private. I am glad to hear that you are going to preach at Leeds on hospitals.[215] And I will try to get up some "ideas." But my advice to you is to dwell with great force, grounded on the experience of the "Herbert Hospital," on the propriety or necessity of organizing insanitary measures to fill the hospitals. Otherwise they will not do us justice.

Editor: The facetious point in the preceding letter refers to the decline of death rates and hospital stays in the better-constructed pavilion hospital.

The intermediary for the following letter was Emmy Carolina Rappe (1835-96), a Swedish nurse who trained at St Thomas' in 1867 to become matron at the University Hospital, Uppsala. The addressee is Jean von Koch, member of the County Council.[216] No further correspondence on the matter is evident.

Source: From a copy of a letter to Jean von Koch, Wellcome Ms 9086/16

June 1869

In reply to the questions forwarded to me through Miss Rappe, from a hospital committee in Stockholm, I beg to state:

1. V. [see] the *new* hospitals are all constructed on the pavilion principle;

2. V. [see] the corridor system, meaning thereby that the wards are all entered by a common corridor along the side, as at page × 37 (Netley) of my *Notes on Hospitals* (a copy of which I beg to forward) has been quite abandoned. The old military hospital at Woolwich was constructed on this plan and it was abandoned for the Herbert Hospital. The result is that the sick remain one third of the time in the pavilion hospital which they did in the corridor hospital. There were out of the same garrison nearly 600 (579) *constantly sick* in the corridor plan. In the pavilion plan (the Herbert Hospital) there are 200 sick. (This amazing improvement is, however, also connected with sanitary improvements in barracks.)

3. The Herbert Hospital, being a military hospital, publishes no reports. But I beg to annex the report of the construction of that hospital.

---

215 Galton's speech at Leeds, to the British Medical Association on 29 July 1869, was subsequently published as a short book, *An Address on the General Principles which Should Be Observed in the Construction of Hospitals.*

216 Précis in Sue M. Goldie, comp., *A Calendar of the Letters of Florence Nightingale.*

4. Workhouses publish no reports. For the same reason, therefore, I cannot, as requested, forward the "last report" of the Chorlton Workhouse Hospital. But I will forward the report of its construction with this packet.

5. If the gentlemen who have addressed to me questions through Miss Rappe decide on the pavilion system, I will do myself the honour of procuring and sending them a set of the plans of the new St Thomas' Hospital. But, as these plans are not published, it is impossible to send a copy of them everywhere. Besides, the Herbert Hospital plans, which I forward, are much more complete, and contain plates of every part of the construction.

The best way, however, to reply to these gentlemen's questions is to descend to first principles:

1. The foundation of hospital construction is the ward. The ward must have windows *on opposite sides*, with no more than two rows of beds between the windows—in the manner shown in the Lariboisière, Herbert, etc. (see pp 150 and 160 above) of my *Notes*, as in new St Thomas' plans. To each ward should be attached a nurse's room, scullery, lavatory and W.C.s, with ready access to warm baths.

2. After the ward comes the pavilion construction. Each pavilion should have only two floors of wards, as shown in the Herbert Hospital plan.

3. Next, there is the question whether the pavilions should be single or double. At Lariboisière and at new St Thomas' the pavilions are all single, i.e., there is only one ward on each floor.

In the new Herbert Hospital at Woolwich, several of the pavilions are double. And this is found to answer very well, that is, there are two wards on each floor, entered right and left from the stair, vide [see] plan. Either the single or double pavilion may be adopted with safety, but with the double pavilion is required a large, well-ventilated staircase, as in the Herbert Hospital plan.

4. Next comes the question regarding the best arrangement *of pavilions*. The pavilion construction is so flexible that it may be adapted to any arrangement of parts in the hospital, provided the pavilions are kept sufficiently far apart from each other to have free external ventilation. In England, they should be placed at a distance from each other equal to 2 or 2½ times their height (but this depends on the length of the pavilion—with long pavilions a greater distance is better).

The pavilions might also be arranged in the form of a square, as at St Bartholomew's Hospital, Fig. 22 (see p 153 above) of my *Notes*, and as at Fig. 23 (see p 154 above), leaving the corners well open for ventilation. But, if the arrangement in square be adopted, the distance across the square should be greater than if the pavilions are arranged side by side.

St Bartholomew's covers too small an area of ground for the height of the hospital buildings. We prefer also that all the wards should be built north and south, to have the sun *on both sides* during the day. This cannot well be done if the pavilions are arranged in a square.

(1) We do not consider therefore the arrangement of building at St Bartholomew's Hospital the best we have in England. The best we have is the Herbert Hospital at Woolwich. It is much better ventilated outside and the arrangement of parts is far better even than at the new St Thomas' Hospital.

(2) Our war hospitals and camp hospitals (and this even in the Crimea, where the thermometer was sometimes 2° above zero Fahrenheit) are generally separate wooden huts. There is a great sanitary advantage in subdividing sick and injured people into small groups or detached wards. But the hospital architect can by his art obtain all the advantages in larger buildings, and by doing this he diminishes the cost both of construction and administration.

(3) The largest number of sick in one double pavilion at the Herbert Hospital is 128. But, as every soldier, however slight his illness, must, in our service, go to hospital, most of the cases are trivial. The largest number of severe cases of disease and accident which ought to be placed in one double pavilion of four wards on two floors is twenty beds per ward (or eighty beds in the pavilion). If the position of the hospital is not well-aired outside, we prefer sixteen beds per ward (or sixty-four beds in the pavilion).

(4) In the report herewith sent on the Herbert Hospital, all the details of construction in that great establishment are given. It is most important to know that *these details have been found successful in practice.*

(5) There is no reason why the construction in small separate pavilions should not do in Swedish climates. The warming and ventilation must, of course, be arranged to correspond to the climate. There is no habitable climate in which small separate pavilions could not be put up for sick and injured. The architect can always adapt this mode of construction to any temperature. And the pavilions can be connected by a corridor for facility of intercourse under cover.

I have myself nursed a hospital in the Crimea, as above-mentioned, consisting of wooden huts [Castle Hospital], *without* a corridor (thermometer 2° above zero Fahrenheit, i.e., 30° below freezing point Fahrenheit). (The death rate in that hospital was *under 3* percent; in the magnificent corridor hospitals of Scutari it was 20 percent on cases treated; and in one large hospital [Koulali] during one month more than half of all the cases died.) . . .

[Enclosures] 1. F. Nightingale's *Notes on Hospitals.*

2. Captain Galton's *Report on Herbert Hospital.*

3. T. Worthington's pamphlet on Chorlton Workhouse Hospital will accompany this letter.[217]

Source: From a letter to Henry Dyke Acland, Bodleian Library, Oxford University, f21

Embley
Romsey
9 August 1869

In your note of 24 July you say, "When I do write I mean to ask you about another subject, the registration of disease in public institutions." And you ask me for "a copy" of our "model forms for this purpose." (I am not sure whether you did not mean me to answer this question at once.)

I believe that I have one or two copies of these "model forms" left (at my house in London). But they are now no longer of use since the new nomenclature came into operation. The only full account of the method is in the 4th edition[218] (Longmans) of my *Notes on Hospitals,* last chapter. But you have a man who is also on the "sanitary commission," Mr Paget, who knows more about all this than any man in Europe. Let him give you a copy of the back St Bartholomew's reports.

The method, described by me and embodied in St Bartholomew's reports, as introduced by Mr Paget, is the only one to give results, subject, however, to the use of the new nomenclature of diseases.

Excuse shortness of words, which means shortness of strength.

Editor: The next letter refers to a debate in the *Scotsman* carried on by Sir James Y. Simpson (1811-70) and Professor (later Sir) James Syme

---

217 Thomas Worthington (1826-1909), architect of the Chorlton Union and Crumpsall Workhouses; his pamphlet was a reprint of the paper published in the *Transactions of the Manchester Statistical Society* (see p 732 below).

218 The third, printed, edition, but the fourth if the original paper given at the meetings is counted; for the table see p 198 above.

(1799-1870), which was later summed up in the magazine *Scientific American.* Syme was in favour of large hospital buildings, relying on disinfectants, especially carbolic acid, to prevent the spread of disease. Simpson, meanwhile, denied their efficacy, claiming that in the two years since their introduction the mortality from amputations had increased from 40 to 53 percent. The article supported Simpson, saying that instead of a large building, with disinfectants and antiseptics, a hospital should have a central building for administrative purposes, with the patients placed in "a series of village hospitals or wards," with "abundance of space, abundance of light and above all abundance of fresh, pure and ever-changing air to every patient in every ward."[219] Nightingale is nowhere mentioned in the correspondence, but clearly her views matched those of Simpson.[220]

Source: From a letter to John Sutherland, Add Mss 45754 f11

Embley
Romsey
7 October 1869

Sir James Simpson's letter in Scotsman. I send you this paper, which has been sent to me with

> I think that the public should be wakened up about the matter of hospitals. Ought not the statistics of hospitals to form a part of Dr Farr's returns, and cannot this be effected? Strong facts must be adduced. Or nothing will be done. There is an opposing interest to that of the patients, doctors and medical students. And practical remedies must be suggested—not interfering too much with existing interests. It is a very difficult thing to retract an error on a great scale.

What shall I say?

Editor: Context for the next letter is lacking. Mary Jones had superintended the maternity ward and training program at King's College Hospital, closed at the end of 1866. Around the same time, she and several other of her nurses left their (Anglican) order, St John's House, to establish their own, smaller community. Nightingale continued to

219 "The Rational Construction of Hospitals," *Scientific American* 21 new series (20 November 1869):329.

220 For Nightingale's correspondence with him; see *Women* (8:219-20).

be in touch both with her and St John's House on re-establishing a training program for midwifery nurses, but Jones never in fact established another one.

Direct correspondence is missing, but a history of St John's House states that Nightingale gave assistance on its new maternity home (date not given), which was not in a new building:

> This work was honoured by Miss Nightingale's sympathy and interest. She inspected the plans (which were based on the newest hygienic principles then known) and gave them her warmest approval.

Nightingale is quoted as having written the order's council, but only this excerpt is quoted:

> I wish you Godspeed with all my heart and strength and shall be proud if we can by maintaining pupils with you follow in your steps and extend among a large number your benefit promised to the poor."[221]

All this may refer to the next letter, but one cannot be sure. The history just cited reported that a maternity home for ten in-patients and the training of midwives, opened in 1877, in Ashburnham Rd., Chelsea (14).

Source: From a letter to Mary Jones, Add Mss 47744 ff196-97

3 June 1870

Lying-in Hospital plans.

Dearest friend, May I trouble you once more with these plans before we go further? I enclose one plan 3A and a statement. I like the sketch on p 4 of the statement—the one occupying three sides of a square. And I propose, after having obtained your suggestions, if you approve it, to ask the draughtsman to make the plans on that *sketch* for one set.

1. Would you also answer whether it will be necessary to provide a small scullery for what he calls the "segregation ward," which you suggested? (V. [see] his last question on statement.) . . .

2. Also, please be so good as to criticize arrangements of pupil midwives' block and kitchen block, as shown on Plan 3A, which will be transferred to the *three sides of a square plan*, if approved.

3. And anything else which may strike you about delivery work, with their appurtenances and bye-wards. Is the bye-ward, which is for extreme cases only, too far?

---

221 *A Record of Sixty Years' Work: St John's House Queen Square* 15.

The worst of it is that I am told this plan will be so violently expensive. And it is even suggested that we should have huts, with a delivery ward (or room) within *each* hut. But huts occupy so much ground. It would be impossible to obtain so much ground in or near a large town. And I suppose a lying-in hospital must be in or quite close to a large town, must it not? for married women *will* not come in, before labour is imminent. And the others, poor things, if you take them in, as the French do, for months beforehand, you alter the whole character of the hospital, and make it in fact a workhouse (though I, for my part, should not exclude single young women, primiparae absolutely—it is grievous to see them mixed up with the most hardened in workhouses).

If it would save you trouble to return me this my sheet of questions with your remarks, please do so. I am shocked to give you so much trouble before coming to you for final revision of these plans. God bless you.

ever truly, *how* truly, yours
F. Nightingale

Derby Infirmary, 1864-69

Editor: The Nightingales were a Derbyshire family, and Nightingale herself continued to regard herself as a "Derbyshire woman," even when the family spent most of its time in Hampshire, and she lived in London. Thus it is to be expected that she would take a warm interest in the Derby Infirmary and any possibility of improvements in it. There is much surviving correspondence on this issue, including letters to and from the main doctor concerned, William Ogle (1824-1905); the chair of the building committee, Francis Wright (1806-73); and her own family. Nightingale had hoped that her father would serve as the infirmary's president, but he never did. In fact, he vexed her enormously by supporting the anti-reform side.

There are seven letters each by Ogle and Nightingale to the other.[222] In his first to her, he introduced himself as a physician to the county infirmary who wanted a "better system of nursing," adding

---

222 Originals in Add Mss 47758 and the Royal College of Physicians of London 2415, published as "The Correspondence Between Dr Ogle and Florence Nightingale," in V.M. Leveaux, *History of the Derbyshire General Infirmary*. Correspondence about nursing at Derby has already appeared, in *Extending Nursing* (13:274-75).

that the hospital would be made available as a school for nursing.[223] One letter of his thanked her for her candour and clarity. He wanted her to be "patroness,"[224] but she would allow only that she would not object to his stating that she would give "the best information and opinion I can on any scheme you yourselves may propose, but in doing so I must clearly be considered as merely aiding you because I am asked." She wished to "inform all sides and to take part with none, but only to give all sides the means of forming a judgment" (see p 709 below).

Dr Ogle's letter to Nightingale of 6 November 1865 frankly related the death of a pneumonia patient who, he had thought mistakenly, had been "properly attended" until another patient described how the man would throw off his clothes, "get out of bed and walk about" unobserved if the nurse were in any other ward. In her reply she pointed to the isolation of the ward and the need for a building design that permitted surveillance of fever patients at all times (see p 712 below).

Clearly there was much dissension on the committee—a usual feature of hospital building committees. The earliest letter by Nightingale available on the subject picks up on this. That there was an "ecclesiastical question" involved is also typical. Here Nightingale affirmed that she must serve all sides, including Jews, and acknowledged having "very strong opinions on religious subjects" (see p 711 below).

Complications on the Derby Infirmary emerged in 1867, coming through connections with the Strutt family. Edward Strutt (1801-80), first Baron Belper and a former MP for Derby, did not want the old building to be interfered with, while Nightingale considered it to be unsanitary and in need of major alterations or dismantling. It turned out that his father, William Strutt (1756-1830), had planned the old building with its faulty ventilation. Lord Belper did not get his way, but Francis Wright, who supported Nightingale's position, did.[225] Nightingale's father, however, supported Lord Belper.

Although the original plan had been merely the addition of a new building, Nightingale insisted on seeing the plans of the existing one.

---

223 Ogle letter 28 December 1864, Add Mss 47758 f108.

224 Letter 30 May 1865, Add Mss 47758 f113.

225 His letters to Nightingale are extant, in Add Mss 47758 ff47-105, but there are no original letters by Nightingale to him. Draft replies by Dr Sutherland are used here. One letter by him is to W.E. Nightingale, about naming a ward in her honour (18 July 1864, f104).

She explained that it was essential to see the whole of the hospital to plan nursing services for it. The defects that became evident were serious enough to convince her that "they had much better build a new building" (see p 720 below). The old centre block could be used for administration, she advised, but not for patients.

Source: From two letters to William Ogle, Royal College of Physicians of London 2415/1-2, partial draft in Dr Sutherland's hand, Add Mss 47758 ff111-12

2 January 1865

Sir, I regret that, overwhelmed with business and illness as I am, I have not found time to answer your note before today.[226] I regret still more that, while the object is in its present immature state, it is impossible to enter into detailed recommendations. After you have people to join, a committee formed, and I suppose I must add, money to work with, I shall be most happy to advise on any points you may wish.

When your society is formed, if you desire to send me the program of your plans, I will do my best to consider them. In the meantime, I will only say that I think experience shows that the superintendent of the nurses to be trained, and of the place where they are trained, should be one and the same person. The training school is of the first importance, the "home" of the second. The "home" should be attached to the hospital—not the hospital to the "home." The superintendent must have herself the highest knowledge of nursing, be herself resident in the hospital, make the training in nursing her first object, and be herself a trained nurse of the highest order.

I send a number of printed papers, in case they should be of any use to you, concerning our training schools at St Thomas' and King's College Hospitals. I also send the last sanitary reports and prospectus of the "Ladies Sanitary Association" in London. They would send you from their office a packet of tracts, report[s], etc., if you wish it, by which you would see what they are doing, and how far you could work in concert with them.

I beg that you will believe me, Sir,
your faithful servant, at any time that I could be of use,
Florence Nightingale

226 Presumably his letter of 28 December 1864, with a prospectus (see p 706 above).

29 May 1865

In reply to your note of 27 May and its accompanying papers, I do not, of course, enter into the ecclesiastical question. I have helped rampant Roman Catholics, rampant Puseyites,[227] rampant non-conformists of all kinds, rampant evangelicals, all as far as I was able to obtain good nurses.

And all local organizations should be left to arrange themselves. You have seen them at Liverpool; an account of its organization will shortly be printed and circulated.[228] There they will have had no difficulty with the ecclesiastical question (although the *rampants* rage in Liverpool more than in any place I know). But on that common ground of nursing sick poor they have met together under the leading of one good man [William Rathbone].

From their paper you will obtain the wisest hints as to a local organization. The first thing you now want, in order to begin, is a good training matron for the infirmary, one who shall not only "have entire charge of the housekeeping and the domestic service," but shall be a *real* trainer and "superintendent" of *nurses.*

The next thing is to lay down the Regulations under which you should train. I send you (confidentially) a paper prepared by me for the Government of India, at their request. (Please return it to me.) Should you find in it what you require, and should you put your scheme in form, I shall be very glad to go over it. Do not make it too rigid. You will find that the system will have, to some extent, to form itself.

Your proposed changes in the Derbyshire General Infirmary are part only of a reform which better nursing will entail on you. The fact is some general principles are required for guidance in all hospitals. If I live, I may perhaps try to do something of this kind—as it is impossible for me to answer in writing all the written questions addressed to me on this administrative matter.

Some of the existing practices you describe, and also some of the changes you propose in the infirmary administration, are not altogether what I should adopt myself. I might even say that I should fancy the gravest mischief would result from some. But it would be unsafe to

227 From the high church, Anglo-Catholic movement of Edward Bouverie Pusey (1800-82).

228 William Rathbone, *The Organization of Nursing in a Large Town,* for which Nightingale wrote the Introduction.

interfere, unless the entire system, including the nursing, were reconstructed: "New wine in old bottles,"[229] etc. (the proverb is somewhat musty).

I should be most glad and happy to go over carefully and criticize for you the plans of the proposed alterations in the building; I can form no judgment about them from description merely.

It would have afforded me great pleasure to have seen you, but I am so feeble that I doubt any good coming of my doing so, in the present immature state of your plans. If, however, you think otherwise, I take so intense an interest in your scheme that I would see you on Wednesday, the day you propose, at 3 P.M. or at 4 P.M. (if you will write me word) at this house. . . . I should not be able to go over the building alterations with you viva voce [out loud]. These, at all events, I must have time to go over by myself.

Source: From a draft letter to Francis Wright, in Dr Sutherland's hand, Add Mss 47758 f140

[c1865]

The question as to the local position and construction of the infirmary is purely a local one, with which the governors and subscribers only have to do, and I could not suggest any special course. I should say that, after the opinions you have sent me, it is very doubtful indeed whether the infirmary is not the reverse of a benefit to the sick poor.

As to the new building, I have great difficulty in naming any architect but Mr [Alex] Graham, Carlton Chambers, Regent St., who planned Swansea Infirmary, would do it justice. I only know him from this and some other works in which he has been engaged. Whoever you employ should have mastered the specialities of the subject.[230] I should like to see the plans which may be sent in.

Source: From three letters and a typed copy of an incomplete letter to William Ogle, Royal College of Physicians of London 2415/3-4, 8 and 6

2 June 1865

Private. I have not hitherto answered your questions as to using my name, etc., because it appeared to me that I had sufficiently expressed what course I am compelled uniformly to take. I can have no objec-

229 An allusion to Mark 2:22.

230 The architects chosen were Henry Isaac Stevens and Frederick Josias Robinson, of Derby, but there is no correspondence with them.

tion to its being stated that I will give the best information and opinion in my power as to any scheme you yourselves may propose, but in doing so I must clearly be considered as aiding, merely because I am asked.

And the reason you will at once see is that I must not, even in appearance, interfere with the entire liberty of judgment and action on the part of your committee and association. I wish to inform all sides, to the best of my power, so as to give *them* the means of forming a judgment and to take part with none.

Suffer me to say that I must also protect myself, or I should be continually dragged in to give my authority, such as it is worth, to schemes which all experience tells us cannot succeed. I will give every assistance in my power whether in the way of training nurses or giving information when asked. But it is necessary, in order to aid every side efficiently, that I should not become "patroness" (a word I detest) of any.

13 June 1865

I am very sorry not to be able to assent to your citing me as an authority. I am most willing to help your committees to the utmost of my power—but to do this effectually it *is* necessary that the committees should ask my advice.

This is not an opinion, or a fear of collision, on my part. It is the result of painful experience. My opinion is asked by and given to one member of a committee. Great injury to the cause follows. I am involved in endless trouble. The committee is convinced, at last, that I am right. The opposition arises from jealousy of the separate action of one member. This is my almost quotidian [daily] experience. And I have determined for the sake of the cause, much more than for my own (for I am used to being skinned alive every day like the eels), to avoid this for the future.

31 June 1865

In obedience to your express desire, but under protestation, I have criticized the enclosed sheet. Such criticisms generally only succeed in alienating those who ask for it. And as the criticizers cannot possibly advance all the reasons for the criticism, it is besides useless labour in general.

To architect's plans this does not apply, and such criticism which I am almost weekly asked for I gladly give. Of course I apologize for the curtness of my marginal notes. Such notes are like telegrams—one cannot go down on one's knees in a telegram.

Also, to avoid all possibility of misconstruction about the ecclesiastical question, it is not from indifferentism I say what I did. I have very strong opinions on religious subjects. But it was only by serving all sides, even Jews, that I could be of any use. I was asked to head a subscription for returning a man with whose *political* opinions I have the strongest sympathies to Parliament. But I declined. I have served the army sanitary administration with both political sides, when either was in power, and it was only thus I could do good.

10 November 1865

Private. I have to thank you for your three notes of 2, 6 and [undated] November. In the first place, I will observe that I completely agree with you that, if the question were asked me whether to extend the old hospital or to build a new one, I should certainly answer the latter. But the question has not been asked me. And you see, like a ghost, I can only speak when I am spoken to.

The fever wing is a nest of holes and corners—equally destructive to health and to nursing. Nothing can be done with it but sweep it from end-to-end, in the way of improvement.

2. I have read your letters with the plans before me. The architect, it is evident, knows his business. And the alterations and additions proposed are very good. I have made a good many suggestions. But I have also said that, to make the building what it should be, it should have two wings (the proposed new one, and the fever one *re*built) and the old centre block should be used merely for administration, etc.

Everything now depends on the course the committee decide to take. If they adopt the latter course I have suggested, I hope they will send me a pencil sketch, when I will go minutely into the details of accommodation for a nursing staff, etc. It is of no use my doing so till *they* have made up their minds.

I return you the enclosed, as you desire. And I should be much obliged to you to *re-return* it to me when the committee have decided. I will then go over in minute detail all these things, and we can then decide whether it will be of any use to the cause your using my remarks on the report. But at present it would perhaps be better to leave the whole matter in the hands of the committee. I have no doubt we shall have plenty of battle to fight afterwards.

I was very much obliged to you for sending me my notes and for your information.

It would be necessary, if I am farther consulted, to tell me the average number of operations in the year:

men, women,
of surgical cases, men, women,
of medical cases, men, women, etc.

It is impossible to arrange the wards and the nursing without knowing these and an infinity of other details.

Oddly enough, sex was not given in the summary sent me of the *proposed* wards. Your pneumonia case undoubtedly was killed by want of nursing, just as much as if he had been killed by an accident. Such cases, neglected in such a way, are all but certain to prove fatal, unless the head nurse's eye *is never off them and the nurses.* If the fever wing had been built expressly to provide for the neglect of such cases, it could not have succeeded better.

I would most gladly have seen you, as you so kindly suggest. But I am completely disabled by illness from any such pleasure, however much I might desire it. I write in haste, because I had not time to write to you on the same day I wrote to Mr Wright. And I would not have you think I have neglected your letters.

Editor: There then was a hiatus in the correspondence while the building committee made its decisions and plans were prepared. Francis Wright duly sent Nightingale the plans, on which she wrote her comments before sending them on to Dr Sutherland for him to add his. The material below consists of her (separate) notes and his draft replies. Neither the original plans nor letters are available. The process evidently went on for several years.

It seems that Nightingale gave the plans one last thorough review in 1869, again with Dr Sutherland also commenting (see p 720 below). Not until then did she finally express her satisfaction. Readers should note that what is called the "new wing" in the correspondence was really a separate building, which in due course was named the "Nightingale Wing."

Source: From three undated draft letters to Francis Wright, in Dr Sutherland's hand, Add Mss 47758 ff58, 60-63 and 89

[1866]

I have read your letter with the plans before me. The alterations and additions proposed are very extensive. I have suggested several changes and pointed out omissions, but I have also stated that, to make the building what it should be, the present wing and fever wards should be rebuilt. Everything now depends on the course the committee takes with my paper. In regard to your using any part of my remarks or the report, it would perhaps be better to leave the whole matter in the hands of the committee, for as they have consulted me formally, I should of course deal with them.

Basement. Deadhouse and post-mortem rooms should be so arranged as to have no direct communication with the hospital. Carry the body outside and into the deadhouse and post-mortem room by doors from the open air. Ventilate each abundantly and make everything in the post-mortem room waterproof: slate, tables, floor, sink, etc.

Accident ward not nearly good enough. You want more light. Windows on at least two sides (as in physicians and surgeons' consulting rooms) and there is no nurses' accommodation for this ward. The surgeons' consulting room would do and the small waiting room would do for the nurses. Or, still better, the museum on the first floor. Put the museum (ground floor) where the proposed surgical ward is and provide a nurses' room.

Ground Floor. Open window in end of No. 3 ward. Place nurses' rooms for wards 2 and 3 where the lavatories are and vice versa. Give each nurse's room a small window into the adjacent ward.

Fever Ward. Query: open the ward from end-to-end as has been done with wards 2 and 3, and block up one door. Each W.C. at the end of the new ward should be ventilated and lighted by a separate window.

Upper Floor. There is no nurses' accommodation in the front of the building where the operation cases are. Wards 9 and 10 have no nurses' rooms. Place nurses' rooms for wards 9 and 10 where the lavatories are, with small windows through to each ward.

Query: convert the scullery and lavatory of wards 9 and 10 into nurses' rooms and provide scullery and lavatory accommodation out of wards 7 and 8.

Fever wards. Query: make into one and close one door.

New ward. Each W.C. and sink require a separate window, Ward 6, a window at end.

These remarks contain the points on which your plan may be improved, but I cannot help feeling that, having done so much, you could do much more. Why not make the wing opposite the new ward into a similar building? Place your lock cases anywhere. The basement is good enough for them. Only give these lock wards quite separate entrances and nursing arrangements. Then rebuild your fever ward separately on a better plan.

If you were to keep the old wing, I should advise you to sweep it clean from end-to-end, including the lock ward, and convert it into a simple ward like the new one. Sweep away the fever wards and complete the opposite windows. Place your lock cases if you will in the basement of this wing.

I don't quite like new wards 2, 3, 5 and 6 they have hemmed in. Why not convert the front angles with wards on the ground and first floor and devote the private rooms in the back angles to nurses' sleeping accommodation, etc.?

The fireplaces in the wards should be no broader across the ward than at present, but the fire grates should radiate heat along the ward and not across it and through the windows as at present. . . .

The proposed arrangement of the central building is costly for the result, but it is the least you can do with to render the central building fit for hospital sick.

The fever wards with their corridor are most objectionable and ought to be cleared away altogether, with as little delay as possible. At the Herbert Hospital the end of [illeg] are warmed by hot water pipes brought from a great central boiler house. Get Captain Galton's report on the Herbert Hospital (a penetrating paper and you will find in it everything you want).

Entrance [illeg] and dead away from the building and invisible convalescent corridor will probably never be used by any *patients.* Work out the architectural points regarding the accident ward.

The best place for an operating theatre is where it can have a large skylight sloping to the north, as well as a window under the skylight in the north wall. It is better not to be in the attic.

Source: From a letter to William Ogle, Royal College of Physicians of London 2415/7

18 May 1866

Private. It would be unpardonable of me not to have answered your kind letter of 30 April, or acknowledge your "letter" to the infirmary governors before, if I had not to urge the ever-increasing excuse of illness and business, and if I had not felt that I could do no good in the way you kindly proposed.

I have never entered into the controversial line, either in politics or in religion. I have given my services to any government who would have them. I have also given my services to any Christian denomination (and even to Jews and Muhammedans) if they were authoritatively asked for. But, if they were asked for to support one "party" against another, though I have been fool enough sometimes to do it, in the interest of the poor and the sick, *never* in the interest of "party," I have always had cause to repent of it—not from the vain trouble which rebounded upon me, and which I did not so much mind, as in the very interest of those poor and those sick which I was advocating.

I rejoice in the great and unexampled progress you have made in public opinion at Derby in the cause of hospital reform—very much owing to yourself. I believe that we shall be able to furnish you with a lady superintendent.[231] (Certainly the lady we propose will now lend herself to the charge of being the "ecclesiastical" head of a "sisterhood." Mrs Wardroper, our matron of St Thomas', and I had a good laugh over that paragraph of your letter, though I did not tell her it was yours.) The lady in question will now return to Mrs Wardroper to be further trained for a few months. And we hope to send you her, and a staff of nurses, by Michaelmas [29 September] or Christmas.

But we hope we shall be allowed till Christmas. You are doubtless aware that I have had much correspondence with Mr Wright. In the present state of the question, I can scarcely interfere in the way you kindly propose; you must fight your own battles, in which I heartily wish you Godspeed—and when the time comes that I am asked my opinion authoritatively, you will always find me ready to give the fullest consideration in my power, or any other assistance as far as health and business permit.

I have already told Mr Wright that any alteration in rules necessitated by having a lady superintendent I would gladly look over, if desired, or any hospital plans. (The India government paper is still strictly private and cannot be used.) In short, in any question either "of construction or of administration," I will do my very best in giving advice, if I am asked authoritatively and not controversially. And, in the meantime, pray let me congratulate you on your success and augur a greater success to you.

Source: From a letter to Douglas Galton, Add Mss 45764 ff32-35

30 January 1867

Burn. Could you find the time to read the enclosed about the *Derbyshire Infirmary* from Mr F. Wright, and counsel me what to do, for this reason that Dr Sutherland told me that Lord Belper had told you,

231 Elizabeth Frances Maria Kilvert (c1828-?), who began work with four trained nurses on 4 January 1867.

etc. From the very confused account that Dr Sutherland gave me of what you did (or did not) say, combined with the information in this letter ("Chinese metaphysics" look out article "China" and article "Metaphysics" in Cyclopaedia and "combine your information").

I opine that the Strutt faction, headed by Lord Belper, have combined to upset the resolutions passed at a general meeting, that it is Mr Wright and I, plus one or two others, against the Strutts, that Mr Wright wants me now to drag him through, *if I can*, and that Derby will have no infirmary. Now it is not the question with me whether the Strutt faction has been factious, whether Mr Wright is right and Lord Belper wrong, but what he asks me to do is simply impossible for me (if the above version is correct according to you). I can't drag a good county infirmary through against the will of the county. If a general committee chooses to ask me my opinion, I will give it as well as I can. If not, not.

However good the man, I can't be made his backer to help him to fight the county, on the turf of my opinion (Mr Wright is in a mess and feels he is so) and wants me to help him out.

2. When does your workhouse committee meet again? Have you heard anything of Mr Hardy's scheme?[232] I devoutly hope that ministers will be out in a fortnight.

3. I will send back your *linen* tormentors tomorrow. It seems to me that our admirable friend, Dr Sutherland, and Mrs Shaw Stewart, both of Celtic blood, are much of the same complexion. There *must* be a debatable ground, which they so much esteem and admire, for the dear delight of getting up a "row" upon. Whereas a respectable old female, like me, who goes plodding on, they *snub*.

Editor: Galton replied to the above letter on the same day, returning Wright's letter, and commenting that some people thought that Wright had taken too much upon himself.[233] The letter Nightingale wrote to her father (the second below) shows him siding with an old friend, Lord Belper.

---

232 Gathorne Hardy (1814-1906), later Lord Cranbrook, the new Conservative president of the Poor Law Board; his "scheme" was presumably the Metropolitan Poor Law Act.

233 Galton letter 30 January 1867, ADD MSS 45764 f36.

Source: From a draft letter in Dr Sutherland's hand, Add Mss 47758 ff96-97

[end January 1867]

Derby Infirmary. The proposed new wards are very good. But as regards nurses' rooms, sculleries, etc., I have thought it better to make my remarks on the plans themselves.

The accident ward in the basement will require to be rearranged in the way I have suggested. What I have said, of course, refers solely to the new additions, but as you cannot judge of the perfection of any animal by seeing only a leg of it, so you cannot judge of a hospital plan without seeing it entire.

There is no information in the plans in regard to the old part of the building which, from what I remember, stood greatly in need of rearrangement and partial reconstruction. All the parts of a hospital hang so much together that, in order to enable a practical opinion to be formed, it is necessary that all the facts should be considered in their connection. Until I see the entire plans, including the old parts rearranged, I can scarcely take it upon me to say that you will, after your new wards are built, have a really good hospital.

So far as the new wards can be considered by themselves, they are, as I have said, very good. The point of my remark about the rearrangement of the old parts of the hospital was not that I wished to see the old plans, but that I could only give an opinion on the hospital as a whole provided I knew what alterations in the old part the committee had agreed to carry out.

Source: From a letter to W.E. Nightingale, Wellcome (Claydon copy) Ms 9002/182

2 November 1867

Derby Infirmary. It was exactly because Mr Wright did not hold the views expressed in Lord Belper's letter that the hospital plans have succeeded. And there is no doubt that all the people who have been defeated consider the plans "very bad."

I am extremely sorry to lose Lord Belper as a valuable ally, and still more sorry for the exhibition of temper he has made. I understand (*not* from the Wright faction) that he, Lord B., has been "very savage," and that Mr Wright has acted somewhat "without judgment." And it is just because Mr Wright has acted "without judgment" (i.e., "without" Lord Belper's "judgment") that he has carried the day for the best hospital improvements that could be effected under the circumstances.

As to the plans being "rash and ill-considered," probably no plans were ever so *well* "considered" before. There are perhaps scarcely twenty people in England who have studied the elements of hospital construction (and of these certainly Lord Belper is not one) and all who knew anything about it were consulted.

I believe, however, that it is not the "Nightingale Wing," as you suppose, which Lord Belper condemns—but the plan to interfere with the old part of the building (which is so insanitary for sick—that we, after *much* "consideration," told the Wright faction that they would really find it better and cheaper to sell the building and build elsewhere a new hospital). This is *not* to be done.

But it appears that the old ventilation in the old building (which is to be gutted) was planned by Lord B.'s father, who put an old man in charge of it, who is dead—since which it has entirely failed. This was told me by a friend of Lord B.'s, *not* of Mr Wright's, as the cause of his, Lord B.'s, ire. We are not to interfere, he thinks, with this sacred plan, which has failed. However, whatever it is (and all sorts of pamphlets have been issued about it) *I* have nothing to do with the quarrel. (And I think, perhaps presumptuously, that I might have prevented it.) From the very first I told Mr Wright that I would consider all plans of hospital construction, as all plans of hospital administration and nursing—but that I never would canvass for any, least of all in my own county, or be made a tool for agitation [end cut off]

Source: From a letter to John Sutherland, Add Mss 45754 ff6-10

Embley
Romsey
2 October 1869

Derby Infirmary. Nothing tries me so much as looking over plans—and therefore for my sins I have plenty of this to do.

Mr Frank Wright came up to London (as usual, without a day's warning) to show me these plans—I should really have asked you to see him at the W.O.—but that before I could receive and answer his (forwarded) letter he was gone. I have now gone over the amended plans, and enclose a few (by no means exhaustive) remarks. Probably many others will occur to you. Will you be so very good as to go over the plans and return them me *with your remarks* and my own? . . .

I enclose a letter from Sir Harry about Derby Infirmary. Please return it.

A few not important remarks. . . .

1. What is the *nurse's room* doing by itself by the "reception room"? She can't sleep out there by herself. If it is a "reception room" for *patients,* the nurse must be in it, not out of it.

2. *Out-Patients' Department.* I believe it is a rule without any exception that there should be no communication between out-patients and in-patients' departments. Here it appears arranged on purpose for the out- and in-patients to have as much convivial intercourse in as jolly [a] way as possible.

3. *Nurses' Dining Room.* I am sure *I* should very much prefer having the nurses dining each lot in their own sculleries, if *I* were matron.

First Floor.

1. *Matron's Rooms.* I think it objectionable to have her closet jammed in in that way between her rooms. A matron ought to wish her store closet to be as public as possible (as to its entrance), instead of as "private" as possible. And if she is ill, poor woman, in her bedroom, then it is exactly as if the stores were kept in the matron's pocket.

2. *House Surgeon's Rooms.* I don't much care about the "cheerfulness" of this "important" gentleman. But I think it hard upon the matron that her only bedroom window should be overlooked by a window of his squinting into hers—I should block up his window in the angle. The surgeon's and matron's rooms are too near as it is.

3. *Convalescent Room.* I don't like them, but I believe it is determined to have them. (a) The proximity of the matron's room is a good thing; (b) I think it objectionable to have *two* doors to the convalescent room—as also to the corresponding ward. (You don't want patients or convalescents to get out but to keep in.) (c) Also, *is* it desirable to have windows looking down the *area* in these two wards? (d) Is the W.C. opening out of the passage (bathroom) good?

4. *Large Ward.* In some respects, the nurses' arrangements, I prefer this to any ward I have ever seen. It is such a capital arrangement to have the under nurses as well as the head nurses sleeping near their work—and I would have them dine in their scullery too. Then the arrangement of the chutes is good. (a) But will the night nurse be able to sleep undisturbed in one of those square projections by day?

Second Floor Plan.

1. *Large Ward.* I have only to repeat the same praise.

2. *Wards in Centre.* These seem well arranged under great difficulties. But I have some criticisms: (a) in front *bathrooms* the W.C.s seem jammed up in corners; (b) the operation wards would only do for patients for a few hours; (c) which is the north aspect? The operating room should be to the north, but then the wards must be cold and dull.

3. *Maniacal Ward.* What an odd thing, to put the poor "maniac" in a "*central*" position? Is it to amuse him or his neighbours? And is the

nurse to be jammed in between him and the "convalescent women"? Or is the "maniac" always to be a woman? (In a provincial hospital maniacal women are rare; men in delirium tremens, alas! not rare.)

4. *W.C. off passage* (opposite "maniac"). Is that right, without a window?

Source: From a letter to Harry Verney, Wellcome (Claydon copy) Ms 9003/119

Embley
7 October 1869

The first real insight I have had about the Derby Infirmary is *your* note. I send you Mr F. Wright's letter, because there is in it a message to you.

I have criticized and returned the plans (alterations in the old building) which he there alludes to—but have added quite plainly the impression which yours has confirmed in my mind, viz., that they had much better build a new building. It will be cheaper in the end. It matters very little how they muddle over the old building, except the cost they are sure to incur, and which will probably in the end have been enough to build a good hospital.

You say truly: "the old building is detestable—W.C.s airing themselves into the passages," etc. They sent bad plans of a bad building for me to criticize. I did so and they say I have sanctioned them. Next, they proceeded to do what was not in the plans and then they made other plans, which they want me also to sanction—and so on and so on until they are in their right minds.

Editor: In the end, sufficient improvements were made to the plans for Nightingale to consent to having the new "wing" (building) named after her. She contributed £150, in three instalments, to the construction. A letter, to either her father or mother, reported: "I have just sent my second third of £150 (£50) to F. Wright (for the Derby Infirmary) by his desire (the new wing called after me is opened) and told him that he may have the *third third* when he likes."[234] The Nightingale Wing was opened on 11 November 1869 by Lord Vernon, president of the hospital.

A report from the *Derby Mercury* on the opening described the "Nightingale Wing" as containing "two spacious airy wards," with

234 Letter 2 December 1869, Wellcome (Claydon copy) Ms 9003/128.

every accommodation for nurses—sculleries, baths and lavatories. There were two thirty-two-bed wards, one male, one female, plus a small ward for separation cases.[235] A report in *The Architect* gives ward size of 108 ft. long, 26 ft. wide and 16 ft. high; male ward on the first floor, female on the second, with a balcony at each end to permit recovering patients the benefit of fresh air. Details of the new kitchen with its conveniences were given, including use of a hydraulic lift to deliver meals. There were special provisions for accident cases, again with reference to use of a hydraulic lift. There was a chapel with "considerable architectural pretensions" attached to the north of the new wing.[236] Clearly Nightingale's requirements were met.

In 1871 an exchange with Dr Sutherland shows concern with the final costs of the infirmary. Nightingale asked her colleague for any comments on what had been reported, enclosing a paper and letter. Dr Sutherland replied that that account showed "the need of studying economy in work. It appears that £300 per bed have been spent in mere building and fitting," or more than twice the cost of the Herbert Hospital; "they build new lock hospitals at 4d a cubic foot."[237]

The infirmary became an issue again for Nightingale in 1891 with the discovery of new defects and the need for rebuilding (see p 918 below).

Workhouse Infirmaries, 1865-68

Editor: The importance of workhouse infirmaries for the care of the sick poor has not been understood in much of the secondary literature. Hospital expert Brian Abel Smith gave a ratio of five workhouse patients to every one in a civil hospital,[238] while data from London show for 1863 more than eight patients in workhouse infirmaries for every one in a civil hospital.[239] Clearly whatever reforms had been

235 Cited in Leveaux, *History of the Derbyshire General Infirmary* 67.

236 "New Buildings and Restorations," *The Architect* 27 November 1869:267.

237 Exchange 23 October 1871, Add Mss 45756 f36.

238 Abel Smith, *The Hospitals* 46.

239 Ernest Hart, "An Account of the Condition of the Infirmaries of London Workhouses," reprinted from the *Fortnightly Review* 16 February 1866 (London: Chapman & Hall 1866) 4.

achieved in the regular civil hospitals did not touch the vast majority of patients, the sick poor. Thus the construction of the first pavilion-style workhouse infirmary, the Chorlton Union Workhouse, was a great step. (Chorlton was not the first planned, which was Blackburn, but whose construction was delayed on account of recession.)

The new workhouse was built at Withington, outside Manchester, to take destitute patients from twelve sections of the city. It was purposely built, on the pavilion plan, and would soon become a model both for regular civil hospitals and other workhouse infirmaries. Later Chorlton was amalgamated with other hospitals to became part of Withington Hospital.

It seems that the architect of the new workhouse, Thomas Worthington,[240] approached Nightingale in 1865—his initial letter is not extant. He sent her his plans, before their completion, for comment. Nightingale's initial reaction was highly favourable, which was very much the exception to her usual response on being sent plans. She told Worthington that it would "be one of the best, if not the best, in the country," and saw only "some small matters of detail" as necessary (see the first letter below).

Another early contact occurred when a consulting surgeon came to London seeking a superintendent of nursing, to arrive at Nightingale's home when Dr Sutherland was there working. Sutherland met with him and wrote Nightingale a note, explaining that the guardians had been trying to get a qualified person to take charge of the nurses, but had failed. They had had much fever and nurses had died. The "nearly finished" new hospital, he explained, was to be completed within an "excessively low estimate." Nightingale wrote back that "there is nothing I would not do to promote such an object, but I can't *invent* a woman. . . . Do you suppose our nurses go about begging? We must have time."[241]

In 1866, Nightingale wrote the Chorlton Infirmary about progress in building (her letter is not extant). The clerk, William N. Edgill, reported back that five pavilions had been built, and that had been one occupied for some time, while the second was then ready. He explained about costs and added: "I trust some day to have the hon-

240 On his work see Anthony J. Pass, *Thomas Worthington: Victorian Architecture and Social Purpose.*

241 Sutherland note 20 November [1865], Add Mss 45752 f71, Nightingale comment f73.

our of showing you the completed buildings and of assuring you how much the guardians are indebted to you for being enabled to provide such efficient hospitals for the sick poor." He evidently also called at Nightingale's home, leaving his Chorlton pamphlet.[242]

Nightingale took the precaution of having two people verify the reputed low costs. She asked Douglas Galton to send someone from the surveyor's office at the War Office, for the hospital was built "on our plan" (see p 725 below). Her other agent, Sir Harry Verney, went himself, reporting back favourably both on the amenities and costs (see p 729 below). Nightingale thanked him for the "news of Chorlton Union, which interests me very much. . . . The inexpensivenss is a model to us."[243]

She again wrote, presumably to Worthington, although the letter is not extant, for the costs of different categories of expense. Dr Sutherland's draft is available:

> I am desirous of obtaining the information as a fundamental fact, based on your experience of a new workhouse infirmary. In London hospitals it is generally considered that £30 per bed per annum includes everything, and what I wish is a corresponding estimate derived from the Chorlton case, which is one of the most important instances of improvement which has yet occurred. This fact, if you could get it, would be a capital foundation for the estimate for London:
>
> She asked for specifics on
>
> administrative expenses
> bedding, infirmary clothing and the like
> food and medicines
> nursing and medical attendance
> any other incidental charges.

The draft asked also that the space allotment of 1200 cubic feet per bed be confirmed[244]

With the prospect of workhouse reform in London under the Metropolitan Poor Law Act of 1867, the Chorlton building was timely. Its low cost was key, for workhouse guardians were wary of raising local taxes, known as "the rates." Nightingale told Worthington (in the letter immediately below) that if he succeeded in building for "anything

---

242 Edgill letter to Nightingale 26 June 1866, Add Mss 45799 f264; Nightingale note to Dr Sutherland 16 July 1867, Add Mss 45752 f187.
243 Letter 18 October 1866, Wellcome (Claydon copy) Ms 9002/66.
244 Sutherland draft 3 January [1867], Add Mss 45752 ff150-51.

like the money, with due regard to the simple sanitary requirements . . . you will have inaugurated a new era in hospital buildings."

When it was clear, in 1867, that the Chorlton costs had been kept low, Nightingale praised the new hospital as "the best and *cheapest* hospital that has yet been built" (see p 732 below). The architect published a pamphlet with the plans, and sent Nightingale a copy. She circulated it widely.

Some of the correspondence in this section deals with the new legislation for the workhouse system in metropolitan London, on which much has already been reported.[245] Nightingale was deeply disappointed that the new law, the Metropolitan Poor Law Act, did not make a clean break, but largely continued "the present system." It was permissive, enabling workhouse guardians to bring in trained nursing and better standards, but did not require them to do either. Consequently, workhouse infirmaries would only be upgraded if there were conscientious reformers who got the support of their boards. Nightingale had to work individually, workhouse by workhouse, both on the introduction of trained nursing and the provision of better facilities.

Source: From a letter to Thomas Worthington, Manchester University, John Rylands Library ENG Ms 1154/1

25 July 1865

I am sorry to have been prevented by illness and business from answering your kind note of 14 July [missing] before. I am deeply interested in "workhouse hospitals" and I am sure that it is a question which will come very largely before the public next year, in relation to London workhouses.

Your hospital plan is a very good one; when completed, it will be one of the best, if not the best, in the country. It might be improved in some small matters of detail, e.g., cutting off more completely the W.C.s and baths from the wards. Still it is capital as it is.

You must provide for the ventilation of the wards by Sherringham's ventilators in each window-pier close to the ceiling and also by shafts in the angles of the wards. Unless this is efficiently done, the three fireplaces will smoke.

I shall watch for the progress and completion of your building with the utmost anxiety. Your estimate is extraordinarily low—even without

245 For material on the initial work and the political context of workhouse infirmary reform; see *Public Health Care* (6:223-506).

the administrative block. If you succeed in completing the buildings for anything like the money, with due regard to the simple sanitary requirements of so great a building, you will have inaugurated a new era in hospital buildings and we shall hasten to imitate you—for you will have set a model to the whole country.

I have not received the number of *The Builder* you kindly promise me. But I had already seen it.

Source: From a letter to Douglas Galton, Add Mss 45763 f198

27 June 1866

Private. I send you a note from the clerk of Chorlton Union about their new workhouse infirmary built on our plan. It appears to be about £50 a bed. Would not you send someone down from the surveyor's office to see it and to verify about the cost? Please be so good as to return me my note at once. . . .

That dreadful M Husson, directeur of the Assistance Publique at Paris, is coming over here again from next Sunday till the Friday after (1 July to 6 July) to see *all* the workhouses and hospitals in London and England in five days (he really terrifies me like a whirlwind or cyclone). Could you send me an introduction to the Herbert Hospital, which he wants to see again, for him?. . . . Would you see him yourself?

Source: From three letters to Douglas Galton, Add Mss 45763 ff247-48, 253 and 254-57

Embley
Romsey
7 November 1866

Poor Law Board Committee.[246] *Burn.* I was convinced at first and have been more convinced than convinced by your letter that it is just waste of time and strength to try to do anything in this matter.

Still, because you proposed to me an amendment on Dr S.'s suggestion, and because he was so anxious, I have written a letter (enclosed), which you said you should "like to be able to show." And I hope that you will think I have done what you wished, viz., "commence with assuming to fix a cubic space and then show that x x some organization, etc., is a necessary sequence." Of course you will do with the letter what you like—put it in the fire. Perhaps the disastrous answer that

246 Galton was a member of the Cubic Space Committee.

was carried to the first resolution (in the printed paper) makes any such letter useless. (Anyone who knows Sir R. Watson[247] could have foretold that that is just the sort of thing he will do, viz., he is led by *any*body—and will say "he had been less well informed when he signed the paper suggesting 1000 cubic ft."!!!)

But I don't agree with you that there is "*no* use" in your and Dr Acland being on the committee. That the committee is "packed" we knew. But what I heard from my old loves at the P.L. Board (yesterday) is this: they know most accurately all that is going on, and it will be his (Mr Villiers's) "duty" to "unmask" Mr Hardy[248] "when Parliament meets," and it will "also be his duty to bring in a bill that shall consign Mr Hardy's patchwork to," etc.

Now, certainly it will be a stumbling-block in Mr Villiers's way if Mr Hardy is able to quote the *unanimous* verdict of a committee of *experts* in his favour. *Both for the cause*, and for the *honour of our side*, I do hope *you* and Dr Acland will make a protest (or a divided report, or something).[249] It will much help Mr Villiers when he comes into action.

I have now read Mr Corbett,[250] and I send you my remarks in answer (he is easily answered) and my remarks upon such clauses of the printed paper as modify the *other remarks*. (Dr S. still wanted me to write you a letter in his former sense. But I was so good as to resist.) It is quite possible that you may think all that I have written needless, in consequence of that vote for "720 cubic ft. per bed." In which case put it in the fire.

I grudge my trouble and your own. I will return the printed questions, and Dr Acland.

---

247 Actually, Sir Thomas Watson (1792-1882), chair of the Cubic Space Committee.

248 Villiers, still an MP, was no longer the minister, replaced by the Conservative Gathorne Hardy. Nightingale considered Villiers, the Liberal, to be the better ally, and hoped that he would be back in office. However, he was not.

249 Both Galton and Acland signed the majority report, but each added a short memorandum. Galton's is particularly strong, listing the main principles of the pavilion system: "Memorandum on the Ventilation of Workhouses and the Construction of Infirmary Wards," Paper No. IX, in Appendix, *Report of the Committee Appointed to Consider the Requisite Amount of Space, and Other Matters, in Relation to Workhouses and Workhouse Infirmaries* (U.K. Poor (Metropolis), Vol. LX Session 5 February-21 August 1867:28-29).

250 Uvedale Corbett, a Poor Law inspector and member of the committee. In 1866 he was moved to London to replace H.B. Farnall, Nightingale's excellent collaborator and informant.

[ca. November 1866]

BURN. I do hope you will make a separate report. Be careful, please, to say nothing, even to Dr Acland, which implies my correspondence with Mr Villiers.

Embley
Romsey
14 November 1866

BURN. I write one line, which I ought to have written yesterday, to say that I have heard again from Mr Villiers—that he would like to see the papers referring to the P.L. Board commission. Mr Villiers is much too much of a man of the world to say that he has seen them—much less that he has seen them through me. Still, I would not send them him without your leave.

I have only Dr [W.O.] Markham's "Suggestions," Mr Corbett's paper, copied by Marianne [Galton]. (If you like Mr Villiers to see the thirteen printed questions—which I returned to you—you must please send me a copy.) I have also Dr Angus Smith's[251] paper on ventilation (your copy). But I am not sure I should like to send that to Mr Villiers, even if you gave me leave. It is so amazingly like Dr Angus Smith—so clever—so full of fallacies. Dr A.S. is immensely more able than Dr Parkes[252] (*vide* [see] e.g., his water analysis paper). But he is like Cornelius Agrippa's[253] Familiar, and can only work under direction. And he makes the most provokingly clever mistakes. Everything in that paper is calculated to do us as much harm as good. Angus Smith has *no practical* sense.

Mr Villiers is extremely angry with Sir R. [Thomas] Watson—he says Watson has given the subject considerable attention and can't say now he was less well informed then—he knew quite well what he was appending his name to on that paper—he has been at different times with deputations to the P.L. Board and has advised Miss Burdett-Coutts (who, you know, in the St Pancras affair, as a large ratepayer, took a prominent part against the guardians). And she and Sir R. [T.] Watson were always supposed to represent our side *in full*.

Mr Villiers says that he believes Dr Acland has very *decided* views upon the necessity of greater space and *separate establishments*. I hope

---

251 Robert Angus Smith (1817-84), chemist, water expert.
252 Edmund Alexander Parkes, professor of hygiene at Netley.
253 Heinrich Cornelius Agrippa (1486-1535), alchemist.

this is true. But indeed I have given up all hope of anyone having "*decided*" views upon anything. I hear from others besides Mr Villiers (people connected with the press, I mean), that it is supposed, if your commission reports *unanimously*, the cause of the reform of workhouse infirmaries may be put off for years—perhaps for a generation. . . .

This note ought to have gone the day before yesterday. But I could not possibly get it off. I wish I were in London. Unless I hear positively today from Dr Sutherland that he comes here tomorrow, I shall come up to South St. on Saturday or Monday. Please *burn*. . . .

One word more: I am terrified to hear that Dr Markham's 60 *superficial* feet makes above 900 (953) *cub.* ft. and not much less than your amendment (*cub. ft.* 966). Because now Sir R. [T.] Watson can say he has *not* ratted. It only shows (what we have always said) that we *must* begin with *superficial area* as a basis, and *not* with *cubic space.* Now, 80 sup. ft. is the *smallest* floor space you can possibly assign with safety, even in properly constructed wards. It would be less objectionable to have 960 cub. ft. with that. But Dr Markham has actually got 960 cub. ft., with only *60* sup. ft. (which is fatal).

Source: From a letter Henry Dyke Acland and Douglas Galton, Florence Nightingale Museum (LMA) H1/ST/NC1/66/18

19 November 1866

We know that the workhouse system is decided upon. *It is to be continued.* If you sign the report you virtually lend your authority to the *continuing* the present system (even if you are satisfied on the questions in the report).

The thirteen printed questions were "*nuts*" to me. What a very fine thing a future (reforming) president of the P.L. Board might make of them in the House of Commons! Here have been all these exposures—all these reports—all this *row.* And it has been fully proved that all the evils proceeded—not from this or from that—but from what? Gross mismanagement of the sick—gross administrative management—not from want of cubic space and the other questions in your paper. These are subsidiary and have only been mentioned as subsidiary, till now. But now all the mismanagement is to be ignored or denied. What a very fine thing the next minister might make out of this!

If you were able to reply to all the questions, you would still have this gross mismanagement left untouched, and you will be smashed, by [the] *Times* and Commons, who will say that the questions at issue were simply mistaken.

I hear (from the very highest authorities) two things: (1) that this commission will be sacrificed; (2) there is no disguising, on the other hand, that if it reports *unanimously* it may put back the reform for years. Therefore, don't sign the report at all, or if you do, put in a special proviso that you give no opinion as to whether the sick should or should not be left under present management.

N.B. Dr Sutherland desires me to quote my "authority" as to cost of Chorlton Union Workhouse against Mr Corbett's contradiction. I have not the clerk of the Guardians' letter to me here. But Sir Harry Verney writes to me:

> 16 October. I passed a good hour at Chorlton Union Workhouse Infirmary for 500 inmates. It seemed to me an admirable institution—rough, to be sure, but airy, clean, sweet, comfortable, roomy. At present about 140 or 150 beds are occupied. The expense has been £47 per bed. But it ought to be reckoned at £50.

Here we have an instance of common sense avoiding all "patchwork" and creating an establishment *de novo* [from the beginning]. Do set your faces against[254] all patching in the metropolis. My afflicted reformers, I wish you a good afternoon and well out of it.

Source: From three letters to Douglas Galton, ADD MSS 45763 ff262-63 and 278-79 and 45764 ff10-11

Embley
Romsey
20 November 1866

Private. Have you seen the *British Medical Journal* on your workhouse commission work?[255] It is quoted in [the] *Times* of 19 November. If anything could prove necessity of your insisting on independent inquiry, this paragraph would do it. These men will sacrifice all hospital improvement for the sake of carrying out their own views (which they have been writing up in this *British Medical Journal*).

---

254 There are several such exhortations in Ezekiel against Pharaoh, for example, Ezek 29:2.

255 Possibly "Metropolitan Workhouse Infirmaries," which related the dispute between Nightingale's man Farnall, who was for the "radical upsetting" of the system, and Edward Smith, who was for mere "reformation." The report concluded that it was the duty of the minister, Gathorne Hardy, to deal with the divergence of opinion (*British Medical Journal* 28 July 1866: 100-102.

I kept Angus Smith to show Dr Sutherland. But, he says, it is now in print. Dr Sutherland entirely concurs with what I have said (enclosed).

Please remember that Dr Angus Smith and I are the very fastest friends. (His water analysis paper passed through my hands—and Dr Sutherland's—fifteen times.) There is a great deal that, in his pros and cons (in this enclosed paper), is good. Because a man like Angus Smith cannot fail to write in his pros and cons, now and then, a good *pro.*

Christmas Day 1866

Private. BURN. *Poor Law "Cubic Space" Commission.*

I have heard from "my side"—I may as well say from Mr V[illiers]—"that the report on 'cubic space' will not be made till the beginning" of the next year, and that "the association" are so satisfied with the scheme hatched by Mr Hardy that they have postponed their own incubation till they know what it is.

Please tell me *by return of post* what you can—what is true and what is not—what you are likely to do, etc. Certainly "my side" is very much up about something. Mr V. sent to Embley (when I was gone) to know if he could see me. And now he has sent here to know if he could see me *this* week. (I shall put it off till I can hear from you.) Mr Farnall has also come up to town with the same request—I am as innocent as a baby. For I really have no scheme at all. Mr V. says "nothing but a *general rate* will do." Please tell me anything you can *as soon as* you can.

Best Christmas love. Tell me how Marianne is. BURN.

18 January 1867

Private. BURN. *Poor Law (Cubic Space) Committee.* My paper has been and come back and gone again to Spottiswoode's for a revise.[256] I expect it tomorrow. Though I have rearranged the matter after the first proof, yet that is all I have not had time to consider the tone.

As you know the temper of the committee, I should much like if you would let me send you a revise, and if you would criticize it severely. But this would prevent it from going to Sir T? Watson *this* week, as you desired.

---

256 "Suggestions on the Subject of Providing Training and Organizing Nurses for the Sick Poor in Workhouse Infirmaries," Report of the Committee Appointed to Consider Cubic Space of Metropolitan Workhouses, Paper No. 16, HMSO (19 January 1867):64-76, in *Public Health Care* (6:367-91).

Ernest Hart[257] who (though a good fellow) is very fond of giving me, mysteriously, "important information," tells me that he hears "with certainty" that your "report will go in *next Thursday.*" Is that true? If so, I must make haste. But I have heard nothing of Dr Sibson's "comparative statement"[258] being ready as yet. I had much rather keep my paper a few days longer for your revision. Shall *you* be out of town *from Saturday till Monday*? Or may I send the paper to you?

Also, Dr Sutherland has absconded and not seen the revise. The paper is slow—not to say funereal. Dr Sutherland took out all my good stories, for fear of you. And I took out all my bad stories, for fear of Mr Corbett, who is the greatest mischief maker and has the greatest "diarrhea verborum" in the three kingdoms. And I was specially warned against him. (He made such inconceivable mischief in the North.)

In short, I think the matter of my paper requires to be very carefully examined and should be very glad if you could give me a few days for your and my own criticism.

I hear that there are to be "changes in the Cabinet," probably "in the first week of February." Is that so?

Source: From a note in Dr Sutherland's hand, Add Mss 45787 f100

[1867]

There is nothing in the objections against the Chorlton Hospital that we are not accustomed to. They were urged against the new army hospitals, but all the suffering here comes to nought and everybody in time gets satisfied.

I was aware of the want of government offices and thought this made the cost per head less than it ought to have been. But probably the building will be found too large for the strictly parish sick, as all our new hospitals are.

The number of continually occupied beds has immediately decreased whenever the wards have become occupied. This is natural and indicates a reduction of the constantly sick, from better sanitary conditions enabling them to get well sooner.

The omission of a lying-in ward is a grave oversight, but even this could easily be supplied in this place by a small additional outlay.

---

257 Dr Ernest Hart (1835-98), editor of *The Lancet.*

258 Francis Sibson (1814-76), member of the Cubic Space Committee and president of the British Medical Association; his "Comparison of Workhouse Infirmaries with General Hospitals," Paper No. XIII.

Source: From three letters to Thomas Worthington, Manchester University, John Rylands Library ENG Ms 1154/2-4

13 April 1867

I cannot thank you enough for sending me your excellent pamphlet, (with plans) on the Chorlton Union Hospital. It is of the greatest use to us, as giving details of the best and *cheapest* hospital that has yet been built. And, in these days when so much attention, wise and unwise, is being directed to workhouse infirmaries (and so little is being really done), the world's gratitude is due to those who have solved a problem in a way which must be a model to the country. For the good and cheap *must* prevail over the dear and bad—though it is by no means so certain that the good and dear will. I shall make use of your invaluable example everywhere I can.

24 April 1867

Might I take advantage of your great kindness as far as to ask you whether you would be so good as to send me (by return of post, if possible) a copy of the account of your Chorlton Union Infirmary (read before the Manchester Statistical Society[259]) for a young Swedish lady [Emmy Caroline Rappe] whom we have been training as hospital superintendent for Uppsala in Sweden, and who returns thither on Friday. If I had twenty copies, I could place them well, abroad and at home. The objection constantly made to me against pavilion hospitals is the construction is so expensive, to which I answer: look at the Chorlton Union Hospital.

9 July 1867

I have felt that you must have thought me most ungrateful in not thanking you sooner for so kindly sending me copies of your invaluable pamphlet on the Chorlton Union Infirmary—which must become a model for the whole country.

I have however made that use of them—which would, I know, please you best—in sending them wherever, not only in this country and in Scotland, but in the colonies and even in the United States I think it possible that people can be stirred up to imitate your example. For, up to your time, the plea put forward for shirking the pavilion principle has always been that it was too expensive.

---

259 Thomas Worthington, "Some Account of the Pavilion Hospital Recently Erected at the Chorlton Union Workhouse, Withington, Near Manchester," in *Transactions of the Manchester Statistical Society* (1867):17-32.

I have sent a copy of your pamphlet to Sydney in New South Wales, where they are building, or rather enlarging, a hospital—to which we send out, at their desire, a trained superintendent and staff of trained nurses.[260] But I am sorry to say that their construction will not be nearly so good as yours. And I fear it will be too late to alter. When I bring out another edition of my *Notes on Hospitals*, I shall make large use of your example—please God to prolong my precarious life so long.

Editor: Nightingale in fact lived for decades longer than the time intimated in the preceding letter, but she never brought out another edition of *Notes on Hospitals*, as she had hoped. Worthington replied to that letter with thanks; he was "pleased" that his pamphlet had "her sanction." He also acknowledged having passed on her "encouraging" letters to his mother, who "felt a mother's pride" in reading them.[261]

Worthington's next letter, on his next infirmary, took up Nightingale's points one by one, such as on nurses not having to pass through the wards to the day room, reducing the number of beds in each room to no more than six (the maximum number she had suggested in her previous letter), the placement of baths and the site itself. He agreed with her as to the "first importance" of superintendence and maintaining proper discipline in the day rooms, and responded to her concerns on baths. Finally, he said

> I feel a more than ordinary responsibility in this work and am anxious that it should be so arranged as to meet as completely as possible one of the great deficiencies of our social organization. As you kindly took a warm interest in the Chorlton Hospital, I shall venture in the course of a day or two to send you a tracing of our wards at the Prestwich Workhouse, now nearly completed, and which, in some respects I think, an improvement on Chorlton.[262]

Prestwich Union Workhouse, in Crumpsall, took inmates from the northern and eastern parts of Manchester. Its infirmary, also called the Crumpsall Infirmary, had four pavilion wards for patients at the back, allowing 1200 cubic feet per inmate. Nightingale sent her comments on the plans without delay.

---

260 The correspondence arranging the nursing is in *Extending Nursing* (13:404-41).

261 Worthington letter 14 July 1867, Florence Nightingale Museum (LMA) H1/ST/NC2/V27/67.

262 Copy of Worthington letter 2 November 1868, Liverpool Record Office 6/33.

Source: From a letter to Thomas Worthington, Manchester University, John Rylands Library ENG Ms 1154/5

7 November 1868

I beg to thank you very heartily for your kind letter and for the plans of the Prestwich Union new workhouse. They appear to me admirable. And, if I ask a few questions, it is only for my own information.

Looking at the depth of the projection, in comparison with the shortness of the ward, would it not be a safe arrangement to place the baths and W.C.s beyond the end wall and behind the fireplace? a separate ventilated and lighted lobby between baths, W.C.s, etc., and ward—all drainpipes going down along outer wall? If the wards were longer, the present arrangement of W.C.s, etc., would be, of course, the best.

I am glad to see the arrangement of one bed to each window gaining force under your authority. In that case I suppose a large end window is unnecessary. Do not the small corner fireplaces rather trench on the beds? Will the scullery be sufficient accommodation for a nurse to sleep in, if necessary?

I shall hail with great expectation your experiment of a Liverpool convalescent building. It is time that this country solved the question of what to do with its convalescents.

Editor: Nightingale was frequently consulted on the planning for the new St Pancras Workhouse Infirmary, to be located in the healthier, higher Highgate area, and hence usually referred to as the Highgate Infirmary. (The Holborn Union Workhouse also built a new infirmary in Highgate, but Nightingale was not at all involved in its planning.) The Nightingale School provided a trained matron and nurses for the new St Pancras Infirmary, but which arrangement did not survive the death of the matron, Annie E. Hill, who was replaced by an untrained person against the strongly voiced objections of Nightingale and the Nightingale Fund Council.

In 1868 W.H. Wyatt (d. 1898), president of the board of guardians of the St Pancras Workhouse, asked Nightingale to comment on the plans for the new infirmary, and sent them along. She agreed to review them and evidently did so promptly. Only one letter by her is available (the first below), but several by Wyatt to her still are.[263] A letter to her later that month commented on the changes she recommended, and

263 Wyatt letters to Nightingale 12 and 18 November 1868, asking for advice, Add Mss 45787 ff156-57 and 158.

welcomed Sir Harry Verney's presence at the laying of the foundation stone.[264]

The lead architect for the new infirmary, John Giles (d. 1900), evidently wrote Nightingale from Wyatt's home, for the letter is on Wyatt's embossed stationery. "Messrs John Giles and Brown presented their compliments to Miss Florence Nightingale" and had "the honour of sending herewith the drawings of the St Pancras Infirmary. If convenient to Miss Nightingale they may be kept a week or ten days." They were pleased to have the opportunity of thanking Miss Nightingale

> for the very valuable suggestions contained in her book on hospitals. She will perceive that, in the report on a fever hospital forwarded to her yesterday, they have endeavoured to overcome some of the difficulties pointed out in her work, especially as regards the position of the staircase. They will be very happy to afford Miss Nightingale any further information on the plans forwarded.[265]

The new infirmary had the merit also of becoming the cheapest workhouse pavilion infirmary built—cheaper even than Chorlton.

Source: From a letter to W.H. Wyatt, British Library RP 2104

17 November 1868

I am extremely obliged to you for your kind note of 12 November and for your offer to let me see the plans of your new infirmary at Highgate "after Wednesday." If it would be possible to let them be sent me on Friday evening, I would return them on Monday to whatever place you might name. I give myself this somewhat unreasonable interval because I am not mistress of my own time, and frequently have business unexpectedly sent me to do within the day. But, if you should deem me too unreasonable, I have no doubt that, if the plans were sent me *by 10 o'clock* on Saturday morning, I could make it possible to return them the same day, or to fix some day next week in the same way.

I do not think that I need trouble the architects to explain the details, as you so kindly propose—though perhaps afterwards, if I find myself in the dark, I might trouble them in writing.

---

264 Wyatt letter 28 November 1868, Add Mss 45787 ff160-61.

265 Giles letter 20 November 1868, Add Mss 45787 f159.

Sydney Infirmary (Prince Alfred Hospital), 1866-69 and 1874

Editor: Nightingale's contact with Sydney, Australia, began in 1866 with a request for her to send a trained matron and nurses—a long and involved tale reported in *Extending Nursing*. When the group finally arrived in Sydney, they were housed in an old building and the matron, Lucy Osburn (1837-91), soon became ill. We pick up the story with consideration of a new building, on which Nightingale eventually gave much advice.[266] She was evidently pressing for a new building early on, dropping information as to the defects of the existing hospital and providing general information on improved construction to Henry Parkes (1815-96) (later Sir), secretary and later premier, of the colony. Parkes had been told of this need by an English-trained surgeon, Alfred Roberts (1822-98), who had emigrated to Australia in 1854. Nightingale felt a particular obligation to assist with the Sydney plans (and nursing) for Australians had contributed to the Nightingale Fund which financed her own school at St Thomas'.

There is much correspondence with Douglas Galton about the infirmary.[267] Nightingale was also in touch with the St Thomas' resident medical officer, R.G. Whitfield, who agreed entirely with her remarks, but feared that it was too late to alter the general construction. There are numerous surviving letters to Nightingale about the infirmary by Edward Deas Thomson, C.B., a surgeon and president of the board of directors of the hospital.

Nightingale eventually approached Deas Thomson directly, despite her preference for first having an introduction. He was keen to work with her, as is clear in numerous surviving letters to her. An improved hospital was a necessity for improved nursing, Nightingale thought, and a nursing team was found and sent quite quickly, although the Nightingale School was in its early days and qualified people were in short supply. However, the hospital authorities did not proceed with either a new hospital building or nurses' home in Sydney, and the nurses and patients suffered unsanitary conditions as a result. The "Nightingale Wing," a separate building, opened in 1869 to house the nursing school, Australia's first, with accommodation for nurses.

---

266 See the plans dated 1864 and 1866, Add Mss 45816 ff12-22.
267 See especially Galton letter 24 January 1867, Add Mss 45764 f18.

An early letter of Lucy Osburn to Nightingale advised that a sister was miserable and ill, having been "poisoned" from "drains and dampness." The fund for building a new hospital had by then reached £17,000. Shortly thereafter Osburn reported difficulties in a ward due to the lack of water (no sink, no tap), and an 1869 letter reported "two evils to contend with": loneliness and rats. Osburn, consequently, took an English terrier into the hospital, which, although not as big as the rats, was large enough, with training, to master them.[268] In 1873 Osburn wrote that the hospital was "flourishing," although not by way of buildings but "thorough cleaning." Henry Parkes, a "true friend," was premier again and evidently the cleaning budget improved.[269]

The correspondence reported here tracks the process of planning from the first letter, in 1866, to 1874.

The Sydney Infirmary, located on MacQuarie St. in the central business section of the city, dates from 1811, and is Australia's oldest hospital. There is much confusion about its name and that of what became a completely new hospital, the Prince Alfred Memorial Hospital, later the Royal Prince Alfred Hospital. Herewith, then, is a brief synopsis:

* On 5 March 1868 the matron and nurses arrived in Sydney;

* On 12 March an assassination attempt was made on the queen's son Prince Alfred,[270] who was in Sydney in command of a ship; he was nursed at Government House by the new nurses; Osburn called in, but did not nurse him;

* On 21 March 1868 a public meeting in Sydney resolved to rename the Sydney Infirmary the Prince Alfred Hospital, demolish the old building and rebuild, with funds raised from the community;

* The prince agreed, and fundraising began;

* In 1873 the Prince Alfred Hospital was incorporated;

* In 1881 the foundation stone for the new hospital was laid and the Sydney Infirmary officially changed its name to Sydney Hospital, and became largely an eye hospital;

---

268 Osburn letters 20 May and 14 July 1868, and 26 February 1869, Add Mss 47757 ff73, 76 and 101.

269 Osburn letter 12 May 1873, Add Mss 47757 f140.

270 Nightingale had herself met the young prince in 1852, with his older brother the prince of Wales, while visiting Birk Hall in 1852, as the guest of the queen's physician, Sir James Clark. While the future sovereign "promised well," Nightingale told her family, Prince Alfred was the "darling," with "higher spirits." In *European Travels* (7:707).

* In 1882 the new and much larger, pavilion-style, Prince Alfred Hospital opened, on Missenden St., Camperdown;

* In 1892 the nurses' home for the Prince Alfred Hospital opened.

Adding to the confusion, Osburn and the nurses immediately started using the name "Prince Alfred Hospital" for the Sydney Infirmary, while Nightingale and her Australian correspondents used the correct, older, "Sydney Infirmary." Osburn objected to the term "infirmary" and often used "Sydney Hospital" instead.

Source: From a letter to Henry Parkes, State Library of New South Wales

24 October 1866

N.B. *not* P.S. I do myself the honour of sending you by this mail the last edition [1863] of my *Notes on Hospitals*—not expecting that you will have time to look into it yourself—but hoping that those who have more immediate business with hospitals will glance over what I have said as to the construction necessary to ensure good nursing and administration. I am sure that it will be a great advantage for our nursing staff, should we be fortunate enough to supply you with one, to work under Dr Alfred Roberts.

I would also say that I am an invalid, entirely a prisoner to a couch, but, I thank God, still able to work! and that no delay shall proceed from this circumstance. I did not receive yours of 21 July till 4 October. But I had already received notice of its advent from Captain Mayne on 21 September.[271] Some little delay, but not much, has occurred in our reply from this circumstance.

Editor: In a letter to Henry Parkes on another subject, Nightingale noted having received the plans of the new north wing, which were, "in most respects, admirable," but they "could have wished that there had been some kind of sketch plan (or even list of wards) of the central building of the infirmary." She made the obvious point about the importance of the physical plant for organizing the nursing. Nightingale added that, as they were not "able to predicate the internal arrangements of the whole animal from seeing one wing, we have not

271 Letter by Captain W.C. Mayne, New South Wales Agency, London, 20 September 1866, Add Mss 47757 f167; there is much correspondence from him, from 1866 to 1867, in Add Mss 47757.

been able to complete our scheme as regards the nursing for this mail, but we hope to do so for the next." She also took

> the liberty of sending you by this mail, though it is more for hospital authorities than for you, a small account of the new pavilion workhouse infirmary at Manchester [Chorlton], the cheapest and the best thing in hospital building we have ever done—480 beds, with 1350 cubic feet per bed, *with every sanitary appurtenance*, at only £60 per bed. Perhaps Mr Alfred Roberts, of Sydney Infirmary, might like to see it.[272]

What Nightingale referred to as the "north wing," it should be noted, was in fact a separate building. It did not, in any event, go ahead at the time. In August 1867 Nightingale told Henry Bonham Carter that she could not understand about the "new wing" being "abandoned." By then she had the "*old* Sydney plans," and the promised sketch of the new had not arrived (see p 742 below). By September 1867 she had concluded that it was "better on the whole" to have given up the planned "new north wing." It would be "a good thing to build anew for the chronic infirm," and it was "a bad thing to connect a hospital and a poorhouse in the same building" (see p 743 below). The poor, infirm elderly were not sick, and Nightingale was keen to keep the healthy, of whatever age, away from the sick.

In the course of deliberations in 1868, Mrs Wardroper returned the plans of Sydney Nurses' Home, which she had gone over with the resident medical officer in considerable detail. While "no expense" had been spared, and the arrangements were of a "most comfortable kind," they agreed with Nightingale on the need for separate compartments for the nurses' bedrooms. She noted that for "our people" this was "customary."[273]

Source: From a letter to E. Deas Thomson, ADD MSS 47757 ff191-97, draft notes in Dr Sutherland's hand f189

26 May 1867

Sir, I am not sure that I am (officially) entitled to address you, as I have not had the honour of any communication from you directly. But as we have now been asked to give a reply on the general subject of the construction of the Sydney Infirmary, as regards the nursing

272 Letter 1 May 1867, State Library of New South Wales.

273 Wardroper letter 29 April 1868, ADD MSS 47730 ff198-201.

proposed to be introduced from my training school in London, I have thought it more businesslike and more respectful to address my remarks directly to you. I need hardly say that I consider our Australian colonies entitled to any service, great or small, any labour which it is in my poor power to give, for nothing that I could do would at all come up to what I owe to them. But, having said this, I will not take up your time with vain expressions of gratitude, however sincere, but go on to the important subject on which I am asked to give an opinion.

I have received the plans of the north wing of the Sydney Infirmary and, by other mails, as you are aware, sundry questions and also information. I could have wished that some kind of short report, or even list of wards and numbers of beds in each, in the south wing and central building had been forwarded to us in order to enable us, with regard to distribution of nurses in those parts of the building, now unknown to us, better to do justice to your requirements and reply to your questions.

I have carefully gone over the plans and all the information which we have received with Mrs Wardroper, the matron, and with the resident medical officer of our training school at St Thomas' Hospital [R.G. Whitfield]. I shall enclose extracts from their memoranda to me of 30 April (but which unfortunately did not reach me in time for the mail, via Panama, of 2 May). I need scarcely repeat that the construction of the new north wing—the beautiful site, airiness and view of the infirmary—are so superior to 99 out of every 100 hospitals in Europe that I can only admire and not criticize. And, if in what follows, I appear to criticize, it is only because, in sending out nurses, I have been desired to enter fully into the general subject of infirmary construction as regards nursing. With regard to the new north wing:

1. You will see that it is contrary to sound practice to put baths and lavatories under wards. (They cannot be kept from causing damp and foul air above in the wards.)

2. Hospital nurses and servants should not sleep (not even in such a climate as the beautiful climate of Sydney) in basements. Their efficiency requires that they have the healthiest accommodation. Stores, dining rooms, boardrooms, may be put in basements, but nothing else.

3. The wall space per bed is too little (5 ft., 6 in.). It should be 2 ft. more at least.

4. The heads of two beds should, properly, be against the space *between* the windows—never under the windows.

5. The cubic space is too small.

6. The wall space between the windows is too small. It should be wide enough for two beds, with 3 ft. between them. (But this is now probably not to be done.)

7. No adequate quarters or arrangements are made for the superintendent of nurses and her staff and for their duties such as we require for our nurses to render their work effectual.

I venture to take the liberty of offering you a copy of my *Notes on Hospitals*, also of a paper on workhouse nursing, written by me at the desire of the Poor Law Board, also of a short account of the best and cheapest hospital (Chorlton Union) which has yet been built. These will perhaps, with less tedium to you than a letter would be, explain what I mean on these points.

Next, with regard to the nursing question more particularly, after careful consultation with my matron, etc.:

1. We think that there must be one head nurse (sister) to each floor of two wards. Two "sisters" would therefore be necessary for the new north wing—two for the south wing—although we notice that there are fewer beds in the latter. In the absence of information about the distribution of wards in the central building, we can scarcely give an opinion. The smaller and the more scattered the wards, the greater the number of head nurses required in proportion, of course. We cannot place the number of head nurses required at less than six, in any case.

Even should you be willing to entertain this suggestion, we fear that we shall be totally unable to recommend more than four head nurses to you by next Christmas for the Sydney Infirmary. We are unwilling, as we never found it answer, to recommend nurses from different training schools to work together. We would, therefore, venture to suggest that—an idea which, I believe, had been previously entertained by you—the nursing staff from England should see, out of the women at present employed in the infirmary, and probably out of the colonial settlers, whether they could not pick out a few who, in time, with additional training, might not become head nurses.

2. We attach great importance to the arrangement that the head nurse should be in command of her own two wards by day and by night. For this it is necessary that her own room should be ventilated and lighted from the outside air—should be such as she can sleep in—and should command both wards.

3. We also attach great importance to the superintendent having her rooms and offices (including linenry) within the building—so that she may visit it at all hours and when least expected, and should

be herself the matron, though with a housekeeper under her. A cottage in the immediate precincts of the building for herself and probationers, *provided* north and south wings and central building are all easily and readily accessible from it—a proposal which has, I understand, been entertained—is by no means inadmissible. The cottage should then hold her office and linenry. In the absence of information, we fancy that the linenry is in the basement of the central building, and that, from the slope of the lawn, it is underground. This is, of course, objectionable for linen, as being damp. But, in our ignorance, we can say no more—except repeat that superintendent's rooms, office, linenry—the more central they are the better for superintendence.

For real efficiency and discipline, there should be but one female head, of course. And as her most important duties are those of superintending her nurses and wards, every material facility should be given her for this. And she should have a person under her to assist in the housekeeping and linen work. Or the housekeeper might also be cook—and the linenry have a separate assistant. We trust that you will agree with us in these things.

Source: From five letters to Henry Bonham Carter, Add Mss 47715 ff35, 39, 59, 68 and 125

19 August 1867

Sydney. I enclose to you Mr Roberts's letter,[274] although I have not had it in my hands five minutes, and although the pencil sketches of the hospital buildings, which he mentions at the end, are not arrived. You will see that what he says bears considerably on what our nurses will have to do.

I cannot understand about the "new wing" being "abandoned." (I thought the danger was that it was so far advanced that our criticisms could do no good.)

20 August 1867

Sydney. I send you the *old* Sydney plans. I have not the sketch promised me by Mr Roberts yet.

16 September 1867

Sydney. This is only to say (à propos of Mr Thomson Deas's letter, which I showed you on Saturday), that, though it seems very odd that, *before* they made the plans, they could not find out whether the new

274 With details on proposed improvements for nurses' accommodation, among other things, and promising a sketch in the next mail, letter 23 June 1867, Add Mss 47757 ff199-202.

north wing would "overlap" the main building or not (but they do much odd*er* things in England) yet, I think it better on the whole that they *have* given up the new north wing.

It is always a bad thing to connect a hospital and a poorhouse in the same building, 200 (and odd) acute cases are quite enough. And it will be a good thing to build anew for the chronic infirm. I only wish Dr Roberts had sent me a plan of the old building, as he promised. But he has not.

28 September 1867

I have not had back from Mrs Wardroper the letter from Sydney which I sent her. I send you the duplicate of Mr Thomson, whose letter you wished to see. Mr Thomson has also sent me by this mail the plans of a *children's* hospital[275]—I shall answer about these by the Panama mail of the 1st. They are very good—much better than anything we have in England. I think it not improbable that Miss Osburn may ultimately be called upon to furnish nurses to this. (Mr Thomson does not however say so.)

2 December 1867

I wrote on the 26th (in your sense) to Secretary Parkes, Deas Thomson, Roberts, at Sydney. Unfortunately, the plans (for the matron's, etc., house) have not yet arrived. But I took the opportunity to say to Mr Roberts that we hoped (giving reasons) that the nurses' and matron's building would not be separate from but connected with the hospital buildings.

I send the list of books I thought should be from me to the nursing *staff*. But, of course, you can charge any others to me you like. (These do not include the books I gave to each nurse personally.)

I have written to Captain Mayne to thank him for his great trouble.

Editor: In 1869 Deas Thomson wrote Nightingale regarding problems with the grant of land for a new building, and the difficulties of taking down an old building and constructing a new one on the same site. He agreed with her (Nightingale's letter on this point is missing) that it would be desirable for an official inquiry to be held on the high

275 The Catherine Hayes Hospital, architect John Horbury Hunt, opened in 1870, and later renamed the Prince of Wales Hospital. No further information is available about it. The hospital's website says that the plans "reputedly" had Nightingale's approval.

death rates in New South Wales, as shown by the Registrar-General's returns. This was a matter which no private individual could take up, but the duty of government, he said, and he already had his hands full. If the opportunity arose, he would bring the matter to government.[276] Deas Thomson sent Mrs Wardroper a photograph of the Sydney Nurses' Home as it then was, which she sent on to Nightingale.[277]

In this next letter we see Nightingale using the name "Prince Alfred's Hospital" for the first time in correspondence.

Source: From two letters to John Sutherland, Add Mss 45757 ff26-27 and 34-35

7 November 1872

Prince Alfred's Hospital, Sydney. I return the whole packet in case you wish to make some further addition. You will see, if you look at "*Details of Ward Pavilions,*" that there is some misunderstanding in your *(5)* and (6). *Only G* is meant for a "*small ward*" (D E F are quite necessary for their respective purposes). But Mr Roberts has a mania for small wards for all that. He wishes "*the broad part A*" to contain *on the first floor* an *operating theatre* and *four small* (single-bedded) *wards for minor operations. Please say what you think of this.* His *cottage block H.I.* with two (single-bed) wards and sister's room *for capital operations* no power on earth will turn him from (and as the difficulty of administration is altered by the fact of their having so few capital operations, I have not tried).

Say what is necessary and healthy *as to sink, scullery, W.C.* for this *cottage block.* (He wished to consult Captain Galton as to *cottage temporary* sections in general—he thinks THIS cottage might be TEMPORARY.) I propose if they at the Surveyor's Department will have the goodness to make a *copy of the* RED *plan* (only the red plan—I will not reopen the question of the others) and of the *two foolscap sheets* to send back by next Australian post all his plans and papers to Mr Roberts of Sydney, *with your remarks, retaining the copies* to obtain the farther information he desires.

This will enable him to send us back (in four months) more detailed plans which, as you justly say, are necessary for us to give him the real advice he wants. Also, please say whether you approve of the *bow window* he has drawn *at the end of ward A A (red* plan). . . .

I will gladly pay for the copies, I need not say.

---

276 Thomson letter to Nightingale 16 June 1869, Add Mss 47757 f262.

277 Wardroper letter March 1869, Add Mss 47731 f33.

Embley
Romsey
19 November 1872

Mr Roberts, P. Alfred's Hospital. Dr Sutherland. Would you kindly look at the enclosed, and return it to me with your *remarks*? I will then forward it to Captain Galton, who now has the plans. Even if I fully admitted Mr Roberts's principle, I do not like this adaptation. It is surely monstrous when or though the hypothesis is that neither patient is able to leave his or her bed, that the only ingress to the scullery for emptying slops, warming food and drink—and for all appliances—is *through* the patient's ward. As Mr Roberts expressly told me that the two wards would generally be for different sexes, it is still more monstrous—so that there is actually a common W.C. or sink and common scullery by entrances *un*commanded by the sister's room to the two sexes (I have never seen this in any, the worst, hospital I have ever known), so that an ill-conditioned Australian bush ranger might actually, *if he chose* to risk himself, reach the woman's ward or meet her in the scullery. Such things ought to be impossible in construction.

2. Also, the sister's room ought to *look into* both wards.

Please return *these* remarks.

Source: From an undated letter to Douglas Galton, Add Mss 45764 ff210-11

[c1872]

Proposed Hospital by Mr Roberts, Sydney. Remarks on proposed plan:

1. The ground will answer.

2. (a) Unadvisable to introduce the Administration Block AAA in a long line between the wards. (b) No objection to the front and back blocks, AA, but the intervening block A joining the two would interfere injuriously with the outer ventilation. No objection to joining front and back blocks by a corridor, but this would scarcely be necessary as access could be secured otherwise, e.g., by the corridors joining pavilions.

3. Ward plan AA good. No objection to proposed bow window at end.

4. Proposed dimensions of nurses' rooms and sculleries, 17 × 14 too large, 10 × 12 sufficient. Yes?

5. One small ward for one or two beds at 2000 c. ft per bed on each floor of ward pavilions.

6. Objection to multiplying small operation wards. (Mr Roberts proposes four small wards adjoining operating theatre in *broad part A*,

besides cottage block HI.) HI with two quite separate small rooms for capital operations as proposed enough, accessible from operating theatre as shown. All other small wards an expense and an incumbrance, not without danger.

7. Cottage block HI must have 2000 c. ft. per room, only one bed in each nurse's room 10 × 12. A scullery ditto with hot and cold water, sink, W.C. sink, small range for cooking (W.C. scarcely needed).

8. Mr Roberts wanted to consult Captain Galton on *temporary* construction for cottage block. *What does Captain Galton say?*

9. Is not the staircase as he proposes in one of the squares in the ward plan difficult?

Source: From a letter to Henry Parkes, State Library of New South Wales

14 April 1874

Private. I agree generally with the whole report as to nursing and management. I do not quite understand—nor, where I understand, do I quite concur with the remarks, e.g., at p 72 about H-shaped hospitals, e.g., the "Middlesex Hospital" in London is an H-shaped hospital, that is, the four legs of the H are four wards, with windows, as the report so justly requires, all along both the long sides of the ward. The sanitary results there are generally good, how much due to *severe* cases being the exception (as much exceptions as in the "London," St Thomas', etc., *light* cases are the exceptions) we will not say, the "Middlesex" being filled chiefly by subscribers' letters and by subscribers' domestic servants as patients, except, of course, in occasional outbreaks of, e.g., cholera.

St George's is neither an H-shaped hospital, in the sense indicated by the report, nor are its sanitary results satisfactory, but very, very, much the reverse. The fault of its wards is that (in many) there are only *opposite* windows, as required by report, for about half the length, besides which, there are all manner of excrescences built just where they ought not to be, on both sides the ward. In some wards it is even worse than this: there are four on one floor with *no windows* at all on *three* of the sides. The result is what may be expected. (One of the two authors of the "Privy Council" report referred to is a St George's man and, I remember, the excellent minister[278] was blamed for his selection of him to write this report.) These little domestic histories of hos-

278 "Mr Lowe was much blamed" struck out. Robert Lowe had been a New South Wales barrister before embarking on a political career in England.

pitals are known to few, seldom but to old nurses like me, never to doctors—or, if known *to* them, are never told *by* them.

With our present experience of sanitary results, no London hospital, or English new hospital of any size, not even workhouse infirmary (although workhouse infirmaries contain few surgical cases, *no* operations or accidents, and chronic cases in large proportion to acute), would be built except in the pavilion form, ends of all wards with large windows quite free, offices on either *side* the end.

The pavilion plan is not necessarily expensive: the Herbert Hospital and new St Thomas' have been expensive from particular reasons; both were on *made* ground. The Herbert Hospital remains the best we have, but the Highgate (Workhouse) Infirmary—which we nurse, 550 beds, is the *cheapest* hospital that ever was built. It is mainly on the plan of the Herbert and also preferable to any hospital I know, far preferable to new St Thomas', which we also nurse, the most *expensive* hospital, expensive chiefly through its *defects,* which are great, and not only through its "made" ground. The sanitary results of the "Highgate Infirmary" are admirable.

If by an H-shaped hospital is meant the taking *two* of the *double* pavilions, e.g., of the "Herbert" (for a small hospital), this would be unexceptionable, provided the "administration" were not crammed into the crossbar of the H, which ought properly, for health's sake to be only an open corridor. But it is destruction to put, as e.g., at St George's, wards in the crossbar of the H. . . .

St G.'s has *not one* ward with windows *opposite* each other *all along* the sides. And, as before said, the sanitary or *un*sanitary results, Mr Holmes non obstante [notwithstanding], are exactly what might have been anticipated. Let me not now add to my shortcomings by giving you a *long* coming more troublesome than my omissions. I wish you Godspeed with all my heart and soul in the noble work of reorganizing your hospital institutions. No one could do the work like you. I cannot express the gratitude which we so deeply feel for all the wisdom and kindness which you have bestowed on our cause.

Editor: In 1880 the nurses at the Prince Alfred Hospital, Sydney, wrote Dr Alfred Roberts, the secretary, to express their "admiration and esteem for Florence Nightingale," and thanked him for the bust of her that was to be sent to the new nurses' home scheduled to be built.[279]

---

279 Letter 18 September 1880, Add Mss 47757 f284.

Sydney hospitals became an issue again in 1882, with another visit of Henry Parkes to London (see p 847 below), and in 1891, on the building of the aforementioned new nurses' home for the Prince Alfred Hospital (see p 935 below). The original "Nightingale Wing," which was, in fact, the nursing school and home of the old Sydney Infirmary (later Sydney Hospital), was renovated in the late twentieth century to house the Lucy Osburn/Nightingale Museum.

Returning to other hospital matters, in 1870 a Plymouth doctor, Henry Greenway, sent Nightingale a copy of a paper on hospital construction he had given and then published. He explained that he had been prompted by Douglas Galton's address on hospital construction, given at the Leeds meetings of the British Medical Association in 1869, to devise a plan that would "secure the advantages of a large hospital without its dangers, and the safety of the hut system without its inconveniences." This was achieved, he claimed, by using glass walls to separate patients from each other in the ward.[280] Nightingale responded to his first communication (letter missing), and he revised his proposal to meet her objections, or so he thought, in 1872. His plan was to have patients monitor other patients who were not being adequately observed by the nurses. His (revised) plan, he said, had been "favourably received" by the medical profession, some of whom wanted him to limit the use of patient monitors to infectious cases only, and to workhouse infirmaries.[281]

Nightingale was appalled by the proposal to use patients to monitor other patients, and thought he had missed her points completely. She argued further that the glass walls would be disturbing to fever patients. An invalid herself, she was well aware of the frustration of a bedridden patient when the best light was at the foot of the bed, instead of behind it.

Greenway referred to his debt to Nightingale in his introduction, for having "bestowed much time and thought on the subject of hospital construction, and to whom I would here beg to express my indebtedness." She commented succinctly in the margin: "And who disapproved this plan." Extracts from his article are given, with her marginal comments, all but one of which were negative.

In 1873 Dr Sutherland reported to Nightingale that Dr Greenway "had been over *new* St Thomas' and considered it a confirmation of his case,"[282] to which neither of them agreed.

---

280 Proposal published in the *Medical Times and Gazette* 24 September 1870:32.
281 Greenway letter to Nightingale 14 June 1872, Add Mss 45803 f11.
282 Sutherland note 10 March 1873, Add Mss 45757 f70.

Source: Extracts from Henry Greenway, "On a New Mode of Hospital Construction," *British Medical Journal* 11 May 1872, with Nightingale's comments, Add Mss 45803 ff13-14

HG: The block is divided longitudinally by a central glass partition, thus forming two rows of compartments, placed back to back.

FN: The back-to-back construction, whether the "partition" be of "glass" or not, is condemned by all experience.

HG: In the main wall there is a large sash window opposite each compartment, which gives light to the corridor and compartment.

FN: Then give the best window light and air to the patient *and not to the corridor!*

HG: As the patient lies in his bed, he sees not only the transparencies, but can look through his glass door and across the corridor at the little garden outside the window.

FN: Is the man wandering in mind? "A pleasing transparency" for a fever case!! (The intolerable nuisance to the patient of having his best light at the *foot* of his bed, instead of behind him—of having a patient *behind* him instead of at his feet—must be known to be believed. It would send a fever patient delirious. It is like being in a tunnel.)

HG: The patient, although plentifully supplied with air, is not exposed to a draught, as the under surface of the bed acts as a screen.

FN: Good.

HG: [On the compartment becoming a type of flue]

FN: So much the worse! Then the patient is not to be in a ward but in a "flue"!

HG: The entire floor to be perforated.

FN: !!!

HG: As regards the oversight of the patients by the nurses, I should say that I propose, in addition to the means already mentioned, employing patrols, who would keep watch in the corridors during a stated period, and then be relieved by others.

FN: !!!

HG: The patients would also to a certain extent watch each other when awake.

FN: !!! !!! !!! Then am I to train not nurses but patrols? A patrol training school!

HG: Not only would ventilation be thus ensured, but infection be destroyed by heat.

FN: Yes and the patients.

FN: [at the end of the article] This plan appears to me to combine all the disadvantages of the hospital with all the disadvantages of the home, without securing one of the advantages of the hospital, without securing one of the advantages of a home.

Influence in Germany

Editor: It seems that Nightingale and Dr Sutherland, at the request of the crown princess of Prussia, commented on the plans of the first city hospital in Berlin, the Städtisches Krankenhaus, built 1868-74 in the district of Friedrichshain, East Berlin. It was the first German hospital to be built on the pavilion principle. It faced much opposition, but was then much followed in other German states and Austria. The Friedrichshain Hospital included a midwifery section, a major source of comment by Nightingale, but it was a general hospital. There were six two-storey and four one-storey pavilions, separated by 160 feet, the pavilions placed north-south, as preferred by Nightingale and colleagues, and which had been demonstrated already in the Herbert Hospital. Isolation wards and administrative offices were well separated, again according to a key principle.

The surviving material is meagre: no direct correspondence with the crown princess or the architects, Martin Gropius and Heino Schmieden, but a copy of a plan with comments (in both Dr Sutherland's and Nightingale's hands) and later references by her to having had contact with the major instigator of the hospital, the eminent Dr Rudolf Virchow.[283] Nightingale referred to him in 1871, when sending him lint he had requested for use in the Franco-Prussian War, as "an old acquaintance of mine through the crown princess (though I have never seen him)".[284] It seems that Nightingale saw his comments on

283 Rudolf Ludwig Karl Virchow (1821-1902), an expert on the relationship between disease and social conditions, then also a state legislator and later a member of the national Reichstag.

284 Letter to Emily Verney 23 January 1871, Wellcome (Claydon copy) Ms 9005/6.

the plans before she made her own, for she noted agreement with him (see p 752 below).

Already in 1867 the crown princess was asking Nightingale for assistance in planning the nursing and a nursing school.[285] The Nightingale School duly trained nurses and a matron, Luise von Fuhrmann, for the training school, and contact was maintained with Nightingale, often through the St Thomas' matron or home sister, until 1893 at least.[286] In 1868 Nightingale had Mrs Wardroper prepare a detailed plan of the staff needed for Friedrichshain, from matron to ward assistants. Wardroper's resulting "paper" is especially valuable, since no direct letter with specifications is extant. It gives precise numbers of pavilions (six), wards and beds per ward, plus details on related buildings for maternity and convalescence.

Lucy Osburn, when she visited Friedrichshain in 1885, described the hospital as having 622 beds in twelve or fourteen pavilions. She also gave Nightingale details of the antiseptic and aseptic precautions taken, including the surgeons and assistants exchanging street clothing for garments of white macanate, which covered them from chin to toes; all then soaked their hands in sublimate of carbolic acid (a disinfectant described as available in different strengths), so that they began the surgery wet. Towels were not used in operations for any purpose. Wounds were filled with gauze dressings saturated with iodoform; cotton bandages not used.[287]

The hospital was thoroughly demolished and rebuilt in the late twentieth century, although the old entrance was preserved. The D.G. in the first note below probably refers to Douglas Galton.

Source: Notes by Nightingale and John Sutherland on the Städtisches Krankenhaus Berlin, Add Mss 45753 ff150-56

[ca. 15-19 December 1868]

It was very kind of D.G. to do that lying-in paper. But it is not of the least use to the crown princess. She says what she wanted was not the statistics of the lyings-in (which after all show a death rate among hun-

---

285 James Clark letter 10 April 1867, stating that the crown princess had telegraphed for a copy of Nightingale's instructions on training nurses, Add Mss 45772 f203.

286 See a letter from Luise v. Fuhrmann to S.E. Wardroper 23 July 1884, Add Mss 47733 f188, and one to Mary S. Crossland 21 September 1893, which recalled Fuhrmann's meeting with Nightingale in 1881, Add Mss 47741 f82.

287 Osburn letter 24 December 1885, 47757 ff148-51.

dreds worse than that among thousands in the workhouses), but the plan and working of the one lying-in hut which you told her had had 800 lying-in cases without one casualty. What's required to tell her what to avoid, she says. . . .

The princess wants to make a training school for midwives—that's her purpose.

What the princess says is this: what I wanted to have is the *plan*, ground plan and *section*, and the working of that one lying-in hut where there were no deaths. It's no use sending me the statistics of all those hospitals and putting at the bottom that out of -- deaths were not from puerperal causes—without specifying *in which* hospitals this were so. E.g., in Chatham, if the deaths there recorded were *all* from puerperal causes, then the mortality there was higher than that of the worst London workhouse with thousands of cases. What I wanted was to take the lying-in hut with 800 cases without a death and learn all about that. *I* can't construct a lying-in hut or plan of working from anything in that paper.

Also, it's no use telling me excessive cleanliness and ventilation. If I were to ask a German midwife, she would say that excessive cleanliness is what she uses.

Brown Plan

JS: 1. The site is close to a lake and also to a canal. I take for granted that care should be taken that the sub-soil on which the hospital is to be built is sufficiently raised above the water level to keep the foundation dry and that the banks of the canal do not generate malaria. The slaughterhouse should be away *from the* hospital altogether.

The wall space of the wards should be better divided. At present two beds are placed close together. These beds should each be 3 feet apart but the wall space should be better divided so that which the beds are placed two and two between the windows each bed should on the nearest side be 3 feet from the adjacent bed.

All the nurses should be placed in the nurses' position at the end of the hospital and the matron's quarters should also be there. Arrangements should be made for separating the night from the day nurses' sleeping rooms so as to ensure quiet for the patient. The nurses detached quarters K [?] on the white plan are too far away from the building and would not therefore answer. The brown plan arrangement of the end [illeg] for nurses is better. [I] concur with Dr Virchow's criticism about the position of the lying-in quarters. It would be better to turn the end to the eastward.

The arrangement of the convalescent cottage appears to be good. The architect who put it, the beds, and the architect who wrote the description appear to have differed in them. Error: one puts in thirty-two beds, not twenty-four.

Then she began telling me about those altars. She said that having seen the wounded recover under sheds, she thought bad fevers or bad surgical cases ought to be moved out under such altars. I, mindful of the disastrous Indian verandas, said I thought it would be better to have a separate hut or shed for such cases.

There are two ground plans. one brown, the other white. The arrangement of the wards is good in both; each has advantages. The single ward pavilions on the brown plan admit of greater distances between the pavilions. The double wards on the white ground plan admit of readier supervision.

The centre block of the brown plan, containing the chapel, kitchen, etc., is better than the corresponding block in the white plan, because in the brown plan the centre block is wholly isolated from the wards. The schlacerie [slaughterhouse] in the brown plan should be recovered altogether to a distance from the hospital plan showing the pavilion is good in its general arrangement.

The crown princess of Prussia is going to build a hospital and has sent us the plans, begging us to criticize them. Each sick pavilion resembles precisely one of the smaller pavilions of the Herbert. Each pavilion is on two floors and contains a ward on each floor. Each ward contains thirty-two beds. There are altogether six sick pavilions connected together as in the Herbert by a corridor. Each pavilion has its own staircase besides. There are thus sixty-four beds on two floors to each pavilion.

And $64 \times 6 = 384$ beds for the main buildings. The matron's and nurses' quarters are placed on a pavilion at one end of the line of corridor. The kitchens, chapel, stores, day room, etc. are placed in the centre of the hospital line, exactly as in the Herbert. The part allotted to the administration in the Herbert, and which contains there the nurses' quarters, is in this present plan reserved for general administrative accommodation. Separate convalescent cottage for twelve beds standing by itself, with nurses' rooms lying-in hut. . . .

[FN:] The princess has begged that these lying-in plans may go down to her by Q. [Queen's] Messenger who calls here on Monday. But what's this [illeg] plan? That's just what I want to learn.

Convalescent and Cottage Hospitals, 1857-74

Editor: Cottage hospitals were a new institution for Britain when Nightingale began her work on hospital reform.[288] The first was opened at Cranleigh, Surrey, in 1859. They were favoured by local doctors as they permitted seriously ill patients to stay close to home, while allowing doctors to continue to attend them. The rigorously empirical Nightingale, however, insisted that cottage hospitals, as much as any other type, be evaluated as to their outcomes. Far from lowering mortality rates, she said, there was evidence that cottage hospitals had actually raised them (see p 764 below). As for the building of any hospital, the question first to be answered was whether or not it was necessary at all.

Cottage hospitals also had the drawback of taking patients away from larger and better county hospitals. To remove patients from "more skilled advice and attendance" would be evil, she wrote. Patients would suffer, and the better county hospitals would lose patients (see p 865 below).

Nightingale's reticence about cottage hospitals was confined to their use for the sick. Small hospitals for *convalescents*, especially at the seaside, were much to be encouraged. As she told people planning one, "every county and every hospital" should have such a "rest [home] as yours" (see p 768 below).

It seems that Nightingale was consulted about the building of the Ascot Convalescent Home, run by the Sellonite sisterhood, but there is only passing reference to the sending of plans (see p 395 above), and no direct correspondence. Nightingale did subscribe to the home and periodically sent convalescent patients to it. Again, as for hospitals generally, French superiority in design was evident, at least in the early years.

---

288 On their background see Henry C. Burdett, *The Cottage Hospital: Its Origin, Progress, Management and Work*; R.M.S. McConaghey, "The Evolution of the Cottage Hospital," *Medical History* 11 (1967):128-40.

Source: From a letter to Sir John McNeill, Florence Nightingale Museum (LMA) H1/ST/NC/SU135

Hampstead, N.W.
13 October 1860

Could you, by means of your inspectors, tell me anything about the enclosed lady and convalescent hospital? Nothing would give me greater pleasure than to help on, as far as I could, such a project. But, as set forth by Miss Wedderburn, there does not appear to be *any* project at all—at least not definite—except that of getting subscriptions.

Source: From a letter to John Clark-Kennedy, Wellcome RAMC 801/92

23 April 1861

We are extraordinarily indebted to you for the trouble you have taken. The report[289] is most excellent and contains the information I had in vain attempted to procure from other quarters, even in Paris.

I am exceedingly struck with the ingenuity of the construction—it can be enlarged with so much facility, if necessary. If convalescents are people who only want to take the air, I cannot conceive a better plan. The French are far ahead of us. At the same time, there are obvious defects in which it would not be difficult to improve on them.

Would you be so good as to tell me where the exact sites of the hospitals are with reference to some known landmarks? E.g., where is this Vincennes Military Hospital . . . [on the] road to Paris? Also, would you please state the total number of beds at each of the two convalescent hospitals (male and female)?

I will apply to you, if you will allow me, should any other points occur in studying the question. I shall be very glad to receive your notes on the female hospital and the plans, should they arrive. I will be careful to return you those which you have already sent me, if you wish it, as I should be quite ashamed of the trouble it has given you, if I did not know that it is a question arising throughout England, civil and military, which we must solve. . . .

It would be as well to recognize that it would be impossible to carry out any discipline or any nursing in this plan of hospital. Now in many cases, e.g., compound fractures, typhus fever, there are, say, two long months between the time when patients are ordinarily dismissed from civil hospitals and that when they would be able to go into such a place as this, during which, too, they require the most unremitting

289 Used in *Notes on Hospitals* (see p 171 above).

nursing, but which ought to be passed in country air. A different plan of hospital would be required for these.

Editor: In 1861 Mary Jones was exploring the establishment of a convalescent home for St John's House, which prompted her seeking Nightingale's advice. Jones and Nightingale had a long meeting on the subject on 27 July 1861, for which the letter immediately following would seem to be the follow-up.[290]

Source: From a letter to Mary Jones, Florence Nightingale Museum (LMA) H1/ST/NC1/61/6, copy King's College Hospital KH/NL/PP16/Jones

Hampstead, N.W.
7 August 1861

I have inquired as to different sites for your convalescent hospital and I find:

1. That the best places to get ground to build are Roehampton Park, near Richmond; Blackheath; Upper Norwood, near Crystal Palace;

2. That Hampstead and Highgate are better places to find *houses* in to let at once for the purpose, but not for land to build on afterwards.

Near the upper end of Hampstead, on the N.W. or S. side of the hill, at the "Spaniard Public House," or near Child's Hill (between West End and Child's Hill)—also towards Fragnell on Finchley. These latter sites are, however, on clay—Hampstead and the ridge towards Highgate and the upper end of Highgate are on gravel. Roehampton Park is sand—Blackheath, sand and gravel passing into clay. There would be much more difficulty in finding *houses* at these places. The best way would be to consult an agent who knows all the districts and then to visit and inspect the houses.

It occurred to me that the house (Mr Jackson's, Upper Terrace, Hampstead) which you saw me in last winter would be the very place for a convalescent hospital, with very few alterations. I would throw the entrance and drawing room into a ward for men, my bedroom and sitting room upstairs into one for women. The exposure is south of these rooms. There is ground to build. But I don't know whether they would let or sell for such a purpose—and the owner and his wife are the most extortionate and hypocritical people I ever had to deal with.

---

290 Jones letter 29 July 1861, Add Mss 47743 f107.

As there is no gentlemen's house adjacent, there would be no objection on that score. I should like to be allowed to help you with money in this way, if I may.

Source: From a letter to Edwin Chadwick, Add Mss 45770 f242

Hampstead, N.W.
19 August 1861

Would you be so good as to return me Colonel Kennedy's notes on the Paris convalescent institutions at your own convenience?

King's College Hospital is thinking of taking a house at or near Hampstead for its convalescents (and ultimately of building) and has consulted me. But it is very poor. Should you know of any (lettable) house for the purpose, I am sure you will tell me.

I am very glad to hear you are at my old home.

Editor: After his death in 1861, Sidney Herbert was honoured by having the Woolwich Military Hospital named after him the Herbert Hospital. His family and friends, however, also wanted a convalescent home to be given his name as another memorial. The Herbert family had earlier funded a small convalescent home in Charmouth, hence the (initial) reference to the "Charmouth Home" in the correspondence here, although the home was eventually built in Bournemouth. The aim was to have a new convalescent institution for forty-eight patients, housed in cottages. This was, in effect, an adaptation of the pavilion model, each cottage being, in effect, a separate pavilion.

Nightingale and T.H. Wyatt worked on the plans, for which James L. Thomas, of the War Office Surveyors' Department, did the actual draft.

Source: From four letters to Douglas Galton, Add Mss 45760 ff57, 65-66, 94-95 and 96-98

22 January 1862

Mr Wyatt's first plan appeared to me *unamendable.* And I don't see that the "amended" one is much better. Though he has adopted the recommendations, he has done some other things quite wrong.

Miss Mayo's, Oakhill Park
8 August 1862

About the "Charmouth Home," of which I understand you are so good as to undertake to make a sketch for Lady Herbert: ten men, ten women among whom a x [ten] of children is the accommodation she asks for. I consider one room for four essential in order to hold three children *and* a "sister," who must sleep with them, three other rooms, each big enough for three, although they may never be filled up, might be provided, although statistically the Military Department would put 2½ into each. This for each side, of course.

18 August 1862

Thanks for the plans for the "Home for Convalescents" at Charmouth. As the best construction for a convalescent hospital is still in nubibus [in the clouds], would you have the kindness to have made a plan and elevation of the rough sketch we sent you? Also the cost, in order that Lady Herbert's committee may be able to compare the structures. The relation of patients and nurses is far more difficult in these than in ordinary hospitals, while the sanitary considerations are easier. I have no doubt that, after a trial or two, we shall strike out something good. . . .

There is no "superintendent of nurses." The staff is two sisters, two maids, one man, total five (quite enough and too much for twenty patients). But it is absolutely necessary that the man should sleep in charge of the men, the sister in charge of the women, i.e., close at hand (when they don't sleep *with* them as when there are children).

And the sisters' day room, if existent at all, must be close at hand to the women's day room, and the man's to the men's. The committee to whom the plans are to be submitted meets early next month (September).

23 August 1862

I will study carefully both the (Charmouth) plans, and if we have any alterations to make, will ask Mr Mennie, if you have no objection, through Dr Sutherland.

Source: From a letter to James L. Thomas, Add Mss 46123A ff1-3

5 December 1862

I hardly know how to express our gratitude for the great trouble expended on these valuable plans for the cottage sanitarium.

I am pretty well accustomed (in my life), as you may suppose, to architects' plans and building arrangements. And I do not believe that there is any architect's office in London which could turn out such as these. The contribution which you have made to the memorial to Lord Herbert may be estimated, judging by other architect's offices, at about £200 or £300 perhaps.

I have communicated with the Wiltshire chairman, being unwilling to entrust such valuable plans to the rail until I hear from him. He and Lady Herbert will, of course, write their thanks themselves.

Would you be so kind as to give a *lump* estimate of what you think the expense will be of building (in those parts) according to these plans and specifications?

Editor: Nightingale showed the plans to Elizabeth Herbert, who also wrote Thomas at the War Office to thank him.[291] Two years later Lady Herbert evidently asked Nightingale to have money from the Nightingale Fund given to the Herbert Memorial Home. Nightingale corrected the misunderstanding in the item below, explaining that the terms of the trust excluded any spending on buildings. Lady Herbert also objected in some respects to the plans (in the second item below) but why is not known as her letter is not extant.

Source: From a letter to James L. Thomas, Add Mss 46123A ff7-8 and 46123B f1

10 December 1863

I have never forgotten your kind wish to have a copy of my new book on hospital construction. But it is only come out today (I have been so busy on India matters).

Also, I wished much to tell you that your beautiful plans for the "Herbert Memorial" convalescent cottages were actually and fairly started. You can have no conception what weary work it is to have to deal with committees. It is only just now that there is a prospect of their actual fulfillment.

Mr Sotheron Estcourt,[292] the chairman, has ordered tenders to be advertised for copies of the working plans, and specifications have been made (for the builders). Mr Wyatt has been down to Wilton,[293] about it. But only imagine that the site, so long talked about, is, so far as I know, not yet purchased!

The originals have returned to my hands, and are to be employed upon a convalescent home (for King's College Hospital) in Lord Brownlow's estate, at Berkhampstead, who gives the ground for it.[294] I

291 Herbert letter 27 December 1862, Add Mss 46123A f4.

292 T.H. Sotheron Estcourt (1801-76), Conservative MP.

293 The elegant country residence of the Herberts, so large as to dominate the village of Wilton.

294 The 2nd Earl Brownlow (1842-67), who had lost a fight to enclose and privatize the commons of Berkhampstead.

very much fear that this will be done the first. But at all events the plans will now be doubly used. Mr Wyatt and Mr Sotheron Estcourt admired the plans extremely.

Editor: Acquisition of a site was finally announced in 1865:

> The committee have purchased a piece of land at Bournemouth, situated on a high cliff facing the south, at a short distance from the town, as a site for the erection of the "Herbert Convalescent Home." The plan, prepared two years ago under the direction of Miss Nightingale, has been placed in the hands of Mr Wyatt, and it is proposed to commence the building during the ensuing autumn.[295]

Source: From a letter to Elizabeth Herbert, Add Mss 43396 ff196-97, with notes 198-99, and two letters 200-01 and 202-03

14 August 1865

Dearest, I don't know what more I can say than in the enclosed. It is absolutely impossible for me to see Mr Wyatt. I cannot talk for ten minutes without a night of agony. And alas, alas, it is absolutely impossible for me to see you. But if Mr Wyatt wants my opinion any farther, I would give it in writing, to the best of my ability, in answer to any questions from him.

I enclose a list of the council of the "N. Fund." If you like to write to them, you have my full consent. But I cannot do it. They would say at once that the trust deed, prepared by Sidney Herbert himself, its founder, makes it expressly illegal, as you are aware, to alienate the funds or any part of them, in the way proposed.

God bless you
ever yours

1. Mr Wyatt's own plans are *exceedingly good* (B and C Plans). (I would keep, however, as close as possible to the accommodation given in the original of Plan A.) The bathroom between the kitchen and the servants' bedrooms, Plan B, should be taken away or reserved for sisters and servants. I think, too, the communication between men's and women's side would have to be [breaks off] Two baths for patients would be required, one for each side.

2. The half of the original plan as proposed by Mr Wyatt, Plan A, would be, of course, preferable. But I do not know that I am even at

295 "The Herbert Memorial," *The Lancet* 12 August 1865:192.

liberty to say this, as even this is above the sum at the disposal of the committee.

3. The plans prepared at the W.O. were fully considered, and have since been most highly approved by medical authority. I do not see how I can make any alteration in them.

4. The style adopted was not essential, but was to make the hospital a worthy memorial.

5. The question is one of expense. The W.O. estimate was, I believe, sent to the committee and was certainly much lower than the one now named. I presume the cost of building has risen 30 percent in the last few years. No better judge could be found than Mr Wyatt. By his decision we must abide.

6. The "Nightingale Fund" was purposely tied up by its originator to prevent any expenditure in building. And the whole proceeds *must* by the deed be devoted to training.

Hampstead N.W.
15 August 1865

It occurred to me that Mr Wyatt may not have seen the W.O. specification and estimate for the convalescent memorial cottages, which was sent with the plans.

The W.O. entirely disbelieve and doubt the statement that the half of that plan (even including the undoubted rise in building prices) can possibly reach "£5000," as stated in the paper you sent me. They say it is IMPOSSIBLE, according to our specification, and that the builder has allowed himself to be led into fears (as to the cost) by the manner of building intended by him being so much more costly than they considered necessary.

Of course, it would be absurd to talk of Plans B and C (which were sent me) being a *memorial*, although the cottages are exceedingly good in a sanitary sense. But I knew not what to say.

Hampstead, N.W.
22 August 1865

I send the original plans and specification. Yes, if you remember, they were expressly sent to me on the ground that they would only be safe (and not lost) in my custody. I was not asked for them before, otherwise they would have been forthcoming. I sent for them to 34 South St. yesterday. And here they are. But, as to the estimate, of *that* unfortunately I have no copy (neither has the W.O., to whom I have sent) illustrating the great propriety of having given the plans and specification into my keeping, which are now forthcoming, whereas the estimate is not. The estimate was written on a separate sheet of note paper, like a private note.

At the Surveyor's Department of the W.O., where I sent to inquire, they cannot remember the exact amount but they state that they are "quite safe in putting the approximate cost at *under* £4000." x x Also that "the rise in materials and work wages" (since the estimate was sent to you) "would make a very small difference indeed in so small a job." They say, moreover, that "everything in the plan and specification was in so complete a state that nothing absolutely was wanted except putting the quantities up to tender" x x for the whole plan. The W.O. begs that, if they, the committee, decide not to build on the plans, they will send them and the specification back to me for use elsewhere.

Editor: The first stone was laid, on 16 September 1865, by Sidney Herbert's eldest son, the youthful thirteenth earl of Pembroke.[296] Douglas Galton was at Wilton House for the occasion, and wrote Nightingale recalling Sidney Herbert's laying the first stone at the old Charmouth Home. In the absence of the marquis of Bath, Galton was asked to propose a toast to the army, for which he had not prepared, and he regretted not having had time to recapitulate all that Sidney Herbert had done.[297]

When finally built, the home was a success, and the same plans were used for the convalescent institution at Berkhampstead. In 1880, Nightingale strongly recommended the Herbert cottage plan to an inquirer planning a convalescent home at Bolton-le-Moors (see p 866 below).

In 1867, Nightingale was approached by Ellen Gorham, of St Alban's, with a proposal for turning lepers' wards at St Cross, Winchester, into a convalescent home. She would serve gratuitously as superintendent, Gorham explained, and gave references. Dr Sutherland's draft response for Nightingale is curt and negative:

> I am an advocate for convalescent hospitals attached to infirmaries. But to be of use they must be exceptionally well planned, constructed and administered. Unfortunately, from what I know of St

296 "The Herbert Memorial Home for Convalescents," *British Medical Journal* 23 September 1865:323.

297 Galton letter 17 September 1864, Add Mss 45762 f204.

> Cross, it is about the last position which ought to be occupied by a hospital for convalescents and the foundation of your proposal would thus be altogether unsuitable.[298]

Nightingale, however, wrote a more diplomatic letter (immediately below), replacing Sutherland's stark "unsuitable" statement with an apologetic question. She also tried to engage Gorham in a more constructive pursuit. Gorham thanked her for the "kind and explicit" reply, and asked if it were possible to start at St Cross.[299] The paper trail ends there.

Source: From a letter to Ellen Gorham, Columbia University, Presbyterian Hospital School of Nursing C87

24 October 1867

Madam, I take really the first ten minutes I have (not of leisure, for I have not known these fourteen years what it is to have five minutes' leisure) to answer your kind and most interesting letter of 19 October.

No words can state too strongly the necessity of convalescent homes for the sick poor. Every county and every hospital ought to have one. But its situation is of primary importance. It should have the best possible air, the best possible soil, the best possible position, either on hills or by the sea, or in some open healthy district. And, besides being exceptionally well placed, it must be exceptionally well constructed (and of course well administered).

Nothing of all this is, so far as I know, possessed by St Cross, is it? So far as I know of St Cross, it is about the last position which ought to be occupied by a hospital, for convalescents or otherwise, but especially for convalescents.

I am afraid you will think me abrupt. But "it is my poverty" (of strength) "and not my will consents."[300] I am an invalid entirely a prisoner to bed, and I never see anyone except on urgent business. Otherwise I should be too glad to accept your kind offer and make your acquaintance. For such a vocation as yours, is it not a pity that it should be thrown away? Would you not utilize it to the highest possible extent? There is so much room for it. If I could be of any use to you in this way, please make use of me.

---

298 Gorham letter 19 October 1867, and Sutherland undated draft reply, Florence Nightingale Museum (LMA) H1/ST/NC2/V40/67.

299 Gorham letter 19 November 1867, Florence Nightingale Museum (LMA) H1/ST/NC2/V41/67.

300 Shakespeare, *Romeo and Juliet*, Act 5, scene 1.

Source: From a letter to William Lavers, Wellcome Ms 5482/80

28 January 1869

The question you have put to me is one very often put to me—and one impossible to answer except by those on the spot.

I could certainly send you the names and regulations of cottage hospitals already established—or refer you to persons, as at Wrington, Warminster, Wirksworth (in Derbyshire), who have established cottage hospitals and would send you their regulations.

This would be the way to rid myself of all trouble and responsibility. But, in each case, the people, and especially the medical men about a place, should first judge of the necessity of a cottage hospital. And then, and not till then, if all are agreed that a village hospital is necessary, let them proceed to obtain the best site [and] the best plans to fulfill all sanitary conditions. Within my knowledge, a cottage hospital has been the means, not of lowering, but of raising, the death rate of the sick.

1. Whenever it is proposed to construct a new hospital, the first and most important question which ought to be answered is whether the hospital is necessary.

2. Hospitals are a hard necessity of an inferior, imperfect, civilization—in which they are (and were) great boons to a certain class of poor persons. But as it is a proved fact that, supply the same medical treatment, nursing and medical comforts to the sick poor at home, these recover better than in hospitals, we may hope that they will be gradually replaced by such a system of district nursing.

3. It is a serious thing to introduce a hospital where, from time immemorial, there has been none—and where no public demand has been made for one—and this for many reasons.

4. There are other great dangers attending the agglomeration of sick in large town hospitals. But these dangers are of course very much less liable to occur in small village hospitals. The chief question in regard to projected village hospitals is the one already put, viz., are they necessary?

5. It may be safely admitted that, in certain districts (principally large mining or pottery districts, where there are many accidents, or no convenient railroad or other communication with county hospitals), a village hospital would be an advantage. But it by no means follows that, in other districts, similar hospitals are necessary.

In the proposed case, is there a necessity which has been pressing on the public notice and conscience of such a nature that the establishment of a village hospital ought no longer to be delayed? To this question a clear and decided answer ought to be given. And, while giving it, the projectors ought to show that the need, if it exists, cannot be met by sending cases to Plymouth or Exeter.

The moral aspect of a village hospital ought also to be considered with reference to the classes for which it is intended. Except in, e.g., severe surgical cases and the like, where all the appliances of a first-rate hospital may be required, is it wise to withdraw the sick from under the care of their families and neighbours, and from under their own roofs, and to have them tended by other hands elsewhere?

6. This is a very peremptory question. Suppose all the circumstances are favourable for establishing a village hospital, the next question is one of position and amount and kind of accommodation the proposed building is to give. It is always dangerous to bring sick poor from very humble country dwellings, where they have fresh air about them, into even better quarters in an unhealthy village. Hence, unless the building be well placed and well constructed, it may become a source of danger instead of benefit to the sick poor concerned. The greatest care should be bestowed on this consideration, if the village hospital is to exist at all.

In short, a mere benevolent desire to benefit the poor in this matter can never exempt from the responsibility of looking at the proposal on every side, and then deciding whether it is best or worst to give effect to the idea.

By the same post, I send you an account of district nursing, as it exists in a large town where, of course, it undergoes many more difficulties than it would have in nursing the sick poor at home in country districts. . . . But, should you finally decide on a village hospital and wish to revise the plans, I will gladly give them all the attention in my power.

Editor: Nightingale was applied to in 1869 for assistance on a convalescent home in Lincolnshire, for twenty patients each of men and women. From the only surviving correspondence, to a clergyman involved, Nightingale was approached by a Mr Fowler, probably James Fowler, who was both an architect and the mayor of the town of Louth. The letter below, to him, was clearly written after Nightingale had seen the plans. An article in *The Builder* a few months later noted not only that "these plans were submitted to Miss Nightingale, and met with her approval," but that the architect promised to return half the usual architect's charges for the plans. Further, "all the living rooms will be lined inside with Portland and Parian cement, as at Netley Military Hospital,"[301] another sign of Nightingale's influence.

Source: From a letter to the Rev F. Pretyman, Lincolnshire County Record Office M.C.H. 1/8

19 July 1869

Sir, I beg to acknowledge your note of 15 July, regarding the proposed plan for a convalescent home in Lincolnshire, which has since been forwarded to me by Mr Fowler.

The plan is good. It will face a fierce wind, very bracing, and not requiring the same amount of precaution and separation of parts necessary in a milder situation. The following points require attention: a sick ward cannot be placed in so isolated a situation. It must be where the nurse or "attendant" can overlook it day and night. In this case the "attendant," if by "attendant" is meant a nurse, is where she is not wanted at night and not where she is. I myself should prefer the sick ward more apart from the convalescents. But you might move the sick ward to the attendant's room side, i.e., leave the bath where it is, and shift the sick ward across to the two windows to the right (and vice versa on the left) and place the two windows between the sick ward and the bath.

There must be an inspection window through the attendant's wall to the sick ward. (If you have two sexes, you will require two baths.) Also, a lavatory on the *men's* side. If there are two floors, the sick wards should be upstairs and the downstairs room turned to some other purpose. (I think your matron should have two rooms—bedroom and sitting room.) Also, a small *light* linen store or press. The central parts should not be raised above one floor.

One can scarcely from present information answer the question how to build. I feel disposed to think that it is better not to begin till one has the money.

Will you present my apologies to Mr Fowler for having returned the plan to you, as you requested, and not to him, as he requested—on the ground of my total inability to write two letters? overwhelmed with illness and hard business as I am.

---

301 "Lincolnshire Seaside Convalescent Home," *The Builder* 16,1392 (9 October 1869):814.

Source: From a letter to an unnamed architect, Florence Nightingale Museum (LMA) H1/ST/NC18/21/68

January 1870

The following are the criticisms on the tracing which you have sent me:

1. No convalescent home should ever be surrounded—or near a body of buildings. Convalescents should always be placed in the open country where they are not likely to be encroached upon by population.

2. The central portion of the block within the day room and wards and containing the staircase is too large, too complicated, too costly.

3. Lavatory should not be *within* the body of the house, but should have its own outer ventilation and be isolated so as to keep the damp out of the house.

4. Superintendence of the convalescents' sleeping rooms and also of their day rooms is necessary—and would be very difficult on this plan.

5. The sick wards are out of the way of all care and superintendence.

Also, they should not be near the laundry. This part of the arrangement for male and female sick with their nurses will have to be reconsidered.

6. It is undoubtedly better to have one dining room for the men and one for the women. Still this is not essential. The men and women may dine separately at a different hour. Or the room might be partitioned down the middle. On the whole, convenience and economy would appear to be best consulted by having one day room which should also be a dining room for each sex.

7. Generally the administrative part of the building appears large and costly, overweighting in importance the patients' part—for whom nevertheless it is intended.

All that is wanted may be done at £150 or £160 a bed, everything included—or less.

Editor: In 1871 Nightingale was approached for assistance (but the letter is missing) on the Glamorganshire Convalescent Home. Her encouraging response follows. When the plans, however, came, in 1874, they proved to be thoroughly disappointing (see p 772 below).

Source: From a letter to Mrs Lewis, West Glamorgan Record Office, Cardiff D/ D Xe 25

London
28 November 1871

Madam, Let me say, first, with what deep sympathy and earnest admiration (which yet I can hardly express) I see such efforts as yours and Dr Lewis's[302] for the benefit of so many, done in the quietest most persevering manner. Other people begin with a prospectus, great names, a secretary, a public meeting and a castle in the air. You begin with a cottage, a few suffering people, who at last number a great many, and your own noble personal exertions and wise practical benevolence.

I shall feel too much honoured in being permitted to help in ever so slight a degree in your plans, believing as I do that no greater benefit could be bestowed on the working people of this country than that every county and every hospital should have such a "rest" as yours.

If you wish (as you propose) to send me the sketch plans of the institution it is now projected to build, I will look them over most carefully, and also procure a good opinion upon them. With your practical wisdom, you will of course, include in the sketch plans your past experience of inconveniences to be provided against in the new building. And any information of this kind you could give me will be valuable. (All cost for mere ornament should be avoided. Good and substantial wood and stone work is what is wanted at the seaside.)

The question about "*officers*" is a difficult one, and in general is best decided by local experience (which I, of course, have not). Nevertheless if, when I know more particulars of your undertaking, I can answer any questions, I will do so, according to my past experience. But people are apt to forget that no amount of official help will do exactly what you have done from sheer love of the work.

Any sketch plans to be commented upon should include a sketch of the *site* proposed. Your letter of the 24th did not reach me in time for post, which must excuse my delay in answering. . . .

May I ask you to excuse any delay in future answers, owing to my being constantly overworked and a constant prisoner to my room from illness? Any letter addressed to care of Mrs Wardroper, St Thomas' Hospital, will always reach me.

302 Dr James Lewis, surgeon and medical officer of health.

Source: From a letter to John Sutherland, Add Mss 45756 f167

Embley
15 March 1872

Cottage Hospitals. H.B.C. sends me the enclosed, but does *not send* me his own letter, which gave rise to this. The conclusion to which he comes is the conclusion of universal mankind, viz., that I must write another letter saying (in this case) "what are the objections to cottage hospitals?" and how to be obviated?

It would very much oblige me if you would give me any general suggestions as to in what cases they are good and what are the conditions for being so, i.e., at a distance from any good county hospital, where there are many accidents, especially machinery operations, as in mining districts, where they are by the sea for consumption or for scrofula, etc., especially of course for convalescents—here they are essential.

Cottage hospitals *are bad* where they *are bad*, i.e., when they interfere with a good county hospital within easy distance with its efficient medical, surgical and nursing staff, where they are expressly urged on the ground of defective lodgers' dwellings, making the fevers, etc., which the cottage hospital is to cure and thus interfering with our first paramount duty of reforming the bad drainage, bad ventilation, bad water, bad crowding, *bad everything* that *can be bad* of (many) parishes and country villages.

To make the people's dwellings fit for sick, or rather such as will *not make* sickness, and not to have a cottage hospital to cure such sickness when it is made, is of course our first duty.

Editor: Dr Sutherland replied with an outline of several basic principles on cottage hospitals. He began with one he shared with Nightingale: "that cottage hospitals, like all other hospitals, ought to be unnecessary," to strike out "in a Christian country." He went on to argue "The same rule holds good in regard to all such establishments, that nothing can compensate for home care and nursing in sickness."[303] Subsequent letters give detailed material on ventilation, flooring, hospital-acquired infections and space for patients.[304]

---

303 Sutherland letter 18 March 1872, Add Mss 45756 f166.

304 Letters 13 and 27 May, 10 and 17 June 1872, Add Mss 45756 ff19, 204, 206 and 210.

The next letter concerns the Yoxall Cottage Hospital in Staffordshire, built and entirely endowed by (Miss) Meynell Ingram, a member of a prominent local landowning family. She is presumably the person addressed in the letter immediately following. Alex Graham, referred to in that letter, was in fact selected as architect. The opening of the hospital was announced in 1874.[305] The hospital was later renamed the Meynell Ingram Hospital. It joined the National Health Service in 1948, and was closed in 1986.

Source: From a letter with the addressee's name cut out, National Library of Medicine Ms CI-NI6

4 April 1872

Yoxall Cottage Hospital.

Dear Madam

If it is decided to erect a cottage hospital at this place, these plans seem admirably suited for the purpose. Mr Alex Graham is indeed an architect for hospitals in whose opinion every confidence may be safely placed.

1. The proposed change in the position of the slop sink should be adopted.

2. As regards earth closets generally, wherever there is water and a drainage outlet, there will necessarily be an outlet for the bath water, sink water, lavatory water and cooking water. Now this should not be allowed to run into ditches. The best way to do with it is to run it over grassland, and if this is done there might just as well be two W.C.s as two earth closets.

Earth closets require great and constant care, which they seldom receive. I cannot give an opinion as to their use unless there is no outlet for the house drainage and it has to be carted away. If so, then earth closets might be tried. If there is an outlet for drainage, then use W.C.s. But an earth closet must be completely cut off from the building by a cross-ventilated passage. . . . Not only must the earth be put in from the outside, but the tank must be removable from the outside.

3. If the closet for earth attached to the washhouse is to be an earth closet, it must be properly lighted and ventilated. *Two* earth closets are undoubtedly necessary.

4. The cellars must not open into the building. They must be reached from outside.

---

305 *The Architect* 28 March 1874:190.

5. Whether for so small a hospital a porcelain *fixed* bath is needed? We could do very well with a moveable bath and a sink.

6. In so small a place, would hot and cold water laid on be necessary? The kitchen is close at hand and one would say a big pan or jug would do everything.

7. No indication is given as to sex of patients. It is very much easier to separate properly 100 men from 100 women, with their separate pavilions, ward appurtenances and nurses, than it is to separate two from two (unless they be for quite young children). The objections are so very great to letting the two sexes use one W.C., one bath, etc., especially as where, in this case, the one sex would actually pass the other's door on the way, that they have probably been considered. (The objections are also great to one nurse between two men and two women, and there seems no provision even for a maid servant to sleep in the house, unless in the "spare ward.")

8. Will not the "spare ward" be rather hot in summer—next the kitchen and with a western? exposure? for a bad case?

9. I could not undertake to criticize an estimate as to expense farther than in the most general manner (as to leaving out expensive ornamental style and the like), which in this case is not needed. Mr Alex Graham is entirely to be trusted—in all these respects—of ability and honour.

10. I quite agree that the steps will be "very inconvenient." . . .

11. The kitchen is so near that the "range with oven" for "nurse's room" might possibly be omitted—provided that in the kitchen there were all conveniences for sick cookery (included facilities for airing and warming linen, for fomentations and the like). . . .

12. A linen room ought to be so thoroughly warm, airy, light and dry that, if it has not a fireplace of its own, I should almost have wished it had been *against* the kitchen fireplace. The kitchen fire is good for the linen and not for the patient. Also, the exposure is east—want of sun has a bad effect on linen—which should have either sun or fire or, better, both. . . .

This is a P.S. 12. Is it not necessary to have a small surgery where the "doctor" can sit down, where he can examine a patient before admission, or even afterwards, and where the few necessary drugs can be kept? It is most undesirable that the "doctor" should have no place which he can use except the nurse's room.

A linenry is not absolutely necessary for so small a number of beds. Indeed I have known a good linen press (not set into the wall) in a dry, light, airy, warm part of the corridor—with a folding dresser made on hinges, to stand out from the wall—and be let down when not in use to fold the linen upon answer much better than the dark closet usually assigned to the linen in small English hospitals. Linen is as jealous as a patient of light and air for its good health. (This criticism is not however meant for the linenry in the Yoxall plan, which is much better than usually afforded) for a much larger hospital. If it were turned into the "surgery," it would require a fireplace.

How would it do to make it both surgery and linenry? It may here be noticed that, for any kind of stores to be kept, or any sort of hospital work to be going on, in the nurse's room is very undesirable.

[continued] 6 April 1872

Also that in planning a cottage hospital, where the nurse's room was *between* a man's and a woman's ward, as in this case, a partition and door (kept locked) entirely cut off the men's from the women's side—the nurse's room had *two* doors, one on either side the partition. And there was, of course, W.C., bath and sink provision for *each* side.

Dear Madam, this "codicil" occurred to me afterwards—after I had written to you on the 4th.

Source: From a letter to John Sutherland, Add Mss 45757 ff240-41

16 May 1874

Glamorganshire Home for Convalescents.

You will remember having before a previous plan for this, from that Dr Lewis.[306] I hardly know how to criticize it.

1. "It is like a *cottage home,*" *because* it is *not.*

2. I think I never saw so much *complication* with so little *accommodation.*

3. It has all high-wrought accessories of a *hospital, without* its means of *supervision.*

4. And it has all the inconveniences of *subdivision, without* its advantages.

5. The *wards* are like the famous *goose,* too *much* (for a *home*), too *little* (for a *hospital*).

6. *If the "central pavilion"* is meant for *sick* (relapses), then they ought not to be separated by *day and dining room* but by a *nurse's room.*

7. Every arrangement seems to be made for *something else.*

---

306 In 1871 (see p 767 above).

8. The appendages are those of *St Thomas'*, the site's plan *wild country*.

9. The blocks are like *pavilions* seen through the wrong end of a telescope and called *cottages*.

10. You might as well diminish the Herbert *Hospital* to one hundredth of its size and say: now I have built a *cottage* for *convalescents* because I have omitted the corridor.

11. The *matron's* room must not be in the *offices* and the *manager's* room must not be by the *sick*. (I should recommend the architect to go and see the Liverpool Convalescent Home built by Worthington—I do not like the plans, but it is far better than this—it has *three-bedded* rooms, like Vincennes, six or eight, I think, besides others. Miss Leslie,[307] a most intelligent woman, trained by us, is its matron. She would frankly tell its success and its defects from experience.)

12. There is *no supervision whatever* for *ground* floors of *side pavilions*.

Editor: Correspondence on other issues resumes.

Source: From a letter to Dr E.J. Waring,[308] Wellcome Ms 5482/96

London
8 November 1872

Sir, I beg to thank you for sending me a copy of your *Hospital Prayer Book*. I am afraid that, overladen as I am with illness and business, some time must elapse before I can do what you ask in the way of examining it thoroughly. May I beg you, as you seem to require an answer, to accept a very brief one for the present?

In all the hospitals with which I am connected, what is recommended in your preface is done, more or less closely. We have great satisfaction from the results of morning and evening prayer, conducted in their wards by "sisters" of the wards (head nurses).

In many hospitals with which I am not connected the same thing is done, each following its own method, very good in many cases. I do not quite understand for whom "Part 2" is intended. If for a "minister," he will certainly choose his own method. If for a "lay reader," as certainly almost. If for a head nurse, a great deal more variety is necessary (and ought to be given in a published work) for *daily* prayer.

---

307 A recruit of William Rathbone's, Lucy Sophia Leslie (c1834-?), who began training at St Thomas' in 1872.

308 Edward John Waring, *The Hospital Prayer Book*.

Omit "General Exhortation" p 78. Omit "Prayer for Bishops and Curates" p 86. Omit "Prayer for Queen and Royal Family" except on Sundays. Give a much larger selection of collects to be chosen amongst, and varied. Have a morning service different at least for Mondays and Wednesdays; Tuesdays and Thursdays; Fridays; Saturdays; and an evening service (different): prayers, collects and benediction, different for each, and even a variety to choose amongst.

Hymns printed too small. *One Hundred Large Type Hymns* (Edinburgh: Taylor) a favourite selection for sick. Excuse the brevity of these remarks, which I understand you to ask for.

Source: From a letter to R. Brudenell Carter,[309] Royal Free Hospital Archives

14 November 1874

Sir, Though somewhat heavily pressed down by business and illness, I cannot forbear writing a line (with my mite to the "Anstie Memorial Fund"), to express—what I cannot express—how great is the loss to our country in Dr Anstie.[310] Had he lived, many thousands of deaths would not have died (if I may use such an expression), which now will fall victims to the want of public health measures of which he was such a devoted supporter. To follow in his steps is the best tribute we can offer him, the only one he would care for.

When we were agitating to improve the new Sanitary Act by giving certain powers of inspection to local boards, we had in view such cases as the place where he laid down his valuable life to serve his country on what is really the battlefield of this day, both in England and India. They would not follow our advice (though they will some day). And there are many, many buildings where similar deaths are now taking place, and will continue to take place from want of this inspection.

In our new army buildings, these calamities are provided against. But the crying fault is that we have a great and costly sanitary organization which cannot touch the most powerful disease causes connected with houses and establishments. And now one of our very best men of this or of any age has been called on to pay the penalty!

I wish I could afford to send 100 times *to* HIS "*memorial*" this petty £5.

309 Robert Brudenell Carter (1828-1912), ophthalmic surgeon.

310 Francis Edmund Anstie (1833-74); Nightingale considered him "the best of all the workhouse reformers," in *Public Health Care* (6:433).

St Thomas' Hospital, 1859-74

Editor: St Thomas' Hospital was the flagship hospital for the Nightingale Fund, the home of her first (and always primary) training school. While nurses at the Edinburgh Royal Infirmary and the Highgate and St Marylebone Workhouse Infirmaries would also be known as "Nightingale nurses," St Thomas' got the lion's share of her fund and her time. St Thomas' had been chosen as the base for the school not on account of its merits as a hospital, but those of its matron, Sarah E. Wardroper, who had begun to reform nursing there in 1853, and of the resident medical officer, R.G. Whitfield, who was a rare doctor who understood the importance of sanitary precautions and had assisted Nightingale on her Crimean War reports. Mary Jones gave her detailed advice as to the requirements of nurses' and probationers' rooms,[311] but Nightingale's letters on this point are not extant.

At the time the Nightingale School opened, in June 1860, the hospital was located in Southwark, on land leased from a railway company that would soon want it for a new railway line and new London Bridge Station. That a move was likely was known even before the school's opening, as an act of Parliament had been introduced to permit the railway company to build on the land. Nightingale (and others) saw the impossibility of a hospital sharing space with a busy railway line and station. Moreover, she always preferred a healthier site in the suburbs. The railway company's need for the site then became an opportunity to build a better, safer hospital. *The Builder*, which had published her three articles on the defects of Netley, again obliged. The three articles she did for it were short and anonymous, stressing the opportunity for a healthier site. She was aware that the medical professors attached to the hospital preferred a location close to the city centre for their own practical reasons. She argued, however, that patient safety was not only more important, but that medical students would learn more by seeing patients recover than by seeing them linger or die. The only part of the hospital that had to be centrally located, Nightingale held, was the accident ward (see p 778 below).

The practical solution was to get the railway to buy up the entire site and for the hospital to use the proceeds to purchase elsewhere and build anew, according to the best architectural principles. Black-

311 Jones letter 28 March 1860, ADD MSS 47743 ff3-6.

heath was Nightingale's first choice, for the purity and dryness of its air, its good drainage and easy accessibility by rail.

After getting press attention to the possibility of a completely new, suburban location, Nightingale's next move was to recruit Prince Albert, a governor of the hospital, to speak for it. She approached him via his private secretary, Sir Charles Phipps. St Thomas', she pointed out, was one of two "royal hospitals," and the queen was a "visitor" to it (see p 778 below). Phipps was evidently against Nightingale contacting the prince (his letter is not extant), and so she had to send another one justifying approaching the prince. What actually transpired is not clear, but by the end of 1860 the prince was quoting Nightingale and Phipps was the intermediary.[312] The old hospital was sold and planning began for a new one.

In the interim, the hospital moved to Surrey Gardens, where it stayed from 1862 to 1871. Nightingale, from her Crimean War experience, had become keen on hut hospitals and hoped that St Thomas' would use "brick huts" as temporary quarters while the new hospital was being built. She even argued that the trial of huts would prove so successful "that a new enlightenment on the subject of hospitals would arise." Obviously, she did not succeed.

By the time the new hospital was under construction, the Herbert Hospital had opened. Nightingale had worked prodigiously hard on getting the best fittings and materials for it, and so wanted St Thomas' officials to see them and demand the same.

It is well known that Nightingale did not succeed in getting St Thomas' built at Blackheath or any other place distant from the city centre, for the hospital (although largely rebuilt after its bombing in World War II) can still be seen on the south bank of the Thames, opposite the Parliament buildings. The design, however, was her preferred pavilion model, and St Thomas' became the "most prestigious" of the early pavilion hospitals in Britain.[313] The new nurses' home, when constructed,

312 Two further letters Nightingale wrote the prince via Phipps are published with other royal correspondence in *Society and Politics* (5:416-17 and 417-18).

313 Taylor, *Hospital and Asylum Architecture in England* 130. For background see also E.M. McInnes, *St Thomas' Hospital*; and F.G. Parsons, *The History of St Thomas's Hospital*, vol. 3.

also was a model of its kind, and was much commented on for its comfort. Nightingale had had to remonstrate considerably to ensure adequate standards for space, privacy and ventilation.

The correspondence begins in 1859, with site the issue. Context on planning and building is given as those issues arise.

Source: From a letter to R.G. Whitfield, Florence Nightingale Museum (LMA) H1/ST/NC1/59/1

21 February 1859

I received your letter with great pleasure on Saturday when I returned to town.

I think that you have the finest opportunity of building the finest hospital in the world, if you do but take advantage of it. I have no doubt that we can help you in bringing public opinion to bear upon your authorities.

The first question I will ask you to inform me upon is, has St Thomas' any property in the neighbourhood of London and if so where?

Source: From a letter to William Farr, Wellcome Ms 5474/5, typed copy Add Mss 43398 f117

25 February 1859

I have sent a *leader* to *The Builder* (which has been accepted) about St Thomas' removal (see p 780 below). I think it best not to try the medical papers because they will be up in arms about their schools! But you know best. On the other side the sheet, you will find the facts about St Thomas' written by Sutherland. Do please put a paragraph into the *Times* or some of the great luminaries. We lost Netley; let us win St Thomas'.

Source: Anonymous leader, "A Chance for St Thomas' Hospital," *The Builder* 17,838 (26 February 1859):154

A railway is projected for connecting the railways to the west of the metropolis. It will pass through the property of St Thomas' Hospital, close to the wards, so close indeed that the hospital will have to be removed from its present site. A public necessity has thus opened the prospect of two great public improvements, namely, the extension of the London Bridge Station, to make it commensurate with the requirements of the vast traffic which passes through it, and the possibility of rebuilding the noble charity which the station would supplant, on a better site out of the noise and traffic and foul air of London. It is to be hoped that the managers of St Thomas' Hospital, who have done so much for the relief of human suffering, will see it to be their duty to remove the hospital to a healthy, dry, suburban or rural site, where they will be able to supply the sick poor committed to them with pure air, the most important of all the elements of recovery from disease, and one which cannot be obtained anywhere within the limits of this great metropolis. Here, then, is likely to be a great opportunity of performing a great duty, the good example of which would do more to improve our hospitals than all that could be said or written on the subject. A magnificent occasion offers itself to the managers of St Thomas' Hospital, and it is to be hoped they will avail themselves of it.

Source: From two letters to Sir Charles Phipps, Royal Archives, PP/Vic/1859/784

7 March 1859

Will you pardon me (Florence Nightingale) for presuming on your old kindness to me to ask you a question? A bill is before the House of Commons this week for carrying a railway from the S.E. Station to Charing Cross. The line passes so close to the north wing of St Thomas' Hospital as to render it useless. The hospital will thus be reduced to its old dimensions and to the buildings which were condemned by the medical officers, as unfit, so far back as 1832.

The hospital is one of our two royal hospitals (upon Edward VI's foundation) and the queen is visitor. The prince consort is also a governor. I have reason to know that a word from his royal highness to Mr Baggallay, the treasurer, would determine the latter. And from the prince consort's well-known interest in all questions affecting the welfare of the people, it has occurred to me to ask you whether it would be proper to bring the matter to his royal highness's cognizance.

If the railway people would purchase the whole site of the hospital, not only would a great injury be saved, but a great benefit gained, for the hospital might then be rebuilt (bodily) in the neighbourhood of London.

I have such ample experience of the injury inflicted on the sick poor by the foul air of London that I know that to move St Thomas' (medical school and hospital) out of the crowded London Bridge district into the suburbs would be a public boon. Blackheath would be a very accessible place and has great facilities by railway. A surgical ward for accidents is all that would be necessary on the present site of St Thomas'. And all the other sick might be taken by railway to Blackheath (or some other accessible suburb) with the greatest advantage to the sick.

Unfortunately, in all such arrangements, the sick are generally the least considered. Pray forgive me for being troublesome.

10 March 1859

I could not for one moment have intended to indicate that the prince consort should in any way interfere with a railway bill. The facts about St Thomas' Hospital had come to me privately, and knowing his royal highness's great interest in all matters affecting the welfare of the people, it occurred to me that it might not be improper in me simply to state to you the facts of the case. This was really all I intended to do, leaving it entirely in the hands of his royal highness. . . .

It appeared to me impertinent to indicate a course for the prince consort's consideration. But as you add "I do not understand exactly *what* you think the prince might do," might I to you in private state the following facts?

On Monday the railway bill goes before the committee, of which the chairman, Mr Ingham,[314] is well disposed to view the matter in the same light we do, i.e., to say that the railway people must buy *all* the site *or none*. If (*after this* bill has passed, if it does pass, should it be improper to do it before), it were considered that the removal of a royal hospital like St Thomas', the second only in antiquity[315] and in usefulness in London, were an event of sufficient public importance for the prince to take the chair at a meeting of the directors of the hospital, his word would be enough, were he to propose that such an opportunity should not be lost for removing the hospital to a healthy site in the neighbourhood and re-erecting it upon the best plan.

(There are not wanting jobbers even in royal hospitals—and two sites are mentioned which governors and cousins, uncles and brothers-in-law of governors who want to sell, have proposed, where the hospital would be far worse off than it is where it is now.) But, if it is not an occasion for the prince to appear as chairman, a message from him to the treasurer of the hospital, a Mr Baggallay, would, I am informed, have the desired effect, should the prince see the matter in this light.

I will, not take up your time with any apology for this long statement.

---

314 Robert Ingham (1793-1875), barrister and MP.

315 The two oldest hospitals in England, both of "royal foundation," were St Bartholomew's, founded in 1546, and St Thomas', in 1553.

Source: From a letter to George Godwin, Wellcome Ms 5482/33

9 March 1859

The subject of the removal of St Thomas' Hospital is one of such public importance that I would fain hope you could find room for some further notice of it in your *Builder*. It is now before the House of Commons committee.

Source: Two anonymous leaders, "London Bridge and Charing Cross Railway, versus St Thomas' Hospital," *The Builder* 17,840 (12 March 1859):185, and "The Removal of St Thomas' Hospital," *The Builder* 17,842 (26 March 1859):223

On 27 June 1832, the physicians and surgeons of St Thomas' Hospital addressed a letter to the governors on the injurious effect likely to be the result of extending the buildings in "the low, close and confined position of the hospital, as it at present stands." And they stated that "after mature consideration, they felt it a duty earnestly to call the attention of the governors to this question, whether instead of the expenditure necessary to keep the present decayed edifice in a state of repair, and increase its accommodation, the rebuilding of the hospital in a more eligible situation would not be a measure infinitely better calculated to promote the benevolent views of the founders and supporters, by rendering it more extensively and efficiently useful." This letter bears the signatures of Drs Williams, Elliotson and Roots, and of Messrs Travers, Green and Tyrrell, physicians and surgeons to the hospital. They were, at least, twenty-seven years before their time, for their wise and benevolent advice has not yet been followed. The works of New London Bridge were the occasion of the representation being made. And the same question, as we stated on the 26th of February, has come round again in another and more important form. The Charing Cross Railway, as we observe on the Parliamentary plan, starting from the Greenwich Station, London Bridge, makes a sweep over the arcade of shops, crosses the north-east angle of St Thomas' ground within about 10 feet of the corner of the new north wing, and bridges the street close to the west end of the wing. Besides the constant noise and vibration from passing trains, the ventilation of the whole hospital will be most seriously interfered with, and no one can doubt that the hospital will be damaged as a hospital, to an enormous extent. Nothing short of removing the institution altogether will meet the case, if the railway is to go on. The question is being battled before a committee of the House of Commons in the usual railway style, and it is to be feared that the interests of those whose interests are most at stake—the sick—will be overlooked in the contention. In the meantime we have heard it stated that the question of removing the hospital has in some sense been discussed, and that sites have been proposed more unhealthy, if anything, than the one the hospital at present occupies. We should rejoice to see a more enlightened view taken of the whole question, and a building worthy of so great a charity erected, say, at Blackheath, or some similar suburb easily accessible by railway, a measure which, in the words already quoted, would be "infinitely better calculated to promote the benevolent views of founders and supporters" than either leaving the hospital where it is, or transferring it to any other populous neighbourhood.

The Lancet of 19 March takes exception to part, at least, of the recommendation we made in the numbers of *The Builder* of 26 February and 12 March, in both of which we advocated the removal of St Thomas' Hospital to a suburban district.

The Lancet agrees with us insofar as concerns the removal to the country of convalescent patients, but it lays down as a principle that, for patients other than convalescents, "It is one of the essential conditions of usefulness for such an institution that it be located in a populous district x x for the reception of the sick poor in the immediate vicinity, and of those suddenly seized with sickness or maimed by accident."

We feel bound to dissent from part of this doctrine, and for the following reasons:

First, the sick poor have to be removed from their houses in any case, and if suitable means of transport were provided, it would, in the great majority of instances, matter very little whether they were carried a mile or two farther, while it would matter a very great deal indeed whether, having undergone the fatigue of transport, they were put to bed in fresh, pure country air, or in foul, damp town air.

Secondly we believe that an examination of the hospital books would show that a very considerable proportion of the cases received are brought from the purer air and quiet of less densely peopled outskirts into the foul air and noise of the present locality.

Thirdly, from inquiries we have made, we are justified in stating that, even after the sick are brought to St Thomas' and other hospitals, and have undergone the risk of transport, a very large proportion of them might be sent off immediately into a country hospital with the greatest advantage.

Fourthly, it is a mistake to suppose that most of the accidents necessarily take place near the hospital which receives them. We find, for instance, that on a recent occasion, out of all the accidents (thirty-five) in St Thomas' Hospital, two thirds (twenty-four) of the whole number came from a distance of two miles and more, and eighteen of them, or half the whole, came from New Cross and beyond. New Cross is nearly 3½ miles by road from St Thomas'.

We suggested Blackheath as a likely place to furnish a good site, on account of the purity and dryness of its air, the porous, self-draining nature of part of its sub-soil, and the great facility with which sick admitted at the present hospital might be raised to the level of the railway, placed in an easy carriage, and landed in fifteen or twenty minutes at Blackheath. Now it so happens that, of the accidents in St Thomas' Hospital at the time we have referred to, fifteen could have been taken to Blackheath in cabs with less suffering than they underwent in being carried to St Thomas' Hospital.

We do not on this account advocate the removal of all accidents indiscriminately into the country. We discussed this question in *The Builder* of 28 August 1858, in which we stated that "even in so vast a place as the metropolis, a few casualty wards, where accidents might temporarily be seen, rooms for the examination and reception of cases, and suitable vehicles for transferring them to the country, would be all that would be necessary to effect the reform."[316] To this opinion we adhere. Let St Thomas' Hospital be removed to Blackheath or to some other equally healthy and accessible locality; let a reception room, and one or two wards for the treatment of accidents, until convalescence begins, be provided on part of the site of the present hospital, and all the rest of the establishment may be removed bodily with the greatest advantage to the sick.

Even severe accidents can be removed with safety at the very beginning, provided ordinary precautions be exercised, and a very small number of accidents would, in reality, require accommodation on the site of the present hospital.

In *The Builder* of 12 March, we showed that the removal of the hospital was advocated twenty-seven years ago by Drs Williams, Elliotson and Roots, and by Messrs Travers, Green and Tyrrell, the then physicians and surgeons, and we have reason to think that their successors of the present day entertain no less enlightened and humane views on this most important subject.

---

316 This is a quotation from Nightingale's first article on Netley (see p 282 above).

Source: From a letter to Harry Verney, Wellcome (Claydon copy) Ms 8998/3, draft Add Mss 45791 ff1-2

7 July 1859

There seem to be three points to be attended to in the compensation (v. [see] St Thomas's):

1. the value of the number of square yards of the hospital land to be taken by the company, which should be the same as the land in the neighbourhood;

2. a sum in the name of "dommages intérêts" [damages and interest] of the hospital property, even if the hospital were removed, for the railway will damage the ground for building purposes;

3. a sum to be paid for the total cost of removing the hospital.

There need be no controversy except about the amount to be paid. It appears to me that an ordinary valuer could settle the point. £30,000 is certainly only a fractional part of what ought to be paid to the charity, *unless* the legislature intend to lay it down as a principle that trust property and private property are to be sacrificed to the schemes of joint stock companies. If you can do anything in this matter, I am sure you will be doing a national benefit. I am doing my best.

Editor: A letter of Phipps to Nightingale thanked her for hers of 21 December 1860, which had been given to the prince. He enclosed a copy of Prince Albert's letter to Baggallay, noting that the prince had used her very words. A letter by Phipps on 27 December 1860 related General Gray's answer from Baggallay. He also conveyed the prince's thanks for her advice and assistance on the Lisbon Children's Hospital.[317]

Source: From a letter to R.G. Whitfield, Florence Nightingale Museum (LMA) H1/ST/NC1/60/7

31 December 1860

The part of Mr Baggallay's letter to the prince [Albert] which *nails* him is this: "The governors" x x "expressing their conviction that the railway is incompatible with the proper treatment and comfort of the sick poor" x x. They can hardly go back from this.

Please to write to me in future at 30 Old Burlington St., although I am not quite sure of the day I shall be able to go there.

---

317 Phipps letters 23 and 27 December 1860, Add Mss 45750 ff1 and 7, copies Royal Archives PP/Vic/1860/6403.

Source: From a letter to Richard Baggallay, Florence Nightingale Museum (LMA) H1/ST/NC1/61/2

7 January 1861

I shall rest more than satisfied in the conviction that your judgment favours the removal of St Thomas', and that, as in the chief hands, so in the best hands now lies its chance of success. No assurance could be more satisfactory than this.

I think that nothing which I have said can be construed to point at more than the irremediable damage inflicted by the *railway* on the hospital. I should perhaps mention to you that three governors[318] (knowing my twofold interest in your noble institution), sent me the "Notice" for the "General Court" of the 24th ult. [last month] at the same time as Mr Whitfield.

I trust that you will be able to make St Thomas' into the first hospital and finest school in Europe.

Source: From a letter to Douglas Galton, Add Mss 45759 ff133-34

7 January 1861

Could you tell me the following: the Charing Cross Railway question as to what it shall pay for cutting into St Thomas' Hospital is to be decided in a few days. St Tom's persists in asking an enormous sum, £750,000 (I think), as a matter of policy. Do you think this is bad policy? Or would the railway be not disinclined to refer it to a jury, safe that the jury would favour them?

Some of the governors of St Tom's are anxious that only a fair sum should be asked, believing that that would be the best policy.

Source: From an incomplete letter to Samuel Smith, Add Mss 45792 ff231-32

[after 2 August 1861]

Mr Whitfield has written me an immense letter [missing], full of mistakes about hospital plans, including that for the removal of St Thomas'. Also the enclosed, as to which please to tell me what I (or anyone) can do. Mr W. is one of my many friends who is always preaching to me to do nothing, and compelling me to do something, and that something 1000 times more harassing than my own business. Would you write and tell him (in civil language) that a great and overwhelming affliction entirely precludes me from attending to any but pressing busi-

---

318 One of them being Prince Albert.

ness at present. (He knows this just as well as you do; how happy widows are, because people don't write them harassing letters in the first week of their widowhood,[319] and yet I know no widow so desolate as I.) . . .

Don't take any notice (to him) about the letter about his son. No wonder he wishes it to be "private." And don't give him my direction [address].

Source: From a letter to Douglas Galton, Add Mss 45760 ff79-80

24 April 1862

St Thomas is shrieking for succour—he has got himself turned out by 26 July and does not know where to go. I have promised that you will help him, though he does not deserve it.

At our suggestion, he is thinking of putting up brick huts to live in till he can build. And I have invited Mr Currey,[320] the hospital architect, and Mr Whitfield, who moves everything (both were here today in the wild hope of finding you or Dr Sutherland or something and found nothing), to come here on Saturday at 3. I promised that you, or if not you, Dr Sutherland, would meet them and give them information about *hut plans*. And I hoped that, at all events, you would send up here some of your best *hut plans* to give them an idea. (I believe they think a hut is a kind of mud cabin.) I told them that you had, I believed, some *hut plans* later and better than any they had seen.

Source: From an incomplete letter and a letter to Harry Verney, Wellcome (Claydon copy) Ms 9000/38 and 52

9 May 1862

The article favourable to the removal of St Thomas' is in the *Medical Times* of 19 April.[321] It is quite within my remembrance since an article (like that) saying that anything but medicine and surgery signified for medical and surgical patients would have ruined a medical paper. And it is inexcusable in the *Times* to be behind a medical paper, which we *used* to think the lowest vehicle of ignorance.

---

319 A reference to the death of Sidney Herbert on 2 August 1861.

320 On Currey see G.C. Cook, "Henry Currey FRIBA (1820-1900): Leading Victorian Hospital Architect, and Early Exponent of the 'Pavilion Principle,'" *Postgraduate Medical Journal* 78 (2002):352-59.

321 "Mr Whitfield on the Removal of St Thomas's Hospital," *Medical Times and Gazette* 19 April 1862:405-6..

Even now, Dr Guy is advocating that dirt is healthy and that King's College Hospital (the worst of all the hospitals) is the healthiest.

20 June 1862

The St Thomas' Hospital Bill is now before the Lords. It is intended to grant the Railway Co. a title to sell the site of the hospital. Nothing can be done until it is seen what the House of Lords will agree to.

Mr Whitfield came here to ask me to speak to Lord Redesdale[322] and to assure him that Mr Baggallay (the treasurer) did not mean to make the Surrey Gardens the permanent site of the hospital, but to move it into the country. Of course I said that Mr Baggallay must be testimony to his own truth before Lord Redesdale, and that, if he were not believed (which indeed I am not surprised at, after his blundering) it was not I who could make his testimony believed.

As to Bethlehem,[323] that site was already discussed by St Thomas' and found to be entirely beyond the disbelieving apostle's[324] means. It is enormously expensive. Besides which, the building would have to be entirely gutted and rearranged. If the hospital is to remain in London, Bethlehem is the best site in those parts, but shares the disadvantages of all the south side of London. But, though I am decidedly for the poor Bethlehem patients being moved into the country, yet, of the two, I had rather give this chance to the patients who are sane than to those who are insane.

The *Times* is excessively unfortunate in all its suggestions about hospitals, which I attribute to those articles being written by [John] Simon (the St Thomas' doctors have issued the most preposterous manifesto). The *Times* once advocated Chelsea Hospital,[325] one of the unhealthiest buildings in London, being turned into a hospital.

---

322 John Thomas Freeman-Mitford (1805-86), 1st Baron Redesdale, chair of committees in the House of Lords.

323 Bethlehem Hospital, abbreviated "Bedlam," was a psychiatric hospital then located in Southwark; in 1936, after another move, the building was made into the Imperial War Museum.

324 A joking reference to St Thomas', from his doubting the resurrection of Jesus.

325 Residence of the Chelsea pensioners, opened in 1692.

Source: From a letter and an incomplete letter to Henry Bonham Carter, Add Mss 47714 ff18-20 and 22

19 July 1862

1. I am very glad Mr Baggallay has lowered his charges. It will keep almost two more nurses.[326]

2. Mr Whitfield sent me the "Surrey Gardens" plans. But I suggested to him that Sir J. Jebb should see those for nurse accommodation, as he did formerly, and make his valuable improvements. It struck me that there was a great deficiency (perhaps unavoidable) of window and window light ventilation.

3. What "Building Act" forbids *huts*? How do they define a "hut"? Better hospital accommodation of a *temporary* kind can be put up than of any permanent kind. Because to build permanently for such as effectually as you can put up temporarily costs too much.

Would this building be a "hut" in terms of the act? I am certain that, if temporary buildings of the *best* possible kind were put up, supposing the act could be evaded, recoveries would be so numerous, deaths comparatively so few, that a new enlightenment on the subject of hospitals would arise. And people would wonder how they could ever have murdered patients in the old hospitals.

[ca. January 1863]

[I] would like to have independent and experienced advice (of men who *can* have no self-interest in the thing, and yet are versed in such matters as facility of access, etc., as well as sanitary things). I believe I could engage that Captain Galton, Dr Sutherland and Mr Rawlinson would visit any reasonable number of sites and report upon them to the governors. I would so gladly help Mr Baggallay, if I could. I had already mentioned this to Mrs Wardroper. If you like to say this from me to Mr Baggallay, pray do.

Source: From a letter to Douglas Galton, Add Mss 45763 f78

Oak Hill Park
Hampstead, N.W.
29 July 1865

Dr Sutherland told me you would like to see the enclosed plans, etc., of St Thomas'. The full-sized plans are at the London Bridge International Hotel.

---

326 The Nightingale Fund paid St Thomas' room and board for the pupil nurses.

Please return me the enclosed (including printed paper) in a day or two, as I have to write to the treasurer.

Source: From undated drafts in Dr Sutherland's hand for Francis Hicks,[327] Add Mss 45799 ff163 and 164-65

[ca. November 1865]

Your letter stresses several of the points in which you can help, e.g., from *experience*, the absolute necessity of any constructive arrangements providing for the supervision of the probationers by the matron, the necessity of bringing all the administrative arrangements within as *narrow* a compass as possible. Mr Currey is preparing a plan for me to see containing the following points:

1. A separate house for forty probationers on the site, set apart in the plans for the *northern* block of office quarters.
2. The matron's house will form part of this.
3. Each probationer to have a separate room and half a window, to the outer air, an area of floor 120 square feet.
4. Home to have a distinct entrance.
5. Three floors of dormitories.
6. Sisters' rooms and room for convalescent house.
7. Nurses' day and dining room, kitchen and all conveniences.

The linen store and matron's office to be on the ground floor of the first pavilion to the north of the chapel.

I have gone over your proposals very carefully and, as I learn from Mr Hicks that you think you might be able to find room for forty nurses, perhaps the way to arrive soonest at an agreement would be to ask you whether you can arrange the plan as follows:

1. A general kitchen, etc., in basement.
2. Dining and day room are sufficient, but the windows should not open into any corridor or passage of communication.
3. Half a window will be sufficient lighting for each small nurse's room.
4. No nurse's room window to open into any corridor or passage of communication, all to open to the outer air.
5. Sisters' day and bedroom to have windows to the outer air.
6. Dormitories can be arranged either round a central hall, open from top to bottom of the building, with balustraded terrace round for

327 Francis Hicks (1821-77), appointed treasurer of St Thomas' in 1864, knighted in 1871 on the opening of the new hospital.

getting at the doors (windows all to open however to the outer air), or the dormitories may be arranged on opposite sides of a central passage, with a door at one end and window to the outer air at the other. In this case, also, all the dormitories to have their windows to the outer air.

7. If the plan you left with me were adopted, it would be necessary to close up the windows of the sisters' sitting room, and also the windows of room 6, 7, 8, 9 and 10 opening into the corridor.

8. Area of dormitories to be 120 square feet. I send your plans with the windows closed and rough sketches to show the kind of arrangement, with a central passage, in the same scale, and with a hall from top to bottom, and a skylight over.

9. Baths, W.C.s, stairs, etc. If you can do without extending your buildings so as to interfere with the outer ventilation, it would be most admirable.

I am afraid you must try to find the accommodation without extending your building so as to curtail the already small distance between the existing buildings in the plan. Every foot is of importance, and we may be injuring the accommodation for the probationers in the very point where it should be kept free in its external ventilation.

Please send the plans back to me with your reply, as I must reply to Mr Hicks by Monday morning and tell him when the committee are prepared to go on.

Source: From a letter to Francis Hicks, Florence Nightingale Museum (LMA) H1/ST/NC/65/26

16 December 1865

I have returned the plans to Mr Currey with a few suggestions. And, as your note of the 19th leads us to expect an amended plan with increased accommodation, I think it best to defer making any observations until I have had an opportunity of going over the amended plan.

I beg to thank you for your kind note, also for giving me occasion to see Mr Baggallay, who has written to me offering an appointment.

Editor: The treasurer, Francis Hicks, wrote Nightingale regarding an agreement with the Nightingale Fund Council for the probationers' home, saying that she was to write on any desired improvements in arrangements for it.[328] Henry Currey's letters to Nightingale about

328 Letter 9 January 1866, Florence Nightingale Museum (LMA) H1/ST/NC3/SU198.

the design begin with a courteous willingness to receive her suggestions (20 January 1866). They continue with sending the plans (4 and 8 May 1866), a request for their return (24 May 1866), an initial response to her suggestions, and questions about heating, water, lighting and probationers' rooms (both 29 May 1866).[329] Mrs Wardroper naturally was also involved in the consultations.[330]

Source: From a letter to Douglas Galton, Add Mss 45763 f171

9 May 1866

Could you give me such a letter to someone in the Herbert Hospital as will enable Mrs Wardroper and Mr Whitfield (of St Thomas') to go steadily over it, seeing all the fittings especially and all the arrangements at their leisure? They wish to go Friday or tomorrow or some day next week. They would be much obliged if the letter (of introduction) left the day open, as Mr Whitfield is ill. If you could send me the letter kindly by return of messenger, I would send it by hand to them.

I am particularly anxious that they should accomplish this visit efficiently, as its purpose is for their own new hospital. Could you also kindly send me another copy of your *Herbert Hospital* book? I have lent mine to them.

Editor: As construction proceeded, the hospital asked Nightingale to be its spokesperson with the queen. She, in turn, used the queen's physician, Sir James Clark, as her intermediary. Her first attempt to get the queen to preside at the laying of the foundation stone was evidently unsuccessful, for both Whitfield and Clark wrote her about further attempts. Nightingale was reluctant to try again, however, as Dr Sutherland's draft response for her to Whitfield explained:

> I am afraid I have done in the matter of the foundation stone all I could possibly do, and that I should newly expose myself to another refusal by interfering further. The only way to have done would have been for the governors to have moved and not the officers. At least this is what occurs to me.[331]

329 Florence Nightingale Museum (LMA) H1/ST/NC3/SU199-204).

330 Wardroper letters 18 and 23 May 1866, Florence Nightingale Museum (LMA) H1/ST/NC3/SU206b-07.

331 Draft letter after 15 August 1867, Florence Nightingale Museum (LMA) H1/ST/NC2/V37/67; James Clark letter 15 August 1867, H1/ST/NC2/V35/67.

Yet she was evidently persuaded to make another attempt, which did succeed. A letter from Whitfield informed her that, "through her kind introduction," and through Sir James Clark, her majesty "graciously condescended to perform [the] ceremony of laying the first stone" of the new hospital on 12 May.[332] Nightingale did not attend, but kept the invitation to the ceremony, which gives 13 May 1868 as the date.[333] The queen obliged again by opening the new building on 22 June 1871.[334]

In 1872, an assistant surgeon, W.W. Wagstaffe, wrote Mrs Wardroper that, since the hospital had opened, there had not been a single case of hospital gangrene in the building: "I do not consider there is any reason for supposing the hospital to be at all unhealthy."[335] Numerous outbreaks of disease Nightingale considered preventible, however, continued to occur. Faults in both design and administration appeared, but Nightingale's fears about the site being unhealthy proved to be unfounded. The epidemics that occurred seem to have been due to faults of design or administration, rather than of the site itself. Letters to Dr Sutherland recount Nightingale and Mrs Wardroper tracking down the source of pyemia at St Thomas' in 1872.[336]

In 1873, after two years of experience in the new building, Nightingale wrote up and had set into print a set of "Notes on the New St Thomas'," tellingly subtitled "Being Simply Those Things Which Should Be Avoided" (the first item below). Many defects are set out, so that it surprises that she described the new St Thomas' as one of the "best-constructed" hospitals, but "indifferently furnished." She sent the printed notes to Dr Sutherland for comment. His response began with a note that her points, with two exceptions, were on matters to be remedied, but which scarcely touched the causes of hospital diseases.

> Under present circumstances, all that can be done is to insist on perfect cleanliness, abundant window ventilation, closing all the existing communications between the air of different wards, and of necessity disusing wards in which pyemia cases appear.

---

332 Whitfield letter 16 March 1868, Add Mss 47742 f215.

333 Invitation to ceremony, Add Mss 47760 f5.

334 *Times* 22 June 1871 12a.

335 Letter, Add Mss 47732 f55.

336 Letters 8 July and 21 October 1872, in *The Nightingale School* (12:211 and 218).

He suggested that she frame her notes as questions, as she had had to rely on the eyes of others. It is not clear if Nightingale sent the notes on to hospital officials, either in this or any revised form.

Source: Note for John Sutherland, with corrected proof, British Library Tab 1281.a2(13).12

13 June 1873

On new St Thomas' Hospital.

These are a portion of the notes I mentioned to you. (I have sheets upon sheets of them in manuscript.) I had *these* printed partly because the labour to me of copying on own corrected manuscript is so great that it is less trouble to me to have it printed—partly because I don't wish my own hand to be seen. *Would you kindly say anything upon these* that is to be said? (The last two notes refer only to our *own* management of course.)

Notes on the New St Thomas's Hospital (Being Simply those Things which Should Be Avoided)

Chutes for Linen

The chutes for soiled linen are too small. They are, however, *never used,* the nurses stating that the linen of the three wards to which the chute belonged became mixed, and the sheets often wet, and wetted the chute. (*A long narrow basket or bag would have obviated this difficulty.*) They are put in the bathroom, under an open window, and removed only four times a week to the wash.

Ditto for Dressings

This chute is *never* used (!) as it was feared that the soiled lint, etc., would "stick to the sides" and make the chute a simple shaft for foul air. (*And yet a bag or small oblong bucket, with lid, running on a wire, would have overcome this difficulty.*)

Soiled Dressings

The "dressings" were, therefore, thrown into a *zinc bucket* (it should be iron, with glazed earthenware lining, and lid of course) which never could be properly cleansed, *without a lid,* kept in the W.C. compartment, and when full the said bucket was carried *through the ward* by the wardmaid twice a day. Bandages washed by wardmaid in the bathroom.

The Lift

Was never used by nurses or students, because it takes too much time, and they cannot work it themselves. (N.B. *Would not* steam *have been less expensive*? It is used in the large hospitals of Holland and Denmark.) Probationers obliged to go up No. 2 staircase only on their way to the wards.

W.C. for Men

These were placed *in* the W.C. compartment, where the nurses had to empty bedpans, etc., and where all soiled dressings, etc., were kept. (*On moral grounds is not this very objectionable?*)

Lavatory and Bath

The hot water pipes gave an insufficient supply of warm water, as they had "to run" a long time before any could be obtained. This was only in the upper wards, however. (N.B. Does not always run hot; hot water has to be fetched from the kitchen.)

Flooring

Is scraped (but scarcely polished) only once in six weeks, should be done every fortnight and dry-rubbed by a man every day. Scrubber now does it. Porters are the *frotteurs* [floor polishers], often called off; a much better polish should be given, and slippers to patients. Floors often dirty. The boards of the wards were stained too dark a colour and looked dirty and uncared for; they were certainly *not* "well-polished." Such is usually the rule with regard to these floors. A highly polished floor may endanger the patients slipping. (*I never knew nor even heard of an accident of this kind at the Val-de-Grâce. But there the men were provided with slippers.*)

Bedsteads

The few "spring beds" that there were struck one as being of an expensive and complicated kind, not to be compared to those in use in the best civil hospitals of Paris. They are wire, only three to each ward. Patients slip down. (No rheoclines.)

Bedding or Quilts

The mattresses were good, but the coverlets or quilts *were* bad, being dark blue cotton, "so as not to show the dirt" (!) They are replaced by grey quilts (of mixed cotton and wool) with scarlet borders. All the quilts were so arranged as to make each bed resemble an "ottoman." The corners (though only at the bottom) being so carefully "pinned over" that no air could pass under the mattress. This arrangement had the questionable advantage of permitting bedroom utensil, etc. (without lids!) to be "out of sight"!! (No, they are not.) Lidless chamber vessels very objectionable, emptied only twice a day (by wardmaid). She goes round with an iron bucket, with lid, and wooden bucket to rinse. Sister's "cross" always to make her do it thoroughly.

Windows

Were difficult to open, and not so well constructed for ventilation as those in use at the St George's Hospital—open in three sashes. Joiner [carpenter] has to be always easing them. Top sash in many will not open at all. Middle sash the one generally opened.

Ventilators

"There *were* some (?) under the flooring," but not above it (i.e., along the wainscoting *to raise* foul air. *Do you consider this desirable?*) Eight gratings, one at each corner, near ceiling and near floor; [one can] hear very distinctly from ward above and below at the grating. Atmosphere *must* communicate from one ward to another. Ventilating tubes from each of the three centre stoves through to roof by stove chimney.

Cupboards

These cupboards at end of the ward had thick wooden doors, and were used for lint, padding, splints, etc. Should have glass doors. (N.B. nurse shuts up her lint from probationers; probationers and dressers extravagant in lint.)

There was not the slightest attempt to *ventilate* (quite true) these cupboards, and there was neither order nor arrangement visible with regard to their contents. (*This is a thing to be always insisted upon with nurses. In France such an "omission of duty" would have met with instant punishment. The crown princess, in her "model barrack," had the doors made of* GLASS. Yes. *For charpie*[337] *and bandages this was desirable, as it kept such things free from dust, but splints, air cushions, etc., are better on shelves, where the air can freely circulate.*) The splints come up clean from surgery, or are cleaned in bathroom. The air cushions should be free to air, but there are seldom more than one or two not in use.

In conclusion, there were no bed tables, nor any other table by the side of the bed for the patient, except in children's ward. The "lockers" were almost the worst ever seen—of unstained, unpolished wood (which had to be scoured once a week, the things being put on the bed, and of course "dry" in the wards, except when dragged into the bathroom by help of a patient to be done there!!), formed like a chair or night stool, acting as a table for the patients, as a chair for their visitors. On the floor was a drawer for their *clothes*, and over *this* was their "store closet" for sugar, oranges, preserves, fragments of bread and butter and other "luxuries," mixed up with work and writing materials, pipes, purses and odds and ends. The smell and flavour of these things can be better imagined than described. In a few cases the men had pinned cork at the corners (under the lid) to prevent the lid shutting down tight, and thus ensured a certain amount of ventilation. Medicines either put

337 Unravelled old linen, used for surgical dressings. The "model barrack" was probably her small hospital at Homburgh, during the Franco-Prussian War, where Florence Lees nursed; see her "The Crown Princess's Lazaretto for the Wounded," *Good Words* (1873):500-05.

behind the locker or on one of the ward tables should be on a shelf at head of bed; also there should be a place for the "card" [chart].

What is done here is not the custom in any other hospital, it is believed, viz., *oiled paper* used for warm water dressings, instead of oiled silk or gutta percha [rubber]. The lint is sometimes single—but, if so, with linen over it—but generally double. Have to make the dressers supply lint sometimes. (N.B. Mr Simon prefers using only lint and cotton wool, no oiled paper or silk.)

There were no bed rests, only "alderman's beds." The bed rest of frame and sacking or bands is best—none of these. Some bed rests of all bars—bad.

The bedsteads had no footboards or headboards. There were no muslin curtains to the beds (or substitutes) for a protection against flies in the children's ward. Sometimes green gauze put over faces of bad cases; muslin curtains very much wanted for such—for wounds in face. There are rings put up, but no poles or curtains. (The few urine bottles that there were—*opaque* earthenware, but seldom used.) A small chamber vessel and a large chamber vessel for each man much better (and always given) for the small chamber vessel will *rinse*. Urine bottles have often to be destroyed—cannot be cleansed.

Still one must add that, with the one exception of the W.C.s in the male wards, this is, with all its deficiencies, one of the best-"constructed" hospitals ever seen, although it is also one of the most indifferently furnished.

"Alderman's beds"

In three partitions of mattress, with iron pan, should be *earthenware* (smell very bad), double incline for fractured spines, always get bedsores on it, mackintosh and linen laid round pan (smell fearful). We put india rubber cushion under the back, but this raises the patient too much and slips; an air cushion should be let *into* middle partition of mattress. Troughs called *water beds* bad, water mattresses better.

Wardmaids

Want "mothering," dine in separate mess, no classes. Sister has much trouble with them; men patients fling their pillows at them sometimes, and get into ways of foul language. (Ringleader once expelled.) This wardmaid sent to female medical (where the sister had but one ward) and did well. Should dine with sister and nurses, but nurses would not like it.

Ward Management

Vide [see] sisters' reports. Probationer has none, unless on staff duty, then to see to stores, to replacing of them, to being methodical, etc., or (nurse off duty every other day from 6 to 8 P.M.) then put probationer on that duty—this is her test in ward management.

At 6, begin worse dressings, go on to less important ones.

At 7, supper for those patients who have supper.

At a quarter before 8, medicine.

At 8, gas turned down.

If probationer does this methodically—if, when she gives the patients their tea she feeds those who can't feed themselves, etc.—then she may be put down as good at "ward management." "I used to make the probationers do it, while I sat by reading to the children—my fingers itching to do it—that I might see how *they* do it."

Source: From a letter to Parthenope Verney, Wellcome (Claydon copy) Ms 9006/51

12 July 1873

Unluckily Wednesday is the "Annual Show Day" at St Thomas', when the governors come to inspect. For three months beforehand, all the wards are emptied of patients (successively) and cleansed and white-washed, etc. (I never knew before of how much use "governors" were—except as governors *à non governando* [not governing]—oh what a good thing are governors.)

But the eve of the show day our nurses can scarcely be spared.

Source: From a letter to Douglas Galton, ADD MSS 45764 ff212-13

10 March 1874

Frotteur [floor polisher]. *St Thomas'.* Could you be so very kind as, through any of your contractors or otherwise, to discover and recommend a good *frotteur*? The treasurer of St Thomas' Hospital has at last (and it is desirable to strike while the iron is hot) sanctioned the engagement, on trial, of a *frotteur* to do *one* or two wards.

The "trial" means that—if it is found to be halfpenny per ward cheaper than the present (porters) floor work, to which erysipelas has been distinctly traced, the treasurer may then extend a real *frotteur* system. (An ignorant boy of nineteen is now their only frotteur, and the porters who clean are stated actually to leave *mud* in the wards.)

Editor: A letter of Nightingale to Dr Sutherland in 1878 asked him to criticize a report on St Thomas' Hospital: "Now is the time if we wish to do anything at St Thomas'."[338] The hospital became the subject again in the 1880s on the building of a new nurses' home (see p 871 below).

---

338 Letter 12 January 1878, ADD MSS 45758 f74.

The next hospital to be discussed is the Edinburgh Royal Infirmary, which became a second "Nightingale school." Very little correspondence, however, survives on hospital construction, although there is much on the first decades of trained nursing and its spread[339] to other Scottish hospitals. Available material from a variety of sources shows that Nightingale had long had her eye on reforming the great Edinburgh Royal Infirmary, which she had first visited in 1856.

The invitation to start trained nursing at Edinburgh naturally prompted consideration of the hospital itself, which was then in the process of being completely rebuilt on a new site. The hospital clerk, James Hope (1803-82), when writing Henry Bonham Carter with a request for a matron and nurses, told him where they stood on building plans:

> The whole plans for the infirmary are completed and we are just going to commence excavating the foundations. A short time ago I spent some hours with our architect in the new St Thomas', where the clerk of works showed us everything. We got some good hints but, on the whole, I think our new infirmary will bear a strict comparison.[340]

The appointment of Charles Hamilton Fasson (d. 1892), a surgeon general from the esteemed Herbert Hospital at Woolwich, as new medical superintendent in February 1872, undoubtedly helped promote reform on both goals of nursing and hospital administration.

Nightingale naturally sought safe living and working conditions for her trained matron and nurses. In the case of Edinburgh, they were to be housed initially in the old fever hospital. A letter in 1872 to Dr Sutherland explained:

> *Edinburgh Royal Infirmary.* We are going to undertake the nursing of this beastly "den of thieves." (Nothing that I have ever known, except the Vienna General Hospital, approaches it in badness—medical staff in both cases *ex*cluded.) The *fever* house (late) is to be converted into a nurses' home for us. Will you kindly tell me whether the precautions enumerated by Mr Fasson are sufficient? Should not the drainage, W.C.s, etc., be thoroughly looked to (overhauled)? . . . Also, any other suggestions?[341]

---

339 In *Extending Nursing* (13:304-78).

340 Hope letter 4 July 1871, Florence Nightingale Museum (LMA) H1/ST/NC18/19/8.

341 In *Extending Nursing* (13:312).

The St-Thomas'-trained nurses, in fact, started living in the old fever house in 1872, and illness resulted.

In 1873, Sir T. Galbraith Logan, then director general of the Army Medical Department, approached Nightingale to comment on the plans for the new infirmary at Lauriston, in the then-suburbs of Edinburgh. The architect of the "new hospital" was David Bryce, but there seems to have been no direct contact with him (Bryce himself died in 1876, before the opening; the work was completed by a relative in the same firm). She evidently did comment on the plans for Logan, for a letter later that month thanked her for looking at them.[342] Any comments she might have made, however, have not survived. Nightingale greatly approved of the magnificent new building and its healthy site, calling it "Christ's palace."[343] Only later did she learn that insufficient space had been allowed between the pavilions for their height, which impeded sunlight from entering the wards. The Lauriston site served for many years until a completely new and larger hospital was built, on land still further away from central Edinburgh, at Little France, opened in 2003.

Wellow School, 1872-74

Editor: Nightingale's father gave the land for Wellow School, near the family home in Hampshire, apparently in 1872. However, no arrangements had been made for building when he died in January 1874. Nightingale turned to the project soon after his death. In the only material dating from 1872, Nightingale's concern was to have a survey conducted of the land intended for the school, prior to any plans being prepared. In 1874 plans were available, which Dr Sutherland reviewed.

There were vexing issues of adequate light, especially given the competing interests, on a small site, of the master's house, the infant school and the main school building itself. On this point she consulted, as well as Dr Sutherland, other "school and sanitary authorities." She noted that light was well known not only to affect health, but the "power of learning," especially for infants (see p 801 below).

The plans were evidently revised numerous times and the process was wearing, with the possibility of contamination from a brickworks, for example, having to be considered.

---

342 Logan letters 10 and 21 May 1873, Add Mss 45803 ff69 and 70.

343 Pringle extract 12 October 1879, Edinburgh University LHB 61. She noted that the hospital opened on 29 October 1879.

Source: From a letter to Harry Verney, Wellcome (Claydon copy) Ms 9005/171

27 December 1872

I could very much wish that you could yourself set on foot the *surveying* of the site offered by my father for *Wellow School* at once.

It is a very small job—could be done, I should think, by the Mr Eggar who is to do the working plans. And I will gladly pay the fee. In all the building operations with which I have been concerned for government offices and public institutions, we should as soon have thought of not *beginning* by having an exact survey of *levels* as of not having a site at all.

You will be doing a great service if you will kindly set this going without more ado. It is really absurd our going on with the plans, without knowing the exact site the school is to stand on, i.e., without this survey of *levels*. Please speak to Mr Empson[344] about it.

Many thanks for flowers and vegetables from Claydon.

Source: From a note to an unnamed family member, Wellcome (Claydon copy) Ms 9006/1

10 January 1873

Kindly inform me what was the result of your visit to Mr Forster[345] about *Wellow School*, as the plans have reached me a second time from Beatrice,[346] aided by the C. of C.'s architect. And I must consult you and Mr Empson.

Source: From three letters to John Sutherland, Add Mss 45757 ff228-29, 233-34 and 235-37, the last with his comments

27 February 1874

Wellow School.

1. Would you be so very kind as to look once more at these miserable plans?

2. They have now chosen a new *site*, to the *north* instead of to the *south* of the *same road*. In some respects this is a great improvement, but if it is to entail the objections I have pointed out (in the four enclosed pages), *which please return to me*, does it not become inadmissible?

---

344 William Henry Empson (d. 1883), vicar at St Margaret's, East Wellow, the Nightingales' church.

345 Probably William Edward Forster (1818-86), Liberal MP and author of the Elementary Education Act.

346 Beatrice (Shore Smith) Lushington (c1838-?), a cousin.

3. Please be so good as to make your remarks and suggestions on *all* these points.

4. *And on any other that may occur.*

5. Also, as to whether the *W.C.s* are not too *near*?

6. (I cannot conceive Beatrice suggesting the *boys'* porch on the *only sunny* side. Some weeks ago, when Mrs Empson suggested it, the *long schoolroom* having—as you will perhaps, I hope, remember—*then two* good sunny aspects, *S.E.* and *S.W.*—the *infants' room* being as in *pencil plan B*—Beatrice violently, and as I thought justly, opposed it.) "Tantaene animus coelestibus."[347]

7. The *coppice* may be *grubbed up*, leaving four or five good trees, a nice addition to the *boys' playground*, but as, unfortunately, the largest of these trees is in the green line *between coppice and school*, this would overshadow the school if placed too near, *and the school* overshadow the playground.

8. On the *other* side the coppice and *road*, but within the seven prevailing winds, there is a nearly used up *brick field and kiln.* They say this will be *extinct* by the time the school is built. Are there any precautions necessary with an *extinct brick field*?

9. N.B. The specifications Mr [James L.] Thomas so kindly overhauled will be almost the same for any alterations we may pass. We shall be truly obliged to you for your suggestions *to cut our knot.*

Please return me all this.

[continued] 2 March 1874

This, and this only, viz., the *two* ridiculously small *windows* to the S.W. in the gable of the general schoolroom (above the lower pitched roof of infants' room), which are all that is possible, makes one think that one must give up Plan A.A. What do you say?

13 March 1874

Wellow School. Could you look once more at these and return them to me tonight? Their last invention (see plan pinned on "Block Plan") appears an unmitigated evil—giving no more sun to *master's house* and cutting off BY *master's house* the whole free line of schoolrooms to the west. But I don't object to the *boys' porch* (I am quite weary of this). Please say. . . .

I send you the *old* elevation for you to judge about roofs. I don't object to master having *a* sun, but he must not have *my* sun.

---

347 Can an divine being be so persevering in anger? from Virgil, *The Aeneid*, 1,2.

Embley
Romsey
10 April 1874

Wellow School. Please let me ask you a last "vero ultimo" [truly last] question about this: Shore[348] and I are really at last breaking ground. The *last* plan, accepted by all the great tycoons, is to build master's house and school *separately*. The question I want to ask you is about the *school. Please answer by return of post.*

We have reverted to this plan. The lie of the ground (in the new site) favours this plan and gives a very good playground on one side and on the other (planted out) yards and school offices. The questions are:

1. Will that *corner* between *boys' porch and infants'* room be *dark*, looking as it does to the *north*? **JS:** Yes.

2. Do you like the *S.W. and S.E.* aspect of *long* room? **JS:** No. or do you think the *S.W. long* side will be hot? **JS:** Yes.

3. Do you think there will be a deficiency in light and air on opposite side of *long* room? (*N.E.* side)? **JS:** To some extent yes.

N.B. We get rid of *passage porch*, which I always thought a nuisance.

Source: From a letter to Harry Verney, Add Mss 68890 ff41-44

13 May 1874
6 a.m.

Pleasley School. You did not remember to give me notice, as you promised, that you stayed Tuesday in London, and when you came on Tuesday afternoon you could not stop. So I can only put on paper the results of my labours. I have done what you wished; I have consulted several school and sanitary authorities, and they all agree with me in this:

1. That it is quite out of the question to build an *infant school* with so little sunlight or indeed window space at all. An infant school ought to have its *two long* sides and one of its short ones quite *open* to the *sun and air*, so that the children may have the sun from the moment they come into school till the moment they leave, *S.E., S.W., N.W.* (closing it to the *N.E.*). It is well known that both health and power of learning depend on this—in infants especially. This school has only *one S.E.* and one N.W. window.

The beautiful *S.W.* exposure is entirely blocked up by *gravel yard* and *large schoolroom* and, worst of all, made pestiferous by "*offices*" into

348 Favourite Nightingale cousin William Shore Smith (1831-94).

which it looks. *Pray do not so much* as listen to such a plan. The only proposition we can make is to slew round the *long* side of *infants' room* to the *S.E.* (putting the master's house somewhere else). See *Plan A.* This plan will be of course objected to because of the length of front (*96 feet,* without the thicknesses of walls). And, without knowing the ground, it is impossible to say whether the *master's house* can be detached, or must be added to the length. (This would be an advantage under some circumstances to the appearance, but if the slope is so great as to place the roof of the master's house nearly on the same level as the floor of the school, the advantage we suppose would be lost.)

If the *infants' school* is under a separate *mistress* and carried on altogether separate from the *mixed school,* as we should imagine from the numbers being so large, would it be possible to detach the *infants' school* and make *one block* of the *infants' school and master's house*? and *another* of the *large schoolroom and classroom*? The only way to give a proper (*S.E.*) aspect to the *infants' room* is either to *detach* the *infants' room and master's house,* it would appear, or to submit to the ugliness of the *immensely long* front.

If it were one's own affair, one would cast about for a *site* that would admit of the former plan, and if it is necessary to have communication between the two schools, this could be managed by means of a corridor or lean-to.

2. The *offices* and walls and gravel yards blocking in the whole corner of the building and completing—not even a square but—*a parallelogram* will be pestiferous. (And people wonder that *country* schools have measles and scarlet fever!!!) The *offices* must be projected far out behind.

3. The *large schoolroom* has a good *S.E.* and *S.W.* exposure, but the *porch must* be moved up to the part of the wall adjoining *classroom.* Else it intercepts sun on winter afternoons.

4. The *classroom* will have *no sun* all the year round: *S.W.* and *N.E.* windows!!! except *summer,* the worst sun, viz., afternoon sun. But I know not how to improve it (and it is of far less importance than *infants' room*). I would however block up *N.E.* window and give one large *S.W.* (*or two*) and one *N.W.* window.

Pray assure Mr Stewart, if he will accept it, of my very great interest in these schools, which must excuse my very strong convictions against parts of the plan (*as it is*) and of my desire to subscribe, if he will allow me. You know how overworked (and underhelped) and suffering I am, so that I am hardly able even to undertake this small extra correspondence. *God speed the schools. . . .* I am writing this *before* my day's work.

Children's Hospitals, 1874-76

Editor: Nightingale's considerable objections to children's hospitals, which had become fashionable charities, have already been made clear in *Notes on Hospitals* and some correspondence. However, when she was actually sent plans for criticism, she gave detailed advice. The first example goes back to 1859, with the Lisbon Children's Hospital (see p 524 above). In the letter immediately following, the hospital in question was in Moscow, directed by the distinguished pediatrician Karl Andreyevich Rauchfuss (1835-1915). Rauchfuss was the founder of the Russian pediatric society, had been director of the St Petersburg Children's Hospital, and was soon to become director of the Vladimir Children's Hospital, Moscow, the hospital at issue here. He was noted for his insistence on the careful separation of infectious cases from other cases.

The timing of Dr Rauchfuss's approach was lucky for Nightingale, for she learned something of winter climate conditions and hospital ventilation from her interaction with him. She then put that knowledge to use for planning the Montreal General Hospital as winter conditions are very similar between the two cities. She was soon quoting "the *Russian*" to the effect that "what the *Canadians* said was *impossible* was *perfectly easy*" (in the first letter below).

The approach to Nightingale was made through a St-Thomas'-trained nurse, Emily M. Gregory (1845-1911), who explained that Dr Rauchfuss, then on visit in London, wanted to consult her.[349] Nightingale evidently provided him with detailed criticisms, of which no record is extant. Indirectly we know that the then home sister at St Thomas', Maria Machin (1843-1905), met Dr Rauchfuss soon after. She wrote Nightingale:

> He asks me, as I told him I was writing to you, to say he is *most grateful* to you for your criticisms, regrets so much he had not better plans to place before you, but had hoped it would be possible to do in person, and thus explain and discuss much that is imperfectly represented in those plans. He will write you from St Petersburg,

---

349 Gregory letter 21 August 1874, Add Mss 45804 f14.

> sending better plans, copious explanations, etc., and answering the questions in the criticism. I think he places unbounded confidence in your judgment and opinions, and as for your *Notes on Hospitals,* says there is no such other valuable book on hospitals existing—a very earnest man he seems, and so deeply interested in the training scheme, etc.[350]

Source: From a letter to John Sutherland, Add Mss 45757 ff261-64

4 January 1875

Moscow Children's Hospital. The enclosed gentleman came to London at the end of August with plans of the above, as he said to consult me. At the same time came two Canadian gentlemen from Montreal with proposals to us to send a Canadian lady we have in training (an admirable one) and nurses to their *old* hospital—*improvements* to be made—at Montreal.

The collision was in the nick of time, since the *Russian* declared that what the *Canadians* said was *impossible* was *perfectly easy,* viz., ventilation by *windows* open—*open* fireplaces.

W.C.s in *outside* wall, apparatus to prevent water and soil pipes from freezing. (Everybody was out of London but me so I made what *strife* I could by myself. You were abroad.) The Russian has now written me the enclosed letter [missing], in answer to my written (August) criticisms. I have from memory put down a slight sketch of one of the eight buildings. There was much that was really beautiful, but the administrative and nursing arrangements were fabulously insufficient.

Proposed Moscow *Children's Hospital,* from memory. One building (out of eight) for "surgical and internal diseases"; (one storey this wing), boys' ward for sixteen beds. Play room for girls and boys. Vestibule, W.C., bath, etc. Two storeys, thirty beds for infants, both sexes. . . .

1-bed operating room
1 bed
2 beds
1 bed
1 bed
1 bed
1 bed

---

350 Machin letter to Nightingale 25 August 1874, Add Mss 47745 f33.

1 bed		
W.C. bath and vestibule		
Girls' ward		Corridor
for 16 beds	Porch and	(Nurses' rooms above
	Entrance	2nd Storey)

(I think there was more *outside* wall in this Moscow plan than in any plan I ever saw.) The advantages of [the] plan were enormous: *outside* windows and ventilation by windows . . . pipes and water prevented from freezing by warm water apparatus. But there was no W.C., bathroom, nurses' room or scullery *to* any of the *wards*. The *one*-bed wards all opened out of one another and into the corridor, which corridor was closed at both ends—at one end by a darkish vestibule (and wing), at the other by W.C.s (and wing). Over the centre building are the nurses' rooms.

One of my criticisms to the most intelligent projector (Dr Rauchfuss) was that *all* the nurses' rooms were away from the wards. He concludes from this that I wish *all* the nurses' rooms to adjoin wards. Like a man, he does not see (all the nurses, it appears are under him at St Petersburg, as under a director at Moscow) the absolute necessity, rather *more* in a *children's* hospital than anywhere else, rather more where *mothers* are admitted to nurse their own children in *one*-bed wards than under any other circumstances, of having a *head nurse* or sister *sleeping off her own ward* in command of her own ward or division day *and night*, and of having a matron.

(It is rather disheartening to be having always to repeat this self-evident axiom.)

Editor: No further correspondence is available on the Moscow (Vladimir) Children's Hospital. Based on the pavilion principle, the hospital was built on a large parcel of land, for a total of 180 beds, well spread out. It was opened on 15 July 1876, the feast day of St Vladimir. In 1878 it was recognized as a model at the Exposition Internationale at Paris, and it was awarded a gold medal as the best children's hospital in Europe at the 1897 World Exhibition in Brussels. The hospital was allowed to fall into ruins during the Communist era.

The next children's hospital on which Nightingale worked was in Staffordshire, for which only one letter survives. This letter, written for public consumption, was read by Dr Godfrey Wedgwood (1833-1900) at a public meeting to consider the establishment of such a hospital and subsequently published in a local newspaper. It shows that Nightingale had not modified her negative views of children's hospitals and children's wards and, moreover, she now also wondered about their nursing standards. She said that she knew of no good nurse training conducted in a children's hospital, which made her doubt the quality of nursing they provided. She regretted that there were no reliable comparative statistics on length of stay or mortality, as between children placed in general wards, special children's wards and children's hospitals.

Source: Nightingale published letter, *Staffordshire Advertiser* 22 January 1876:3

I wish I could answer your question with regard to children's hospitals, and children's wards in general hospitals, with more satisfaction to you and myself. I have not "modified the opinion" to which you refer in my *Notes on Hospitals*. Rather do I see reason every year to be confirmed in it. But every "view" is to be "modified" according to its modifications (i.e., mutatis mutandis [with appropriate changes]). A local district wants according to its local wants. A local arrangement is modified according to its local modifications. I can only explain this by giving illustrations, and I will give none but actual facts coming within my own experience, e.g. (1) an experienced matron or head nurse, whose "opinion" is really valuable, tells you "never put sick children in an adult ward; they disturb the other patients." You inquire, and you find her experience to be that of a ward of forty beds, where throughout the winter there have never been less than twenty severe children's cases, chiefly burns, and twenty "heavy" adult cases, all of them too serious to think of anything but themselves, or to be able to take any other interest in a child than to be disturbed by its moans and cries. It is obvious that here the very object of treating children amongst adults is lost by their being treated amongst adults. If, added to this, the head nurse has not that peculiar power, which seems almost a gift, of soothing children, so that the most suffering cases will not cry, but will quietly lie patient or even happy, you have certainly the most imperative of all conditions for treating your sick children apart.

Crying children do not so much disturb one another as they disturb women seriously ill or in a state of prostration. Children's cases must obviously bear a certain proportion to adult cases in the ward, and not only this but to severe adult cases, if their presence there is to be a benefit to themselves and the other cases. If they exceed this proportion, there must be a children's ward for the excess of infants and very young cases. But I think I would never put this children's ward into a building so separate that the same current supervision cannot be extended to it. And I would add that a great medical school of students, and a great training school of nurse probationers ("lady" and otherwise), materially diminish the danger of children being left to the mercy of one or more nurses, for you bear in mind that children cannot complain like adults.

But I would also say that I know at present in England hardly any one children's hospital or children's ward in [a] general hospital, which gives a good training to probationers, and when I see this I extremely doubt the quality of the nursing or supervision. I wish my children back in the general wards.

Now take the other side. (2) An equally experienced matron or head nurse whose "opinion" is as valuable as that of No. 1 tells you, "Never put your sick children except in an adult ward; they do the other patients so much good, and the other patients nurse them." You inquire, and you find her experience to be that of a ward of thirty-two beds, with five or six (or even more) children in it, a clever sister (head nurse) placing each next [to] an adult whose own woes are capable of alleviation by alleviating the child's. You see, e.g., a young unmarried man of twenty (who has not been over sober or over good in times past) taking the entire charge of washing and amusing and feeding a troublesome, naughty child of three, who will be good with no one else but its impromptu nurse, whom, however, it has never seen before. What good influence can replace this for either man or child? The man, even when in the progress of his disease, too seriously worse to leave his bed, has the child's bed wheeled up to his with doctor's and nurse's joyful consent, and both continue their care of each other, and both recover.

A little mombey of two, a lithotomy case, swore frightfully in a children's ward, and with two nurses, one by day and one by night, to itself, was almost unmanageable. It was placed in an adult ward; it was quite quiet and good. Where there is a good sister (head nurse) you rarely, if ever, hear swearing in a man's ward. But everything depends on the head nurse.

I might multiply instances, but everyone can do it for himself. I despair of seeing anything like a children's hospital with proper adjuncts in England. May I add that, in your case, I should feel more inclined to have the roughest children's convalescent home by the sea, of about twenty-four beds, than to put them in the kind of building you describe. The difficulty of getting a really good *children's ward* head nurse ("sister") I believe to be immense. I have known but few in my whole life. "L'art fait un cuisinier; on est né rôtisseur";[351] art (training) makes a hospital nurse; one must be *born* a *children's* hospital nurse. If I have said nothing satisfactory to you, may my good intentions stand in lieu of deed. I would gladly help your case if I could.

I have kept this open several days hoping to get you some additional information. It would be exceedingly interesting to find out the relative rate of mortality and duration of sickness in children's cases, otherwise *similar*, placed in "general" or "children's" wards or hospitals, but unfortunately hospital statistics are not sufficiently well kept to ascertain this. I am (perhaps more than ever) under pressure of illness and business.

Editor: It seems that Nightingale and Douglas Galton were consulted about a new building for the Norfolk and Norwich Hospital in 1875. According to a history of the hospital, Galton visited it in February 1875 to ascertain its defects, put forward Nightingale and Godwin's ideas, and advised on costs.[352] However, there is no surviving correspondence between Nightingale and Galton for 1875, so details are lacking. Nightingale had received what she considered to be inadequate statistics from a doctor at the hospital in 1864 (see p 658 above). A later analysis of mortality data from this hospital shows that its rates were not decreasing, and that those for 1860-79 were slightly higher than those for 1830-59.[353] The hospital duly had plans prepared by a local architect and later mayor, Edward Boardman, with T.H. Wyatt, beginning in 1876.

The new two-storey hospital was built on the pavilion principle, with wards of twenty-two beds,[354] in short, closely heeding the advice of Nightingale and Galton. It was closed in 2003 and replaced by the new Norfolk and Norwich University Hospital.

351 From a French proverb that does not translate well: a man can make himself into a cook, but one must be born to grill well.

352 Jeremy Taylor, *The Rebirth of the Norfolk and Norwich Hospital 1874-1883: An Architectural Exploration* 6.

353 S. Cherry, "The Role of a Provincial Hospital: The Norfolk and Norwich Hospital 1771-1880," *Population Studies* 26,2 (July 1972): 291-308.

354 Taylor, *The Rebirth of the Norfolk and Norwich Hospital* 10.

Montreal General Hospital, 1874-76

Editor: When Nightingale was asked to supply a matron and nurses for the Montreal General Hospital, there was good reason to be concerned about their health and safety. A new, improved, hospital building and nurses' home were intended, she was told, but she wanted firm assurances, "in black and white, i.e., in plans" (in the first letter below), before deciding on sending a team. Nightingale urged the selected matron, Canadian-born Maria Machin, not to agree to go until such assurances were given, but Machin had already signed a contract. As it turned out, construction for neither the new hospital nor the nurses' home had begun, due to a serious unforeseen economic downturn in Montreal. The material here, then, relates advice that was not acted upon.[355] The advice itself was influenced by information Nightingale had only recently acquired about cold-weather climates from Moscow (see p 803 above).

Officials at the Montreal General sought Nightingale's views on their building proposals even before they had any actual plans, again not the way to proceed, she thought. There were numerous misunderstandings in the correspondence, for she did not like to propose an architect, although she sometimes compromised and did. She offered to criticize the plans when drawn up. The hospital evidently sent Nightingale the plans of the existing building, which she needed to plan the nursing for it. She gave them the "most minute and careful study," to conclude that there were "no improvements or alterations" that could make the present building into "a good hospital." It was "hopelessly unhealthy and inconvenient," so that "it would be throwing good money after bad to attempt it." It would be "far more economical to obtain convenient ground for building a new hospital" (see p 812 below), a point she would often make in criticizing hospital plans.

The matron and nurses duly went to Montreal in 1875 to a defective building, and suffered for it, as did the patients and doctors. One of the six nurses sent out died, as did the doctor fiancé of the matron.

---

355 On the complicated history of the planning and building of the Montreal General Hospital see H.E. MacDermot, *A History of the Montreal General Hospital*; W.F. Hamilton, "The Montreal General Hospital: Its Organization, History and Management, with Plans of Surgical Pavilions and New Operating Amphitheater,"in *Papers and Discussions in the International Congress of Charities, Correction and Philanthropy* 404-14.

Several further nurses were sent out but, in 1878, Machin and all her nurses quit and returned to England. Alex Graham's plans for a new hospital were simply dropped as too expensive for the time, as is explained in an aptly titled article "The Hospital that Never Was."[356] A new nurses' home was not built until 1897, when Lord Lister laid the foundation stone of what became the Jubilee Nurses' Home.[357]

In due course, a second English-speaking hospital was planned for Montreal, the Royal Victoria Hospital, which took the pressure off for expansion at the Montreal General. Nightingale did a great deal of work on the plans for the Royal Victoria (see p 891 below).

Source: From two letters to Maria Machin, Thomas K. Fisher Rare Book Library, University of Toronto

26 August 1874
5 A.M.

I do most solemnly say, don't commit yourself to Montreal on any such understanding as this, "that if your demands are within reason, they are ready to do everything, etc." Have the *plans* of what they consent to do sent here to you (I will show them to the War Office). If they are what WE think "within reason," then and not till then consider their proposal for yourself and nurses.

I will not write to Mr Bonham Carter without your leave, but I do most emphatically say that, in your interest and in that of the nurses, I consider it our duty to decline letting them have our nurses till we see in *black and white what improvements in accommodation and construction* they propose to make, i.e., in PLANS. I am quite sure that Mrs Wardroper and he are of the same opinion, and I charge you to let Mr B.C. see this note before any interview takes place between him and your vice president. No time for more. God speed you. . . .

When I see what sanitary arrangements they propose as feasible in a much severer climate like Russia, I think it simply impossible to let nurses go to that Montreal Hospital till we know what they will do to improve it.

---

356 "E.H. Bensley, "The Hospital that Never Was," *Pages of History* (reprinted from *Dominion Illustrated* 12 January 1889).

357 Taylor, *Hospital and Asylum Architecture in England* 82.

14 April 1875

I think you know full well (almost as well as I do myself), how near my heart lies a good new *model* hospital at Montreal for you, and that I need not repeat what I have already said full often, that I desire and am anxious to look over any plans and to obtain for you the best opinions in England on them.

But I do not quite know what "advice" I can give now that would be of use. All general conditions needful I have stated many times in print. Any particular specification offered by me for that particular piece of ground (though in looking over the plans, an accurate ground plan is of course a first essential to enable one to come to a correct judgment) could only end in disappointment and failure. They must draw their plans; we revise them.

You inquire for an architect—I have always declined to recommend architects. But the man whose work I thoroughly knew to be good at the War Office, and who afterwards set up as an architect for himself, was Alex Graham, Carlton Chambers, 4 Regent St.

You did not enclose the letter you proposed, but anyway I do not see that I can say more than repeat what I have so often said and ever felt, that I rejoice beyond anything of the prospect of a model hospital for Montreal, which must be *new*, and that nothing that I can do to be of any use shall be wanting.

Editor: W. Whiteford[358] wrote Henry Bonham Carter with thanks on his own behalf and that of Peter Redpath (1821-94), president of the Montreal General, for the "very clear statement," which he and Machin had found "to include all the requirements." He asked Bonham Carter to procure Galton's "invaluable suggestions" as soon as possible. This advice, "fortified by the authority of Miss Nightingale and of Captain Galton, may enable Mr Redpath to prevent the adoption of a less complete plan by the board of management in May or June." However, he misunderstood Nightingale's intentions by referring to her wish to see the ground plan "now," to which Bonham Carter added "No," explaining that Redpath was correct in his understanding of her willingness "to revise the architect's plan when sufficiently advanced."

Whiteford clearly saw the broader importance of the Montreal project for the then Dominion of Canada. He closed with: "I know

358 A James W. Whiteford is listed in the *Annual Calendar of McGill College and McGill University*.

the enthusiastic gratitude with which the Canadians, at the connection of Miss N.'s name with the endeavour, to extend to the dominion the system with which she has blessed other portions of the world."[359] As we know, however, the nursing experiment came to an unhappy end and the planned hospital was not built.

Source: From a letter to Henry Bonham Carter,[360] Add Mss 47719 ff107-10

1 May 1875

Montreal plans. I have before expressed the opinion, after the most minute and careful study of the plans of the existing Montreal Hospital, and giving a most elaborate criticism upon them, that no improvements or alterations could make the present building into a good hospital, hopelessly unhealthy and inconvenient as it is, that it would be throwing good money after bad to attempt it, and that it would be far more economical to obtain convenient ground for building a new hospital.

In this opinion I entirely concurred with Captain Galton's, as I do in what follows, namely, that by far the best and most economical plan, and the only healthy one, would be to acquire at once the whole site bounded by Dorchester St., St Dominique St., St Constant St. and La Gauchetière St., which would form, as far as can be judged from imperfect materials, a most excellent and spacious site for a hospital of 400 beds. I also agree with Captain Galton that, if infectious blocks are to be built, they should be on the ground already possessed by the hospital N.W. of Dorchester St., and that in the meantime, that is, till the whole site south of Dorchester St. can be obtained, these two suggested pavilions might be used for the general hospital accommodation now wanted.

N.B. Referring to *Mr Whiteford's* letter, there must be some mistake. F.N. wrote almost the converse of what he says, namely, that she could not undertake to suggest a plan for their ground, and that, even if she could, it would be most undesirable that she should take that responsibility, *that they should themselves select an architect, give him a ground plan of their site to be acquired,* and *he* should make their plans for that site, *the best that could be obtained,* and that she would then, if desired, care-

359 Whiteford letter 21 April 1875, Thomas K. Fisher Rare Book Library, University of Toronto.

360 Nightingale sent a letter the same day with much the same content to Maria Machin, in *Extending Nursing* (13:532-33); two further letters to Machin are in the same volume (13:536-38).

fully make, upon the architect's plans, any suggestions in her power (as she has often done before). They desired her to recommend an architect; she declined, but at their request mentioned the address of Mr Alex Graham, whose hospital work she had known for years at the W.O. . . . Either Mr Graham or Mr T.H. Wyatt would be a competent hospital architect.

Captain Galton and the Army Sanitary Commission, etc., *are* the experts whose opinion F.N. promised to obtain.

Editor: The architect selected, Alex Graham, wrote Nightingale the next week requesting a meeting with her on the plans.[361] Nightingale had to make the case, again, that nurses should not have to use the patients' toilets, especially in a hospital with smallpox and fever patients (see p 815 below). Nurses and probationers should have their own washstand in their rooms, and not have to use a common lavatory. The matron's rooms should not be near the furnace room. The post-mortem room should not be under the nursing superintendent's room—nor anywhere else in the building—but in a separate building. Graham apparently obliged by making substantial changes in his next set of plans.

Source: From a copy of a letter to Maria Machin, Florence Nightingale Museum

2 June 1875

Montreal Hospital plans. The plans were left late last night here and I have given them one careful looking-over this morning and written one criticism.

I think them admirable, but (as you ask me) I say most definitely that I do NOT "consider it wise to send them as they are over to Montreal." We quite agreed, if you remember, that they were to receive all kinds of suggestions from experts, when they were sketched. These are only sketch plans.

I was all packed up to leave for Norwood with my mother on Friday, but I will stay till Monday if it will be any comfort to you, that I should put forward the criticizing of these plans and look them over with you. I have Sir George Campbell[362] coming today, my mother's

---

361 Graham letter to Nightingale 8 May 1875, Thomas K. Fisher Rare Book Library, University of Toronto.

362 Sir George Campbell (1824-92), governor of Bengal.

solicitor tomorrow, so could not see you till Friday or Saturday. [I] will at once send to see if the Army Sanitary Commission will look at the plans today. But please remember that professional men are not like us—and keep plans for as many days as I do hours.

Source: From a letter to John Sutherland, Add Mss 45757 ff284-93

2 June 1875

Montreal General Hospital. Could you kindly look over these plans and make any suggestions? I enclose a few of mine (very imperfect, as yet). We are requested to make haste, but this should not prevent the most careful scrutiny. I am staying on purpose. . . . .

Will the *private paying patients* come, unless their wards are in a *separate block* or cluster from the mass of patients?

General Hospital. I conclude that this hospital can be so *warmed* as to admit of *open fireplaces, open windows,* of the *W.C.* and other pipes *not freezing* and hydraulic machinery ditto, and so *ventilated* that when windows can't be opened there will be *fresh air* provided.

Out-patient department. It is certainly undesirable to have this *under* the wards, though it appears well cut off.

Accident Receiving Wards. Doors too narrow and an awkward turn for carrying in patients, *if from corridor.* Or are they to pass *through in*-patients waiting hall? Undesirable to have *stores under wards,* though kitchen being under chapel is well contrived.

Where are *nurses, probationers, to dine?*

Please say whether it would not be undesirable to place *another storey (for probationers)* OVER the *ground floor buildings* one storey) of entrance hall, etc.

Fireplaces. Is it not intended to give *open* fireplaces to lady superintendent's rooms, day rooms, medical officers' rooms?

Smallpox and Fever Hospital.

1. I should not like to be the *private paying patient* in the *small polygonal wards*—they are terribly built in, with *only one corner* squinting out to open air, and *smallpox and fever* ought, if possible, to have the open air ALL ROUND, them as in bathroom. I had much rather be in *bathroom* jutting out at end. Also, I should have thought *private, paying, smallpox and fever* would peculiarly have objected to not having *their small wards* in clusters to themselves. Anyhow, they must have a *W.C. and W.C. sinks* to themselves, as there *is* strong objection to carrying all their W.C. slops THROUGH the wards.

2. And the *nurses* ought *not* to be required to use the *patients' W.C.s*, especially in smallpox and fever patients' *general hospital*.

(1) This objection occurs elsewhere in the hospital. The *lady superintendent* must have *a private W.C.*, and *the nurses* of the *men's* wards at least *a private W.C. on each floor*. And all these *W.C.s* so contrived so that the pipes shall not *freeze*.

(2) The provision of *baths* for the nurses is good. They should also have a *housemaid's closet* to the dormitories.

(3) I think the dormitory for the *seven-day nurses* would require *a W.C.*, or they would so disturb the *sixteen-nurse dormitory* in passing through.

(4) The *windows* of all the dormitories should be so constructed that one woman could *open her half without opening her neighbour's half*.

Ground Floor.

1. *Probationers* (*and nurses* in general) should never be compelled to use *a lavatory*. A *neat washstand* in *each compartment* essential, and the *compartment* must be *large enough* for this.

2. How are the *nurses' compartments to be warmed*?

3. *Lady superintendent* must have *an office*, and also *matron* should not be near furnace room.

4. *Post-mortem room* should be *quite removed from hospital*. It is almost under the *lady superintendent's room* and the *nurses' day room*; *another window* looks down upon its roof.

1st Floor. Not desirable to have a *private paying ward adjoining night nurses'* dormitories; preferably one *nurses' sick ward* may be required, e.g., for a lady probationer who does not like being warded.

Operation Room. Two operation beds may be useful, but (generally) carry your patient *back to his ward* as soon as possible.

1st Floor. Private paying wards off night nurses' dormitory would require a *W.C.*, or all slops would have to be carried *through* either the dormitory, which is impossible, or the female ward, which is undesirable. The objection applies to all the *P.P.* [private paying] wards and *no P.P. patient* would go *through* a ward to his/her W.C., supposing him/her able to use it. Nor should it be required. They should have a *private W.C.*

Editor: Graham wrote Machin a detailed letter on the developments, which she forwarded to Nightingale:

> You may have heard that all "the hospital" plans and documents were despatched to Canada yesterday. I succeeded at the last in making a third design, which I think is fairly successful. It appears

> to meet all the difficulties of the site and the many reasonable objections raised against the original scheme by my generous critics. I do think it would meet with Miss Nightingale's approval.
>
> This third scheme is for 282 beds and eighteen paying patients, exclusive of fifty-eight beds in the infectious wards on the smaller site. This gives a total of 358 beds, without overcrowding on the smaller site. I have also placed a suitable laundry and the entire ophthalmic department, as well as that objectionable little edifice called the deadhouse.
>
> When you see Miss Nightingale, would you kindly tell her how largely I feel indebted to her for all her generosity towards me. Such kindness is never forgotten. Now that Mr Redpath has such abundance of information upon hospital arrangements, I hope he may induce the committee to take some definite action before long, and that when you leave England in August you may have the satisfaction of hearing that the days of the present little disreputable hospital are numbered and all your wishes in regards the new hospital to be committed to your care fully realized.[363]

For (financial) reasons above-noted, the "little disreputable hospital" was not replaced for many years. The last letter in this section reports the death of one of the nurses.

Source: From a letter to Dr Campbell,[364] McGill University School of Nursing Alumnae

11 April 1876

I regret indeed very deeply to lose this opportunity of making your acquaintance, and of hearing news from your own lips of the future prospects of Montreal General Hospital, in which I am so much interested, and of my dear friend Miss Machin.

But alas for me! it is not possible in my state of increasing bodily weakness, and at a time of year when the over pressure of business is particularly heavy, to see you at such short notice, on any day you offer me. But I did not lose a moment after receiving yours in sending to my cousin, Mr Henry Bonham Carter, the secretary of our training school and Miss Machin's friend, who has doubtless written to you before this, who is as anxious as I am for Montreal.

Excuse my pencil writing. I trust that this trip to England will entirely set up your health, and am only sorry not to be able to profit

363 Graham letter to Machin 25 June 1875, Add Mss 47745 ff59-66.

364 Dr George William Campbell (1810-82), dean of the Faculty of Medicine, McGill University.

by your presence on this side the water, which I should so have wished myself.

Source: From a letter to Douglas Galton, ADD MSS 45764 f235

9 May 1876

Montreal: You remember your verdict on the old *hospital* and the proposed new one, and what you were kind enough to write. Greatly against my will, we sent out nurses to the *old hospital*; seven months from the day of their sailing, one, the noblest of them all, a young nurse whom we cannot replace,[365] died of *typhoid* (a public mourning to *us*) and ten of the nursing staff were under medical treatment for various forms of *hospital filth* disease.

I don't like to say much more about it for Miss Machin, our admirable superintendent there, is so terribly cut up; she is a Canadian.

Editor: Correspondence on other issues resumes.

Source: From a letter to Edwin Chadwick, University College, London ff110-11

6 October 1875

I have to thank you for two kind letters and your admirable proof. It is quite perfect, except that at *p 3* (italic type beginning "water supplies").

1. Is it not certain that water should *not* be conveyed into *every living room*? Would not the houses be uninhabitable?

2. Is it not a fundamental principles that no sink pipe should be connected with a drain? Should it not open *over it* in the open air?

3. Should not a W.C. pipe be carried up *open* to above the roof?

I think that these are probably only oversights? In many hospitals it is now the custom to place the sinks on the outside wall in such a way that they can be got at by throwing up a window, and then completely isolated by drawing down the window.

You give a great many excellent hints, especially about non-absorbent materials. (The exact quantity of water a brick holds is 12½ oz., a piece of cement of same size only ¼ oz. or 1/25th as much, is it not?) This is of immense importance in the warming of a house.

Will "the reward of the architects," which you propose at the end, viz., credit, tempt them to do much, or keep them alive long?

365 Martha Rice (c1853-76), who began training at St Thomas' in 1874.

Editor: The identification of the proposed midwifery institution in the letter immediately below is not clear, nor if it was ever built. Architect Stephen Salter (1825-96), a pupil of T.H. Wyatt, was the architect for King's College Hospital.

Source: From notes, Florence Nightingale Museum (LMA) H1/ST/SJ/A44/1

[January 1876]

Mr Salter appears to forget that in "trying to assimilate" his "plan" to that of "lying-in women's own homes" he has omitted *the most essential* condition, viz., that in any room inhabited by the same couple, *a second delivery* CANNOT *take place within* ten months, and may not take place for years. *This I believe to be the real secret of safety at home.*

The nearest approach that can be made for her is to have *two delivery wards to each floor,* one of them always standing empty month and month about.

It would be impossible to nurse this, in many respects *admirable construction,* with only *twelve pupil midwives,* even were there *three qualified training midwives,* as there ought to be (and for the first year, two qualified nurses besides). Nor could there be any *training* worth the name in such a case: *see note at back.* With *twenty-seven* occupied beds, there might well be *twenty-five pupils,* or with *thirty-six,* three [illeg] and there *must* be a thorough, sufficient and completely organized, and thoroughly qualified TRAINING MIDWIFE *staff.* (I do not think one midwife to every six or eight pupils too much—this is roughly speaking, for the *staff midwives* are, of course, not "told off" in this way.)

There should also be a *classroom.* . . .

The architect states that *three beds* only out of each set of four are to be occupied at the same time. If there are *delivery* wards, it would not be necessary to have one ward out of four always undergoing cleansing (i.e., each empty for three months), especially as *one block* out of four must be always undergoing a thorough cleaning, scraping, limewashing and standing empty for rest and aeration.

Are there not too many windows and draughts (through a fault on the right side) to the *wards*? . . .

Ward ventilation, is not this open to some question? The architect proposes to combine Tobin tubes with the ventilating grate. He says the Tobin tube is intended to clear out the air from the stagnant corners of the room, but in one half of the room he places the tube in the corner close to the door, where the opening of the door would prevent stagnation. Would not the long channels for these tubes soon become foul and be difficult to clean? Moreover the inlet for foul air, thus proposed, would it not prevent the action of the ventilating grate when the fire is lighted? In warm weather it would only act provided there are adequate means for the removal of the air as well as for the admission of fresh air. The Sherringham ventilators would scarcely suffice for the exit, and moreover would allow the foul air to pass into the upper wards.

On these grounds is it not essential *to provide shafts carried from a little below the ceiling of each ward* SEPARATELY, *to above the roof*, the lower part of the shaft to be terminated by a louvred opening, so that, in case the action should be reversed, there should be no down draught? The bottom of the shaft should be capable of being removed to admit to easy cleaning. The shafts should be placed in the corner of the room on the same side as the ventilating fireplace. The proposed ventilation would differ for admission of fresh air.

As regards the *corridor and passages*, if these are to be closed (by ventilating division windows to open and close by a handle) and warmed, it should be by coils of pipes in each, heated from a central boiler, and fresh air should be admitted through the coils so as to ensure the ventilation of each corridor and lobby separately.

Editor: Nightingale's involvement in 1876 in the design of Johns Hopkins hospital was evidently considerable, but the correspondence is largely missing. The Quaker businessman and philanthropist Johns Hopkins (1795-1873) gave the money, then the largest philanthropic gift in the United States, for the university, hospital and associated medical and nursing schools. He had set out instructions for the new hospital, and bought the site, before his death. No plans had by then been drawn up, however, and the project was handed over to John Shaw Billings (1833-1913) for realization.[366] Billings, an army doctor, not an architect, nonetheless did the design himself, which had to be redone many times.[367] The philanthropist's instructions had set the size of the hos-

366 John S. Billings, *Description of the Johns Hopkins Hospital*; see also Zachary Cope, "John Shaw Billings, Florence Nightingale and the Johns Hopkins Hospital," *News, Notes and Queries* 367-68; Henry M. Hurd, "Description of the Johns Hopkins Hospital, Baltimore," in *Papers and Discussions in the International Congress of Charities, Correction and Philanthropy* 429-43.

367 Annmarie Adams, *Medicine by Design: The Architect and the Modern Hospital 1893-1947* 9.

pital at 400 patients, who were to be mainly free patients, and admitted without regard to sex, age or race. He left open the possibility of expansion. There was to be a convalescent hospital and an orphan asylum as well. The hospital should "compare favourably with any institution of like character in the country or in Europe." The grounds were to have trees and flowers and "afford solace to the sick" and be no less than "an ornament" to the city (see picture on p 496).[368]

In 1876 Billings wrote Henry Bonham Carter asking for hospital reports, rules and regulations. Bonham Carter put him in touch with the St Thomas' matron, Sarah E. Wardroper, who in turn passed on to Nightingale his request for assistance on the plans. Billings duly sent Nightingale the information and asked what she thought: "They are only sketch plans and I desire criticism before going farther."[369] Nightingale apparently consulted Douglas Galton first, as she usually did, then sent Dr Sutherland the plans, along with Galton's comments.

When Dr Sutherland advised Nightingale of the safe arrival of the plans, he regretted the trouble to her by people taking "nobody's opinion but their own." He called the plans "somewhat old acquaintances of mine." Further, they had been:

> sent to me along with others by someone in England, and I saw in a moment that not one of the plans ought to receive one word of sanction from me. I simply said that the architects had taken every proposal they had heard of, and strung them together without any attention to economy or necessity.
>
> When any dyspeptic patient came to Abernathy he used to take his fee and dismiss him with a recommendation to read his book. I should feel disposed, if I were you, to commit yourself in no way to these plans, but to say that you were thoroughly aware of the requirements of hospital construction and that, if the plans admitted of criticism, you would gladly have helped to perfect them. Such, however, not being the case, you beg to refer them to your book on hospitals, which contained an amount of those fundamental principles required to be embodied in hospital plans. As it is, one might suspect, from the plans, that they were intended as a mauvaise plaisanterie [bad joke] to show how the sick might nurse the attendants. I have sent the plans to Captain Galton.

---

368 Johns Hopkins letter to Trustees, in Alan M. Chesney, *The Johns Hopkins Hospital and the Johns Hopkins University School of Medicine* 13.

369 Billings letter to Nightingale 23 October 1876, Add Mss 45804 f169, typed copy Royal College of Surgeons Box 3(1).

Another letter by Sutherland to Nightingale advised that he was returning the plans, with Galton's remarks, with which he concurred.[370] She then brought together all this material in a twelve-page report, dated 2 December 1876, but not extant. Billings's reply acknowledged the extensive advice:

> Your remarks shall be laid before the trustees as soon as I return to America, and I feel sure that they will be very greatly interested in and influenced by your criticisms. The labour and expense of conducting a hospital built on this general plan I fully appreciate, as also the complications which arise in trying to cut off all service rooms from the ward.

He explained that no less than five different plans had been made, the first of which, he thought, avoided her objections. He agreed with her that only one or two blocks should be built at first. He Would "not attempt now to comment upon your notes, nor indeed do I think it probable that I should do otherwise than agree with them."[371]

There were then serious delays in building owing to the substantial drop in value of the railway shares in the Hopkins bequest. The hospital eventually opened, partially finished, in 1889, reduced in size but still very much in accordance with the principles of its benefactor. It was in the pavilion style, but with three storeys rather than the preferred one or two; the toilets were well separated and ventilated; and pathology was located in a separate building. Billings gave very careful attention to ventilation.

The separate fever building went further than other hospitals at the time in isolating patients and nurses. Each patient had a separate room, independently ventilated, and there was a vestibule between it and the corridor. Rooms for nurses were provided in the building so that they would not carry infection into the regular nursing quarters. This is in line with Nightingale's advice, but goes beyond it with the vestibules and rigorously separate ventilating shafts for each room.

The first matron at Johns Hopkins, appointed in 1889, was Canadian-born Isabel Hampton Robb (1860-1910), whom Nightingale mentored. The assistant matron was the British-born Louisa Parsons (1855-1916), who had trained at St Thomas' and who, like Robb, went on to a dis-

---

370 Sutherland letters 14 and 18 November 1876, Add Mss 45758 ff52-53 and 54-55.

371 Billings letter 4 December 1876, Add Mss 45804 f173, typed copy Royal College of Surgeons of England Box 3(1)/Ms 0261/4.

tinguished career as a nursing leader. The nursing school opened on 9 October 1889.

Nightingale's involvement (presumably on both nursing and the plans) was evidently appreciated, for the hospital had a statuette of her prominently displayed. A letter of the university president to Henry Bonham Carter in 1893 encloses a photograph of it, with the information that the statuette itself was then on display at the Chicago Exhibition.[372] Henry Mills Hurd (1843-1927), the hospital's first medical superintendent, wrote Nightingale as late as 1910.[373]

Correspondence on other matters resumes.

Source: From a letter to Henry Graves, Columbia University, Presbyterian Hospital School of Nursing C116

29 January 1877

I am extremely indebted to you for your note of the 25th with reference to the verse of the hospital hymn. I should like to have one done after the present sketch (returned), viz., on "drawing paper" in "black letters" with the *capitals* in *colours* as here indicated, and also "*brightened here and there with a little colour,*" as mentioned. "And mounted on a strainer, price £2.10." It has been suggested to me that the *words* might be a line or two more *apart,* without or scarcely lengthening the whole. If this one succeeds, I shall have at least one more copy done, with your kind permission. I will ask leave to be allowed to decide whether to have them *framed,* after I have seen the first "mounted on a strainer."

The beautiful engravings gave the most affecting impression and immense pleasure at Edinburgh Infirmary. They beg to return their truest thanks.

---

372 Letter 18 October 1893, Florence Nightingale Museum (LMA) H1/ST/NC18/28/26.

373 Letter of acknowledgment by Nightingale's secretary, to an invitation to send a message to the graduating class, with a copy of Dr Hurd's address at the graduating ceremonies, 29 July 1910, Johns Hopkins University.

Source: From a letter to John Sutherland, Add Mss 45758 f56

15 February 1877

"*Art in Hospitals.*" *Dr Lawrence-Hamilton.*[374] I wrote to this man declining to be on his committee—telling him that "bric à brac," "old armour," etc., in wards would not do and the reason why.

Would you revise the enclosed extract from my letter telling him *what you would do*, and say what *you* think *would do*? And would you also tell me whether you think I should let him publish it? And would you also send me, *for myself*, not for publication, a sentence of yours which you sent me, about three years ago, for Miss Lees,[375] defining the evils of hospital dust: what it includes, viz., flakes of skin, and what is the beau ideal [perfect way] of removing it, from bedclothes, etc., to which we are to come as near as we can in practice?

Source: From a letter to Harry Verney, Wellcome (Claydon copy) Ms 9007/96

19 April 1877

Parthe's birthday

In answer to your question, a *hospital* architect requiring special study, experience, knowledge of requirements and innate talent, I know no one who unites these qualifications, except Douglas Galton, so well as Alex Graham, 4 Regent St. I know no class of murderers who have killed so many people as hospital architects. At this moment (1877) there are many diseases less fatal in their most wretched homes than in hospitals, i.e., hospitals secure a higher mortality. Medical men with few exceptions have not turned their attention at all to hospital requirements as buildings.

Editor: It seems that Douglas Galton asked Nightingale in late 1877 to review plans for a new building for University College Hospital. The notes with the letter immediately below are the result, but there is no other surviving correspondence on the request. She was appalled that the post-mortem theatre was placed in a regular ward, next to the outpatients' department, knowing that the high death rate of the midwifery ward at King's College Hospital was at least partly the result of its proximity to the post-mortem room (see p 824 below).

Alterations and enlargement took place, but what influence Nightingale might have had on them is not clear. The hospital reopened in

374 J. Lawrence-Hamilton, "Art in Hospitals," *The Lancet* 109,2789 (10 February 1877):219.

375 Florence Lees (1840-1922), later Craven, district nursing leader.

October 1879, but it was not until 1904 that a completely new building for University College Hospital finally opened.

Source: From a letter to Douglas Galton, Add Mss 45764 ff237-38, and notes, Add Mss 45820 ff5-9

7 July 1877

University College Hospital. I have done my very best, though at the last moment of business, with these plans, which I return to you with seven pages of notes upon them.

The most ample or even excessive cubic space can be of no avail where *post-mortem room* is in one ward and *out-patients* in another. I do most earnestly hope that you will warn them in time. Do you know, among all the plans, both Continental and British that have been sent me to criticize for twenty years, this is the first I have ever seen with the *post-mortem room* in a *ward.* Surely we have terrible experience enough of post-mortem rooms in much better positions than this revenging themselves upon their hospitals to make this impossible.

(I began work before 6 this morning to put on paper my strong conviction about this to you—without delay.) They will disgrace themselves forever if they do it. If you *could* prevent it . . . !!

University [College Hospital]: to persons about to—Don't. Pavilion principle of course an improvement, but this [is] as bad as it can be. If it is a necessity to build a hospital and out-patients department on this site, then it is a necessity to have increased death rate, increased average time in hospital and fewer recoveries—very much increased percentage of hospital disease. Out-patients department and W.C.s *under* wards, in fact, in place of a lower ward, absolutely inadmissible. (Are male and female out-patients to be in same waiting room—and out-patients' W.C. to be under patients' larder?) The out-patients' department, and more especially the W.C.s, though nowhere *under* the wards, a perpetual nuisance and source of hospital disease at St T. This is denied by none.

Post-mortem room and mortuary inconceivable over a ward. This is far worse than at King's[376]—yet what a destruction that made.

376 Nightingale concluded that a major factor in the high rate of puerperal fever was the post-mortem room in the basement, with an open staircase facilitating communication of disease, such that "the smell of the post-mortem theatre" was "quite perceptible in the ward." In *Women* (8:193).

Kitchen over wards, servants' hall and lecture theatre!!! over ward. Should never be in same block. What a noise overhead, much more objectionable to patients than under their feet.

How are the patients to be got down from operating theatre and through that narrow corridor? Operating theatre should be on same level as principal surgical wards, with a broad corridor between and staircase.

Does he call that "larder" an "adequate provision for storing provisions in connection with the wards"? I wish the "occupants of the mews" would "raise an objection" to having the hospital there altogether, as the hospital won't raise an objection to having the mews there altogether.

Private wards looking into mews. Preserve the patients—they had much better be in public wards. W.C.s not sufficiently outside, and access from centre wards inconvenient. At least put door of adjacent private room in corner farthest from W.C. Is there to be no slop sink, bath or scullery for all those private wards? Are those in public wards to be made use of? I don't see where erysipelas wards are.

No nurse's room all over the building. Where is a nurse to retire? What supervision over night nurses?

Scullery must have a fireplace for heating things for patients. Nothing could be kept in that larder. Bad plan to raise up W.C. and lavatory. Are male patients to pass through bath to get to W.C.? Bath should be on one side, W.C. on other, scullery and nurse's room on each side doorway.

Then dead, the outside people and the live patients mixed up, intolerable.

Are there any dust and dirty linen chutes?

Basement beyond criticism. Coals in an objectionable place and patients' lift adjoining.

No possibility that out-patients' effluvia will be drawn off by furnace.

Dead lift, inquest room, coals, chaplain, baths and splints all mixed up together indescribably. And that horrid mews behind, all with "tenements" of the most inferior description. You cannot criticize a building where out-patients are in one ward and no nurse's room, post-mortems in another anywhere, and kitchen and servants' hall in another. End of blocks ought to be free—as you say—not with that bank of private wards before them.

Editor: The hospital in question in the next letter was presumably the Brompton Hospital for Consumption, for a letter a short time later announced Nightingale as being able to recommend a matron for that hospital. In it she remarked, "I earnestly hope to hear, for *their* sake, that, at yesterday's 'general committee,' Mr Graham was appointed architect for the proposed new wing."[377] (In fact another architect was appointed, T.H. Wyatt.) The "new wing" was a separate building from the old Chest Hospital, connected by tunnel under the Fulham Rd.

Nightingale's high opinion of Graham can be seen also in a letter fragment which mentions his "great success and ability in planning sanitary hospital constructions—so rare in an architect."[378]

Nightingale and Galton each did two articles for Quain's *Dictionary of Medicine*, discussed in the letter below. Because of the lag in publication for such a large work, the articles appeared only in 1882 for Galton's ("Hospitals") and 1883 for Nightingale's ("Nursing," a later volume). Nightingale's articles are published in *The Nightingale School*; the item below concerns Galton's on hospitals, which very much reflected Nightingale's views on all nursing matters. Other correspondence then resumes.

Source: From a letter to Douglas Galton, Add Mss 47719 215-16

Lea Hurst
Cromford, Derby
30 October 1877

Dr Quain's articles: he proposes that the article *Hospitals* should take the form Hospitals:

1. Construction } by Captain Galton
2. Organization }
3. Nursing } by F.N.
4. Nurse Training }

(does not wish for a "special list of books").

Captain Galton's proposed Dr Quain's articles, sketch of article on *hospital construction*, included in packet, all remarks on nurses' *accommodation* to come under this head. He says, if so, some supplementary remarks required on his part. He thinks, does not wish to exclude *reasons.* (*Male*) *administration* part still remains *undone.*

377 Letter to Harry Verney 4 May 1877, in *Extending Nursing* (13:156).
378 Letter fragment 12 May 1869, International Museum of Surgical Science M1957.397.

Source: Published letter, *Times* 27 March 1878:11d

Dear Duke of Westminster, You were so good as to speak to me about the subject of your committee on intemperance once, and to send me your Blue Book. "God speed" with all my heart to your "Coffee Public House Association," with all the heart of an old nurse like me, appalled with the diseases of hospitals, and especially of workhouse infirmaries, where the young men patients—at least a very large proportion—come in from "the drink," and worse, come in again and again from "the drink," knowing that it will be "the drink" again which brings them there, and will bring them there as long as they live, helpless and hopeless to save themselves, knowing that they are caught and will be caught (like Hindu ryots [peasants] in the moneylender's clutch) in the same desperate trap, which, like the Indian moneylender, extorts a higher and a higher rate of usury every year—another pound of flesh—to their dying day.

Almost all the unmarried men and some of the married ones (away from their wives to be near their work) in these infirmaries tell the same story:

> I live in a miserable lodging where I am not wanted, and may not poke the fire (the definition of a comfortable lodging is to be allowed to poke the fire) or even sit by the fire. I have nowhere to go but the public house, nowhere to sit down, often nowhere to take my meals. We young men lodgers all often sleep in one room, with two or even three generations of the same family, including young women and girls, unless, indeed, we can get into the model lodging houses. Coffee houses might save us, model lodging houses might make model men of us; nothing else would. As it is, here we are, and here we shall be, in and out of this same sick ward, "every man jack of us," till the last time, when we come to die in it.

This is the story told with every shade of feeling from tears to desperation or callousness, sometimes mixed up with a pitiful love story, sometimes with a theft story, or worse, of thousands.

Yet these men are so far from "all bad" that, if the nurse of the ward is a "trained" nurse, which implies a character and education to carry some weight and influence, they will scrupulously respect their nurse's property, and even her feelings, and will send her word if they have "kept straight," how seldom! or when they have got work.

The children of these men are as much born to the same lot as the children of English are born to be English.

The excellent medical officer of a workhouse infirmary which we nursed used to say to all such patients, "Now, my good fellow, do drink coffee for the rest of your life." Where are they to get it?

Thousands and tens of thousands will, I am sure, bless the Coffee House Association, especially if it could be made to include lodgings. What these men want is a place where they can have coffee, read the newspapers and play games (without temptation to gambling), also a place where they can eat and have decent sleeping accommodation.

Have you seen "Our Coffee Room," two volumes, by Miss Cotton, now Lady Hope?[379]

I must not even ask forgiveness for this long letter, filled with hope at your making this subject your own, yet ashamed of taking up your time, and of asking your grace to forward this little cheque to its destination, and to believe me

ever your grace's faithful servant

Florence Nightingale

Editor: The above letter was read, with Nightingale's permission, at a public meeting.

Also in 1878, the new county hospital at Lincoln opened, for which Alex Graham had done the plans. An article in *The Builder* gave details, beginning with the elevated site, central administrative block and two pavilions, with a covered way between. The ward floors were of English oak and the walls finished in Parian cement and painted. The walls of water closets, baths and lavatories were lined to the height of 5 ft. with white tiles. The corridors and passages were paved with tiles on brick arches.[380] All these details show decided Nightingale influences. She and Galton both saw the plans, but there is no correspondence from the time on them.

A hospital history notes the invitation to Douglas Galton to inspect the hospital, moving on to the development of plans by Alex Graham. The appointment of a new matron from the Nightingale School, Elizabeth Vincent, was noted.[381]

In 1879 Nightingale, with Galton, looked at plans for a lying-in cottage hospital at Ravensworth House, Balham, but complained that the tracings sent her were not adequate to judge by.[382]

---

379 Elizabeth Reid Cotton, daughter of India expert Arthur Cotton, and spouse of Sir James Hope: *Our Coffee Room*, 1876, and *More About Our Coffee Room*, 1878.

380 "Lincoln New County Hospital," *The Builder* 37,1999 (5 July 1879):747-48. See picture on p 494.

381 Thomas Sympson, *A Short Account of the Old and of the New Lincoln County Hospitals* 27 and 45.

382 In *Women* (8:375).

The item immediately below consists of an article Nightingale had set in print for publication in a journal, but which was never published, for reasons unknown.

Source: Florence Nightingale, "Hospitals and Patients," *The Nineteenth Century* (September 1880):1-4

Do we care for the patients in hospitals? Hospitals were made for patients—not patients for hospitals. Yet sometimes it would seem as though the patients were the only things left out of the consideration: the play of *Hamlet* with the part of Hamlet left out.

What is the "new system" of hospital nursing for? Is it to find a career for educated women? as if the sick existed for "the ladies," not "ladies" for the sick; is it that "so many ladies who want a livelihood, etc.," may find one? that God's great world has sickness awarded in it as the consequence of breaking certain laws? or is it that we are to learn how to do the best for the sick, how to advance the methods for doing this best, how to educate men and women, the physicians and nurses, for the sick, how to advance science and practice for curing and preventing disease and smoothing the path of the dying and the incurable?

If so, then let women and "ladies" be trained so that they *shall* be for the good of the sick, if "ladies" are to be among their nurses—all nurses to be trained of course. Doctors and nurses seem to be getting into an excited state. If this keeps out of the nursing profession some "ladies" who look upon it in the wrong way, i.e., for themselves and not for the sick, so much the better.

Such nursecraft, if any such there be, is guilty of high treason against nursing—guilty of taking one of the noblest arts of life, noblest because it is to be of use to living bodies and souls—in a mean spirit of "ladyism," that is, falsely ladylike exclusiveness—devotion to a fantastic guild, and not to helping the suffering, or not to this as a first object.

Times have been when statecraft has stood up wrongly for a prerogative of the crown, so nursecraft sometimes may stand up for a false prerogative of the nurse, where "ladies" enter not as a privilege, to do the more good, but as claiming privileges on account of their class.

2. What is true nursecraft? What is true nurse training?

The essence, the object of all training, is *intelligent* obedience to medical orders, to teach the nurse how to obey intelligently, so that the orders which are for the good of the patients shall be carried out so as to be for the patients' good.

What possible meaning can be attached to military discipline or training—to the Prussian, for example, of which we have heard so much as being the highest standard, but to obey orders with the utmost intelligence and perfection of detail, which details must have been taught beforehand, but now they must be carried out not by an automaton, but by an intelligent human being who has to do with matters of life and death.

A branch of the German military service is called safety service (*Sicherheitsdienst*). What is more truly "Sicherheitsdienst" than the nursing service? "The disciple is not above his Lord";[383] the soldier is not above his military officer; the nurse is not above her medical officer in the treatment of his patients.

If "trained nurses" are less obedient to the medical authorities than charwomen nurses, it is not from training but from *want* of training—from defect in (so-called) training: *lucus a non lucendo*;[384] it is as if we said, they are "trained nurses" because they are *not* trained. As well might we say that an educated physician knows less than the old village crone or bonesetter. What possible meaning can be attached to the word "training" if it were otherwise?

But if it *is* otherwise, if the doctors were to talk as if they had a sympathy with Mrs Gamps,[385] then may it not be the fault of the nurse trainers and the "ladies"? Somebody has mistaken her calling. The whole object and essence of training has been missed.

Ought not the nursing staff to hold much the same relation to the medical officers that the building staff does to the architect? That the nurse should know her business—that each individual employed by the builder should know his business, is of the first, the most essential importance to the physician or surgeon, as it is to the architect. It is indeed the sine qua non [without which nothing]. And how can either know his or her business if he or she is not trained to it? But then she must be trained to do her business, and *not not* to do it.

3. It follows that to pit the medical school against the nurse training school is "worse than a crime," it is a blunder.[386] It is to pit the

383 A paraphrase of Matt 10:24.

384 To shine in a dark grove.

385 Sairey Gamp was the stereotypical bad nurse in Charles Dickens's novel *Martin Chuzzlewit*.

386 A reference to Napoleon having a royal duke executed in 1804 to frighten the royalists who opposed his rule, but which emboldened them instead.

minute hand against the hour hand of a clock. The training school for nurses can only be at its best there where there *is* a medical school. This is almost a truism, most truly felt to be so by the best nurse.

It is not a cricket match that we are playing, with patients as balls, and students as one eleven against nurses as the other. The object is far other than this: it is that the whole building, civil administration, medical staff and school, nursing staff and training school, matron and all, shall be one great and organized whole to be worked and harmonized for one purpose—that purpose the good of the patients—that which doctors and nurses alike are there for.

It is again a truism, that the more the free outer air of public opinion is brought into the hospital the better, in order to keep up the highest standard of care, including nursing care, of the patients. The [medical] students are thus an advantage to the nursing, as a highly educated element among the trained nurses undoubtedly is to the students. Free public opinion does look so sharply after everybody's errors but its own. And this is so wholesome.

The worst nursing in Europe is perhaps that of *sisterhoods* where no civil administration or medical school is admitted. The worst hospitals in Europe are undoubtedly those where no matrons or nurse training schools are admitted, but only nurses under the direct disciplinary (matron-al) authority of the doctors—where the doctor himself is matron, in short. It cannot be otherwise.

The female element is universally admitted to be an essential element of nursing. And women must be under a woman for discipline. The architect cannot supervise the bricklayer or plumber. The nurse deals with far more valuable and delicate material than the builder's man. The nurse's daily life—and without a good daily life there can be no good nurse—cannot be organized or supervised by doctor or man at all. This will be agreed on all hands.

As there is certainly no question in the great civil hospitals of going backward to a period when there were no medical schools, we may happily leave the subject. For that matter, they had no nurse training schools till long after medical schools. The time will soon come when the public, including especially "the doctors," will consider a great hospital as incomplete without its training school for nurses as without its medical school for students. Let us do nothing to prevent that good time coming.

By public opinion we do not precisely mean the airing of personal piques in the press. As for this kind of grievances, medical or nursing school and hospital are something like man and wife. They cannot be unmarried. If friends want to reconcile them, it is not exactly by putting their personal squabbles and recriminations, their incompatibilities of temper, into the newspapers that it will be done.

4. We cannot enter here into technical points of what constitutes a good training school for nurses—what constitutes a failure. But there are two or three common-sense points and common sense applies or ought to apply to all things which non-technical people may enter into. And everyone can say whether they *are* common sense or not. One is: nothing can be more wholesome (for the patients) than a friendly rivalry between one ward head nurse (sister) and another, as to the respective merits of the visiting physicians and surgeons. If every head nurse thinks her physician or surgeon greater than any other, so much the better. Don't silence her. It follows from this, and all common sense, that ward sisters and nurses should not be moved about, like probationers, from ward to ward, by way of "training" them. The sisters and nurses *are* trained or ought to be when appointed to the wards. The training is done beforehand during their probationer's year. They are now there to nurse, not to learn nursing (although they do learn every year, or they are no nurses), to train, not to be trained, although every year *is* a training, not only to the probationers, but to themselves also.

The convenience of the matron is a misnomer. The good of the patients *is* the convenience of the matron, of course, and of every official there.

It follows that the whole regulation of the nurse's life, including her hours of recreation, is to preserve a human being (who is not a piece of furniture) in such health of body and mind as will enable her to do her duty best for the patients in carrying out medical orders. For this purpose she must hear them. The sister and nurse *always*—the "probationer" would think herself much aggrieved if she too were not of the party—must be present at the medical visits. This is an essential part of any organization or system (much ill-used word, which often means a no-system). It is also one of the most instructive times of the hospital day, that, in short, which the organization is there for is the regulation of the nurse's life to make and keep her capable of nursing.

Nothing can be less unwholesome than the "breezes," provided they do not become tornados or dust storms, which occasionally sweep through the best-regulated hospital—the free air which freshens all the atmosphere—the good-humoured rubs between administrative, medical and nursing heads of staffs, with the public opinion belonging to each, provided the rubs are not blisters. It makes the difference between a prison and a public school.

But we must not expect if we sow the "wind" not to reap the "whirlwind."[387] And "whirlwinds" are indeed unwholesome and destructive.

Do we care for the patients first and foremost? That is the last and the first keynote. The alpha and omega is, do we wisely care for the patients?

Source: From undated notes, Add Mss 45820 ff1-2

Great saving of human life would be effected if hospitals, instead of being crowded palaces with layers of sick, were iron villages of cottages, with one or at most two patients in each room—taken down and rebuilt, if possible, being iron, every few years . . . little gardens to provide means of recreation and exercise for patients.

Mortality in lying-in hospitals, both as to mothers and infants, higher than among women confined at home. The larger the hospital (of any kind), the greater the rate of mortality, according to our present mode of building, where the impure air of any one ward diffuses itself by corridor and staircases through the whole hospital. . . . chance of recovery at home much greater.

Ceilings and walls to be painted and highly varnished in order to prevent the imbibition by the plaster of efflorescing, which happens with limewashing, and to allow them to be the more readily cleansed, discharging shaft in the wall, [illeg] by a sliding cover, by which all dressings, etc., are at once passed to the wash cellar.

Hospital System of London. Workhouse infirmaries ought to be more liberal, hospitals less extravagant.

London	4000 beds	40,000 patients	£175,000
Paris	7000	90,000	£165,000

French centralization, however, too much praised as beneficial. But London hospitals might be rendered at least twice as useful.

387 An allusion to Hos 8:7.

Source: From a letter to Harry and Parthenope Verney, Wellcome (Claydon copy) Ms 9009/4

19 January 1882

Bucks Infirmary. Two additional wards.

I did not answer Sir Harry's printed paper about the extension to this infirmary, because I could not understand it without the plans, though I have no doubt he was right.

But nothing is more risky than adding to an infirmary—you may entirely spoil the sanitary advantages. Surely it would be better to have the highest sanitary advice (professional). If you will send me up the plans, including ventilation, drainage, etc., I will have them overhauled by the Army Sanitary Commission, and overhaul them myself, if you please.

I see the meeting at the Bucks Infirmary is to be held on *1 February*.

Editor: In 1882, Nightingale was sent the plans and sketches for the Whatstandwell Coffee and Reading Rooms, by Thomas G. Iveson. An extract (the letter is not available) shows that she showed them to her cousin, William Shore Smith, and sent back detailed comments. "We earnestly trust that all will prosper and succeed," she wrote, and "that all will go well and be a blessing to many."[388]

Source: From a letter to Douglas Galton, ADD Mss 45765 f109

12 May 1882

Sir Henry Parkes asks me (for Sydney) to recommend any documents or books concerning the administration of civil hospitals—provision for the health of towns, management of *country* hospitals. I have sent him a quantity of Local Government Office plans, documents and works and Army Sanitary Commission ditto, recommended your *Healthy Dwellings*, but can find no books about the *management of hospitals*. Can you recommend any?

Is Dr Quain's *Dictionary* out? And could I have your article on the administration of hospitals? There is plenty written about the *construction* of hospitals, but such a *dearth* of anything about their management.[389]

---

388 Catalogue note, Sotheby's 22/6/99.

389 Galton's two entries in Quain's *Dictionary of Medicine* were on construction and administration, respectively.

Editor: Sir Henry Parkes visited Nightingale again in 1883, when he was out of office. Nightingale hoped to see him, but she was then taken up with nursing her sister, and hoped that he would see Henry Bonham Carter.[390]

Typhoid Epidemic in Bangor, 1882

Editor: In 1882 William Rathbone asked Nightingale for her advice on the fever epidemic in Bangor, referred to variously as typhoid or enteric fever (the newer term). She searched out relevant reports and sent them to him.[391] The bacillus that causes the disease had been identified in 1881 by a German bacteriologist, C.J. Eberth, but this information is not referred to in the material related here. The epidemic raised practical questions as to the source of the disease, and who or what department was responsible for prevention and remedy. Reference to a general "fever epidemic," part of which passed into "enteric fever," shows Nightingale's continued adherence to the "miasma" theory of causation, as opposed to germ theory, which specifies different diseases caused by different bacilli. Nightingale came to accept germ theory roughly two years later.

Vigorous disinfecting methods for houses are given. There are comments on centralization and decentralized public health regulations. Nightingale saw Bangor as a typical instance of what could go wrong with an imperfect sewer system. Her last comments are on the prevention of similar epidemics.

Source: From five letters to William Rathbone, University of Wales, Bangor, 37616-20, typed copies Liverpool Record Office ff70, 71-72 and 78, all from Lea Hurst

21 September 1882

I am so sorry to be out of London. But I have written to London for "books" and "information" and "advice," if anyhow I could be of the least use in the terrible Bangor epidemic to you.

And let me not lose this opportunity of thanking you most gratefully for your everlasting kindness (which I do scruple to accept) in send-

390 Letter to Parkes 8 October 1883, New South Wales Archives.

391 On the issue see "Dr Barry on the Outbreak of Enteric Fever at Bangor," Medical Reports to the Local Government Board, *Medical Times and Gazette* 9 December 1882:701.

ing me the beautiful flowering plants, which I stopped on 26 August, and for five weeks previously when I was away. I cannot be grateful enough to you for this unceasing kindness. But I must not encroach upon it any longer.

Joy that the war in Egypt is over. Mr Childers[392] says that the troops, "thanks to sobriety and plenty to do," have actually been "more healthy than in England." You know perhaps that we sent out nurses.

22 September 1882

Private. I have asked "advice and information" of our Army Sanitary Commission in London relative to the Bangor typhoid.

The best book about English enteric fever, Dr Sutherland says, is Dr Murchison's treatise on continued fevers,[393] which states cautiously one side of the case. And therefore I have sent it from London, as you asked for books, though Dr Murchison's (which I make a standard book among our *nurses*) treats the thing far too medically for your purpose, I think.

I am also desired to send you, which I do by this post, the latest and by far the best information on the subject in Dr Marston's[394] paper in the Army Medical Department Report, Appendix No. 2, p 238. But again the same objection holds, I think, because the Bangor epidemic belongs to the Local Government Board work, and it is better for the Army Sanitary Commission, and also for yourself, not to appear to interfere with their responsibility. I send this volume as from myself to you.

If we may advise, ask for the inspector's report to be sent to you, and also for an account of any sanitary measures adopted after the inspection. We mention this because *our* custom is to direct the works *pari passu* hand in hand] with the inspection, and not to wait for the report. (In our last case at Dublin, after summing up at the end the works required, our last paragraph said that, of these measures, all had been either taken or were in the process of being carried out. And there has been no more fever.)

To *you* it is superfluous to say that it is a great mistake to wait to draw up a fine report, for the whole object is to save life, and the inspector ought to direct the measures on the spot.

As to the water poison theory, that must, of course, be proved by proving the transmission of the enteric fever poison, *not* by the occur-

---

392 Hugh Culling Eardley Childers (1827-96), secretary for war.
393 Charles Murchison, *A Treatise on the Continued Fevers of Great Britain.*
394 Jeffrey A. Marston (1831-1911), later deputy surgeon general.

rence of typhoid fever cases. (In India not a single enteric fever case has been traced to enteric fever poison, either in or out of water, and as there are no sewers, there is no sewer gas.)

One of our army sanitary commissioners, who has been several times at Bangor, says that, supposing the water theory unproved, he would feel disposed to look very carefully at all the house closets and pipes, and also to the street drains, *and whether the sub-soil is dry and clean.* If, quietly between you and me, you would think well to communicate to me such facts as these, and allow me to get you an opinion from such authorities in London, I should be only too happy if I could be of the least use.

This Bangor typhoid is so disastrous a thing that we are thankful you have gone to the spot. It is like yourself.

2 October 1882

Bangor typhoid. PRIVATE. The papers you kindly sent me about Bangor are intensely interesting. Any remarks that I venture to make on them must, of course, rest solely on what the facts are and on nothing else.

1. Up to a given date, there seem to have been 141 cases and eight deaths, or one death to 17½ cases. The usual mortality of enteric fever is about 1 in 6.

It would be impossible, without an accurate record of the cases, to say whether or not all were enteric fever. All we know is that it is so stated, but judged by the mortality, we should say that it is not an enteric fever epidemic but a fever epidemic, part of which has passed into enteric fever. If this be correct, the Bangor fever outbreak resembles many others which have broken out in badly cared for towns.

2. The inspector's notes show local causes quite enough to account for the facts, which might be arranged in the following order: the people in Bangor and in the district have been living in neglect of the most ordinary precautions; they have all been more or less undergoing slowly and unknowingly certain important functional degradation; at last, possibly from some climatic reason, fever appears in single, then in multiple cases, and a certain proportion of them put on the typhoid condition, and of these the usual proportion die; the evil is not yet exhausted, because all the *pre*disposed have not yet suffered.

3. But what a state of matters the inspector's (dated Bangor 23 September) notes reveal! With such a state of administration, might not anything happen? Not one of the defects stated in the notes ought to have existed, and the real practical question is *whether such things can be prevented elsewhere*?

(In the old Board of Health days, the view was that the sanitary administration should be special, uniform and skilled, and by consequence more or less centralized. But the House of Commons decided that the administration should be decentralized, and consequently not special but local—not uniform but multiform—not skilled but medical. And might not this unhappy Bangor fever be almost called one of its typical natural results? Probably the best way would have been to have continued the central action until every town in England and Wales had been reported to Parliament as having been improved, and by that time the central administration might have educated the local authorities. Now all that can be done is to send an inspector to help (?) the local authorities after the people have suffered.)

4. The only remedy in the Bangor case would be the one we always adopt, were it practicable, namely, to remove the people out of every house where any indisposition had shown itself, then to put all the drainage and water supply in order, then to scrape all walls and ceilings and limewhite them with quicklime (we have done this for officers' rooms). And when floors, woodwork, etc., had been thoroughly cleansed, and doors and windows left open for a week, to return the people. We ought scarcely perhaps to say more except that the loss by sickness and death is simply another instance of the cost of dealing with such cases after the penalty has been incurred and the "bill" has been sent in.

I may add that I have consulted my "colleagues" in London on the subject of this answer. Many thanks for letting me see a copy of your most admirable letter to Mr Dodson.[395]

N.B. I ought perhaps to add that the Parliamentary principle of decentralization is undoubtedly the true one, and in large towns with enlightened local authorities no doubt already works well. But in small *localized* places, the ignorance of which we don't want to be "*represented*," works deplorably.

13 October 1882

Bangor. Typhoid. Private. Thank you for your frightfully interesting papers.

These July Local Government (Whitehall) Board letters are simply astounding. They seem to afford almost sufficient reason for passing over the medicos altogether, do not they? The whole of these papers leave the matter *just where it was.*

---

395 John George Dodson (1825-97), president of the Local Government Board.

The case now is more of an *engineering* one than simply a sanitary one, is it not? *In answer to your question,* is not the only man connected with the board whom we could advise for a report *Mr Rawlinson*? He would trace the evil in its relation to *engineering* and *household* causes, and I am sure would do his best. Mr Rawlinson is the man Bangor seems to want. He might be obtained either by yourself, through the office, or the Local Board might write to ask for him at their expense. I have consulted the medical standing member of our Army Sanitary Commission, who thinks the "doctors" have failed and that it is now an *engineering* case, about this, but of Mr Rawlinson's return to London I did not know till this morning (through the said medical standing member).

I venture to enclose a letter (or the beginning of a letter) to you ten days old, but which I did not send because I was afraid it would be of little use. I return these (truly terrible) enclosures with many thanks. May Bangor be an example for good to others and to itself! And may your efforts succeed as they always do. God bless you. . . .

Bangor is such an important case, so terribly typical for itself and for others, that we wish you doubly success!

7 May 1883

Bangor. I return these most interesting papers and letters. As you say, while not materially altering the former position, they make an end of the enteric fever poison hypotheses, which never had any support from the facts in the original report.

This is what the authorities to whom I submitted the original documents, and to whom I have submitted these, draw as a conclusion, and they add that the case appears to stand as follows: from time to time there occurs in every locality a tendency to certain classes of blood diseases, just as at certain seasons there is a tendency to inflammatory chest affections. We know nothing of the *why*, but it is our duty to use every effort to diminish or guard against this liability. In the case of chest diseases, we clothe more warmly and keep from exposing ourselves to damp or cold or change during the period. In the case of blood diseases, we depend on sanitary works and measures. If, during an inflammatory period, we leave off clothing, we suffer. And if, during a blood disease period, we intermit sanitary precautions, we suffer.

Bangor was furnished with a good sewage system, and with a good water scheme, provided the sewer system had been completed up to the houses, and provided the water supply had been properly protected and properly connected with the drainage. All the sewers required ventilation, and all the lines flushing, and at the same time the usual cleansing work thoroughly organized had to be carried out, including the absolute abolishing of all sources of nuisance within the board limits. In short, a proper system of improvement complete in all its details, and under constant supervision is necessary.

There were, as you know, some missing links in the administration as well as in the work, and in order to prevent a recurrence of the evils, they must (for the main thing is what should be *done*):

1. Complete the whole scheme, including protection of water sources, ventilating sewers, flushing sewers at very short intervals—several times a week at least (there is a special apparatus for this)—house drainage.

2. They must provide for constant supervision. The officer of health is quite unfitted for this. The work is of an engineering character, and must be continuously seen to by an engineer.

The board complains that the doctors did not tell them about the fever. The reason is obvious. The great bulk of the fever cases were simple enough, and only a proportion of these were enteric fever, which is *presumed* to be contagious, and to be forcibly reported. But all this is a mistake; the mischief was all done at Bangor before the fever showed itself. The engineering inspector ought to have forestalled the fever. The object of sanitary work is not remedy but prevention.

St Marylebone Workhouse Infirmary Nurses' Home Addition, 1882-83

Editor: Workhouse infirmary reform was long a priority for Nightingale. However, opportunities to bring in trained nursing were slow in coming, and the first two attempts, at Liverpool and Highgate, worked out badly thanks to the untimely deaths of their respective matrons. When Sir Edmund Boulnois (1838-1911), the chair of the St Marylebone Workhouse, sought trained nurses for its new infirmary in 1882, Nightingale jumped at the opportunity. The school sent an excellent matron, Elizabeth Vincent (c1841-?) and a team of nurses. A nursing school was the logical next step and planning for it then became an issue.

The increased numbers of nurses, as well as the need for classroom space, led to the decision to add a building. The hospital did not want to build a full "nurses' home," but simply additional accommodation for the nurses and superintendent and a classroom (a full nurses' home would have included a living room or lounge, dining room and kitchen). Since the Nightingale Fund was contributing financially to the training school, Nightingale had some leverage in demanding high standards for the new building, and Boulnois was a good ally throughout the process. He was asked to join the Nightingale Fund Council in 1890, which he did, and became chair in 1900.

The architect for the new St Marylebone Workhouse Infirmary was Henry Saxon Snell,[396] and Nightingale considered him to have done it "very well" (see p 874 below). It is not clear if she examined the plans for the workhouse infirmary itself, for her surviving comments are confined to the addition, on which she found more than the usual failings. Nightingale saw an initial set of plans late in 1882, and sent lengthy and detailed criticisms of them (immediately below). She also consulted Mary S. Crossland, the person in charge of the nurses' home at St Thomas', for advice (the second item below) and the St Marylebone matron, Elizabeth Vincent, who gave her comments on the plans via Henry Bonham Carter.[397]

A year later, Nightingale received a second set of plans, but found them virtually unchanged on key points. She sent them to Douglas Galton for another opinion: "They seem to me so formidably bad that I hesitate without your verdict to give such a sweeping condemnation" (see p 848 below). These second plans were bad enough to preclude her fund from sending probationers to St Marylebone, she told him. Specific complaints include the need for a "living room" for the nurses, even if they took their meals in the infirmary, and a lack of windows to the outside. A "home sister" or instructor of the probationers also had to be provided for, and the resulting required living space for her as well.

Source: From a letter to Henry Bonham Carter, with his comments, Add Mss 47720 ff173-74

5 February 1882

St Marylebone Infirmary. *Proposed Home.* I have the plans here. I heard with delight from Miss Vincent that you were to have a conference on Friday last with Mr Boulnois. It is because I suppose you may have something to tell me about it, the home's, proposed scope that I trouble you with my criticisms. I have to return the plans *tomorrow.* The "home," it appears, is merely to have SLEEPING accommodation, a *classroom* and home sister's rooms.

---

396 On the plans see Henry Saxon Snell, *Charitable and Parochial Establishments.*
397 Vincent letter 7 March 1882, Add Mss 47720 f187.

1. There is not enough bathroom, W.C., etc., accommodation. And there are no housemaid's sinks at all. I very much deprecate the place of the W.C.s between bathroom and nurse's room. Surely it should be beyond the bathroom so as to have *end* windows, one in W.C., one in the present wholly unventilated lobby, which can be ventilated only into the passage, this is quite inadmissible.

HBC: Possibly might place W.C.s in a projection with ink.

FN: 2. The rooms and large windows are very nice. But it will be extremely difficult to keep these rooms healthy, being as they are in two rows, one on each side a narrow passage, with a window only at its each extreme end (not built round a "well"). I fear epidemics. There is no large airy open hall or staircase so that the building can be swept with fresh air from end to end, from top to bottom, from back to front. The front door is so small and leads directly, not to a hall, but to the dead wall of the "lecture hall."

3. I think there should be (1) sick room, (2) small kitchen for ditto, (3) at least one servant's room, (4) and offices at least for coals.

4. The "lecture hall," I presume, is to be classroom: how is it to be warmed? And is it to have a skylight? It is in a most unfortunate position, blocking up the front door little hall. Would there be any possibility of a covered corridor to infirmary?

5. Is it proposed ever to make it more of a self-contained home and training school? I will not send in my criticism till I know from you what line you, from your interview with Mr Boulnois, propose to take, and advise my taking? Please return me *this* tomorrow MORNING *with your advice.* I will then add what proportion of bathrooms, etc., is necessary or desirable to (so many) rooms (nurses') to this. . . .

HBC: You can send in your criticisms on that plan as it stands without reference to the ideas of extension.

Source: Letter/draft/copy to Mary S. Crossland, ADD MSS 47738 ff242-47

5 March 1882

I was just thinking of writing to you about the plans for the new "home" (Miss Vincent's) when your letter came.[398] The plans are here.

1. Supposing you could have what you like, *to what number of nurses'* (or probationers') *rooms* would you have? *One bathroom, one W.C., one*

398 Crossland letter 4 March 1882, which reports her assessment, ADD MSS 47738 ff240-43.

housemaid's sink and closet to *five?* to *six?* to *eight,* nine, to *ten* probationers? (there is no harm in planning).

2. They will want a first-rate home sister to keep those rooms in rows in the healthy state that you do yours. Would they could have been built round a "well," lighted and aired from the top with galleries! Even our "well" is too dark for my mind, but then you keep it (and the "housemaid's sinks") so beautifully.

3. There appear to be no *housemaid's sinks* at all, and I rather dread the W.C.s unventilated lobby between nurses' rooms and opening into their passage.

4. The front door is so small and leading to the dead wall of the "lecture room." There is no wide-open airy space from top to bottom or from front to back—no thorough draft through the building in *any* direction to sweep it from end to end. I should be rather afraid of any epidemic spreading.

5. Ought there not to be a *sick room*? But perhaps one of the larger nurse's rooms, first floor, could be set apart for this. I quite agree in the need of a *small kitchen.* But must there not be room for at least *one servant,* for the home alone? Do they mean to scrub it with the infirmary scrubbers, and not only this but to serve it entirely with the infirmary housemaids and servants? Surely the home sister should have at least one resident servant.

6. The "lecture hall," I presume, is exclusive for the women and for [the] classroom as well. Have you any hints to give us as to this? There seems no means of warming it—is it to be warmed with warm water? And there should be a skylight. And I wish it did not block up the air opposite the front door. (I like the porter's lodge W.C. much better than the nurses'.)

7. I conclude that all meals are to be taken, all dining rooms and sitting rooms to be, in the infirmary buildings. It will be rather serious crossing the road at rising and going to bed, and to all "classes" in all weathers to and from the home. But, on the whole, it is perhaps better than having to cross for all meals.

8. If you were asked, what should you say was *the main defect of our* home? Is it anything we could avoid here?

9. The little rooms and large windows are very nice here. But should it expand into a regular large training school, of thirty-forty probationers, I think they will want to make it more of a self-contained "home."

10. Do you want a *fireplace in a bathroom*? There is none shown here. I should very much prefer the W.C.s being at the end beyond

the bathrooms, with windows *at the end* in both lobby and W.C., instead of being between bath and nurse's room.

11. Some kind of kitchen offices there must be, if only for coals for forty rooms.

12. If I do not receive your kind answer to this by the 9 o'clock post tomorrow (Monday) morning, I will send messenger for it by *10 tomorrow morning*. So sorry to hurry you—please only answer the principal questions and please be so good as to *return* this (my) *letter* with it. (It will save you trouble and me too.)

Please go *out* every day to have fresh air. You must need it. God bless all those who will ever be in those forty rooms and God bless all those who are, and have been and ever will be in *our* rooms, including always their dear matron and home sister. . . .

One nurse's room is shown without a fireplace. W.C. might possibly be placed on the staircase, though not a good place for the night.

Source: From a letter to Henry Bonham Carter, Add Mss 47720 ff219-27

7 March 1882

Proposed New Accommodation for Nurses. St Marylebone Infirmary. It is understood that this building is merely to contain *sleeping* accommodation for additional nurses, classroom and rooms for a superintendent of nurses, and that it is not contemplated to make it a nurses' home or training school for probationers, for it lacks the essential characteristics of a "home" self-contained? This being understood,

Sleeping rooms:

1. The small rooms with large windows and with fireplaces are very good. . . . The partitions between the rooms are doubtless all *walls* and not wooden partitions (which let the least sound pass and are cold). The sleeping rooms being only on TWO floors is very good. But will it not be extremely difficult to keep these thirty-six rooms healthy, being as they are in two rows—one on each side a rather narrow passage, with a window only at each extreme. . . .

2. There is *no* central airy open *space* or *staircase*, so that the building can be swept with fresh air from end to end, from top to bottom, from back to front. The front door or porch is small and leads directly not to a hall but to the dead wall of the "lecture room." (Had it been possible, it might have been suggested that the rooms on the first—second—floor should open on a gallery, or at least the two rooms in the centre—thus throwing a space open to the top—with a ventilating skylight. But this does not appear to be possible, so narrow is the passage.)

Doubtless it is intended to have *ridge ventilation* all along the upper storey and a ventilating *skylight* in the middle—with good *ventilating windows* at each *extreme end* to secure fresh air by night and by day. Perhaps it is meant to set aside the upper storey for night nurses with their two night superintendents. In that case the gallery system would make it noisier for night nurses, but it also renders supervision easier.

3. To every *eight* nurses (or probationers) at *most* there should be *one bathroom with fireplace, one W.C., one housemaid's sink.* This would render *five* for forty necessary. There appear only to be four bathrooms and six W.C.s. But I should hold this sufficient.

4. The place of those *W.C.s* which are *between* nurses' rooms is very much to be deprecated, also of those W.C.s which are *not* in a projection. The W.C. *lobby* appears to be wholly unwindowed and unventilated, or to draw its light and air only from the passage, which is quite inadmissible. Could not these W.C.s be placed with and *beyond* the bathroom next the outer *end wall,* with *end* windows, one in *W.C.*, one in *lobby*? It is true this would make a great deal of passing to and fro', and be too far from the boiler. Possibly the W.C.s might be placed in a *projection* with sink?

5. In each *bathroom,* there should be a fireplace, a slab to make poultices on, a cupboard where two or three saucepans, tow, linseed meal, etc., would be kept, a roller behind the door for a towel. (Among thirty-nine [or] forty nurses there are certain to be trifling ailments, which a ready application of fomentation or poultice by a careful home sister would prevent from becoming serious ones. And there are certain to be occasionally serious ailments with every care.) There should be a good *housemaid's sink* (with brush for cleansing slop pails), best in a compartment of its own. And let it never be forgotten that the housemaid's sink is often the means of poisoning the whole house, if not well constructed and carefully looked after. Doubtless there will be hot and cold water laid on to all the bathrooms.

On the first floor plan, there are *six W.C.s, but only two* and four *bathrooms* (to twenty beds). The centre W.C.s are made as little objectionable as possible by being on one side, but not in a *projection,* and by the *un*windowed *lobby* of two opening opposite the *stairs.* And doubtless there is a ventilating *skylight over* it. Still they *are* objectionable; their doors opposite two nurses' rooms are very objectionable, or, better still, if they could be on the staircases?

6. *"Lecture hall" and classroom.* Is it not in an unfortunate position, blocking up the air opposite the front door? It is to be hoped that it looks north. If it is to the south, it will take the sun from several

rooms. If it is to the south, ought it not to have also a south window, besides the two and the skylight?

7. The *staircase* windows are good, the staircases not very roomy. It is to be remarked that, perhaps, an object is to isolate a wing with all its rooms, by doors. . . .

8. Will not a good *sitting room* be ultimately required? even though they do take their meals in the infirmary? It might be found over the lecture and classroom by sacrificing the skylight of lecture room. But two storeys are bad. Even with sitting rooms in the infirmary, this may be wanted. A *"home" sister* is of course wanted.

9. There should be an isolated room in case of sickness, "handy" for the "home" sister, for a *sickroom.* And there should be a *small kitchen.* But if *no* kitchen is granted, as the nurses are to have all meals in the *infirmary,* then *fireplaces in bathrooms* become absolutely necessary, and good-sized bathrooms. Should there not be at least one resident *servant's room* and *coal cellar,* etc.? *This is not shown.* Would it be possible to devise *a passage straight through* from front to back with lecture room on one side and kitchen on the other (which would be better than having it *under* the lecture room) without interfering with the light and air of the *nurses' room windows?*

10. Would there be any possibility of a *covered corridor* to the infirmary? It will be trying early morning, and late at night, crossing to and fro' to bed in all weathers.

11. I wish the *aspects* of the proposed building had been marked.

N
W ┼ E   They are so now.
S

12. I do not gather whether the two nice *bow-windowed rooms* on either side the front door are the *bedroom and sitting room* of "home" sister (or assistant matron), which if there is a *probationers' school,* they certainly ought to be, or whether they are merely two bedrooms for two upper female officers.

N.B. The bow windows have disappeared in the present plans and this is a sensible change for the worse. . . .

Training School for Probationers. As it is understood that it is *contemplated* to establish a school for probationers, it might not be amiss to set down the essentials in a building for such a *home" and training school.*

1. Rooms for a "home" sister of the home, where she should live entirely—having her sitting room so placed as to command a view of all coming in and going out.

2. Good sitting and dining rooms.

3. Classrooms.

4. Kitchen, etc.

5. Servants' bedrooms all complete, if possible *not* underground, so difficult of supervision.

6. Sickroom.

7. Bathrooms, W.C.s, housemaid's sinks, *not less than one* of each to every *eight* nurses' rooms.

8. Nurses' (probationers') sleeping rooms, each with fireplace, partitions to be walls, not wood, etc.

Editor: The next letter shows Nightingale making arrangements for Sir Henry Parkes, who was visiting from Sydney, to see both the St Marylebone Infirmary and St Thomas', the latter with its architect.

Source: From a letter to Sir Henry Parkes, State Library of New South Wales

14 April 1882

Many thanks for your kind note, just received. Mr Currey, the architect, will have the greatest pleasure in showing you the construction and ventilation of St Thomas' Hospital tomorrow (Thursday) morning—to meet at the matron's office at 11, as arranged. The treasurer, who is the official head, is, I am sorry to say, away till Saturday or Monday—I am sorry because *he* will be sorry not to do you the honours of his hospital, but he would be the first to say that he has little or no practical knowledge of the details you wish to see.

Mrs Wardroper, the matron, will show you the nursing part. And I hope you will also see Miss Crossland, the trainer of our probationers, under Mrs Wardroper. I have also informed Mr Bonham Carter, the secretary of the Nightingale Fund, who hopes to have the honour of meeting you, too, but is afraid he will be prevented by business.

2. He is writing to Mr Boulnois, the chairman of St *Marylebone* Infirmary, to communicate direct with you as the best way of making an arrangement suitable to you. And I will write to Miss Vincent, the matron, that this has been done. I informed them of your "mornings" extending up to "Thursday week," but said you wished the engagement to be made by tomorrow, Thursday, afternoon.

Source: From a letter to Henry Bonham Carter, ADD MSS 47720 ff215-18

7 February 188*3*

The plans now sent me are so similar to those sent exactly eleven months ago that the observations then made may be repeated almost word for word: 1, 2, 3, 4, 5, 6, 7, 8, 9. Perhaps the scullery, which now appears on the first floor between head nurses' rooms, is meant for the sick kitchen. But in case of much slight sickness, this is in an inconvenient position for poultices and fomentations, etc., and would not at all obviate the necessity of *each bathroom* being fitted up in the manner aforesaid:

a. It is extremely undesirable to have the lecture room where it stands, blocking up light and air. It would be of course much more undesirable to have it in *two* storeys.

b. There appear to be doors on the ground floor shutting out the staircases and shutting in a space perfectly airless and dark except for the front door, which will thus be a reservoir (for the whole block) of foul air.

c. As far as appears by the ↓ the long sides of the building look north and south, therefore half of the whole of the rooms will look only north, and this aspect will be marked by the sickness of the nurses in it, i.e., we shall be able to tell who have the north rooms by the greater proportion of ill health. Does the *north* side include the superintendent's and head nurses' rooms? This does seem objectionable. And the south side the lecture room with no window to the south!!!

d. And [I] would at least pierce a window at the end of the four nurses' *end* rooms looking to the *north*, placing the fireplace on the inner wall, if the bathrooms are to be kept where they are, which probably must be the case, on account of the boiler room (though it was not so in the former plans).

e. The extreme objection to the W.C. door (for nine people) opening exactly opposite a nurse's room door, over a close passage 5 ft. wide, and apparently without any lobby, need hardly be pointed out. In the former plans the W.C.s were in projections. Now they are in none. Two W.C.s on the first floor are between bedrooms; still they open on the staircase space, have lobbies, probably ventilated and lighted from above. The W.C.s on the ground floor seem all that is objectionable.

f. I would venture again to repeat the extreme danger of having thirty-nine persons in a building of this form, i.e., in two rows, along a close passage, on each side. All the best modern nurses' homes are built lighted and ventilated on the four sides of a well-lighted and ventilated well, as far as I am aware.

Source: From a letter to Douglas Galton, ADD MSS 45765 ff203-04

8 February 1883

St Marylebone Infirmary. I should be extremely obliged to you if you would kindly give your verdict upon the enclosed plans, by Saxon Snell—a supplementary nurses' home for the new St Marylebone Infirmary at Notting Hill which, as you perhaps know, we nurse. They seem to me so formidably bad that I hesitate without your verdict to give such a sweeping condemnation. *We* have a voice in them, *because* we are to contribute (money) to their proposed training school, for which this additional accommodation is necessary. And, therefore, they are obliged to ask for our approval.

The plans were sent to me a year ago, and I enclose a copy of the criticism I then made, and a copy of the letter which I made our matron, Miss Vincent, then write. *It* dropped for a year, because the Local Government Board would not give its consent to the rates being employed for a training school. *It* has now revived, but the plans have "revived" in a "deadlier" state than ever, in my opinion.

The four sheets in pencil, which I enclose, are my *this* year's criticism—last year's being almost as applicable now as then.

I hope I shall not be giving you much trouble in saying whether *my* alteration could make this form of building healthy. Supposing a nurse were attacked with scarlet fever or erysipelas, what would be the consequence? (In our St Thomas' Home, we have not had one case of *spreading* in what are called "infectious" diseases, but we are built round a well—though I am by no means satisfied with it, and have a most energetic "home" sister.)

Source: From a letter to Henry Bonham Carter, ADD MSS 47720 213-14

9 February 1883

St Marylebone Infirmary. The present plans have all the blunders nearly and a few more of those of last year. They appear to me so formidably bad that I can neither see how it is possible for us to sanction our probationers being placed in them, nor how they can be rendered healthy without entire remodelling.

I send you my remarks on those of last year, a copy of Miss Vincent's letter written after reading my remarks, both which I have got back from her for your purpose, and my pencil remarks on the present plans. But I was unwilling to send such a sweeping condemnation without first consulting Captain Galton and asking him to suggest improvements in [the] present plan. He writes as follows:

> 8 February 1883. I think the cutting off of all south light and air from the central corridor on ground floor is very objectionable. The impossibility of getting fresh air into lower central corridor, the placing of all principal nurses' rooms on the north, the putting the W.C.s downstairs in the least ventilated part of the building, the position generally of W.C.s, close to head or foot of stairs and opposite nurses' rooms, the darkness of ground floor corridor, all make it impossible to suggest improvements in present plan. It wants *entire reconstruction.* I should say I cannot add anything to your remarks, which are ALL TO THE POINT. (signed) Douglas Galton.

I am frightened at being unable to say anything but "Don't."

Source: Notes on the St Marylebone Infirmary New Nurses Home, ADD Mss 45820 ff19-20

[December 1883]

Understood that there are two invalid rooms on first and second floors, with door of communication; two bathrooms (instead of nurses' rooms, which will not "do" there) on *ground* floor as well as other floor; kitchen on ground floor; rooms all divided by *walls*; corridors warmed by hot water pipes.

Should this not be *especially* at the end lobbies opposite W.C.s, so that the in-draught of air in cold weather should rather be from the corridor to W.C. lobby than from W.C. lobby to corridor? If more ventilation is wanted in nurses' bedrooms (but with a fireplace and window and door opposite, it appears sufficient), one of Boyle's small-size mica flap ventilators close to ceiling and entering through wall into room chimney.

Lift? Salary of "home" sister?

Source: From a letter to Douglas Galton, ADD Mss 45765 ff235-36

19 December 1883

Infirmary: *New Nurses' Home Plans* (with Dr Sutherland's criticism). Do you remember being so good as to look over these plans very early this year? They were then two storeys of *streets* of rooms on each side a very narrow corridor, and W.C.s very badly placed. We condemned them and the present *three* storeys' plans were substituted—rooms only on one side corridor.

I am afraid the building is *too far advanced* for any but questions of *internal building arrangements* to be yet *open.* Could you be so very kind as to glance at the plans? Do you approve them?

The criticism which stares one in the face is that there must be *bath-rooms* on the *ground* floor, and *not* two nurses' rooms instead (at each end) opening *out of W.C.* Could you kindly criticize the internal arrangements?

Source: From a letter to Henry Bonham Carter, Add Mss 47720 ff236-37

19 December 1883

St Marylebone Infirmary. I send you the present plan of the nurses' building, as sent me by Mr Boulnois at your kind suggestion, Dr Sutherland's and Captain Galton's suggestions, and the old papers for reference. Could you kindly tell me whether *that* is the best that could have been made of it, referring to your *sketch* at the back of the old papers? I presume that the windows of the nurses' rooms (and not of the corridor) do look *south,* but under the high carmelite wall.

I still think that it would be most desirable to have a *class and sitting room,* but over the lecture room seems the only place, [and] that the *bathrooms* should have *fireplaces.* (*We* feel this want so very much.) And there *must* be *bathrooms* on the *ground* floor and *not* nurses' rooms *opening out of the W.C. places.*

I also enclose the *Rules for Probationers* which Mr Boulnois has sent me. Please *criticize* them for me and *Mr Boulnois.* Could you be so very good as to let me have the *whole* back, if I send *tomorrow* (Thursday) *morning* at 10, with your hints as to what I should urge on *Mr Boulnois,* who is coming to see me?

Please say particularly whether you are satisfied that all has been done that could be done with their narrow strip of ground. (I presume they showed you the present plan) and what you think I may *urge* on Mr Boulnois and what it is *useless* to urge.

Are the *partitions* between nurses' rooms walls of wood?

Editor: The training school at St Marylebone opened in 1884. The infirmary was renamed the St Marylebone Hospital in 1923 and then the St Charles Hospital in 1930. In 2012, when I went to see it, it was still functioning, with other buildings on the site, but now as an out-patient centre. There is a Nightingale building on the grounds.

Children's Hospitals, 1879-81

Editor: When the grand duchess of Baden took on the establishment of a new children's hospital for Heidelberg, she sought Nightingale's advice. Nightingale, however, had long been sceptical that children's hospitals were a good thing. In her correspondence with the grand duchess, Nightingale diplomatically confined her remarks to doubting that England had been "successful in her children's hospitals," and assured the grand duchess that she would endeavour "to procure and forward" the material wanted.[399] Nightingale then went to an enormous amount of trouble to find good examples. She wrote to a number of children's hospitals for information—to the matron if she knew her—otherwise to a hospital official, but most of these letters are no longer extant. She did, however, find some plans already published in *The Builder*. By the end of the process a considerable number of plans had been amassed: two for London (the famous Great Ormond St., in central London, and the Shadwell, in East London), and one each for Liverpool, Nottingham, Belfast and Manchester.

Only the Lisbon Children's Hospital, on which Nightingale herself had done much of the work, and the Manchester Children's Hospital, in nearby Pendlebury,[400] met the standard. All the others proved to be, if not thoroughly inadequate, to have some serious defect. They were either risky to health or unconducive to efficient nursing, or both.

Nightingale sought Douglas Galton's advice on the plans before she sent them off. She had, more than once, to ask if the plans should be sent at all, they were so bad. In the case of the Belfast Children's Hospital, where she knew the matron, she was initially enthusiastic (see p 854 below) but, on careful review, thought the hospital was more to be avoided than a model (see p 858 below).

In the course of the collection process, the grand duchess of Baden came to London and a visit to Nightingale was arranged. It was their first (probably their only) meeting and Nightingale was enormously impressed. The grand duchess, for her part, took the advice Nightingale gave and had the plans for her hospital revised, although not thoroughly enough, in Nightingale's view.

---

399 Printed letter to the grand duchess in *Women* (8:839).

400 By architects Pennington and Bridgen, but without any involvement by Nightingale; see "Manchester Children's Hospital Competition," *The Architect* 17 September 1870:161-62; the hospital closed only in 2009.

Source: From a letter to Douglas Galton, Add Mss 45764 ff248-49

5 April 1879

Could you tell me anything about the plans and construction, sanitary and to be recommended, or the reverse, of the *children's hospitals* in London? the Evelina? the Victoria in Chelsea? the East London in Shadwell? the old Great Ormond St., now that it is enlarged, or any children's hospitals in England that you could recommend, either as to be imitated or to be avoided? (I would gladly pay for the copying of any plans that you recommended.)

I am told that there is a good new one at Nottingham. Do you know the Liverpool one? The grand duchess of Baden (we have had a good deal to do with her training schools for nurses, as well as with Princess Alice's[401]) has written to ask for "some plans of the best children's hospitals" in England. She wishes to "know of any new progress in the different parts" and "to see some English plans." They are going to build a new children's hospital at Heidelberg. I dare say you know all about it.

I wish they would send us the plans to criticize. You very much doubt our having any model children's hospitals here, I believe. But our sending plans might lead to their sending theirs for our revising, lead, at all events, to my proposing it. Please give me all the information and advice you can.

3. You did us and the world great good service about the York Road Lying-in Hospital—very many thanks.[402]

Source: From a letter to Harry Verney, Wellcome (Claydon copy) Ms 9007/208

Easter eve [12 April] 1879

Would you not think well to get for the grand duchess *plans* (tracings) of every children's hospital? Does she not ask in her letter to you distinctly for *plans*?

Would you tell Miss Mackenzie[403] that the tracing has not *yet* reached me of her hospital?

---

401 Princess Alice (1843-78), grand duchess of Hesse-Darmstadt, daughter of Queen Victoria.

402 Further letters on the faults of the York Road Lying-in Hospital is in *Women* (8:381-84).

403 H. Mackenzie (later Goodall), matron of the Children's Hospital, Shadwell, who had trained at the St Marylebone Workhouse Infirmary.

Source: From a letter to Douglas Galton, Add Mss 45764 ff250-51

15 April 1879

Great Ormond St. Children's Hospital. How much obliged to you I am for the report and plans of the Great Ormond St. Hospital, which are just what is wanted by the Baden-Heidelberg people.

You are so very good as to say that you will have the plans copied for me. And I am only too thankful to return them to you for that purpose. May we have the description also copied? And in that case do you not think it would be desirable to send that also to the grand duchess?

Could you have it copied without much trouble—well understood at my expense? But I am giving you a great deal of trouble. The construction of the wards seems good. Of course having the out-patient department *under* the in-patients (more especially as they are children) is an enormous error, probably unavoidable in London.

But I do not see any provision for an adequate quantity of baths, which would form perhaps nearly half the whole out-patient department and fight half the battle in a Paris children's hospital, and to which in-patients and out-patients would alike be admitted, but at different hours. (Do you know the "Enfant Jésus" at Paris?) Also I see no adequate provision of W.C.s in the out-patient department. And are there any particular kinds of W.C.s for *children*?

I think there ought to be sisters' rooms off the wards, more particularly in children's hospitals. Or there can be no real supervision.

Source: From a letter to Jessie Lennox,[404] Glasgow Royal Infirmary HB95 12/2/3

21 April 1879

Many, many thanks for your letter.[405] I take the liveliest interest in your new children's hospital and I give you joy, and your little patients joy, and Belfast joy of this extension of a good work.

I am going to ask you a favour—could I have tracings of the *plans* of the ward floors (storeys), the administration floor and the out-patients' department? Also sections of any particular baths (fixed) or W.C.s more expressly for children's use? I need not say that I would joyfully pay for the tracings that may be kindly made for me from any plans.

---

404 Jessie Lennox (c1839-c1941), who had trained at the Nightingale School, was matron of the Belfast Hospital for Sick Children. On it see H.G. Calwell, *The Life and Times of a Voluntary Hospital: The History of the Royal Belfast Hospital for Sick Children 1873-1948.*

405 Lennox letter 5 April 1879, Add Mss 47751 f162.

Your excellent secretary, Mr Herbert Darbishire,[406] would, I believe, further my wish. My reason for this request is not only that I could not write to the ladies' committee (as you desire, but as I very much deprecate, feeling unfit for such an honour) without seeing the plans—but also because they will be really useful. In Germany they are going to build a new children's hospital at Heidelberg (Baden) and the grand duchess of Baden, who has done a great deal in training of nurses, has written to me for *plans* of the best new children's hospitals in this country. I am collecting and having plans and tracing of plans made to send her, and I should be very glad to add to them the new Belfast Children's Hospital.

Thanking you again for your letter, and again giving you joy, pray believe me dear Miss Lennox,

ever sincerely yours

Florence Nightingale

Thank you much for telling me about the Belfast Ladies' Society for giving work to poor mothers. Again I say Godspeed the children's hospital. Under severe strain of overwork and illness but

ever theirs and yours

F.N.

Since I wrote this, I have received your newspaper slip; it is very interesting, but makes me wish all the more to see the plans.

Source: From a letter to Harry Verney, Wellcome (Claydon copy) Ms 9007/218

22 April 1879

Have you had a communication from Miss Mackenzie and the secretary of the Shadwell *Children's Hospital* about *plans*? I should like to see the plans.

Editor: The matron of the Shadwell Children's Hospital duly sent the requested plans to Nightingale, who wrote back that neither they nor any of the "other many plans I had collected were worth anything as model plans to the grand duchess of Baden for the proposed children's hospital to be built at Heidelberg."[407]

---

406 Herbert Darbishire (d. 1908), honorary secretary and major founder of the Belfast Children's Hospital.

407 Letter to Mackenzie 19 July 1879, in *Extending Nursing* (13:194).

Source: From two letters to Douglas Galton, Add Mss 45764 ff252-53 and 254-55

22 April 1879

Children's Hospital, Great Ormond St. I am very much obliged to you for your note and the two numbers of *The Builder* with plans, elevation and description of the Children's Hospital.

I think they will answer the purpose, if you would be so good as to have copied a drain ventilation section, which, if I am not mistaken, was in the "cahier" [notebook] you sent me after the page on which the plans are. (This section is not in *The Builder*), that is, IF *you* think it of consequence to a German architect. Should the copies you kindly have ordered be, however, near completion, I would still have them finished and send them to Baden.

2. Do you know whether there are in *The Builder*, or other architectural paper, plans of *any other children's hospitals*? I have written for tracings of *Shadwell* Hospital (which we nurse and where we have just lost a young trained head nurse[408]), of *Belfast* (Children's) Hospital just finished, of *Liverpool* ditto. Though none of these I believe to be good, not very good Victoria *(Chelsea)* I understand to be merely an old house adapted, rooms opening out of one another.

3. To return to *Great Ormond St.*, *The Builder*, dated 1872, gives the ward plan, with two excrescences or wings (very bad) opening from each *end* of the ward floor, as "not yet built." They were not yet given in the plan (cahier [notebook]) you sent me. Do you understand that they are still "*not yet built*"? I hope not.

28 April 1879

I am so very glad that your Chatham sanitary lectures are being done into a book. I am afraid I am a poor critic, and I am undertaking far too many things. But if you are kind enough to let me see them before going to press, I would gladly do so.

Thank you very much about the Great Ormond St. Children's Hospital. I have seen a quite rough sketch of a floor of the (Chelsea) Victoria Hospital. It is hard for anything to be worse in these days of outcry for progress. And they have had fatal typhoid arising in hospital.

408 Ruth Owen (c1851-79), buried on 16 April 1879.

Source: From two letters to Harry Verney, Wellcome (Claydon copy) Ms 9007/220 and 224

28 April 1879

Is this a hospital from *not* being a hospital? This plan is of course not of the slightest use, from having *no wards*. Where is the *ward plan*?

As there is haste, I will see you today "between 5 and 6" (though overcome with work) if you will be so good, and will return to you those melancholy performances you sent me. If they will send us tracings of the *Rhyl* Hospital and the *Nottingham* Hospital (the slightest sketches), that will be of use. Of course what they have sent is not the least use.

6 May 1879

I return [the letter of the] grand duchess. I have written for divers children's *hospitals plans* in London (perhaps you could do Nottingham and any others) and I will send them her. And perhaps you could advise her to *send us* her Heidelberg *sketch plans* to review, when I will have them carefully revised by the highest authorities here. I very much doubt *our* having any model children's hospitals here, but I think we could do good by revising the Heidelberg sketch plans.

Source: From three letters to Douglas Galton, ADD Mss 45764 ff256-57, 258 and 259-60

10 May 1879

I cannot thank you enough for the copy of the plans and description of the Great Ormond St. Hospital, which are all that is wanted. (Please kindly to tell me what to pay for the copying.)

2. I have received the enclosed tracings of the plans of the NEW Belfast Children's Hospital, just finished. Would you kindly tell me whether you think they are worth sending to the grand duchess of Baden? To me they seem rather what ought to be avoided than what ought to be imitated: the great square ward with only five windows, leaving two adjoining sides of the ward quite windowless for seventeen beds; the corridor apparently without light or air; some bedrooms, kitchens, receiving rooms and lavatories with no outside window and numerous other defects (there are INside W.C.s) so glaring that one thinks the mistake must be in one's own understanding.

Mr Herbert Darbishire, the secretary, wrote to me before sending them that "the building had been entirely constructed after" the rules laid down in my *Notes on Hospitals*. And the matron [Jessie Lennox], who came from us, has asked me to write to the committee a letter of approval on the plans.

What do you advise me to do? I mean about sending them to Heidelberg. And would you kindly tell me what you criticize?

15 May 1879

Children's Hospital Plans. Very many thanks for your decision and criticism concerning the Belfast Children's Hospital, *not* to send it to the grand duchess of Baden. Would you be so very kind as to look at:

1. Shadwell Hospital, *two plans and elevation* enclosed. (This hospital we nurse.) It seems good. Would you kindly look at the plans and say whether I shall send them to the grand duchess, also give me the benefit of your *criticism.*

2. *Nottingham Hospital, one pencil plan, two letters? What do you think of this?* Is it worth sending to Heidelberg?

24 May 1879

Liverpool Children's Hospital, Manchester Children's Hospital. I am very much obliged to you for your criticism and advice on the last two plans I sent you (for sending to the grand duchess of Baden). I hope this is the "*vero ultimõ*" [very last] time I shall trouble you.

I send two plans of the Liverpool Hospital, which is a new one. Its merit is that the out-patients department is built quite separate from the hospital (there is an entrance to it under cover). The dispensary is in the out-patients' department. But I am surprised and disappointed at the wards entering from one another, etc.

Do you think the plans are good enough to go to the grand duchess of Baden? (Germans are so fond of small wards that they might be deterred from them by seeing this.) If you think they are worth sending, would you kindly write a criticism to go with them?

2. I enclose a report of the *Pendlebury* Hospital near Manchester, with a plan in it. It seems to me by far the best I have yet seen. And we understand that there is but *one floor* of wards? Is this printed plan *sufficiently explicit to send* her? Or should I write to Pendlebury and ask for more elaborate tracings? (N.B. The [Lisbon] plan by Mr Humbert in my *Notes on Hospitals* is also good (see p 175 above). That and this are really the only very good ones, I think.) What do you say?

Editor: The Humbert plan referred to in the above letter was Lisbon. A ward sister at St Bartholomew's, Helen Blower (formerly at the Montreal General) obtained plans of a children's infirmary, which she hoped would not be "too late to be of service to you." The architect, E.H. Bamner, she said, was "very glad to show it to you."[409]

---

409 Blower letter 23 May 1879, Add Mss 45805 f206.

Source: From a letter to the Children's Hospital, Royal Manchester Children's Hospital Website

31 May 1879

To the Secretary of the Children's Hospital, Pendlebury and Carlisle Street

Sir, The glimpses that I have had of the plans of your hospital lead me to think that it must be one of the best constructed in Europe.

Might I trouble you to send me a copy of the report for 1879, which I think has a plan of the building in it? And might I ask you kindly to put the address of the architect on the enclosed letter?

Source: From two letters to Douglas Galton, Add Mss 45764 ff263 and 270

3 July 1879

I took your advice and have asked the architects for a ward plan or tracing of the *Pendlebury Children's Hospital.* There have been delays upon delays. But the chairman came to my help. I hope to have it soon, and send it to you before sending it and others to Baden.

24 July 1879

Plans for the Heidelberg Children's Hospital. After a month's delay, and calling in the help of the "chair" of the Pendlebury Hospital, I have got in the accompanying packet. There is, as you will see, a tracing of the ward (in the long envelope) and there are the photographs of the interior of the wards. What do you think is desirable to send to the Baden grand duchess? Do you think *the photos* are of any use? And if so which?

(I enclose a copy of the report in this cover for reference to the general plan.) Do you think we ought to keep a copy of the ward tracing for ourselves? (We shall never see it again.) You will see that the architect does not forbid its use abroad, but does at home. We must keep it to ourselves. If you think it desirable that we should have a copy of the ward tracing made, could you be so very good *as to have one made*? Messenger shall call tomorrow at 10 for your instructions.

I was so very glad to see you again, and so very grateful for your visit.

O that the Zulu War[410] may be now at an end, but *O O O* that they may learn from it a lesson.

---

410 Nightingale assisted with sending nurses to the Anglo-Zulu War, which was fought from January to July 1879.

Source: From two letters to Harry Verney, Wellcome (Claydon copy) Ms 9007/249-50

24 July 1879

I have at last received the plans for the grand duchess of Baden and hope in a few days to send off these weary (children's hospitals) views, photographs and tracings.

6 August 1879

I was just doing up the plans for the grand duchess of Baden, when on Monday Mme E. Bunsen called here to ask me to see the grand duchess on Tuesday, who was in London for one day. I did so. And she stayed a long, long, while. I think I never saw anyone in any class who struck me so much.

I have a great dislike to doing things for the big. I had so much rather do them for the little. But for this woman I could do anything. We had a very long talk. I am sure she is of the "manifestations" of the daughters "of God." And my "earnest expectation" would always "wait upon" her.[411]

She asked most cordially after you. She has gone today to Eastbourne for her daughter's health, to stay. She seemed to have true genius, the genius of good.

Source: from a letter to Douglas Galton, Add Mss 45764 f272

6 August 1879

I cannot thank you enough for your great kindness about the plans for children's hospitals for Baden, your care in criticizing them and your goodness in having them copied. (I wish you would let me remunerate somebody for this.)

It is like days gone by. Just as I was putting up the selected plans for Baden, arrived a lady to ask me to see the grand duchess. She was in England. So I was able to explain them viva voce [out loud]. She is, as you know, a most intelligent woman and has done a great deal both in training nurses and in hospitals.

411 A paraphrase of Rom 8:19.

Source: From a letter to Harry Verney, Wellcome (Claydon copy) Ms 9008/23

23 February 1880

I send you the grand duchess of Baden's letter,[412] which I happened to have here. Please return it to me as it is one of the heaps of letters of which the *non*-answering pulls me down to Hades. I have not answered it.

If you like to look at her "plans" (which I am ashamed to say I have not) they are *two cahiers* [notebooks] in a square shallow frame *box* (*not* in a "*portfolio*") on the floor in my dressing room in the corner next the window. The maids will give them you. Please return them when I return.

Source: From two letters to Douglas Galton, ADD MSS 45764 ff329 and 331-32, both from Lea Hurst

16 November 1880

Are you returned from America? and how are you?

You will remember how last year you most kindly helped me in collecting, choosing from and having copied children's hospital plans for the grand duchess of Baden, who was about to build a children's hospital at Heidelburg, which is to be a supplementary hospital for the (medical) university at Heidelburg. (This is not an advantage, but a necessity.)

Your labour has not been in vain. And the grand duchess (who has just given us a lady probationer[413] to train at St Thomas' as a superintendent) has sent me by her the plans of this hospital "to criticize freely" before they begin to build.

Would you have the *great kindness*, if I were to send you those plans to look them over with critical carefulness, and make your severest remarks, with your earliest convenience? I have made a few, but would like to await yours.

24 November 1880

Child's Hospital. Very many thanks for your kind offer to look at the plans for the proposed *children's* hospital at *Heidelberg*. I had already sent them to Dr Sutherland, and he will forward them to you. Pray be so good as to return them to me here, when you have done with them, WITH YOUR REMARKS.

---

412 Letter to Nightingale 12 August 1879, Wellcome Ms 9030/63.

413 Fräulein von Cornberg, daughter of the minister of war of Baden.

Source: From two letters to Harry Verney, Wellcome (Claydon copy) Ms 9008/101-02, both from Lea Hurst

2 December 1880

I do not quite understand Mme Bunsen about *Mlle de Cornberg.* She came, introduced to me by the grand duchess, with whom I have had the most detailed correspondence about her. I got her into St Thomas' at my own expense. The grand duchess and I have settled together, I submitting a program to her, of what "institutions" she is to see when she leaves St T. And I shall of course see Mlle de C. as soon as I return. (Mme Bunsen asks you to "introduce" her to me.) . . .

The grand duchess has sent me the plans for the proposed *Heidelberg Children's Hospital,* and I have gone over them with much labour and made Dr Sutherland and Captain Galton in London do so too. (They are not very good.)

How *would you advise me to return them to the grand duchess at Baden?* They are in a *box.* (It is rather a job for me "toute seule [all alone]" *to dispatch a package to Germany.*)

4 December 1880

I find that the grand duchess of Baden would like to have the plans returned to her *as soon as possible,* as she "was particularly anxious to obtain our criticisms thereon before any work was begun." I should therefore be extremely obliged to you to "*write* AT ONCE," as you so kindly propose, "to *Sir Charles Dilke*[414] to ask if a *Queen's Messenger may leave them as he passes* at Baden on his way" somewhere. *Must I send the box up to the Foreign Office? and with what address?*

Source: From a letter to John Sutherland, Add Mss 45758 ff143-44

24 May 1881

Children's Hospital. Grand Duchess of Baden. The grand duchess of Baden begs her best thanks to you for your kindness in revising the sketch plans of her proposed Children's Hospital at Heidelberg. You know that I obtained for her the plans, among many others, of the Pendlebury Children's Hospital at Manchester, by far the best there is. Would you read the enclosed letter?[415]

---

414 Sir Charles Dilke (1843-1911), 2nd baronet, Parliamentary under secretary, Foreign Office.

415 The letter is not in the Nightingale files, and the name of the sender is not known; it is probably the architect.

I thought the things he so wisely mentions were now acknowledged everywhere, and that they were in my *Notes on Hospitals* and every book on the subject.

1. What shall I say to her? and
2. Should I warn the grand duchess's architect on these points?

Whether they are acknowledged everywhere or not, it is certain they are not acted upon. Would you believe it that, in the new Edinburgh Infirmary, the drainage of especially the nurses' quarters, and, worst, the quarters of our invaluable *Miss Pringle,* the lady superintendent, *are* so bad: steam pipes, wastepipes, soil pipes all intercommunicating, ventilation, so-called, forcing the sewer gas *into* the rooms instead of *out,* that typhoid has arisen, even in a visitor, and her, *Miss Pringle's,* health has been almost ruined. A lady called the R. sanitary inspectors, did it, re-did it, inspected it, and now *report* on their *own inspection.* And *no* radical reform is made. What is to be done?

Please return me my own note with your answer. Pray give my kindest love to Mrs Sutherland. It is long since I have heard from her.

Editor: The hospital in the next letter, the Chelsea Hospital for Women, was the first to be built specifically for women's diseases. Founded as an establishment for distressed gentlewomen and the deserving poor, it was then in the course of constructing new and larger quarters, in Fulham Road. The foundation stone was laid in 1880 and the hospital opened in 1883. The papers noted by J.S. Wood, the secretary, are missing.

Source: Letter to J.S. Wood, Northwestern University

London
18 May 1881

Sir, I am truly sorry to be compelled to decline the honour that you do me, by asking me to write my name on the papers you enclose for your most desirable Chelsea "Hospital for Women," that I am fain to explain how I am always under the severe and ever-increasing pressure of overwork and illness—how I am beset, like others, with similar applications from all parts of the world—but how unlike others it would be impossible for me to carry on the duties I have undertaken, were I to answer these applications, and how in order not to give offence I have been unwillingly forced to take notice of none. If I were to make exceptions, I should of course receive applications which I could not decline.

Pray accept my regret, which is greater than yours can be, and allow me nevertheless to wish Godspeed to your hospital. . . .

I have been interrupted over and over again, even while writing this short note.

Editor: The meeting of the International Medical Congress, in London in August 1881, brought a visit by a distinguished American doctor, Joseph Meredith Toner (1825-96), a former president of the American Medical Association and editor of the *Journal of the American Medical Association.* Toner had been instrumental in starting nursing in Washington, D.C., just prior to the Civil War, with the Sisters of Charity of Emmitsburg. It is not clear, however, to what nurse training school the next letter refers. Nightingale met with Toner on 8 August, but her notes from that meeting concern the Washington Training School, which had no home, nor hospital, but used hired rooms.[416]

Source: From a letter to Dr Toner, Library of Congress

6 August 1881

I thank you a thousand times for your great kindness in bringing me your books, the photographs of the nurses, and the china manufactured for the Nurses Training School—all things which I shall value so much.

I cannot bear that you should leave England without my seeing you personally on a subject so interesting to us both. But I am so overworked (and always a prisoner from illness) that I can only say, could you give me a few minutes on *Monday* at *12:30,* or on *Tuesday* at *12:30* or at *5*? Please let me have a word in reply, and for the nursing cause, pray believe me,

ever your and its faithful servant
Florence Nightingale

Convalescent and Cottage Hospitals,[417] 1877-89

Editor: In 1877 Nightingale flagged the lack of convalescent facilities in England, especially compared with France, in a letter to Harry Verney:

416 Letter in *Extending Nursing* (13:512-13).

417 On cottage hospitals see Meyrick Emrys-Roberts, *The Cottage Hospitals 1869-1990: Arrival, Survival and Revival.*

> No one knows as I do the difficulty in England of getting anything between a private family house and a hospital. In France there would have been a good "Pensionnat pour Malades" or "Maison de Santé Municipale" at every one of these places, so much recommended by doctors, good and cheap. However, we have, an't please God, hit the right thing at last: at an infinite profit to Post and Telegraph Offices.[418]

According to a note in her diary later that year, Nightingale sent her criticism of plans for a convalescent hospital in Eastbourne to Douglas Galton, but neither the notes nor any correspondence about the plans are available.[419]

By the late 1870s, alternatives to cottage hospitals (not for convalescents) were becoming more available. Some workhouse infirmaries at least provided care similar to that in regular civil hospitals. The state-funded fever hospitals were now an option, and did not have the stigma attached to the workhouse infirmary. District nursing, that is, with trained nurses to visit patients in their homes, had been established.

The first item below was evidently written in response to a request by the bishop of Truro, but his letter is not extant. The letter notes many of the drawbacks of cottage hospitals, but wishes him well in his project, about which no further information is available.

Source: From an incomplete letter to Bishop Stubbs,[420] Hampshire Record Office 61M 88/20

[ca. late 1870s-early 1880s]

In very many instances when cottage hospitals have been built, they undoubtedly are the means of withdrawing patients from the county hospital, and thereby diminishing its usefulness. Cottage hospitals are very convenient for the local medical men: they save their time, centralizing cases, many of which would be visited without remuneration. They also afford them opportunities of performing operations, and of experience which country practitioners do not otherwise obtain. If the hospital is thus the means of withdrawing patients from the advantage of more skilled advice and attendance, it is of course insofar an evil.

Then the cost—most important—depending mainly on the average number of legitimate cases which the district supplies—usually *very few*

---

418 In *The Nightingale School* (12:332).

419 Note 27 June 1877, ADD MSS 45847.

420 Charles William Stubbs (1845-1912), bishop of Truro, Cornwall.

in an agricultural district. The workhouse infirmary meets the demand to a great extent (and to improve workhouse infirmary nursing is one of the things to which this present time is awakening, and in London and the great towns with some success).

A cottage hospital should at any rate require a minimum payment for every inmate (to be remitted only exceptionally after due inquiry). It is not suitable for fever cases, for which the parish authorities [local government] are responsible. A qualified hospital-trained district nurse, at a cost of, say, £100 a year, may be sufficient to meet the larger part of the requirements to the district. In a populous district, both hospital and district nurse may be usefully combined. Effective supervision, whether of cottage hospital or of district nurse, is difficult. The advantages and disadvantages are a question of degree, and local circumstances and sound conclusions can hardly be arrived at by a stranger.

May the highest success attend the carrying out of this work (and the decision arrived at be the just one), and all your works is the hearty wish of,

yours ever sincerely

Florence Nightingale

Pardon dryness—*not* of good wishes. I am sorry not to be more definite. Should a cottage hospital plan be ultimately decided upon, and you care to send me the *sketch plan,* I would have it carefully considered and criticized by experts.

Editor: The following letter provides the only information on Nightingale's involvement in the founding of a convalescent home near Bolton-le-Moors, Lancashire. Nightingale was evidently contacted by Mrs Blair (letter missing) and a short time later by a Mrs Harrison Blair in Kent, presumably a relative. Nightingale sent this second Mrs Blair her own copy of *Notes on Hospitals,* as the book was out of print. From an announcement in *The Lancet,* it is known that a legacy of £30,000 was left for the purpose in 1870 by a Stephen Blair and a site acquired.[421] A "Blair Convalescent Hospital" opened in 1887 in Bromley Cross, some three miles from Bolton-le-Moors. It closed in 1991.

421 *The Lancet* 9 August 1884:253.

Source: From a letter to Mrs Blair, Florence Nightingale Museum (LMA) H1/ST/NC1/80/61, typed copy Add Mss 45806 ff40-42

24 June 1880

Madam, You have my deepest interest, my deepest sympathy, in the matter of the convalescent hospital which you wish to build near Bolton-le-Moors, and of which you already have the site.

I am sure that the benefits of convalescent homes are only second to those of hospitals, and indeed that no hospital is complete without its convalescent adjunct. So few patients leave hospital able to return at once to their work and their poor homes. And this dooms them sooner or later "to the parish" [workhouse] in too many cases, i.e., to be dependent on the poor rates, to a life of infirmity.

Not only do I think "small" convalescent homes admissible, but I think it better to begin with a small building which can be enlarged. You ask me "where to see the *working* of a small convalescent hospital?" Would it not be better to see several? You have probably seen (1) Miss Hawthorn's, St Agatha's, near Beckenham.[422] That is in a private house and for children only. Have you seen the (2) Dover Convalescent Home? (3) the Ascot Convalescent Home, near Brecknells, Berks, kept by "sisters."[423] One could hardly recommend the *building*, but the "working" is excellent, that is, for women and children. (4) Have you seen the Convalescent Home, Black Rock, Brighton (Miss Marsh's)?[424] (5) the Eastbourne Convalescent Home? (6) You have of course seen the Memorial Herbert Home at Bournemouth? that was built on purpose for its object, viz., for *convalescents*. But before building on any large scale, you will probably see those near Glasgow, in North and South Wales, and others. But I strongly recommend the *cottage* form, like that at Bournemouth.

You ask to see me. How gladly would I do so in such a cause, but you only give me from today, Thursday, when I received your note, till Saturday. It is quite impossible. I could not even name any time *before* the *week after next*, alas! Mrs Wardroper will have told you that I am under the severe pressure of ever-increasing illness and overwork and

---

422 Isabella Hawthorn (c1835-?), who had trained at St Thomas', opened a convalescent home for children, which the Nightingale School used also for nurse training.

423 A convalescent home run by the Anglican Sisters of Mercy of the Holy Trinity, on which see p 395 above.

424 Run by philanthropist Catherine Marsh (1818-1912); correspondence with her is in *Women* (8:814-15).

entirely a prisoner to my room. And, I might add, to show you how gladly I would see you if I could, that my doctors order me to talk only half an hour every other day, which in *practice* is *every* half hour *every* day.

My time is entirely filled up with overwork—persons leaving London or England who appoint themselves for weeks beforehand, among the rest. I am scarcely able today to write this note. If you would have SKETCH *plans* of your proposed "small convalescent home" made, and sent me, I would give them all the attention in my power, and consider every detail. And I would obtain valuable opinions from the Army Sanitary Commission, etc. But I must have the permission to keep the plans at least a week for criticism, as I cannot command my own time. God speed the future "Blair Convalescent Home" is the earnest prayer of

ever your faithful servant
Florence Nightingale

Source: From two letters to Douglas Galton, ADD MSS 45765 ff266 and 269

6 June 1885

Could you be so very kind as to tell me what advice to give about her hospital building to this old "hospital" sister of ours? And also whether Burdett's *Cottage Hospital* book is worth her having? They are quite sure to choose the worst plan in it, if there are bad plans, you know. I have not seen the book. What is the best-planned cottage hospital you know?

Please forgive my troubling you.

12 July 1885

You remember a small hospital to be built at Haydock, in Lancashire, about which you were good enough to advise me—the sketch plan has now been sent me. Would you kindly criticize it? May I send it you?

Shall you be in London this week? Might I hope for some afternoon?

Editor: Nightingale prepared a twelve-page critique for Mrs Hayward, superintendent of the above-mentioned cottage hospital, but only a brief excerpt is still available:

> 14 July 1885. I have shown your plan to one of, if not the greatest authority, on hospital construction, and he very much approves, as I do, of the general arrangements. x x By all means keep it all as a healthy "cottage," and not as a miniature hospital. The working

> people should see how, with furniture like their own x x and appliances like their own, . . . the clean and comfortable arrangements can be produced, and by them imitated. x x Success to the Haydock Cottage Hospital![425]

There is then a gap in information until 1890, when Mrs Hayward wrote Nightingale with a report of their last five years' work in the cottage hospital. The place was "increasingly useful," she said, and they had had "some very interesting cases." They had not been hampered by lack of funds; rather, help had been beyond their expectations.[426] The hospital closed in 1978 after ninety years of operation.

Source: From a letter to Amy Hawthorn,[427] Add Mss 45776 ff187-90

16 March 1886

Dearest Mrs Hawthorn, I am quite heartbroken about this result of little Frank McGee's going to the convalescent hospital with whooping cough still hanging about him. Of course I have written no excuse, for no excuse is possible—or will undo the mischief. I have merely written that if proper accommodation can be found in the neighbourhood for the "permanent" inmates who have not had whooping cough, it is to be done immediately, at my expense.

It is terrible that children patients, and adult ones too, for that matter, should have been kept out of the convalescent hospital by this disaster. I have written that the two poor little mites should be placed at my expense *wherever* they can be taken in, when they can be moved, if they live. But that is the difficulty, *where*? Everything is so complicated for patients by this extraordinary weather. What could the doctor have been about who gave the certificate, not to ascertain whether the whooping cough was over? Every doctor must know that it would be almost as pardonable to send a bag of dynamite as a child with the remains of whooping cough in with other patients and children patients. It is a frightful calamity.

Would you, please, return the poor superior's letter and help me, as you have so often, to find out what is best to be done? Has the mother [superior] been imposing again (on anyone) with her "dates"?

---

425 Excerpt from a blog, Alan Whalley 21 August 2008.

426 Letter to Nightingale 20 January 1891, Add Mss 45810 f168.

427 Amy E. Hawthorn, wife of Colonel Hawthorn, R.E., and cousin of Charles George Gordon, also R.E., who alerted Nightingale to the bad conditions of Zulu War hospitals.

I am so very glad that Mr Campbell-Bannerman[428] means to continue provision in payments for the lock hospital at Chatham and elsewhere. You see Mr Stansfeld's[429] motion for tonight and Sir J. Kennaway's[430] amendment.

With regard to the poor private soldier, Harding, now at the Hampstead Hospital for Consumption, I have not forgotten about getting him into St Thomas' if possible. I think the better plan would be, if you would kindly let me know about *a week* before 6 April—I think you said that day his time at Hampstead would expire—what his state is and, if possible, send me a certificate from the Hampstead medical officer what the progress of his disease is, *and whether he would be benefited* by a general hospital.

Of course now all medical wards in general hospitals are crowded with acute diseases, the result of cold. I am afraid they ought to require such a *recent* certificate before admitting him. But I hope they will admit him, if benefit can be had for him, *and* if they have room.

Editor: In 1889 Nightingale was invited by the marchioness of Dufferin and Ava, a colleague on India issues, to "be present at the laying of the foundation stone of the Queen Victoria Convalescent Home . . . at Newtownbreda on Thursday 19 September at 3 o'clock.[431] She did not attend.

Correspondence on other hospital matters resumes, beginning with a letter updating Sir Henry Parkes on the literature on both hospitals and towns.

---

428 Henry Campbell-Bannerman (1836-1908), Liberal secretary of state for war, and later prime minister.

429 James Stansfeld (1820-98), later Sir, the leading MP opposing the Contagious Diseases Acts. The motion was for repeal of the acts, enforcement of which had been suspended for several years. Nightingale elsewhere praised Stansfeld for appointing the first woman, Jane Senior, to the civil service (Sybil Oldfield, *Jeanie, an "Army of One," Mrs Nassau Senior 1828-1877: The First Woman in Whitehall* 180-81).

430 John Henry Kennaway (1837-1919), Conservative MP. The amendment added provision for the maintenance of the lock hospitals for voluntary treatment, which failed, but the main motion passed.

431 Printed invitation of the Belfast Hospital for Sick Children 11 September 1889, Add Mss 47751 f205.

Source: From a letter to Henry Parkes, State Library of New South Wales

9 May 1882

I am afraid, after this long delay, I have yet to make a most unsatisfactory return to your request for books. As relates to "health provision for towns," I send the following documents and plans:

1. Copies of by-laws prepared by the Local Government Board;
2. Suggestions as to sewerage by Mr Rawlinson;
3. Report on treatment of sewage, and copy of lectures and papers, also by Mr Rawlinson;
4. A set of detail plans for manholes, etc., for main sewerage. Also a copy of our "*Indian Suggestions*," but these, I may say, are now under revision in order to be made much more complete.

You should take back with you a copy of Captain Galton's book showing the principles of construction of *Healthy Dwellings*.[432] As regards hospital management, there is a singular dearth in such books. I have inquired in vain. Part 2 beginning at p 14 of the Regulations for the Army Medical Department (which I send) may be of some use to you. I wish I could send better. Please excuse—I have done my best. . . .

P.T.O. Mr Rawlinson sent some of those papers I now enclose to the municipal authorities of Melbourne and Sydney some time ago.

Editor: Many faults in the new St Thomas' Hospital became evident soon after its opening in 1871.[433] The next correspondence concerns those found much later.

Source: From a letter to John Sutherland, Add Mss 45758 ff191-92

[23 January 1885]

It seems to me that one must always repeat the most elementary notions of sanitary things again and again. Do you know that in one week we have eighteen!!! probationers at St Thomas' "down" with diarrhea and sickness "and in a typhoid condition"? Today we completely empty our "home," send all the really sick probationers into two special sick wards, send all the *well* ones into an empty ward fitted up in haste for them, send the convalescents to their homes, and then thorough inspection.

---

432 Galton's *Observations on the Construction of Healthy Dwellings, Namely, Houses, Hospitals, Barracks, Asylums, etc.*, 1880.

433 These appear in *The Nightingale School*, for example, with pyemia in 1872 (12:211), and several diseases in 1872 (12:257).

It is believed that the same cistern supplies drinking water and sinks. It is believed that the wastepipe of the sink goes straight into the drain, without being cut off. It is known that the tap for the drinking water is over a sink and Mr Currey is our architect! and Dr Bristowe is sanitary officer!!! to the hospital!!!

I think *I* ought to be hanged and Dr Bristowe, Mr Currey, his builder and plumber shut up in a sink!!!

Source: From two letters to Douglas Galton, Add Mss 45765 ff259-61 and 264

25 February 1885

Could you be so very good as to look over the report and recommendations of the "sanitary protection" inspector on the drainage, wastepipes, etc., of our probationers' "home" at St Thomas', the defects in which occasioned the epidemic outbreak among our nurses, of which I told you, and you were so good as to dictate to me certain general recommendations, which are all adopted. Also the proposals of the architect, Mr H. Currey, upon the report of the sanitary man. If I may send you these papers for criticism, where may I send them?

The same defect will have to be dealt with all over the hospital, which makes it the more important. N.B. In minor matters, we asked for the "slop sinks," but it would be very inconvenient to have them in the "bathroom," as proposed by Mr Currey. The only convenient place would be where we put them in the "home" of St Marylebone Infirmary, viz., in the lobby to the W.C., but there the lobby had an outside window. This, I am afraid, is not the case at our "home" at St Thomas'.

2. One of the W.C.s in the basement *must* be abolished. The other, Dr Smith, resident physician, says cannot be either properly ventilated—Foreman says it *can*.

3. We modestly ask, could there be any warming by hot water of the *north* rooms of our probationers, which are *very* cold? All this, however, is but as the "mote in the eye"[434] compared with the great defects and recommendations you will see in the report, on which I hope for your criticism. The treasurer has already sanctioned the necessary expenditure, and our "Fund" will do the rest. He is quite aware that the remedial works will have to be extended to the *whole* hospital. (The pyemia, erysipelas, etc., and outbreaks in the children's ward *may* now be accounted for.)

---

434 An allusion to Matt 7:3.

20 March 1885

We were exceedingly obliged to you for so kindly helping us with your valued criticism on the two sanitary reports upon the defects of drainage, etc., in the home for probationers at St Thomas' Hospital. They are now at work there, but I fear they will not reconstruct the drainage of the whole hospital as they ought.

Liverpool Royal Infirmary, 1882-85

Editor: Nightingale was asked in late 1882 to recommend an architect for the new Liverpool Royal Infirmary. Typically, she consulted Douglas Galton for a name, and even hoped that he might be willing to do it himself. In the end, the contract was given to Alfred Waterhouse (1830-1905), a prominent Gothic Revival architect.[435] Both Nightingale and Galton met with him (see p 876 below).

The new building was to follow the pavilion style. Nightingale's concern then was that the pavilions be far enough apart to ensure sunlight in the wards, recognizing that at the great Edinburgh Royal Infirmary, pavilion style as it was, insufficient distance had been allowed between the pavilions. In the case of Liverpool, adequate space had been allowed for, but the women's pavilions were cut up. The "separation" wards for highly infectious cases like erysipelas were close by other wards, when they should be in a separate block entirely: Nightingale's early belief that infectious patients could be mingled with others had long been abandoned.

Correspondence shows that the amount of cubic space considered necessary in an acute-care hospital, such as the Liverpool Royal Infirmary, had gone up by 1885 to "never under 2000" (see p 877 below). The Edinburgh Royal Infirmary here was a positive model, for it had 2300 to 2500 cubic feet per bed.

The circular wards planned for the Liverpool Royal Infirmary posed a number of problems. Nightingale objected that patients could not look out the window opposite their bed, for the distance was too great. Some beds were too far from the fireplace. Both fresh air and sunlight were lacking at the centre. The circular wards also failed to provide enough space around the beds for the "swarm" of medical students who accompanied doctors on rounds (see p 877 below). No

435 On his work see Colin Cunningham and Prudence Waterhouse, *Alfred Waterhouse 1830-1905: Biography of a Practice.*

nurse's room for the management of the circular wards was provided, and the combination of circular wards with the pavilion style made for difficulties in allocating nursing staff.

To his credit, said Nightingale, the architect had allowed for six rooms for sick nurses, but no toilet, bathroom or slop sink (for emptying bedpans) for them. She wondered if the sisters' rooms were large enough to be comfortable as bedrooms. The space given to the twenty-four maids was too cramped.

Alex Graham, who had been so much praised in 1875, was now off the recommended list of architects, for not having done well at Lincoln. Precisely what was unsatisfactory is not clear in the letter immediately below, beyond being mentioned as such. On the Liverpool Royal Infirmary there is a surviving letter to the architect himself and notes for him, with comments co-ordinated with those of Galton.

Source: From three letters to Douglas Galton, Add Mss 45765 ff172-73, 174-75 and 176-77

12 November 1882

Private. Thank you very much for a copy of your admirable address at Newcastle.[436]

Whom do you think a rising hospital *architect*? They want to rebuild the Royal Infirmary at Liverpool—they *don't* want "a great architect, who would want his own way and aim at making a handsome building, instead of a commodious one." They want "to know what has been done lately, and who are the best men to choose from." They want "a young man of ability, who would visit any hospitals worth seeing, and try to make the Liverpool one, which is now a beast, the best thing done yet, without unnecessary expenditure."

I think Saxon Snell did the new Marylebone Infirmary at Notting Hill very well. Is he an expensive man? But I don't know the rising men. Please tell me and please give me any general hints about hospitals and sites to give them (Liverpool) when you tell me *whom you would recommend.* I have to see them this week. . . .

Graham, whom we used to recommend, did not do very well at Lincoln.

436 Galton's inaugural address as president of the Sanitary Institute of Great Britain, held at Newcastle-upon-Tyne, and published in its *Transactions.*

28 November 1882

Rebuilding Liverpool R. Infirmary. Private.

I took immediate advantage of your kindness in mentioning hospital architects for Liverpool R. Infirmary (rebuilding) and I now enclose a letter of further inquiry.

Saxon Snell—I sent them a splendid book[437] he gave me, but told them he was not considered "amenable."

The first name you gave me I gave in: *James Osborne-Smith.*[438] I said what you had said of him, and said (privately) that you would be so good as to overhaul his plans, if he were chosen. I did not "back" him, for I never heard of him, but said that I should be most happy to do my "petit possible" working under you, upon Mr J.O. Smith's plans, if desired. *Rogers:* Dr Sutherland gave this name, which of course you know, and said that the Army Sanitary Commission would criticize any plans he proposed, if desired. I thought it best to give in this name, as they wished for names "to choose amongst." Upon my being asked whom I should choose, I replied that I should choose *Captain Galton* as the best hospital architect in existence, leaving it to be implied that the next best was the man whom *he* would supervise.

1 December 1882

Liverpool R. Infirmary. Were you serious in saying that you might be willing to offer yourself as architect to the Liverpool R. Infirmary? I cannot say whether they *would* "select" you, for people are queer, queerer and queerest. But I do say it would be the most magnificent offer ever made.

Editor: Galton evidently made an expedition to Liverpool about the infirmary, for a letter Nightingale wrote him in 1883 on another matter trusts that the visit was "successful." There is a break then in the correspondence until 1885, when Nightingale recalled to Galton how he had "very kindly . . . inspected and advised about the proposed new Liverpool R. Infirmary."[439] The first item below reports a meet-

437 His *Charitable and Parochial Establishments* contains numerous drawings and plans of workhouses.

438 James Osborne-Smith (1847-1928), architect, not selected.

439 Letters 5 August 1883 and 21 January 1885, Add Mss 45765 ff219 and 242.

ing Nightingale held with architect Alfred Waterhouse. He evidently made many changes to meet her criticisms.

Source: From a letter to and notes for Alfred Waterhouse, of the same date, Lea Hurst RSAS and ADD MSS 45820 ff87-100

15 December 1885

You were so very kind as to wish to see me to explain the "lie" of the ground for your proposed Liverpool Royal Infirmary buildings before I trouble you with my "suggestions."

Unexpectedly I find that I could see you, if you would do me that favour, today, Tuesday 15th, 5 or at 6 in order to ask my ignorant questions. If you find it possible to come this afternoon, I will keep your plans till then, with your kind leave. A verbal answer, please.

Liverpool proposed new R. Infirmary. Private and Confidential.
PRIVATE. Please *return.*

The pavilions appear far enough apart and not high enough to shut out sun from one another—a point of great importance. (In the most recent and largest pavilion hospital, Edinburgh, the pavilions are too near, 88 ft. apart, and the walls too high, 63 ft., and they shut out sunlight.)

The fact that the Liverpool wards are to be on only *two* storeys is a most desirable fact. The pavilions being to the *south* of the circular wards, it must be ascertained that they will shut out *no* sun from the *circular* wards. On the score of discipline, there should be *one* entrance only.

The out-patients' department, though it is understood to be, as it ought, only for those going into the hospital or who have been in the hospital, should be as much as possible detached from the hospital. And care must be taken that no nuisances arise from its W.C.s, etc., to the hospital proper. Should it be thought very desirable, it might have its separate entrance, only to be opened at out-patients' hours.

Administrative block. Nurses' floor. A great desideratum that their windows should not have a N. aspect, that each nurse's room should have a fireplace; a very small scullery, with fireplace, is desirable, though not necessary (a poultice or warm drink might be wanted at going to bed, which would prevent a cold degenerating into an illness). Two baths, two W.C.s, two slop sinks necessary for the nurses, beside the superintendent's W.C. and bath. It is undesirable having the great kitchen over their heads, and there is a prejudice in favour of having a kitchen for a great hospital *on the ground,* but this seems overruled by the circumstances of the ground.

It is understood that the night nurses, night superintendents, probationers, (wardmaids?) sleep in nurses' home and the sisters in sisters' rooms, that the nurses, etc., dine in their mess room on the same level as the kitchen? Do they take *all* their meals there? That there is a covered way for the superintendent and nurses from the *administrative* block to the hospital (the superintendent's office and linen room in the hospital are good), that there is a small central room for the two night superintendents in the hospital, that the floor of the nurses and superintendent is cut off as completely as possible from the medical officers' floor—in *administrative* block—that there is also a covered way from "nurses' home" to hospital—is there an entrance for nurses?from this home?

Proposed new R. Infirmary Liverpool. Circular Wards (18 beds)

56 ft. diameter
13 " height
112 " to each bed superficial area
136 " taking in *whole* of ward, which is not fair
1668 cubic feet to each bed
9 ft. from head to head of beds from *middle* of bed
7 " from foot to foot of beds from *middle* of bed
4 " from foot to foot, from *side* to *side*. This is too narrow—especially taking into account the swarm of students eating up the air. Diameter too great (56 ft.) for centre of ward ever to be flushed with outside air or to be reached by sun.

Pavilion Wards. (32 beds), 28 ft. width, 13 ft. height, 112 ft. superficial area, 1456 cubic space to each bed:

8 ft. from middle to middle of bed
5 " between the beds
3 ft. 6 inch window.

It is understood that all the cases are acute or severe. In Edinburgh R. Infirmary, where this is the case (the latest built hospital on a large scale), there are 153 superficial feet to each bed, 2300 to 2500 cubic feet.

(Cubic space should never now be *under* 2000 ft. for *hospitals* proper. And as this must not be taken out of an undue height or width (or diameter) of ward, it shows what the superficial area should be.

Circular Wards. The objections to these appear unchanged, to wit, the centre of the ward must always remain unsunned and unswept by fresh air from opposite windows—the space in central area is too large—between beds too small—a large amount of superficial area exists which cannot be reckoned for patients—they are too far from the fires (the four open fires are good. It is understood that hot-water warming besides is necessitated. The windows are good—down to 2 ft. 6 inch from floor—and up close to the ceiling), but too far for patients to look out of opposite windows.

It is quite a walk for the nurses from centre of ward and from tables round centre to beds. But the very serious objection is that there is no sister's room and scullery, both with inspection windows into ward—there may be six if these were added, a window high up, admitting southern sun *over* sister's room, etc., I understand, into ward. Would a circular ward be as easily supervised if there *were* a sister's room and inspection window from it as a pavilion ward? . . .

Wards: It appears that the "instructions" of the medical staff were to each visiting surgeon:

some 32 men surgical patients
some 18 women " "
the whole under one sister to each visiting physician
some 18 men medical patients
some 14 women " " the whole under one sister (exact numbers not vouched for).

The objections to dividing up the women's medical pavilion wards are considered farther on.

N.B. There is a great objection to having a man's and woman's ward under the same sister, for obvious reasons. No excuse of any kind should be afforded for anyone, except the medical staff, to communicate between men's and women's wards. If a sister belongs to both, an excuse may be made to fetch her from the other ward. In well-ordered hospitals, the nursing staff is never allowed to go into any but its own ward.

Liverpool first floor. Operating theatre on basement seems awkward for patients—the surgical men patients having to go up two flights. Is the entrance to surgical ward wide enough?

Thornton Ward Block: W.C. and bath lobbies, seem very good. Administration in nursing matters of this block very difficult. Circular (surgical) ward appears included under same nursing staff. The "sister" is divided from circular ward by corridor, lift, chapel—from Thornton Ward by three *separation* wards. No supervision of circular ward, either by night or day, is possible except by a person actually *in* the ward. It is separated from main corridor by quite a length of rooms. Its scullery even is at a certain distance. The *same thing* must be said of the *Thornton Ward.*

The same thing may be said, only more strongly, of the next (middle) block. The sister and nursing staff have to pass through a ward of fourteen beds (and a lobby), which ward thus becomes a passage room, to reach the further ward, which is inaccessible to supervision and which will, in its turn, become a passage room to much that will have to be carried to the further bathrooms, lavatories and W.C.s (although there *is* a bath just opposite the lift).

It is sometimes preferred that the scullery and separation room first floor should change places (in the pavilion block), because then the ward can be overlooked from the scullery. (At the same time there is an advantage in the sister's ward and scullery being like sentries, on opposite sides at the mouth of the whole ward and appurtenances, so that no one can go in or come out without the sister's knowledge. But nothing of this can be available for the circular ward, and is of little avail for the broken-up pavilion ward.)

Of the farther block, the same must be said: six rooms for sick nurses (a most desirable provision) incapable of being supervised themselves (a nurse would almost be required for each room) and forming an undesirable street—cut off all power of supervising the farther medical ward. Then there is no bathroom, no slop sink, no W.C. to the sick nurses' group of rooms. In that respect they would be worse off than the medical ward—and had almost better be warded there.

The distance of circular ward from all supervision remains the same—separated by corridors and patients' clothes. This multiplicity of "patients' clothes" rooms seems an evil.

Second floor. *Male surgical* PAVILION wards—thirty-two beds are best for purposes of supervision, nursing, etc.; they are not cut up and they have the requisite ward offices. Circular *wards* have no sister's room and only a scullery separated by a neck. They are separated by 100 ft. from the pavilion wards, though supposed to be under same sister. Are the "sister's rooms" large enough to be comfortable bedrooms?

Third floor. Day rooms at top of circular wards in outside (first and third) blocks so absolutely isolated from all supervision nearly as much as if they were in separate buildings. Are they for the nurses? This is not the case with nurses' mess room. Central block—that is nicely placed.

Fourth floor administrative block: twenty-four maids seem rather closely packed. Scarcely *room for a washstand* each!! Apparently no fireplaces—will be very hot in summer—between kitchen and roof. Windows not indicated. Housekeeper's bedroom appropriately placed there, but rather hard upon her to have W.C.s and baths both sides. Otherwise W.C.s and baths well placed.

Source: From two letters to Douglas Galton, Add Mss 45765 ff281-83 and 284-85

16 December 1885
7 A.M.

Private. I am most anxious to know that you are seeing Mr Waterhouse's plans for the proposed new Liverpool R. Infirmary. I did not dare to ask him. Is it *today* or *tomorrow* that you are to see them? I have seen him and the plans, and I want to be in the same voice as you. May I send you my criticisms that you may bring them into accord with yours?

He is a very alarming man, because he is so good-natured. He proposes to embody my suggestions and then to discuss them as MINE with the Liverpool committee. Now this, it is needless to say, will *not do at all.* Except with Mr Rathbone, he must only discuss them *as his.*

I did not mean to discuss them with him (Mr Waterhouse) at all till I had seen yours. But he came last night for two hours and it all came out. The main faults are (1) want of superficial area, especially in the circular wards, (2) want of the commonest principles of supervision and nursing. (The pavilion wards cut up into lengths and small wards and the circular ward completely isolated and divided by a 100 feet from the pavilion ward, though one sister is to have charge of both.) (But I think one or two of his proposed remedies are worse than the disease.)

The doctors have given him instructions—thinking only of themselves, and neither of patients nor of nursing.

May I send you my notes? I should not like them to arrive while Mr Waterhouse is with you. But I should like you to see them before he comes to you. . . .

Private. Burn. Please not to let him know that I am in consultation with you—we should be like "pickpockets in a crowd."

16 December 1885 [later]

Liverpool Proposed Infirmary. Private. Many thanks. I send you my notes which I am afraid you will hardly be able to read.

1. I have not meddled with *drainage* at all with Mr Waterhouse, though after our terrible experience at St Thomas', I am doubly anxious that you should. But my opinion, second-hand from you, would add no weight to yours.

2. *Circular wards.* I have not withdrawn from my notes what I had said generally against these. But you have seen them *at work* and may perhaps have modified a hostile opinion. And it seems impossible to substitute any better form of ward on one side the corridor in that pernicious bit of ground.

3. The doctors each want (the surgeons, as I understand, each thirty-two male surgical and eighteen female [patients], all to be under one sister, the physicians each eighteen male medical [patients] and fourteen female, all to be under one sister). This is pure doctors' whim. And to prevent the doctors fighting in the wards, he has ruined his female pavilion wards by cutting them into three compartments, two wards of fourteen beds each, thus making them into passage rooms, and a lobby. And what is still worse, he has divided two other pavilion wards, one into a street of six nurses' rooms and a ward of fourteen beds at the end, one into "separation" wards (i.e., erysipelas, etc., which ought not to be in the block a[t] all but in a separate block) and a ward of fourteen beds at the end.

Pray help him with this. But don't betray me. (Perhaps he may have modified somewhat before he comes to you.)

Source: From a letter to Douglas Galton, ADD MSS 45765 ff296-97

28 August 1886

In pursuance of your advice that we should urge the union of the local military sanitary officer's duties with those of the local military statistical officer, so as to make every district a miniature of the central officer, based this on your statement and advice that I should quote the civil "medical officer of health" of the civil district *who gets* all the disease statistics of the district," I was asked at once *where does he get them from?* and was very anxiously told that *infectious* statistics and *death* statistics are reported to him, but who reports to him disease statistics? It would be of the utmost importance if you, by *return of post,* would kindly *enable me to answer this.*

(I am going to see an important officer once more before he leaves England.)

Your gist of course was that the sanitary officer ought to have the same functions as the civil officer of health, in order to be useful in collecting statistics, and that I might urge the civilian as a model. But they ask, where *are* these civil *disease statistics*?

Thanks for returning my letter. But I wanted them to go through with you.

Source: From a draft letter to G.V. Poore,[440] Add Mss 45809 ff47-48

15 November 1888

Private. Sir Douglas Galton encourages me to trespass on your great kindness to answer a question which none could answer so well. But still I am unwilling to trouble you, though I hope it will take you, if you are kind enough to answer it, but a few minutes. It is briefly this: is there a chair of hygiene, of public health and sanitary science and practice taught [at] the great London medical schools? not in the sense of there being a course of lectures, which there is almost everywhere on these subjects, but in the sense that Dr Parkes, whose name is now so knit up with yours, was professor of hygiene and sanitary matters at Netley?

And should you, might I ask confidentially, be satisfied with such teaching generally? . . . and with chemical analysis as now universally taught in the civil medical schools? of London? as also with the work taught in the physiological laboratories for practical instruction in the great London hospitals? And are facilities (including the now favourite bacteria) for the study and teaching given in the great London hospitals? But hygiene and sanitary things, the first part of my question, and not bacteria, is the matter of vital importance for us so much.

I see my questions have swelled to three. My object in troubling you is not merely to gain interesting information—I will not trouble you to make any inquiry for me—I know your time is too valuable. I only ask for such information as you have ready in your full head. But the answer will affect questions likely to arise for army medical schools. . . .

May I ask is hygiene a part of the regular medical *students'* course at University College Hospital?

Carlsruhe Hospital, 1886-87

Editor: While earlier correspondence with the grand duchess of Baden concerned a children's hospital at Heidelberg, the subject of the next set of letters is the grand duchess's "clinique," a general hospital with a nurse training school, for Carlsruhe.

Yet again Nightingale had to argue for more bathrooms and toilets—four baths would not be too many for thirty-one nurses, and they should be separate from patients' facilities. There is no subsequent correspondence to indicate whether any of Nightingale's advice was taken.

---

440 Dr George Vivian Poore (1843-1904), Royal Hospital for Women and Children, general secretary of the Sanitary Congress.

Source: From a letter to Douglas Galton, Columbia University, Presbyterian Hospital School of Nursing C170

22 May 1886

Professor Weinbrenner, who will present this letter of introduction to you, as the greatest authority on sanitary and administrative hospital building here, is the very distinguished architect and professor of the Polytechnic School at Carlsruhe, who has undertaken the plans of the "Clinique" to be erected there, and comes to England on a mission from the grand duchess of Baden to see the "specialties" of hospital building here, "inside and out," as regards health, administration, distribution of wards and offices, etc. Will you kindly tell him the best hospitals to see, and the best way of seeing them, and perhaps introduce him to some of the best hospital architects? He also wishes to see the "specialities" of building of other institutions, schools, etc., and English houses "of the English Gothic style, sloping roof, bow windows, etc.," as the grand duchess calls them.

Source: From a letter to Harry Verney, Wellcome (Claydon copy) Ms 9011/160

17 August 1887

I wrote to the grand duchess yesterday [letter missing] about the plans not having arrived. And now this morning they are come. Shall I telegraph? It will do at 3 o'clock, I think?

I am glad I wrote before the plans came; they are hopelessly bad. No Englishman would look at them. What shall I do?

Source: From a letter to and notes for Douglas Galton, Add Mss 52427 ff89-91

28 August 1887

Carlsruhe Proposed Hospital. By your kind leave I send the grand duchess of Baden's plans for Clinique and Training School for your criticism, and also my notes, which are merely a nurse's notes. I hope that, however tiresome, you will be so good as to read them—as they must have your criticism as well as the plans.

What *you* will do is to show how these great defects can be avoided or diminished. . . .

The first two pages, 1, 2, are extracts from the grand duchess's letter, necessary for understanding the plans; A to H are mine. The plans were posted today to your address.

Training School Upper Floor

Left-hand Wing

	9 beds	3 Windows	too little air for health
Supt	1 bed	1 "	good
	4 beds	1 "	not good
	13	*staircase*	large window good

Private Patients: are they for *men* or *women*?

6 beds in 4 wards It seems good, but same remark applies as to three-bedded ward, viz., want of ventilation—not even opposite window in passage.

Is not a scullery wanted here?

W.C.: nurses one, patients one (if men, they must have one and women one).

Centre:

18 pupil nurses appear to sleep here in 6 rooms, 3 each with only one window, and *not* an uninterrupted, windowed, corridor opposite.

13

31

Ample W.C. and bath and lavatory accommodation should be provided for them (certainly four baths to thirty-one nurses), no part of which of course should be used by patients. Ample slop-sink accommodation also. It is considered better for each nurse to have her own washing apparatus, if possible, near her own bed, and for this purpose each bed to have a window and curtains to make a compartment round each bed, to be drawn far back in the daytime. It is better still for each nurse to have a room to herself, however small, with a window to herself if possible.

Women's Hospital, Euston Road, 1888

Editor: By 1888, more women were being accepted into medical schools in England, only to find upon graduation that hospitals would not appoint them. Hospitals run by women for women were an obvious solution. The Women's Hospital, Euston Rd., started as a modest dispensary in a house, with Elizabeth Garrett as the major force both for the hospital and for women's medical education. The correspondence here begins with plans for a new, purpose-built hospital. The architect chosen was John McKean Brydon (1840-1901), who was said to be a minor Butterfield for temper (see the second item below).

Nightingale, with Douglas Galton, assisted considerably in criticizing the design. It seems that the original plans had at least the usual faults: one-bed wards with no means of oversight, inadequate space for nurses—hardly anywhere for them to sit down—and no rooms for night nurses to sleep in. Without better accommodation, Nightingale pointed out, the hospital would not get "proper women" to apply for posts. The wards were described as a labyrinth and a "rabbit warren," while the matron was said to have been "secluded from the scene of her labours." Nurses would have to make a journey to find her (see p 888 below).

A comment in passing refers to improved precautions for ovarian surgery, and specifically that gynecologist Spencer Wells had brought in better sanitary procedures.

Source: From four letters to Douglas Galton, Add Mss 45766 ff89, 98-101, 102-03 and 148

17 June 1888

Private. Might I send you the sketch plans of the new (proposed) *Woman's Hospital* in Euston Road—*not* finished, like the Gordon, nor yet begun—which I have been asked to criticize, a criticism nearly completed, which I should scarcely have undertaken without hope of your help. Are you in London?

20 June 1888

New proposal. *Women's Hospital Euston Road.* I send you the plans (three) according to your kind leave, with one elevation and one site plan of this "valuable estate," and eleven pages of mine which "do make that darker which was dark enough before,"[441] and one page of building committee. Do you approve of "*Mr Yuill*" as sanitary engineer for "drainage"?

2. Do you think the great *staircase* with single window sufficient to air and light this most intricate hospital—which requires Fortunio's telescope[442] which could see round angles? O that it could be swept

441 Perhaps a paraphrase about a Norman keep enclosed by a quadrangle, "which almost entirely darkened what was dark enough before," in Bernard Burke, *The Historic Lands of England* 158.

442 Fortunio Liceti (1577-1657), a pupil and advisor of Galileo.

from end to end with air! You see it is to be filled with the cases which, of all others, require sanitary precautions, and it is to be a women doctors' medical school!

3. The estimate is for £10,000. *Brydon* the architect—who built small hospital for stone in Henrietta St.,[443] said to be a minor Butterfield for temper. Do you know him and it? "Large air shaft or well for ventilating W.C.s and bathroom at end" said to be successful at stone hospital. "Varying lines of foundation and walls and roofs" said to make the "elevation expensive."

4. My chief anxiety is, as you see, that the ward floors are like a rabbit warren, one-bedded wards without direct inspection—hardly anywhere for anyone to sit down, nowhere for anyone to sleep besides the poor patients, who may all be bad cases. Third, or nurses' and servants', floor still more like a rabbit warren, and so unhealthy. *Must* have better accommodation for head nurses, or they won't get proper women. And how can they nurse that labyrinth with six nurses? They could hardly nurse it with twelve.

The "private" wards, I understand, are for ladies.

5. The "shops" in the white space to the right may be built up to any height—they cannot prevent it. I was told that the tall (pink) houses 144 to 136 cannot be pulled down because they cannot afford to lose the rents. But 144 to 136 must be pulled down, because you see the hospital fronts on Euston Road. I was told the *height* of houses would be given me—but it has not come.

Now we await your criticisms with the utmost anxiety—I am told to "aim high" in order to get *some*thing. The ladies' committee beg us to send our alterations *as soon as possible,* because they want the plans to be remodelled accordingly, in time for a lord mayor's meeting when funds are to be collected. *When* may I send for your kind criticisms? . . .

I am afraid the air will be always losing its way through these intricate rooms and corridors.

Claydon House
Winslow, Bucks
8 July 1888

New Women's Hospital. Thank you exceedingly for your most able letter on the plans of this (Euston Road) new Women's Hospital, which determined their "building committee" to have the plans entirely remod-

443 St Peter's Hospital for Stone (stone is a kidney disease).

elled, according to your advice. They ask, do you know the new *Great Northern Hospital* or the *Miller Memorial Hospital*, built by *Young and Hall?)* architects?[444] The committee (on which is Alice Bonham Carter[445]) would be glad to know whether *you would recommend them? the architects? Or what small hospital you would recommend* as a *safe model* as to *ventilation* and *sanitary condition?*

I would remind you of Lincoln, Aylesbury, Blackburn, Swansea, Oldham, all which plans and a great many others passed through your (and my prentice) hands—merely as to whether you would recommend any.

And there was a *man*, Graham, I think, and one or two others whom you used to recommend as having built *good small hospitals*. But, do you think that that *site* can ever come to good? Can "any good thing come out of Nazareth"[446]?

31 August 1888

New Women's Hospital. It was delightful to me to read your remarks—as noted down by Alice on the Tadpole. But I fear it will be a poor concern—that out-patients' department underneath!!!

Thank you for writing to me. Alice sent me the plans afterwards and I made some notes.

Source: From undated notes, Add Mss 45808 ff126 and 138-40

[c1888]

One's experience of hospital obstetric cases is that, in a ward of, say, twenty beds, there will be a very great, large number of minor operations performed in the roomy lavatory, to the very great advantage of women [medical] students and women's nurses if present. There's nowhere here where these minor operations could be performed. And if there were, not a mouse could creep in to see.

Eye cases among out-patients: what is the average of eye cases in wards? This makes a considerable difference in number of nurses wanted.

Will not criticize ground floor (but it is always a misfortune when out-patient department is not entirely disconnected from hospital),

---

444 Keith D. Young and Henry Hall, architects of the Miller Memorial Hospital, Greenwich, the first circular hospital in England.

445 Alice Bonham Carter (1828-1912), sister of Henry Bonham Carter, cousin of Nightingale.

446 John 1:46.

except that the matron seems to be carefully secluded from the scene of any of her labours, and must make a journey from them to her own bed or sitting room, where she cannot overlook anyone, either patients or nurse, for there is no one to overlook, and she will be overlooked, for they must make a journey to see her. Is she to overlook medical institute? . . .

[I] do not understand remark about eye cases, must have 22 feet first and second floors, two beds for eye cases, twenty [for] obstetrics. Plan most ingenious. Pelvic cellulid, pneumonia, cancer of larynx, hysterical. These are all women's cases. . . .

What is the average of obstetric cases, what of ovariotomy, for which the wards marked private or operations are doubtless intended? . . .

It must be remembered that, of nurses, the precautions against blood poisoning, or by whatever name it may be called, are as urgent as or even more urgent than in midwifery cases, which are really the most "infectious" cases going, that Spencer Wells has completely changed the whole aspect of ovariotomy (for the better) by insisting on sanitary precautions.

The patient is to be operated on for ovariotomy in her own ward. Between each case the ward is to be thoroughly purified and stand empty, so that the patient enters as it were a new and thoroughly clean ward. It should be airy and in a measure isolated—have at least two windows, quiet. A nurse is of course with patient night and day, and after the first two or three or four days may sleep in the ward. Is 12 × 12 enough for two people? not to mention that women [medical] students will be present during the operation. The operator and her assistant, patient and nurse, etc., people are the very least of course that can be present during the operations. I do not understand the sink or W.C. in corner of ward 12 × 12, or is it a lavatory basin? We do not like even a fixed basin.

Is 15.6 × 15.6 (by 13?) even enough? The patient must be transferred from the operating table to her bed by the surgeon and her assistant. All the private wards would be better if large enough to have two windows and door, not wastepipe opposite.

I conclude you will think that the staircase gives sufficient light and air to the corridor, which seems narrow, and at one end there are 9 ft. without any direct light or air.

I cannot agree with the remark that one duty room would be enough for the floor. On the contrary, I was going to remark that two, and such small, duty rooms were scarcely enough, one 9 × 9, one 12 × 9.

You have no ward kitchen, and there must be a small range in each where drinks, light food, poultices and fomentations, especially at night, must be made, flannels made hot, etc. You have four one-bedded wards without direct inspection, each of which, if all occupied by critical cases at once, might require two nurses, one by night, one by day. You have, besides, two wards of eight beds each, each of which will require a night nurse (there must be a night superintendent of nurses). No one apparently sleeping on the floor.

As this hospital is expressly for women students to see women's practices—the cases will probably all be grave. But in one obstetric ward with twenty beds, and a small ward with two, there are a large lavatory where minor operations are performed—impossible here—large ward kitchen and sister's room and the advantage of four and even five good-sized ovariotomy wards in different parts.

You can hardly fetch and carry for the four private or operating wards to and from the W.C., sink and lavatory of the twenty-eight bed wards, which besides is very small accommodation. Must there not be one W.C. at least outside?

I was going to beg for large window at end of eight-bed ward to the east, but fear that that abuts only on a tall house. I should agree with the "alternative" ward offices in a projection to north—as it takes no good sun away—and space between each and next house. Might we not have a window at end of N.W. eight-bed ward on each side projecting ward offices?

I think the sink and bath should not share one window. This often turns out awkward. It seems to me that more lavatory accommodation is necessary.

"Lengthen east ward and put another small window facing south." Yes, "and two towards east (coloured)," "operating room to be enlarged."

Third floor. Has a calculation been made of what nurses you will want? The six rooms are small enough for one—impossible for two. Where do your night nurses sleep? Are there no rooms for them to sleep quietly in by day? Where is your head night nurse's room?

Your six rooms from 10 × 9 to 12 × 10 on each side a narrow passage, doors opposite each other, are not very nice.

Will not the passage more than 30 ft. long be close, notwithstanding the end window and staircase, but is not the number insufficient? Is not one sick room wanted? And also will the dining room, which is cheerful, do also for sitting room?

Windows of nurses' bedrooms, N.W., rather dull, S.E. better. What is the height? Kitchen stuck in rather higgledy-piggledy? Assistant surgeon only divided by partition.

One operation room. Operating wards fixed basin?

3 Operating wards downstairs
5 Private " "
3 or 4 ovariotomies or abdominal scales
2 Gynecological wards upstairs, not on ovariotomy
2 operating rooms
Operating in general
12 × 12
Ovariotomy ward, 2 windows
1 in 3 Mix Obstetric qualified cases
Gynecological ward
8 beds
Small ward
Minor operations
Windows projecting

How do you propose to nurse the hospital? To each floor two (eight-bed) wards, four (one-bed) wards, one head nurse (or sister).

2. There is no sister's room to each floor. You must give better accommodation to a head nurse fit to take charge of such a floor.

1 staff nurse}
1 night " } in a space which is like a divided dormitory

It does not require hospital experience to see that the supposed nursing is wholly inadequate. Indeed, the servants' accommodation is almost better than the nurses'.

Editor: After comprehensive revisions were done, Nightingale gave her support to the fundraising campaign and made her own donation. Her public letter set out the need for a women's hospital, flagging the failure of the regular hospitals to give posts to women doctors, and the special needs of women patients.[447] On the death of Elizabeth Garret Anderson, the hospital was renamed in her honour. It remained in use for more than a century. It was then acquired for offices by a nursing union. The old building was partially demolished for new space, part gutted and renovated so that the fine exterior can still be seen at

---

447 In *Women* (8:63-65).

130 Euston Rd. The (to Nightingale) deleterious features are also evident: a building five storeys high, with small rooms that would be difficult to nurse. Nearby University College Hospital, also rebuilt in the early twenty-first century, has an Elizabeth Garrett Anderson Wing.

Royal Victoria Hospital, Montreal, 1888-89

Editor: Nightingale's first efforts towards the construction of a new hospital and nurses' home for the Montreal General Hospital came to nothing (see p 808 above). The issue was rejoined in 1888 on the building of a second hospital for the English-speaking population of Montreal, to be located on the airier "mountain," in contrast with the old hospital, which was in the lower city, near the St Lawrence River. (The Montreal General in fact later relocated to the mountain, not a matter covered here.) The new hospital, with an entirely separate board and administration, was called the Royal Victoria Hospital, although Nightingale called it the "Montreal Hospital" in the correspondence here. See picture on p 496.

The architect of the Royal Victoria was one Nightingale knew: Henry Saxon Snell, who had done good work on the St Marylebone Workhouse Infirmary (but not its nurses' home). She made copious notes for him on the new Montreal building, but only parts of their correspondence survive. One substantial document that still exists is in Saxon Snell's handwriting, but has points that repeat Nightingale's known views. It is possible that he extracted these points from a (missing) letter from her.

The benefactors of the new hospital were Scots in origin, and the Edinburgh Royal Infirmary was their model. It was accordingly built in the Scottish baronial style, with "Nightingale wards" that were joined by bridges to the central administrative block, and with a fine view over the city. The original plan was for a larger hospital than the one that was actually built.

Nightingale was highly critical of Saxon Snell's plan, saying his ward unit was "the worst I ever saw for a modern hospital" (see p 903 below) and that she would not send a nurse there. Again she had to make the point that nurses must have private bedrooms. The lengthy notes immediately below were largely reiterated in a letter a year later to Douglas Galton,[448] not reproduced here.

---

448 Letter 16 October 1889, Add Mss 45766 ff275-80.

There were delays and problems stemming from lack of funds for the main hospital. Additional wings were built, but not a whole new hospital.[449] A new floor provided better accommodation for nurses, but still proved to be inadequate.

Source: Notes, Add Mss 45820 f133-41

17 January 1888

Saxon Snell. Montreal Hospital: position of bathrooms; duty room is as far from the ward as it can be. In fact should be called off-duty room. Separated by passage to W.C.s and bathroom from ward; no one in duty room can exercise smallest supervision over ward or over anything but day room, and that not much from its shape.

Objection of hospital authorities to day rooms—patients play tricks, not under supervision, and do themselves hurt. Door must be half glass that everyone may see in and see into every corner of room. I entirely agree with the sanitary reasons you allege.

Sister's room absolutely essential overlooking ward. . . . But where is the sister's room? W.C. for sisters and nurses in male wards. There is no sister to supervise for there is no sister's room. The duty room must be a kitchen as well as nurse's room and the sister must have a room to herself.

Bathroom not in effect used by the small wards. Separation patients not generally bathable. And if they are—portable bath. In effect much more supervision exercised by sister and nurses if bathrooms and lavatory. There must be a lavatory, W.C. and W.C. sink at further end of ward. Then if sister sees a patient not in the ward, she knows that patient must be in lavatory or bathroom or W.C. Besides, nurses are constantly traversing lavatory and W.C. sink and see after the patients—all this is lost if at entrance of ward—patient may have gone to day room or kitchen.

All being equal, huts are undoubtedly more healthy, sanitary, than two or three-storeyed buildings. We always prefer one storey, for sanitary reasons. In war hospitals, even in climates with *almost* the same extremes as in Canada, experience has proved that even winter mortality is much less, even in pneumonia, in huts than in two or three-storeyed buildings. To your question, is "the one-storey (hut) system adopted in the design the most desirable," I should undoubtedly answer Yes.

---

449 See Description of Plans, Royal Victoria Hospital, with plans and drawings, Add Mss 45816 ff25-31.

But then comes another question—the huts I speak of had none of the appliances of civilization. How did you propose in such a climate as Canada to warm the air, to ventilate, to lay hot and cold water all over the building, to render the pipes unfreezable, to arrange bath, lavatory, W.C., appliances. . . .

The multiplying corners in itself is objectionable, while in an administrative point of view the position to secure command. The beau idéal [ideal type] of ward offices is sister's room, kitchen, separation ward on each side entrance door. Bathroom and lavatory, W.C.s and sink on each side further end window.

Do not you think that, if the first plan is difficult of administration and supervision, the sketch with the double corridor and divided wards is almost impossible, without any commensurate sanitary or other advantage? All the personnel would have to be doubled. The administration building is at best a weary way off. No matron could supervise it, while every ward must have a responsible sister, because the essence of supervision is that the sister should see her whole ward from one point. . . .

In a civilized country like Canada, however, we cannot do without the appliances, as we do in war hospitals. And would not this make an essential condition in any plan adopted?

2. With regard to the second question, "dividing the large wards, having two fourteens instead of one twenty-eight, and having the offices in the centre of each pavilion," our answer would be, I believe, unhesitating: it is easier to keep a ward of twenty-eight beds in a Montreal ward unit.

First principle: all ward offices to be self-contained within one door, commanded by ward sister's room, so that at any moment she may know where every patient is. Where are the W.C.s and W.C. sinks of the patients? If in (see large thin paper sketch of ward unit) the large lobby beyond the bridge, it makes control of patients impossible. Also there is but one W.C. and the sink is too far for the patients' secretions to be carried. Where too are the patients' secretions to be kept?

3. W.C.s and one ward sink necessary for thirty patients. (It is a matter of experience that the gravest irregularities occur if the patients' W.C.s are outside the ward precincts and ward control.) At the same time, the W.C. indicated would be a very convenient one for nurses. Bathroom and lavatory ought to be useable for small operations, especially in this necessarily intricate building.

Great care must be taken that accessibility by wide doors and passages from surgical wards to operating theatre may be made as little difficult as possible. This is not clearly indicated on principal floor. Is it necessary to sacrifice one of the best positions for ward offices?

Fire escape stairs? In the plan of floors, the ward offices are in this lower. . . .

The ideal, as well sanitary as administrative, of the ward unit is lavatory and bathroom at the further end of ward on one side the end window, W.C.s and W.C. sink on the other. (It is not marked on the ward plan what the compt corresponding to fire escape stairs contains.) Where is the lavatory?. . . .

Ward kitchen on the other side and lift or linen place. But it is not so objectionable, the linen being outside the bridge and the W.C.

In one famous hospital and medical school, a doctor's room was imperatively asked for and given. But it is found that multiplying rooms belonging to ward is very undesirable. And the M.O.'s room could hardly be separated from head nurse's bedroom by only a partition. The one window of the separation ward is very small. Is this desirable for a ward which generally contains the worst cases? Also, it should not communicate with the bathroom.

Plenty of time for suicide and murder if you depend on electric bells. Is there to be a staff of nurses kept up? . . .

Principal floor: officers' mess room and scullery should not be in the midst of the nurses. First floor. Bathroom appears where it should be, instead of fire escape. Stairs and ward kitchen where it should be.

Children's ward at the top. A children's ward demands publicity more than any part of the hospital, because children cannot and ought not to complain. It should be in the most frequented part of the hospital and nearest the superintendent. Up there it could have neither superintendence nor publicity.

The superintendent must have an office, easily accessible. The night superintendent's office, too, should be as much in the way as possible. Night supervision will be difficult.

Source: From a typed letter to Douglas Galton, Add Mss 45766 f206

31 December 1888

I am delighted that Mr Saxon Snell asks me to name a sum for my services on his hospital plans, but "I never goes away under £1000, though his plans put my eyes out" (as the organ grinder in the street said, when he was offered sixpence to go away: "I never goes away under a shilling"). But I think you are quite wrong not to charge for your services—you who do so much for other hospital architects in overlooking their plans.

Editor: On the same point, Nightingale joked to her sister:

> By the way, I think the world must be improving, for I was asked by a hospital architect to "name a sum" as my "fee" for doing his hospital plans. How dead the world must be never to have offered me one before![450]

Source: From two letters to Douglas Galton, and a list of questions for the architect, Add Mss 45766 ff275-76, 285 and 286-88

16 October 1889

Anent [regarding] S. Snell's Montreal plans: they are extraordinarily ingenious. But without your paper I could have nothing—and I shall be able to do nothing more till I come to London. As you said you could work at them now, I return the plans and your paper and two note sheets of mine (for yourself) on what seems to me simplest and most necessary: the *ward unit*, the *not* putting *children* at the top floor, and the enormous difficulty of superintendence—not to say impossibility by night.

I could write a good deal more for Mr S. Snell, if you like it. But my eyes are hardly equal to following the intricacy of the plans. And as to the superintendents following the intricacies on floor, or the patients reaching the theatres or, etc., it seems hopeless. Simplicity of plan and publicity are the sine qua nons [without which there is nothing] of hospitals—are not they? Let me see the plans and your remarks again, with you, and my own mean remarks.

1 November 1889

By your kind desire I enclose questions for Mr Saxon Snell. But I also trouble you with my notes (four sheets) to make them intelligible, if readable . . .

Perhaps Miss Washbourne would kindly make an intelligible copy of the questions for Mr S. Snell. Please return my rude manuscript to me and let me see you on Monday.

Montreal Hospital Plans. Questions.

What is the proposed number of beds?

Surgical }
Medical } may be classed together
Eye }

450 Letter to Parthenope Verney 6 January 1889, Wellcome (Claydon copy) Ms 9012/81.

Private
Children's
Infectious, etc.
What is the proposed number of *nurses* in each of these categories?
What number of probationers for all?
What number of *superintending* staff?
Bedroom and sitting room for each? (1 lady superintendent?)
Central offices for 3 or 4?
1 lady superintendent
2 day superintendents
2 night superintendents
1 for probationers
1 private wards and
1 infectious
8 or 9
What average number of *students? Medical school* upon this depends so much of arrangements.
What building for medical school, museum, etc.?
What number of RESIDENT medical officers in *hospital*?
" " " students in medical college, if any?
Two? Three? operating theatres, of *easy access*, best on principal floor. Minor operations to be done in lavatory? if to be big enough, but where is lavatory? Ovariotomy to be done in lavatory, never in theatre, or in patient's own small ward. If small wards near theatre (but theatre *ought* to be accessible to surgical wards) they must have offices and supervision?
System of electric bells?
Separate building accommodation for probationers with their assistant superintendent.
Night nurses apart from *day* nurse? To sleep by day quietly with superintendent.
What and where W.C.s and W.C. sinks for wards?
What and where W.C.s for ward nurses?
Nurses' accommodation should be *quite* separate and by a different stair from medical officers.
What baths, W.C.s, dining rooms, etc., for nurses? Each should have a separate bedroom.

Source: Notes for Henry Saxon Snell, ADD MSS 45820 ff143-44

[14 November 1889]

"*Questions.*" I trust the questions to matrons will be answered so as to be of use. As regards "Question 4" *second paragraph* (and also Mr Saxon Snell's letter to Sir D. Galton), it may be observed that "a head nurse when on duty" is "always in and about the wards." And it is *to enable her* to be so that her own room off the ward is necessary.

In a high-class hospital, where probationers are carefully selected (without "interest") from the most suitable classes, are trained *morally* as well as professionally to be approved nurses, it is a thing unknown for them to shirk their ward duties. You would find them at their post at every minute they ought and are supposed to be there, and a great many minutes besides, if there is a press of work.

And if a head nurse wants to put on an apron or take a cup of tea, is she to be running off to the home every time, losing five or ten minutes on each way? *That* is instead of being "*on duty*" taking her "*off*" "duty." A head nurse must breakfast and tea in her own room. Dinner may be taken in the nurses' dining room. Even so, she is often unable (with anxious cases) to leave the ward for her dinner, and must have it brought to her an hour or two afterwards, so with supper.

Those nurses who cannot be kept "on duty" except by *not* having a room of their own, should not be in a hospital at all. The head nurse's room should have an inspection window into the ward, a medical officer's, if any, *not. Neither* should be entered *from* the ward. The objection to *two* separation wards is the insufficient supervision and difficult care. It is impossible for the head nurse's room to look into *both.* It will need two extra nurses for each separation ward, where the head nurse has a sitting room that has to look into the separation ward. And there must be an additional bathroom.

The multiplication of all these small rooms is so very objectionable for supervision, cleanliness, discipline and order.

Source: From notes by Henry Saxon Snell, with Nightingale comments and emphasis in bold, ADD MSS 45820 ff145-58

[late 1889]

PRIVATE. PLANS OF PROPOSED MONTREAL HOSPITAL. ***Rough Notes.* On the information so kindly sent me by Mr Saxon Snell (written for my own use).** Please return to F. Nightingale.

Sister's Rooms. To one of such remarkable talent and experience in HOSPITAL construction, it is needless to lay down the principles of the necessary ward accommodation for nursing. It seems only necessary to say what is one element of the great improvement in the social character and education of all nurses, but especially of head nurses during the last twenty or thirty years in Great Britain. To neglect these elements of improvement carries us back to the days when nurses were neither respectable nor sober, under the sistership or the matronship **of medical officers** had to be always in the wards in order not to be idling or flirting or drinking elsewhere. No one now would wish to give up the strong infusion of **trained** gentlewomen or educated women who are now found in all hospitals of note, especially as head ward nurses (or "sisters"). To secure these, accommodation and modes of life are now given in all the best hospitals such that no mother would object to see her daughter in hospital work, and no educated woman would regret to find herself in it. I have taken unusual pains to make special inquiry as to the present feeling about these sisters' accommodation, especially at Edinburgh, and find that matrons and sisters more and more feel the necessity of a sister's room on one side the entrance of the ward door, in which she is to sleep **some have a second room, a sitting room** and so be in command of her ward night and day.

Opposite to this is the ward kitchen, where the nurses and probationers prepare things for the patients and have themselves command of the room **under the sister**. (Medical officers would themselves tell us that they have nothing to do with the administration of the nursing department, which is entirely under the matron, who is responsible that the sisters and nurses should be such and under such arrangements as to carry out, with intelligence and faithfulness, every order of the medical staff.) In so complicated a building as that proposed for Montreal, the sister's room is one of absolute necessity, if there is to be discipline at all.

With regard to the night nursing, it is apparently intended to have a large room, to which electric bells or telephone would be carried from the various wards to summon assistance in emergencies, but **this is no substitute for the sister's room** suicide or murder **homicide** by **suddenly** delirious patients would be easy before the bell could be answered. Indeed, even where the sister is in her room, and the night nurse at her post, such accidents have hardly been escaped **in the intervals of the night superintendent's rounds**. Is there to be a staff of nurses kept up all night in the electric bell room? Supposing there were only two, and these two called away, and there is a third call? But more, it is the daily, hourly, discipline which necessitates the arrangements of sister's room and ward kitchen. At Edinburgh, indeed, a sister has bedroom and sitting room of her own off the ward. Is an educated woman to have nowhere to sit down except in a male surgical ward, and no conscience but the necessity of being seen ***there***? If her only other footing is in the nurses' home, which in this building not easy of access, she will probably sit up half the night with her anxious cases, for educated sisters, and indeed all the trained nurses now, are only too anxious about their patients.

Montreal plans. Nurses' accommodation. In the "possible distribution of nursing staff," there appears to be no sister assigned to the "general surgical children," for whom a sister is, of **all** other wards, most necessary. It seems rather unintelligible to mix up the lock and gynecological patients. The general surgical wards of thirty-two beds each are rather scantily provided for by one sister, one day and one night nurse, and two probationers. We should give three probationers and ***one extra nurse***, not necessarily attached to the ward.

Should not the erysipelas ward be placed separately from the general building in the infectious ward building? ***Probationers*** should hardly be attached to such a ward at all, and the nurses of these wards should ***not*** go backwards and forwards to the ***nurses' home***, but have their sleeping and eating arrangements all in the infectious branch. A "general medicine" with thirty-two patients is put down without any nurses of any kind whatsoever attached to it.

There must be some (copying) mistake here. With regard to the "pay patients," they require a very much larger nursing staff in proportion than the general wards. It is doubtful whether *probationers* should be allowed in *these* wards.

May I ask, into what sized wards these "pay patients" are distributed, whether in single-tended wards, or single-bed compartments? **or how?** May I say that it is often preferred to keep the probationers' accommodation separate and together under their own assistant superintendent, for their own classes, etc.?

Extra Nurses. Again, it is necessary to recur to the important question: is the proposed Montreal hospital to be a hospital for acute cases in the same sense as a London or Edinburgh hospital? If so, what accommodation for "extra nurses"? It is rare in a first-class London hospital if an *extra* nurse is not required for the night (*besides* the staff night nurse), either for a special case or the small ward (*separation*). And this again brings on the question of the multiplication of separation wards. Twenty extra nurses is not too much for about 400

beds, with *one* separation ward to each large ward. But it might happen that you might require two extra nurses—one by day and one by night—to *each* separation ward. And accommodation for extra nurses must be provided. (They are not moved about from their own sleeping rooms as they are moved about from ward to ward as their cases require.) . . .

Montreal Plans. Medical Officers' Rooms.

1. Upon the size of the medical school **partly** depends whether a medical officers' room off each ward should be there. At Edinburgh there are 1800 medical students, and it appears that a medical officers' room off the ward is considered necessary for examinations and demonstrations and analyses, but great inconvenience arises therefrom, as will immediately be understood, when it is stated that **besides these**, either in the medical officers' room or the convalescent room off the ward, out-patients may be seen. At St Thomas' Hospital, there are only 300 or 400 students and the necessity of a medical officers' room off the ward is never felt, but on the other hand the bathroom and lavatory is a most commodious place, and even minor operations are performed there. The ward bathroom is so small in these **Montreal** plans that there is not room even for a lavatory. In Montreal Hospital the number of medical students is not stated, but as there appears to be surgical theatre accommodation for 200, medical theatre accommodation for 150, pathological theatre for 100, we may perhaps place the number of students at not more than 350. For such a school it would appear wholly unnecessary to give the medical officers a room to each ward.

In a famous London hospital, where there are many more students, and very many more beds than in St Thomas', a medical officer's room is never thought of.

With regard to resident medical officers, it is only stated that there will be a medical superintendent who will have a house of his own. But nothing is said about the resident house surgeons and physicians, who must each have a good bedroom of their own.

In Edinburgh there are or were sixteen, in St Thomas' a much smaller hospital, 380 beds, there are ten **or more**. In Montreal, there appear to be beds proposed for 323. How many residents are proposed?

The resident doctors have of course constantly to be summoned at night in the ward or lavatory.

It would be very desirable to know whether the character of the patients in the proposed Montreal Hospital will be a preponderant

number of acute disease, acute surgical cases and accidents and operations, as in a stirring London general hospital, or of chronic cases, as in a Poor Law infirmary. It makes so much difference in the arrangements, constructive and administrative.

Ward Unit. The first principle of ward offices is to be self-contained, within one door, commanded by head nurse's room, so that at any moment she may know where every patient is. The bathroom and lavatory on one side near the window at the further end from the ward door. This lavatory and bathroom to be large ***enough for minor operations***, especially in this necessarily intricate building. On the other side, the end window, the W.C.s and the W.C. sink—all with cross-ventilation—these should be, if possible, where the "fire escape stairs" are indicated in the enlarged ward plan on thin paper. In the enlarged ward plan on thin paper it is not marked what the compartment corresponding to the "fire escape stairs" is to contain. (If the **patients'** W.C.s are to be on the other side the bridge) indicated to the large lobby, it is scarcely necessary to point out to persons of experience that the gravest irregularities have been known to occur from these being outside the ward precincts, and outside the ward sister's control.) On one side the ward door, the head nurse or sister has her bedroom with her inspection windows into the large ward and into the separation ward. On the other side the ward door is the ward kitchen, also with an inspection window into the large ward. The ward kitchen or "duty room" should have a small range, etc. Here the staff nurses and probationers go **on duty**. (There ought to be a small W.C. **somewhere near the ward** for the women, especially in men's wards.) The head nurse's room should be a **good**, light, airy room (what kind of women can be expected for nurses and head nurses if there are no proper arrangements for health, decency and efficiency?). If the medical officer must have a room off the ward, he must be at all events separated by something stouter than a partition from the head nurses or duty room.

I may mention that in one well-known London hospital, there was a difficulty, if not an impossibility, of getting good ward head nurses to stay, because they had nothing but their ward and their "home."

It should perhaps be asked whether this is to be an infirmary with infirmary patients, like St Marylebone Infirmary in London, or a hospital with hospital patients like the Edinburgh Royal Infirmary (though called an infirmary)? It makes a great difference, both in the accommodation required for nurses off the ward, and for the medical officers.

But it may be concluded from the amount of theatre accommodation that Montreal is to be, strictly speaking, a hospital with hospital cases, that is, acute surgical and medical cases (with few chronic) and accidents.

I have said nothing at all about the infectious block, and the nursing for it, as no particulars are given. **These as a rule are very different from the general wards.**

Principal floor plan. Easy access by wide doors and passages from the surgical wards to the operating theatre is essential, especially in a building necessarily intricate. There are three operating theatres at Edinburgh, all on the principal floor. There is no room in the ward lavatory for minor operations. There are two operating theatres—one for men, and one for women—in St Thomas'. Both are on the principal floor and extremely easy of access. There is room for minor operations in each ward lavatory. Ovariotomy is generally performed in the patients' own ward. At St Thomas' the strictly pathological work is all done in the museum building, at Edinburgh **some** in the doctor's ward room. This is found to be very objectionable.

Can the operating theatres of Montreal proposed building be considered easy of access? I may mention here that, in some of the largest hospitals with most operations, a "recovery ward" is considered objectionable. The anesthetics are administered in a small room adjoining the theatre, so that the patient is carried in unconscious, but is conveyed straight back again *unconscious* after the operation to *the patient's own ward*—it being considered better for the patient to find himself on recovery of consciousness in his or her own bed. But then of course the operating theatre is placed so as to be of the easiest access.

First floor plan. In this plan the bathroom appears in the best place for it, instead of the fire escape stairs, and the ward kitchen is also in the place considered best for it. What are the baths, W.C.s and dining rooms for the nurses' home? One bath and one W.C. to each eight nurses is not at all too much.

To every sixteen nurses (some day, some night) two W.C.s. One slop sink *most* important (W.C. sink), one housemaid's sink, one or two baths.

For every ward of thirty beds, three patients' W.C.s and one W.C. sink are not at all too much. These do not appear to be indicated in the plan. Indeed only one W.C. and one W.C. sink for the patients appear to be indicated on *the* OTHER *side the bridge* from the ward.

This also depends on the proportion of acute cases. In a general London hospital there may be only one patient out of five out of bed.

The slop (W.C.) sink is then of most importance—two W.C.s would be enough for thirty beds. Where there are a great proportion of chronic cases, out of bed, the case is different.

It is hardly considered perhaps enough how very much morality among the patients depends on these arrangements—how it devolves upon the nurses, who are always there to maintain the moral tone of the ward, how it is in the only position where a woman is in real charge of grown-up men, and how the ward is actually now, with the improved character of nurses, a moral school for the patients, where they learn lessons of conduct which often they never forget, instead of being **the reverse**. The time is not very far distant when it was an *im*moral school both for nurses and patients.

I have dwelt upon Edinburgh (in these notes) because it is from the Edinburgh doctors at Montreal that Mr Saxon Snell says he has to take some instructions, and upon St Thomas', because he quotes that hospital. But the ward unit is the recognized ward unit at all modern or considerable hospitals. There are London hospitals quite antiquated and condemned, and many, many provincial hospitals. My notes must be read in connection with Mr Saxon Snell's letter of 6 November to Sir Douglas Galton. Mr Saxon Snell's building of St Marylebone Infirmary is quite admirable for its purpose.

Source: From a letter to Douglas Galton, ADD MSS 45766 ff301-02

14 November 1889

This is dreadful. I have waited all the week for you, and put off everybody tomorrow ("Friday"). And now I am to wait till "Tuesday" for one 3/4 of hour, which however I accept ("3:45").

Montreal. I hope you will be able just to glance at my notes in connection with Mr S. Snell's letter to you (also enclosed, with his papers), which I will send for tomorrow, and tell me how I am to go on. *I* cannot surrender the ward unit, upon which all depends, and upon which all hospital authorities are now agreed.

Whoever gave Mr S. Snell his "Instructions" (I believe the young Edinbro' doctors at Montreal) knew nothing of [the] administration of nursing. His ward unit, as to the offices and rooms, is the worst I ever saw for a modern hospital. *We* would not send [a] nurse there. Now, what am I to do?

I have taken great pains to ascertain the opinion at Edinbro', and it is what I state in my notes. This is, however, but a small part of what I had to ask you.

Source: From undated typed notes, corrected by Nightingale, Add Mss 45820 ff159-67 and 174-77

[ca. November 1889]

Accessibility for nurses and medical officers from their respective quarters to their own wards direct, short, covered. No "up and down" more than necessary. No "holes and corners," least of all in large, intricate hospitals, nothing which prevents easy supervision, or renders punctuality and strict order difficult.

Some of the difficulties of administration to be considered in the Montreal proposed hospital:

1. Emergency cases by night, how to deal with the nursing of them.

2. Not only the best arrangements, but *what use* will be made of them has to be considered. This especially in the multiplication of small rooms outside the ward door, in long, not-well-lighted corridors and tortuous means of access. The fewer places in and about the wards the better. In long, badly ventilated corridors, kitchen smells accumulate, mount staircases and are distinctly perceptible at a distance, perhaps in the wards. So with foul air.

3. The children's wards: what arrangements are to be made for sufficient supervision of these?

4. If there must be fire escape stairs, what arrangement will still keep the four corners of the wards for its offices and appurtenances?

5. *Extra nurses:* number required depending on the *kind* of hospital accommodation required, one bedroom or at least compartment, with window, to each, same as other nurses or better, extra nurses being most experienced.

6. Food for patients seems to have long and circuitous journeys to perform. So with the stores.

To recapitulate:

7. Operating theatre: accessibility to above every other department, its position in proximity to wards (surgical) without turnings or narrow entrances. Anesthetic room before operation necessary. But *not* recovery ward, if theatre in proper position.

8. No corridor or bridge, especially no want of air and light between ward and its most important "office" (W.C.s and W.C. sink).

1. Recovery ward to a patient's theatre not necessary. The p[atient] should be put under chloroform or ether or whatever anesthetic is used in the little entrance room to the patients' theatre, so as to be unconscious when taken into the theatre and not to see the crowd. But it is far better that he or she should be taken direct to his or her ward after the operation still in a state of unconsciousness, and the patients' theatre should be so placed that this can be done. It is better

that the patient should be in his own bed, quiet when he recovers consciousness, and not be moved after it.

2. We do not like a store for patients' clothes to each ward, and generally speaking the fewer places there are in and about the ward the better. The patient's dirty clothes should be put, each lot in a net marked with the patient's name, and carried away to a store elsewhere in the hospital. The clean clothes should be put in the locker by the patient's bedside and this locker should be designed so as to be perfectly sanitary. The few outer clothes necessary for a patient who gets up for a short time in the day may be kept in some room off the ward. But in making the very best arrangements, you should always consider what use will be made of them, and where there is a patients' clothes' store off the ward, you would be surprised to find the things which find their way in there, including butter.

3. For the accommodation of nurses, there is much to be said for the nurses' home under the hospital roof and, of course, much to be said for the other plan, of the nurses of the block sleeping over the block of wards to which they are attached.

First, the comparative ease of supervision is a great argument in favour of the nurses' home; on the other hand, the dormitories, with a little sitting room for each block of wards, may be made very comfortable, and it attaches the nurses to their sister more. They are more completely a little party to each sister, but the little sitting room should be made comfortable with couches and bookshelves, and there should be adequate appurtenances, which there very seldom are. . . .

There should be two W.C.s for sixteen nurses and a slop sink, and all, of course, with separate doors, otherwise it really is difficult for nurses to empty their slops, which, of course, they must not do in the housemaid's sink, for emptying their basins, and making themselves comfortable before the very early time when they must be at work. A part of these sixteen would be, of course, night nurses; they would get up at a different time and they must have rooms in which they can sleep quietly by day. One bath is perhaps enough for the whole number, because they do not take their baths at the same time, but still it requires management, and two baths would, of course, be better. It is so very desirable each nurse should have a separate room and a separate large window to herself, that every nurse should be able to take a bath once in the twenty-four hours..

The compartments in the dormitory: each partition should go up to the ceiling and each have a separate large window. Each nurse of course has washing convenience in her own room. These women must not have to go to a common lavatory.

4. W.C.s for patients. In a great busy London hospital so few patients are able to get up, perhaps not one in five, so that really you may say that the proportion of W.C.s for patients should be from one to fifteen to one to ten. In the workhouse infirmaries, so many are able to get up that the larger number is necessary, but the *slop sink* is really of the *first* importance in the busy general hospital for the majority of patients. There must, of course, be especially for the nurses in male wards, a W.C. at hand. It is the custom in female wards to keep one locked for the nurses; this plan, though not exactly objectionable is not so good as having a separate one for them in the vicinity of the ward.

Almost always two night nurses to each ward, one on special duty. Twenty extra nurses at St T., but these are not moved about from their own dormitory.

Probationers' home has this advantage: home sister has only to housekeep for them and has time for classes, etc.

Source: From a draft letter to Henry Saxon Snell, Add Mss 45809 ff241-42

[c1889]

How long it is since you in your great kindness sent me an admirable carriage clock I dare not inquire. Nor how long it is that I have delayed my thanks on paper, though not in my heart.

It was on the eve of your departure for Montreal, and you wrote saying that you were leaving for Canada the next morning. And you kindly sent me two views of your new design for the proposed hospital. I trust that you have concluded to your satisfaction this great work, designing the building according to true sanitary principles adapted to the Canadian climate.

I shall always be deeply interested to hear how it is going on. I will not weary you with reasons, alas for me too true, including illness/overwork, putting off writing till your return, but beg you kindly to receive my reasons and my thanks at once.

Editor: The following two notes, which come from Nightingale's files but are not in her own writing, are typical of her data-gathering process. She routinely took copious notes in her interviews with matrons and ward sisters on matters on which she could not gain direct information herself. Sometimes she asked the person to write her with further details.

She then used the information in later letters and publications. In the first note below, a nurse from an unknown hospital (one with children, but not a children's hospital), outlined problems of inadequate separation of laundry, food and other supplies, and the inadequate length of time allowed after a doctor's visit to an infectious patient before seeing another. These are all issues on which Nightingale gave increasingly more specific advice.

Source: From a note not in Nightingale's hand, Add Mss 45809 f173

26 July 1889

Diphtheria broke out among the children in hospital—we lost everyone but one. Two nurses and one sister had it—all caught in hospital, and I had it. The hospital had to be closed for two months. The drains were thoroughly examined and no fault whatever was found in them. But, after strict investigation, we found the following errors of management, which had, it appeared, been under my predecessor.

The whole of the patients' linen and bedding was washed together, so that the children and patients who were in the hospital for other medical or tropical diseases received the garments from the diphtheria ward, with all the little diseases and fluffs adhering to them, and so with the sheets. It appeared certain that this was the main cause of the disastrous outbreak. Another cause apparently was that the milk and beef-tea and other things for the children were kept in the lavatoire of each ward, and appeared to have been contaminated by the [illeg] of the children. It was a terrible time.

Another thing is that the sister and nurses were the same over the diphtheria ward and over the nearest ward, and went in and out from one to the other without changing dress or anything, and it was in this adjoining ward that the greatest number of diphtheria cases appeared. The doctors also. The diphtheria cases arising in the hospital were most virulent and were almost all operated upon for tracheotomy. Another thing was that much depended upon arrangement of a gas pipe in the hutch, where the evacuations of the poor little things were put for medical inspection, which gas pipe was to heat the air and carry it up by a tube above the roof, appeared really entirely useless. The smell *was* terrific and in fact the thing had to be abolished.

All this has been altered now: the diphtheria ward is separated by the garden from the rest of the hospital. It has its own nursing staff, its own linen arrangements, its own everything, and the doctors go to the ward after they have done their other patients, or if called in suddenly for a case of tracheotomy, they must be a whole hour before they re-enter the other wards. We have not had a single case of diphtheria arising *in* the hospital since—but we must not sing till we are out of the wood.

Truly we must say that the first thing in a hospital is to do the patients no harm. The out-patients' department was under the wards and communicated with the wards by the staircase. We had at that time a very great number of diphtheria cases, their mothers of course bringing them into the out-patient department. I regret to say that, both under the old building, which is only fourteen years old, and under the new wing now to be built, there will be the out-patients' department. We have ground to build it separate, but it will cost £1200 more, and this, the economical but active and shrewd vice chairman, who is not a doctor, objects to.

Editor: In the following exchange, the questions are in Nightingale's hand, the answers by an unknown person, indicated in bold.

Source: From a note, Add Mss 45820 f109

5 September 1889

Buckingham Cottage Hospital. Number of beds? **Eight and two cots**.

Average number of patients? **Four.**

Number of nurses? **Two.**

Number of private nurses. **None.**

Are the private nurses under the hospital matron? Is the private nurses' home in the hospital? Matron's salary? **£40 inclusive of uniform.**

Matron's post advertised as vacant—is it filled? **Yes.** The name of the matron? **Mrs MacDonald.**

"Hospitals" in *Chambers's Encyclopaedia*, 1889-90

Editor: Nightingale was approached in 1889 by Robert Cochrane, the editor of *Chambers's Encyclopaedia*, for a new article on hospitals.[451] She saw this as an opportunity to get the right views out in such a well-used source, but hoped to get Douglas Galton to write it. Two letters ask him (see the two letters immediately following), but it seems that he declined and Nightingale took it on herself. A second letter from the

451 Cochrane letter 25 September 1889, Florence Nightingale Museum (LMA) H1/ST/NC2/V62/89.

editor told her that she had six weeks to do the article.[452] Galton later had the article typed up for her, for Nightingale wrote him "A thousand thanks, and will you thank Miss Washbourne, for the article for Chambers?"[453]

Nightingale felt that the existing article said all the wrong things, even that "no part of the social economy of European countries is so perfect in its organization, so purely humane . . . as the institution of public hospitals or infirmaries." Nightingale dropped that point, and also the claim that "a leading peculiarity of medical hospitals is their good order and cleanliness." Her new wording laid out the problem starkly, stating that until the middle of the nineteenth century, nursing and hospital management, both for Britain and most of Europe, was, "except in some few instances, extremely defective" (see p 912 below).

Her new text set out three principles, on which Nightingale made her usual points: construction (to ensure pure air in and around the building), administration and nursing. The new text also omitted the previous author's complimentary remarks about religious orders, "these women's unselfish and useful labours," said to have been gratuitously done. Nightingale did not approve of unpaid work in hospitals and had serious reservations about nuns in hospitals.

Only the opening paragraph remained as it was. Nightingale then edited wordings and added sections to bring in more recent examples of hospitals, including American ones. The resulting article gives a succinct statement of her views on hospitals late in life. There is now no insistence on building in the suburbs, but on the pavilion principle she was as firm as ever: more than 100 patients should never be under the same roof, and less is better; no more than two floors for patients, and only one floor was "now universally recognized as best." More than three would be "insanity." She insisted, as usual, on natural ventilation, by windows, with no more than two rows of beds in the ward.

A short statement on lying-in hospitals stressed their dangers and noted the lower death rates in workhouse infirmaries, while birthing was still safer at home. Improvements in Paris lying-in institutions, where they were most needed, were outlined, which amounted to radical changes both in construction and administration.

---

452 Cochrane letter 16 October 1889, Florence Nightingale Museum (LMA) H1/ST/NC2/V69/89.

453 Letter to Galton 3 December 1889, Add Mss 45766 f304.

Children's hospitals were treated positively, albeit with the demand for special measures for bathing, play, exercise and nursing superintendence. "Every child's hospital should have a *convalescent* branch at a distance, if possible by the sea."

Nightingale repeated her view of close supervision of children: sick children could not be left alone for a moment: hence, mixing them in with adults, judiciously placed, in general hospitals was a "better way." Separate children's wards in general hospitals should be kept only for "infants" (see p 917 below).

Source: From two letters to Douglas Galton, Add Mss 45766 ff267 and 281-82

Claydon House
Winslow, Bucks
[ca. October 1889]

See (2) Chambers of Edinburgh has written to me to ask me to "revise," and if necessary "entirely to rewrite," the article on "Hospitals" in his *Cyclopaedia.* I don't think I can undertake it—I have no eyes—no hands. Yet it is a pity to let slip the opportunity of enforcing sound doctrine (I hear of new small hospitals built within the last two or three years embodying all the faults).

Would you undertake it? It would not cost you much trouble. You have already enforced the sound doctrine so often and so well. May I write to Chambers suggesting you? (I have already kept his letter rather long.)

19 October 1889

Article in Chambers's Cyclopaedia. I send by your kind leave the "old article" on "Hospitals" which the editor sends us to "revise," or if necessary to "rewrite." He can give us "*six weeks*" to do it in and he begs us to "keep it about the size of *the old article, that is, two pages or so.*"

As far as I can read the abominable print, it seems to have nothing in it that it ought to have according with modern knowledge and all that it has to be what it ought not to have. It seems to have been written a century ago when a hospital was a box to put sick people into.

Thanking you exceedingly for what you are kindly willing to do and regretting I can help so little.

Source: Florence Nightingale, "Hospitals," in *Chambers's Encyclopaedia: A Dictionary of Universal Knowledge*, new ed. London and Edinburgh: William & Robert Chambers 1890 5:805-07

Hospitals are so called from the medieval *hospitia*, or more properly the class of hospitals established very generally for the reception and relief of lepers, whose malady was one of the scourges of Europe. These leper hospitals were very commonly in England and in Scotland called "spitals," hence the frequency of such names of places as Spital, Spitalfields, etc. The leper hospitals and other kinds of the old hospitia disappeared with the improvement of society, and substitutes for them on a broader scale began to be established in the modern form of hospitals. Of public establishments under this general designation there are now, as is commonly known, three distinct classes: hospitals for the reception and treatment of the sick and hurt, hospitals for the board and education of children, and hospitals for the reception and permanent board of poor old persons of both sexes. Hospitals of these several classes are numerous and on a munificent scale in Great Britain, where they take the position of leading charities in the country. As in the present work the more remarkable hospitals receive some notice under their respective heads, we need here only offer a few general observations.

Hospitals for the sick and hurt are in some parts of England and Scotland termed infirmaries. Under whatever designation, institutions of this kind are now established in all parts of the civilized world. They are supported in most cases on a principle of charity, but in some special instances from the funds of the state or the civic municipalities. The primary or more important object of all such institutions is to mitigate bodily suffering, whether that arises from natural or accidental causes, in which respect they are indispensable as a refuge to all who are unable to pay for private medical or surgical aid, or as a convenient means of succour on emergencies to persons of every rank and degree of opulence. While such is the main object of these benevolent institutions, they are also serviceable as schools for medicine and surgery; as such, no university at which these and kindred branches of learning are taught can be said to be complete without the adjunct of a well-organized hospital, where professors can practically educate their pupils by pointing out varieties of disease and injuries, and exemplifying methods of treatment. Hence the best specimens of hospitals are found in university towns, as in London, Paris, Edinburgh and some other cities famed as schools of medicine and surgery. The older of the London hospitals are St Thomas' (1553), St

Bartholomew's (1546) and Bedlam or Bethlehem (1547), to which may be added the Westminster (1719), Guy's (1725), the Lock (1746), St George's (1733), the London (1740), the Middlesex (1745) and University College (1833).

A considerable accession to the number took place in the reign of George II [1727-60], when society became alive to the value of such institutions. It was at this period that the Royal Infirmary of Edinburgh was established (1736). The antiquity of British hospitals sinks into insignificance in comparison with that of some institutions of this kind on the Continent. The Hôtel-Dieu in Paris, which is alleged to be the most ancient hospital in Europe, was founded in the seventh century and, long known as the Maison-Dieu, received the benefactions of successive sovereigns.

In London, Paris and other large seats of population, besides the general hospitals, there are now lying-in hospitals, ophthalmic hospitals, consumptive hospitals, children's hospitals, etc., each with its peculiar accommodation and staff of officials. Convalescent hospitals (q.v.) are a valuable adjunct to ordinary hospitals for the sick. Independently of these there are hospitals for the treatment of mental maladies, of which Bethlehem and St Luke's in London, and the establishments in Paris known as hospices, are examples. To this class of institutions belong lunatic asylums (q.v.), also asylums for the reception and treatment of naturally imbecile children, these last, though in operation for some time in France and Switzerland, being but of recent establishment in Great Britain. To these must be added the isolation hospitals for the treatment of smallpox, scarlet fever and other forms of infectious diseases, which have been established in recent years by every energetic sanitary authority out of the rates. Besides these institutions under civil administration are those hospitals which are maintained by the English, French and other governments for the military and naval services. In the United States, where every medical college has its own hospital, or the right to teach in the wards of public institutions, there are also many hospitals or asylums for inebriates (see Inebriates), for opium users and those addicted to the use of other narcotics (see also Foundling Hospitals, Ambulance).

Until the middle of the nineteenth century, the organization and management of hospitals and the nursing of the sick in Britain and in most parts of Europe were, except in some few instances, extremely defective. Public opinion was then aroused on the question, and certain principles were laid down on hospital construction and hospital nursing which have been recognized and adopted to a greater or less extent since that time. These principles may be briefly summed up as follows under the three heads: (1) construction, (2) administration, (3) nursing.

(1) *Construction.* The first object is to obtain pure air in and around the building. The purity of air around will depend upon the site. The soil should be clean and dry; the position should admit of free circulation of air untainted by surrounding sources of impurity or damp. The number of sick who can be placed on a given site depends on the form of the buildings in which they are to be placed. It is now considered that more than 100 patients should never be under the same roof. And less is better. This has led to the pavilion form of building being adopted, blocks connected by corridors. *Two* floors only of patients' wards are admissible, but hospitals with only one floor for the ward accommodation are now universally recognized as best. More than three is insanitary.

Hospital buildings consist (a) of the wards for the reception of the sick, and their appurtenances; these necessarily form the basis of the design; subsidiary to these are the operating theatre, etc.; and where there is a medical school instructional accessories have to be provided; (b) the buildings for administration, i.e., for lodging the staff, the kitchen, stores and dispensary should be always subordinate to the question of the accommodation for sick. In some hospitals extra outpatients' departments are provided. These should never be placed under the same roof with the wards for the sick.

(a) The first principle of the ward unit is that the ward and ward offices should be self-contained within one door commanded by the head nurse's room, so that at any moment she may know where every patient is. The size of the wards has to be somewhat guided by economy of administration, so as to enable the largest number of patients to be nursed by a given number of nurses. The limit of the ward is practically the number who can be efficiently nursed under one head nurse. Each ward may have subsidiary to it one or two small wards for bad cases.

The ward appurtenances consist partly of nursing accommodation and partly of offices for patients. The nursing accommodation includes a bedroom for the head nurse; a serving room in which food can be warmed, drinks and extra diets made, and linen kept and aired, hot water obtained, poultices, etc., made; also a nurses' water closet near. The head nurse's room should be so placed as to enable the nurse to exercise constant supervision over the ward and the patients. The offices for patients comprise a lavatory for the patients, a bathroom with a movable bath, which bathroom and lavatory should be large enough for minor surgical operations, and water closets in the proportion of about 3 to 10 percent of the number of patients—the general hospital for acute cases, mostly in bed, requiring the lesser number—one or more slop sinks, a place for keeping ejecta of patients for medical inspection. These appurtenances should be cut off from the ward by ventilated lobbies, and should be always warmed and ventilated independently of the ward.

The form of the ward should be such as to enable the air to be renewed with the greatest facility. Experience in this climate shows that the windows are the best appliance for complete renovation of the air. For this purpose they should be on opposite sides of the ward, and the wards should not exceed from 20 to 28 feet in width. There should not be above two rows of beds between the windows. The rectangular form enables these conditions to be best fulfilled in the case of large wards. Where the wards are not intended to contain more than from four to eight patients, a circular form of ward has been in some cases found unobjectionable, but as it is a principal object in hospital construction to provide a large wall space in proportion to the floor and cubic space per bed in the wards, and as the rectangular form affords the largest, and the circular form the smallest wall space in proportion to the area of the ward, it is evident that the rectangular form is that best adapted to sanitary requirements.

(b) The subsidiary accommodation should be so arranged as not to interfere with the purity of air in or around the wards. The fewer places in and about the ward the better. Not only the best arrangements, but what use will be made of them, has to be considered. The sleeping accommodation for nurses should be so placed as to ensure purity of air in the dormitories, and complete quiet for the night nurses to sleep by day.

(2) *Administration* is intended to enforce economy so far as it is consistent with the provision of requirements for the sick. It is usually in the hands of a governing body, which issues all regulations after consultation with professional advisors; it controls the expenditure and raises the funds to support the hospital. The governing body acts through its treasurer, secretary and steward for the general discipline and control of expenditure. The well-being and cure of the patients is directed by the professional staff of medical officers, which consists of

visiting physicians and surgeons and of resident medical officers who control the treatment of the patients under their direction and in the absence of the visiting medical officers. The nursing of the sick is under a trained matron or lady superintendent, who should be the head of all the women employed in the hospital.

(3) *Nursing* the sick and injured is performed usually by women under scientific heads, physicians and surgeons. Nursing is putting us in the best possible conditions for nature to restore or to preserve health, to prevent or to cure disease or injury. The physician or surgeon prescribes these conditions; the nurse carries them out. Health is not only to be well, but to be able to use well every power we have to use. Sickness or disease is nature's way of getting rid of the effects of conditions which have interfered with health. It is nature's attempt to cure—we have to help her. Partly, perhaps mainly, upon nursing must depend whether nature succeeds or fails in her attempt to cure by sickness. Nursing is therefore to help the patient to live. Nursing is an art, and an art requiring an organized practical and scientific training. For nursing is the skilled servant of medicine, surgery and hygiene.

Nursing proper means, besides giving the medicines and stimulants prescribed, or applying the surgical dressings and other remedies ordered, (1) the providing and the proper use of fresh air, especially at night, i.e., ventilation and of warmth or coolness; (2) the securing the health of the sickroom or ward, which includes light, cleanliness of floors and walls, of bed, bedding and utensils; (3) personal cleanliness of patient and of nurse, quiet, variety and cheerfulness; (4) the administering and sometimes preparation of diet (food and drink); (5) the application of remedies: in other words, all that is wanted to enable nature to set up her restorative processes, to expel the intruder disturbing her rules of health and life. For it is nature that cures: not the physician or nurse. See Nursing.

Poor Law Infirmaries. Since 1870 Poor Law or parish infirmaries for sick and infirm, who used to be harboured (not treated) in workhouses and nursed by paupers, have been built in London and the United Kingdom; these fulfill also more or less the requisites of good hospital construction, and are served by trained nurses. Some difference exists between the essentials for general hospitals and for Poor Law infirmaries, the latter having no medical schools, no visiting or resident medical officers, except the resident medical superintendent and his assistant, no accidents or operations. The large majority of patients in them are chronic, not acute, cases, and incurables. A smaller nursing staff in proportion is needed. Some few of the best and largest have now training schools for nurses. Since 1875, Metropolitan Board asylums, supported also by the rates, have been built near London for fevers, for smallpox, for idiots and imbeciles, etc.

Lying-in Hospitals. The lying-in hospitals require special consideration. The continuous use of wards for this purpose appears to be very dangerous to the patients. Indeed this would seem to be the reason why there are fewer casualties from this cause in workhouse infirmaries than in the ordinary lying-in hospital, and why the lying-in at home is safer than either.

In Paris, where this subject has been much considered, two forms have been tried with good results. In one each patient has a small ward to herself, with its scullery or service room attached, opening through a covered porch into an open veranda. After each confinement, the ward is cleaned and lime-whited before further occupation. In these wards fatal results have been very rare. Another form is to have a ward which can hold two or more beds, in one of which the patient is brought for the delivery, and after a few hours she is wheeled out in the bed into a large ward, where she remains with other patients who have also been delivered. With this plan, also, where the delivery ward is cleaned and lime-whited at short intervals, and where two delivery wards are in use alternately, one always standing empty, fatal results have been rare. Instances of both forms of lying-in hospitals are not unknown in the United Kingdom. But it would be well if they were more universal.

Children's Hospitals must be provided with establishments for bathing, playing indoors and out, large garden grounds, gymnastic grounds and halls, in and out of doors; the gymnastics should be under a professor, and out-patients should be always admitted. A "sister" must superintend each of all these places. Singing in chorus is to be taught. It is a matter of universal hospital experience that intermingling of ages is essential. If you have a children's hospital, let the age of admission include fifteen years, especially on the female side. In all hospitals (in a child's hospital much more than in others) the patient must not stay a day longer than is absolutely necessary. Every child's hospital ought to have a *convalescent* branch at a distance, if possible by the sea. Sick children can never be left alone for a moment. One might almost say a nurse is required for every child. This is why in a general hospital it is much better for the children to be mixed with the adults; and, if they are judiciously distributed, it does the woman in the next bed as much good as it does the child, or the man as it does the little boy. If there *must* be a children's ward in a general hospital, let it be for the infants.

Convalescent Hospitals must be as like a home and as unlike a hospital as possible. A string of detached cottages is the best, admitting of extension by the addition of similar parts. Convalescent wards in a general hospital are not good, nor are day rooms. Healthy open position and climate must be carefully selected. The convalescents are only to sleep at night in their rooms, while in the day they are "out and about" or occupying themselves—the men in the garden, the women at household work. But there must be strict discipline. There must be two small wards for relapses, next the "sister's" room, in the centre cottage. The convalescent beds may be divided by curtains, to be pulled far back in the daytime. A wash-hand stand to be permitted within, no lavatory. Three or four beds a good number for each convalescent room. Men and women should have separate cottages, and only meet at meals. Every hospital should have its convalescent branch, and every county its convalescent home.

Hospitals for Incurables should admit all diseases certified by competent medical judges to be hopelessly incurable, except mental diseases, which require special arrangements. One well-known hospital for incurables excludes epilepsy because it frightens the other patients; avoids, if possible, congenital and infantile disease; prefers patients of and above middle age; and excludes children and all under twenty years. The cases treated by incurable hospitals are principally cases of chronic rheumatism, gout, paralysis and various affections which cripple the limbs, etc. These hospitals, while treating cases within their walls, are no doubt productive of great benefit to the community, but the system of granting pensions from the hospital funds to out-patients is very questionable.

A Samaritan fund is generally provided to assist poor patients leaving hospitals who may be deficient in clothing or other necessaries. In public *Dispensaries* (q.v.), at stated hours, medical advice and medicines are given gratis to applicants; in recent years provident dispensaries have been established, supported by subscriptions, entitling the subscriber to advice and medicine. Valuable establishments are those called in France *Maisons de Santé*—private hospitals for the reception and treatment of patients who are able and disposed to pay a small sum for board and medical or surgical attendance.

Hospital Sunday: On one Sunday in the year it is the practice for churches of almost every denomination in London and throughout the provinces to have special collections for the support of the hospitals of the country. In London the movement originated in 1873, its author being Dr Wakley, editor of *The Lancet*,[454] and the gross total collected there in 1873-89 was £512,476.

See Mouat and H. Saxon Snell, *Hospital Construction and Management* (1884); J. Clifford Smith, *Report of Conference on Administration of Hospitals 1863*; Douglas Galton, *Construction of Hospitals* (1870) and also his report on *Herbert Hospital, Woolwich* (1865) and his article on "Hospital Administration," in Quain's *Dictionary*; H. Saxon Snell, *Charitable and Parochial Institutions*; Florence Nightingale, *Notes on Hospitals* (1859, new ed. 1863) and *Notes on Lying-in Institutions* (1871) and, amongst Blue Books, the reports and commissions on the sanitary condition of barracks and hospitals (1863), on *Regulations Affecting the Sanitary Condition of the Army and Organization of Hospitals* (1858) and on smallpox and fever hospitals (1882).

Derbyshire Royal Infirmary, 1891-94

Editor: A typhoid epidemic in 1890 at the Derby Infirmary, considered to be the fault of building defects, led to the demolition of the building in question by decree of the mayor and its replacement. The correspondence opens with Douglas Galton informing Nightingale that he had seen the plans of the new Derby hospital and thought them "very good," but that he had suggested to the architect, Keith D. Young, that she see them, as her criticism would be "*most valuable.*" Young would call on her if she agreed.[455]

Nightingale duly went over the plans and met with Young for two hours. Her opinion was that the new infirmary would be "excellent" in its sanitary points, but "unworkable" in its nursing organization (see p 920 below). Young she found to be "noisily complimentary" but "silently obstinate" (see p 920 below). The labyrinths and "holes and corners" were his "pet plan," and she did not think he could be talked out of them. He had no regard for the extra walking nurses would have to do. She mentioned the lack of a place for a nurse to sit down for a break. She also noted that the matron needed a sitting room, but that it should not be next to her office. A large staff would be needed to nurse the hospital, given the layout.

---

454 Dr James Goodchild Wakley (1830-86), son of the founding editor of *The Lancet*, who succeeded his father as editor in 1862.

455 Galton letter 2 April 1891, Add Mss 45767 f2.

Evidently the defects of the plan were resolved adequately for Nightingale to give her approval.

In 1891 Nightingale advised a previous nursing matron, Rachel (Torrance) Norris, then widowed and unemployed, that the new hospital would require a matron. That same letter noted that the queen would soon be laying the cornerstone, which she did on 21 May 1891, making the hospital, previously the "Derbyshire General Infirmary," the "Derbyshire Royal Infirmary."[456]

At the hospital opening, in 1894, Nightingale sent a supportive letter to be read, which was acknowledged with thanks: "It is indeed good of you and very helpful to our infirmary to send us such a kind letter for the opening."[457] The letter itself is not extant.

Source: Undated typed notes, corrected by Nightingale, ADD MSS 45820 ff103-08

[3 April 1891]

Derby Infirmary Nurses' Home: so far off, not a well, where probationers? How many? Night nurses apart? Dining room. Kitchen. How many meals will there be in dining room? Classroom. Matron's room. Is she to supervise the nurses or the house surgeons? Supervision difficult by day, impossible by night.

Nurses' Home. Three W.C.s to twenty rooms wanted (only two). Two sinks, one housemaid's sink. All these nurses are up by 6:30. Where do they breakfast? How many nurses in dining room?

Gynecology scullery on opposite side of corridor.

Linen press and dresser in duty room.

You will never get a really good *class* of charge nurse if she has *not a room of her own to sit down in. Do sisters wish to sleep away? Do they wish breakfast and tea away?*

Wards. Query in Ward Kitchen.

Linen, patients' clothes, holes and corners harder. No sister's room. How in the world is the *night nurse to get help*? Wards divided by stairway.

Children's wards of all others should be *in* the way, are *out of* the way. Children should be then scattered among adults.

Gynecological very good, but how in the world to be nursed or supervised?

---

456 Letter in *Extending Nursing* (13:55); Norris did not apply for the position.
457 Letter of Mary Boden 6 July 1894, ADD MSS 45812 f160.

Duty room is what we should call ward kitchen—*must* have a small range; *night nurses breakfast there*, but not charge nurse.

Night superintendent: where does she meet her assistant? She is in charge of her night nurses—*where do they sleep by day?* What arrangements for night nursing, hand-washing, *electric bells*? Lavatory for washing hands?

Source: From two letters to Douglas Galton, Add Mss 45767 ff5-6 and 7-8

6 April 1891

Private. Derby Infirmary plans. I had a curious and rather unsatisfactory two hours' talk with Mr Keith Young on Saturday. He was noisily complimentary and silently obstinate. I doubt his adopting any suggestion. (He is attached to the Middlesex Hospital, one of the few that has still a laundry under the wards, etc., and he swears by Miss [Godiva Miriam] Thorold, the matron, who has never been a trained nurse.)

This hospital, excellent in sanitary points, is according to our ideas perfectly unworkable, but *you* are going to speak at the county meeting at Derby on *Thursday*! And this appears to me *the only chance* of getting any alterations now made. I venture to send you my notes—of which I wrote the first eight pages before I had seen him—the last four after I had seen him. I send them, in case you should be able to look over them. And I kept his two plans, in case you would like to look at them again with my notes, and for me to send them you.

I did not have the advantage of hearing *your* criticisms. Mr Young is not going down to the Thursday meeting. His knowledge of what a woman and a nurse is was conspicuous from its absence.

I will send tomorrow (Wednesday) morning the two plans. . . . The holes and corners, the labyrinth of rooms at the mouth of each ward are obviously Mr Young's own pet plan. And he won't give it up. Help me if you can.

8 April 1891

Derby Infirmary plans. Private. I send you Mr Young's two plans, which I kept for you as my only chance of getting this beautiful hospital, as I believe you think it, free from extraordinary blemishes; I allude particularly to

1. the honeycomb of small rooms at the mouth of wards *and* without (the play of *Hamlet* with the part of Hamlet left out), namely, no accommodation for the queen bee, the industrious charge nurse;

2. the honeycomb of the children's ward—with no accommodation for nursing;

3. the absurd device of the nurses' home—80 yards of space to run over in pelting hail and sleet. It is just what we had to run over to the "Redan"[458] under a murderous fire, *and failed*, etc. But the want of any idea that the staff consists of human beings who have to be provided for is conspicuous all over the plans.

I feel this so keenly that I would even, contrary to all my usual practice, submit my written criticisms to anyone you would name at Derby, provided this could be done with courtesy and justice to Mr Young. But *I hope in* you—will *you* not undertake this criticism tomorrow *yourself* at the Derby meeting, if you agree? (I think Mr Young an extremely nervous man. Besides this, he sent his "partner" [Henry Hall] instead of himself yesterday to Derby.)

Source: Notes and questions for the architect, ADD MSS 45767 ff9-23

[April 1891]

Derby Infirmary plans—Mr Young's April 1891.

1. Simplicity of plan—not one unnecessary hole or corner—too intricate;

a. Put linen press and dresses in duty room (ward kitchen); very little ward linen;

b. Patients' outer clothing BETTER downstairs in nets, baked under clothing—washable—in lockers;

c. No larder because no food—butter in duty room, eggs in locker;

d. What is "rooms"?

e. Must there be two "coals"? every day?

f. Nurse's W.C. very nice. But sister (charge nurse's) room absolutely essential—one side ward door; educated women wanted—won't get them without—you can't have a woman who will throw off all at a stated hour—it won't be *her* ward. Is she to have nowhere to sit down but in the home?

Then—night service. Holiday's a holiday—throw it all off then. Day's holiday. Nurses: sometimes all good undone by extra work next day for another. Relief nurses and sister. Nurses in a state of chronic fatigue. Nurses and sisters don't improve after their year's training. Bacilli to eat. Humble because so learned—Dr Bristowe.

What is to be done in the duty rooms? *Duty room* must have a small range (scullery), (ward kitchen), washing up and cleaning, ward cookery—drinks, fomentations, airing linen, night nurse's tea, etc., in mid-

458 A battle in the Crimean War when the British were repulsed, with great losses, by the Russians in their well-fortified bastions.

dle of night. Doulton's sink, hot and cold water laid on. Advantage of linen press and dresser in "duty room" is to be in a room with a fire.

Gynecological scullery (lying-in?). Fireplace, sink. Linen press and dresser and, in another compartment, bath sink, slop sink, W.C., stove. A gynecological scullery on opposite side corridor an advantage.

Night service: what electric bells intended? Where is night superintendent's central room? by night? for her to meet her assistant—to leave word for superintendent or where she is to be found—to have her little meal in, etc.? What are the arrangements for night service? for emergencies? for sudden delirium to summon help? What are the latest improvements in electric bells and organized services?

It would appear as if everybody were to sleep at a distance in this hospital, and it *is* distance in truth—then wards separated by broad staircases—great difficulty of calling anybody or getting anybody, anyhow, within fifteen minutes:

Electric bell into porter's lodge indicating ward
[ditto] into doctors' rooms " "
[ditto] into central room " "

Porter and doctor—not nurse wanted. Porter must communicate with doctors' rooms.

The D.T. porter must be there night and day; ingenuity wanted. What communication contrived with all small wards night and day? Probationer three months to every night staff nurse. Little girl saved S. George. Sisters and nurses don't improve and enlarge in character *after* year's probation. Nurses get hard. Rarely patients well enough to help. A bell by day would be a convenience. These excellent pavilion hospitals want ingenuity about this more than the old hospitals.

Matron: is she to supervise the house surgeons!!! or the nurses? Could her office be over nurses' dining room?

Supervision difficult by day, impossible by night, i.e., for the night superintendent. Why put porter's sitting room (and bedrooms) in that central position—first floor—would not matron's office be better there with a small staircase from nurses' dining room? After meals they each have their interview with matron—on their way to wards.

Matron's office to be central—look south or S.E. or S.W.; her office should be large, her sitting room smaller and not next it. Assistant matron's hospital linen; gives classes to probationers.

Nurses' home. Corridor between rooms—communicating all their foul air, *not a well,* long corridor with only one window at one end too far off. Is there to be a covered way?

Where are the probationers? how many? classroom
" " " night nurses? how many? should be apart with their superintendent of nurses, where they can sleep by day;
" " " charge nurses?
" " " assistant " how many?
" " " female servants " "
and wardmaids

To twenty rooms—how many W.C.s wanted? (fourteen nurses to pass each other to W.C.). Three, only two on the first floor, slop sinks, two in separate compartments. Housemaid's sink? Are they in HMC? These women have all to be up at 6:30 A.M. (except the night nurses), wardmaids half an hour earlier. Where do they breakfast? in the dining room? Bedrooms: *bed place* should be marked; where bed? wardrobe? table? washing apparatus. Doors should not be opposite each other.

Lavatories only to be used for washing hands in daytime. None of these rooms. . . .

Ground floor: bedrooms opposite sitting rooms, only corridor between—not nice.

Reading and writing rooms? = classroom. Is the charge nurse to have nowhere to go but the duty room and the far-off home? . . .

Slop sinks not good to pass W.C.s to sink (nurse by men). Sink in compartment of its own—high, large, deep, round, pierced earthenware basin—large hole—cock to reach far over enough to send stream into middle of utensil to be emptied and cleansed. *Lavatory basins* to be not near enough for patients to elbow each other. Are all the utensils to be carried through from small ward into large ward offices to be emptied?

What proportion of patients in hospital bedridden? Makes great difference as to amount of slop sink and W.C. accommodation. How is foul linen disposed of?

Gynecological wards admirable, but how to be nursed by night or by day and how supervised? Gynecological wants a scullery beyond any other—roomy lavatory where smaller operations performed. Ovariotomy performed in its own small ward. Nurse never leaves ward day or night. Is all to be carried through to W.C.s in larger ward? What proportion of gynecological patients in bed?

Anesthetics—take them back to ward to recover.

Casualty ward—where will nurse be?

Are *corridors* closed? How do ward *windows* open? Too intricate.

Children's wards, which ought to be more than all others *in* the way under supervision are here beyond others, out of the way, beyond supervision. If over the matron's office, so that she hears every cry, so much the better. Where do the children's nursemaids sleep? How much better to distribute the children over the adult wards?

Infants under six months only rationale for children's wards. Children's hospitals: *not* wards—good. Infectious children to be in infectious blocks? Or may these children's wards be for infectious cases?

Children's balcony N.E. There seem to be conveniences for the children, their linen, their clothes, but none for the nurses, the nursemaids, the charge nurse, except one wretched little duty room, which rather shuts them off from the children. . . . Are the children in the north ward to look after each other? If they are infectious, they ought to have a kitchen, scullery, etc., to themselves.

Is charge nurse, nurse, nursemaids to be all pent up in that duty room?

Nurses' dining room: how many meals will there be in the dining room? Twelve maximum.

Laundry: Ought infectious linen to be washed within hospital boundary? Importance of a good laundry to hospital. But *no* inevitable infection in infectious laundry unless small, dark, wet, unventilated and overcrowded—and full of steam loaded with organic matter. . . .

Floors. What are to be floors, walls, ceilings of wards? Theatre, no corners, glass shelves for instruments.

Surgeons in smocks. If the charge nurses are not to have rooms off their wards, neither by night nor by day, then they must have sitting rooms *in* the building—*not* eighty yards off—and bedrooms *in* the building—that is considered a *sine qua non* [without which nothing] even by matrons of infirmaries who do not approve of rooms off wards. Nothing would persuade charge nurses to use the sitting rooms in a home at a distance—covered way or not.

2. What is to be done in the duty rooms?

3. What electric bells are intended for night service? What night service?

4. What matron's rooms?

5. What proportion of acute cases? (railway) accidents? night? operations? night? Night superintendent can't be spared for night operations.

Derby Infirmary: this small hospital, beautiful in the sanitary point of view, is almost unadministrable, and it may perhaps be said perfectly *un*supervis*able*, at least without a nursing staff large enough for the largest hospital.

It appears that the south wards are half a storey different in level from opposite wards, which of course increases the difficulty of supervision—no couple of wards being on the same level. Are the children's wards on the same difference of level? If so, they are perhaps the most intricate nest of rooms existing in any hospital—and to manage them there is only one wretched duty room, which will be in a crowded bustle from morning to night and night to morning.

The radical mistake appears to be in a misapprehension of the position of matron and nurses (charge nurses). The matron is not a person to have her office (and rooms) near the gate, to receive visitors to the hospital and inquiries. Nor are the "charge nurses" persons to bustle about for a certain number of hours of the day with nowhere to sit down—and then to adjourn to a "home" eighty yards off in the open air in all weathers.

The "charge nurses" (sisters) are the key to the situation—and through them the matron, who is the head of all the nursing—must influence morally, and practically, the nurses, wardmaids, probationers, patients,[459] the night superintendent and the night nurses. *For this* the matron must have an office, *not* looking north, in a central part handy to all the wards. She probably receives the night superintendent's report in her bedroom in the early morning. And it is better that her own rooms should not adjoin her office.

For this, too, the "*charge nurse*" must have a room of her own, so as in some measure to allow her to consider her ward as her home, her "charge," her family, morally and practically. Her room should be on one side [of] the ward door, so that no one should go in and out without her knowledge. And from her door she should be able to see down the whole ward.

If she cannot sleep, she may have a bedroom in the home. . . . But I may add from large experience that I have never known a trained sister in a large *hospital* who did not consider her room off her ward necessary to her work, or who did not refuse a sistership in those few *hospitals* where there is no such room. And the sisters are rare indeed who did not wish to sleep in it. (It is extremely seldom, not perhaps once a year in medical wards, where the night service is well organized, that the sister is called up.)

Have you railway and other accidents—sometimes by night? and operations? The surgical sister must be called up for such. And for such must sleep in the hospital, even if not in her room off the ward.

---

459 Struck out: and even junior resident staff.

P.S. It is to be regretted that the matron of this hospital is also the steward. But she must have a housekeeper besides the assistant. It is also to be regretted that this beautiful building, it is said, will be little more than a convalescent hospital, which had so much better be by the sea. It is hardly too much to say that the building and organization of a convalescent hospital should be, in nearly every respect, almost the very reverse of those of a hospital for acute medical and surgical cases.

In conclusion . . . I find that each nurse and sister is to go backwards and forwards to the home . . . with no covered way in all weathers in CLOGS, CLOAK AND BONNET. This is a mere man's chimera. Under such terms, the sitting rooms, the reading and writing rooms in the home, will never be used. And many will be the colds caught in their going unwillingly to bed there. No sitting rooms appear in the hospital and the dining room, which will have from seven to twelve meals daily, will certainly not be resorted to by any charge nurse to sit in. One must remember these are educated women.

Do not put sick nurses (in the single-bed wards) in the gynecological ward. If you have ovariotomy patients, these will be wanted for them. Put the sick nurses in the home, with a kitchen. But the home in its present form and place is a mistake altogether, which is a pity. . . .

Have you ovariotomy cases? Have you many acute medical cases? typhoid? cerebral? sudden delirium?

In London workhouse infirmaries, where there are comparatively few acute medical or surgical cases, and *no* accidents, few or *no* operations by night, though a very thorough night organization is wanted, the charge nurses (sisters) are not supposed to sleep off their wards by night, or even to have rooms off their wards by day, but they have dining rooms and sitting rooms (for sisters and nurses apart) *in* the building and bedrooms *in* the building, though away from the ward blocks.

Editor: When this editor visited Derby in 2010, the hospital building Nightingale had influenced had gone through another major rebuilding. The "Nightingale Wing" had been renovated for day patients and an up-to-date, much larger new building opened for regular hospital patients. The old "Nightingale Home," which had become a maternity unit, was boarded up and abandoned. The statue of Nightingale that had been in front of the (demolished) main building was moved elsewhere on the grounds. The stained glass window of Nightingale in the chapel was moved to St Peter's Church in the city centre.

Metropolitan Fever Hospitals, 1893-95

Editor: The Metropolitan Asylums Board was established in 1867 by the then Poor Law Board, which was itself replaced in 1871 by the Local Government Board, to manage the various fever hospitals, insane asylums and workhouses of London. This enabled the gradual raising of the standards of publicly funded hospitals to those run by charitable trusts. The "fever" hospitals often referred to in this volume were institutions under this board. Nightingale's major ally on improving their nursing and bringing in training was the Hon Maude Althea Stanley (1833-1915), daughter of the 2nd Baron Stanley of Alderley. Stanley was a member of the Metropolitan Asylums Board for thirty years, and a manager from 1884.[460]

Source: From a letter to Douglas Galton, Add Mss 45767 ff104-05

16 December 1893

Mr Scovell. Metropolitan. Private. I know you were in the chair at the Engineers yesterday, and I have no doubt have little time for me. But it was you who introduced me to this. (Is there an "asylum" for idiots? or at least for "abnormal" children? Take a bed for me.)

Mr Scovell[461] has sent me, through Miss Maude Stanley, the same paper that you showed me, with quantities of erasures. And he also says the "instructions" to "the architect" are *different* from what the *present* paper is!! *Are these instructions* in *conformity with yours*? The paper *with* the erasures seems worse than the original one. *Can I go over it with you?*

For one thing, the work thrown on the matron should be done by at least three heads to give the matron any time for discipline of the nurses or real nursing duties of supervision.

I *will* send you a "revised" "Notes," as you desire. But these people, Miss Stanley, Mr Scovell and Co. ought to go and *see Miss Vincent at her St Marylebone Infirmary.* They will never do anything without a *training school.* For they don't know a nurse from a dressmaker. (In one respect, Miss Vincent differs from me and is on their side. So much the better.)

---

460 There is further material on contact with Maude Stanley on nursing issues in *Extending Nursing* (13:173-78); however, Nightingale's letters to her are not extant.

461 Augustus Charles Scovell (1840-1924), later Sir, later chair of the Metropolitan Asylums Board.

Source: From undated notes, Add Mss 45820 ff39-42

[c1893]

Metropolitan Asylums: Nurses' Accommodation.

1. The first "accommodation" to the matron must be one or two trained assistant matron[s], or one and a housekeeper. It is perfectly impossible for a matron (who has laundry, stores under her, besides 128 nurses of all sorts under her) to do her duty to the *nursing*, to be a real superintendent of nurses, without one or two assistants. And she ought not to have the disinfection to do, but the housekeeper. It is an enormous charge. (And yet they propose, do they? to put her at a distance from her work.) There must be a "home sister" to the nurses' home, who should have a bedroom and office, probationers and night nurses to sleep in the home. The housekeeper in the home should be decidedly under the matron. No end of troubles arises from the contrary.

The laundress, of course, must be under the matron, who has the laundry. But should not all the women servants be under the matron? It is a poor place where women servants are not under the matron.

Offices: matron's in the centre of her work, with assistant matron's and linen room (and perhaps charge nurses' sitting and supper room) all together; two night superintendents: senior and junior, with one office, where they meet in the night. . . . A superintendent should always be present at a death.

Matron needs no dining room. She should dine with charge nurses. As the kitchen is not under her, it is doubly necessary that she should see their food. Assistant matron sits at the head of nurses' table. But the two matrons change about. All dine, in two relays of course. Many good superintendents of nurses prefer that the two tables should be in *the same* dining room. But this is not imperative. Should there be a nurses' kitchen? under matron? Yes, for the sake of providing variety. But the kitchen (general) might be under the matron.

Charge nurse's room off ward. However high your wages, you do not get the same class of woman unless you make her ward a real mother's charge to her. You must have quite other motives than that they have "no other place" to sit down in to keep them in their wards. The charge nurse is the key to the whole position. The superintendent of nurses has to influence, through her, the staff nurses, assistant nurses or probationers, patients, wardmaids or whatever answers to them, and to keep up the tone of the whole ward. If the charge nurses are turned on like water from a cock, or like charwomen, they cannot do this. The whole tone of their minds is different. Even if the charge nurses sleep elsewhere for health, they must (this is *must*, not may) have their own little rooms off the ward, and they must be allowed to have a cup of tea there—they can't always get away to tea or their bedrooms, which besides are so *small*. And every woman requires the recreation of being alone for a minute sometimes. They work all the better.

This is rather more necessary in fever asylums than elsewhere, e.g., general hospitals and Poor Law infirmaries. Nowhere else is there such an immense proportion of children or of acute cases (fever and diphtheria). Nowhere else is there such a strain upon the charge nurse.

Sitting rooms. Give a sitting room to charge nurses, with a piano, and one to nurses, too, if you like it. They will probably take tea and supper in it. But again I must repeat, more than one of our best sisters (charge nurses) left our best Poor Law infirmary for no other reason than that she could not have her little room off her ward.

Isolation wards	4 Wards [with]	1 bed	=	4
	8 "	4 "	=	32

very difficult to manage. They should be under one charge nurse or even two, each having *her own room near* her ward. (Charge nurses don't dislike this isolation), though perhaps they should not have it for too long a term.

In St Marylebone Infirmary, three two-bed wards to each pair of wards. Noisy patients may be put there. But there is a good ward kitchen to each pair. Do the assistant nurses do wardmaids' duties?

Are any probationers? or equivalent?

Charge nurses: where do they breakfast and take tea?

Night nurses: where do the night nurses have their (good, meat) breakfast, say 9 P.M. before they go on duty? i.e., at night. Where do they dine, say 10 A.M. when they come off duty? The two night superintendents preside at their meals. We must remember that the whole staff of day and night nurses are not in the dining room at once. The assistant matron presides over the dormitories.

Day rooms for patients are objectionable unless under strict supervision *of their own*. Patients play tricks and retard their recovery.

There seems no supervision or discipline for the mob of nurses out of the wards. St Marylebone Infirmary has more good supervision and moral discipline than any but the very best hospitals. It is no use training at *any* hospital that will take them.

Telephones: glad to see them named. At Edinburgh they have telephones for fathers and mothers coming to inquire after their children after their day's work at a distance. Telephone is set to work. And a charge nurse attends behind a bar to give them news.

Matron's Rooms: Some matrons like to have their own rooms near the entrance, their office always central. A large pavilion hospital is such a strain when it has, as it ought to have, only two floors.

Editor: The Eastern Fever Hospital, at Homerton, was a major Metropolitan Asylums Board hospital that was opened in 1870. Over the years it employed numerous St-Thomas'-trained matrons and nurses. In 1893, Nightingale met with the medical superintendent, E.W. Goodall, at his request, an encounter she dreaded.[462]

Source: From a letter to Henry Bonham Carter, Add Mss 47725 ff171-73

30 December 1893

Dr Goodall. *Confidential, etc. Homerton Hospital. L.G.B. Organization of Hospitals by*

1. The *medical superintendent* is called so: Medical à non Medicando. He told me himself that he was "never in the wards." He had no time. (The doctrine was entirely done by his three assistant medicals.) It appeared, however afterwards, that he did go into the wards two or three times a week to show a case clinically to his medical students, to whom he lectures. Of that more anon. He was exceedingly strong against the students "roaming about the wards," because he thought I was shocked by their having students "roaming about the wards." No. But privately I think that a medical school, under proper discipline, where "sisters" and ward discipline are what they ought to be, is a very great advantage to nursing—medical and training schools keep each other in order, actually raise the tone and let in light on one another. But of course [medical] students at fever hospitals are not my business.

2. *Medical superintendent à non superintendo.* He appears to know less about nursing than even doctors in general. It is to be doubted whether he knows how scarlet fever children look *by night,* or what *night* nursing they want. He is "patient of his limitations" to an astounding degree.

Confidential. *L.G.B. Rules.*

3. Medical superintendent, i.e., *non-medical secretary*—he told me himself his whole time was taken up by correspondence and the like.

---

462 For correspondence with him and his account of the meeting, see *Extending Nursing* (13:181-85).

4. *Product.* He has seen absolutely none nor wishes to see any infirmaries or hospitals with training schools, hardly heard of any—never seen St M[arylebone] or Brownlow Hill [Liverpool], though he went down on purpose "to ask Miss Stuart[463] "a question," i.e., whether she would train for them, but "did not go into the wards"!! nor Manchester, nor Edinburgh R. Infirmary (though it leaked out what use "certificates" are): they had taken a charge nurse with an Edinburgh R. Infirmary good "certificate," who had turned out badly). "Several years"!!! had elapsed between her leaving "Edinbro' (with her certificate) and her coming to Homerton"!!! (O wonderful is man. F.N.). He had never seen St T., never heard of Highgate.

He would like to have the Blue Book with the "Suggestions" [on cubic space], etc., but he will not even take the trouble of going to see St Marylebone. He is a Guy's man—so I asked him about Guy's training. But he knew nothing. N.B. The principles upon which he was appointed medical superintendent are unknown. . . . is a young man—not a gentleman—and appears younger than he is from his self-confident, positive, know-everything, schoolboy manners, put on I believe to conceal shyness—hardly intelligent, but *honest,* and I feel sure would help us in future. (I took special care, in consequence, not to offend him now.) He *can* help us *now* by incensing us about pitfalls with committees and boards, whom he really seems to understand.

He is afraid Miss Stanley's motion will be lost (which comes on on Friday), or carried because they will think a training school too easy, or lost because they are prepared for nothing of the kind, and need preparation. He says the committee do not like "outside criticism."

He himself is *committed* to the other plan, of getting other infirmaries to train for Homerton as, he says, Miss Twining[464] does. She gets (does she not?) a year's training from Brownlow Hill and other places for the association's nurses? I did not like to say anything in opposition, because you told me that "*Miss Twining* had done a great deal of good." God forbid that I should be even a fly to scotch that wheel. Especially now that, from their own showing, we see what the metropolitan asylums are. (You know what they want is an Agnes Jones to go and live in one of them.)

---

463 Mary Stuart (c1860-?), St Thomas' trained, then assistant superintendent at the Liverpool Workhouse Infirmary.

464 Louisa Twining (1820-1912), philanthropist; founder of the Workhouse Visiting Society in 1858 and the Workhouse Infirmary Nursing Association in 1879.

Confidential. Matron. Miss Jones[465] trained at Northern Hospital, Liverpool, came to Homerton from Middlesborough—a small fever hospital appears to be an old-fashioned almost non-entity—not at all the sort of person to help us.

Editor: In 1891, legislation expanded the scope of the Metropolitan Asylum Board hospitals to include non-pauper patients, which made them in effect free state hospitals long before the establishment of the National Health Service in 1948. The need for more fever hospitals was prompted by fever epidemics in 1892 and 1893. The correspondence below concerns a new hospital built at Shooter's Hill, Woolwich, which also was the site of the Herbert Hospital. This was the Brook Hospital, although it is not named in the correspondence. The architect was Thomas W. Aldwinkle, but there is nothing to show that Nightingale was ever in touch with him or consulted on his plans. That her principles were fully adopted is clear in a report on the hospital in *The Builder*: pavilion design; careful separation of fever cases; three separate buildings for staff, including separate space for night nurses; ample windows and southern vistas for nurses' sitting and dining rooms; fireproof stone staircase. "Each nurse has a separate bedroom with fireplace." The hospital foundation stone was laid in July 1894; it was opened on 31 August 1896.[466]

Source: From a letter to Douglas Galton, Add Mss 45767 ff116

11 January 1894

I hear from one of the managers that they have had a long discussion as to the expenditure of *£220,000* for a hospital at Shooter's Hill for *500 patients*, which brings the expense to *£440 per bed*, allowing a staff of *300* for the *500 patients*!!! I do not give you this for information of course—rather I crave your information. What, in the name of wonder, do they spend £440 a bed for, and what are the *300* for 500 patients to do? and under what *organization* are they, *the 300*, to be? what the supervision?

One of the delightful peculiarities of the "Regulations" is that they are to report *in writing* (I mean the day and night superintendents)

465 Possibly May Jones, matron of the Holborn Union Workhouse.

466 "The Brook Hospital, Shooter's Hill," *The Builder* 71,2792 (8 August 1896): 121-22

everything, including the number of minutes she has been in each ward at night, to the *medical superintendent.* I should guess each day would require thirteen hours' writing. (This was the calculation Macaulay made for Clarissa's letters.[467])

You know we, the vulgar, thought that the superintending *nurse* was to *nurse,* i.e., that she should correct the faults in nursing and teach the nurses on the spot.

Editor: Nightingale next urged Douglas Galton to stay on the board so as to "instruct" the people on fever hospitals at their meetings.[468]

Miscellaneous Last Work on Hospital Reform, from 1890

Editor: Nightingale continued to work on bettering hospitals to the end of her working life, and she had the pleasure of seeing many improvements achieved. Nevertheless, her call, from her 1863 preface to *Notes on Hospitals,* that a hospital should as the very first principle "do the sick no harm" still needed to be heeded. Social administration expert Abel-Smith commented that by the late nineteenth century, although not before, hospitals provided a positive net benefit, that is, that they did more good than harm.[469] This last section of correspondence covers a wide range of concerns from Nightingale's last working years.

Source: Notes from an interview with Dorothy F. Solly,[470] Add Mss 47763 f233 [c1890]

Miss Solly. Hospital Diseases.

In one of the upper wards, Clayton, we remember how much illness there was arising in the ward; they had to clear out the ward three times in one year, owing to pyemia among the patients. Everyone seemed unaware of the cause of the disease, till a workman discovered an escape of sewer gas (in the pipe of the W.C.). The first sister, Miss

467 Thomas Babington Macaulay, a reference to Samuel Richardson's novel of letters, *Clarissa.*

468 Letter 24 January 1894, in *Extending Nursing* (13:187).

469 Abel-Smith, *The Hospitals 1800-1948* 1-2.

470 Dorothy Frances Solly (c1848-93), who was considered for the matronship at St Thomas', but did not get it.

Tatham, was always ill, and the present sister, Miss Carter,[471] has been ill more than once, but since the sewer gas escape was discovered, and of course entirely remedied, there has been no hospital sickness among the patients, or among sisters and nurses, although the ward is often too crowded.

([FN comment:] This is not quite true; Miss Tatham has just been ill at Cheltenham, owing to overfatigue, from a very slight outbreak of typhoid fever).

Source: From a letter to William Rathbone, Florence Nightingale Museum (LMA) H1/ST/NC8/91/6

3 June 1891

About *chaplains:* is it not the case that, in the large hospitals, the chaplain does not "*deteriorate*"; he is *bad to begin with* and bad to end with. He is generally a "job" [patronage appointment] an elderly man, put into a "snug berth" by some governors? (as a matron used to be put into a workhouse infirmary, say a "greengrocer's widow," "second cousin" to one of the board?).

As for the man at the London Hospital, did he not *begin ill* and end ill? not "deteriorate."

Source: From a letter to Douglas Galton, Add Mss 45767 37-40

22 July 1891

Congress. I see *St Thomas' Hospital* is not included in the list of buildings to see which "special facilities" are to be given. I *hope* the foreigners[472] will take as a model Bartholomew's, which does not know if it has any drains, or *if* it has *where* they are, the "London," dirty and detestable in its wards, and other old hospitals which *are* included on the list—St Thomas' is far from perfect but it is better than these. And of course I think its nursing, though not perfect, is better. But I like the esprit de corps which makes each hospital say its own nursing is the best.

However, to return, I asked one of your delegates, one of the senior physicians of St Thomas', why that saint had refused "facilities." He said, "Refused!? Why, St Thomas' is the very one they ought to see!

471 Katherine Elizabeth Tatham (c1860-1932) and Mary Helen Carter (c1857-?), both St Thomas' trained.

472 Attending the 7th International Congress of Hygiene and Demography in London, chaired by Galton.

We can't have been asked." Do pray *ask St Thomas* to give "special facilities" and put him in the list.

Editor: The next short items concern the nurses' home for the new Prince Alfred Hospital in Sydney. The hospital building itself opened in 1882, but the nurses' home did not open until 1892.

Dr Alfred Roberts had written Nightingale in 1889, recalling her efforts (which began in 1866) to get the five nurses they had started with at the Sydney Infirmary (in 1868), reporting on progress made in nurse training since Osburn left (in 1884), and enclosing a syllabus for the nurses' school at the new Prince Alfred Hospital. He regretted to say that the nurses' quarters were scattered over different parts of the hospital, that they were struggling to get the £1000 required to erect a "nurses' home" in the grounds.[473]

Source: From two letters to Douglas Galton, Add Mss 45767 ff33 and 35

6 July 1891

Do you remember being so good as to look over and criticize the plans (very bad) of the nurses' home at Sydney, N.S.W.? I have now their reply—letter from chairman—letter from architect to chairman and a more elaborate tracing. I fear it is a bad job.

Are you so kind *as to look over it again*?

11 July 1891

Are you so good as to look at the Sydney Nurses' Home plans, returned to me after considering your criticisms?

Editor: In 1892, Henry Parkes wrote Nightingale about a new hospital on the old Sydney Infirmary site.[474]

The item immediately below refers to drainage issues in Truro, Cornwall. Its mayor, architect Silvanus Trevail (1851-1903), had a strong interest in the issue. He sent Nightingale seven papers, referred to in the next item below, but there is no further correspondence on the subject.

---

473 Roberts letter 24 July 1889, Florence Nightingale Museum (LMA) H1/ST/NC2/V45/89.

474 Letter 13 November 1892, Add Mss 47757 ff58-59.

Source: From an undated note to Frederick Verney, Add Mss 68887 f101

[c1892]

"Silvanus Trevail" has sent me his papers (seven), which I thought admirable. I answered by asking him to send them to you and by sending him a health pamphlet. I must write today, under cover of sending him Dr De'Ath's[475] pamphlet "Organization of Village Sanitation," to say I know you have his papers.

Editor: In 1893 Nightingale received a letter from William Alfred Pite (1860-1949), architect of the new King's College Hospital, who was then designing "a small London hospital." This, in fact, was the London Homeopathic, on Great Ormond St., later the Royal London Hospital for Integrated Medicine. He asked for advice as to the lining of the walls of the wards and the relative merits of Parian cement and ordinary plaster. Nightingale underlined points in the letter, but no reply is extant. The hospital opened in 1895.

The letter following concerns a nephew of St Thomas' matron Sarah E. Wardroper.

Source: From a letter to Henry Bonham Carter, with his reply, Add Mss 47724 f227

15 January 1893

Also, that a "nephew of Mrs W., an architect at Ipswich" writes to offer his gratuitous services as architect. He seems to think there will be a building. Must I answer?

HBC: I do *not* think you need. If he, the nephew, writes to you, send me the letter to answer.

Source: From a letter to Douglas Galton, Add Mss 45767 ff108-09

18 December 1893

Nurses' Accommodation. Your plans today. Thousand thanks for your visit.[476] You said you were going to do plans today. Please remember the *fireplaces* in the *nurses'* bedrooms—a minor detail, but most important.

2. Where there is no little room for the "charges" (ridiculous name—do call them sisters) *off the ward,* the bedroom must be made large enough, light enough, warm for the charge nurse (we call her

475 George Hanby De'Ath (c1862-1901), medical officer of health, Buckingham.

476 Galton visited the previous day, but it is not apparent for what hospital the plans were made.

sister) to sit in, read in, write in. (Her fire is laid for her, and she has leave to light it whenever she likes.) The sister (charge nurse) has actually more responsibility than the *hospital* sister. And you cannot get the sort of intelligent, devoted woman you want to spend her day between the din (bustle) in the ward and the din in the dining and recreation room. She must sit in her own bedroom when she likes when off duty. . . .

3. The nurse has also a fireplace, but is not allowed to light it, except in the event of any trifling illness, for which she is not warded.

4. There must be [a] good little *ward kitchen* to each ward or pair of wards, where the charge nurse (sister) and nurses take a cup of tea *before* their dining room tea. Excuse this long dissertation, because you listened so kindly. . . .

The *assistant matron's bedroom* is adjoining to the nurses' bedrooms of whom she is in charge.

Editor: In 1895, John Shaw Billings, the designer of Johns Hopkins Hospital, wrote Henry Bonham Carter in his later capacity as librarian (a founder both of the New York Public Library and the library of the National Institute of Medicine). He asked for copies of "announcements, rules and regulations or circulars of information relating to the Nightingale Fund for Training Nurses," giving a London address to which they could be sent; "any expense incurred will be cheerfully met."

Nightingale wrote a fundraising letter for St Thomas' Hospital both in 1895 and 1896, addressed to the treasurer, J.G. Wainwright, each announcing her own contribution of £100. The first campaign, in aid of reopening closed wards, was evidently successful, for the reopened wards were duly announced in the second letter. Henry Bonham Carter did a draft for her for the 1895 letter. She also asked the advice of the wife of Sir Edmund Verney, Margaret Verney (1844-1930), a capable author. Lady Verney gave Nightingale several suggested amendments, which she adopted.[477] The 1895 letter has already appeared in *The Nightingale School* (12:461-63). The 1896 letter follows.

---

477 Bonham Carter undated draft, Add Mss 45813 ff161-62; Margaret Verney draft ff159-61. In April that year they were working on the Derby plans.

Source: From an open letter to J.G. Wainwright, Florence Nightingale Museum (LMA) H1/ST/NC5/3/45

14 February 1896

It gives us all joy, and patients especially, of your reopening of two much wanted wards lying empty for want of funds through no fault of their own. These wards also contain some of the latest improvements. And I hope that all the money still wanted which you desire and deserve will come in.

I beg to send my £100, wishing it were much larger, for the benefit is great, not only to the bodies of the patients, but towards rendering those bodies able to tread a nobler, more useful course in life by the practical lessons they learn in the wards of order, kindness and moderation or self-discipline. This is especially the case with the children.

It is delightful when a hospital is a school of good morals to the patients as well as a training school for nurses and for [medical] students. And such is St Thomas' Hospital.

We rejoice that our president, the duke of Connaught,[478] is to perform the ceremony of opening the wards.

Source: From two letters to Frederick Verney, ADD MSS 68888 ff104-05

4 October 1895

I am so very sorry to hear (half an hour ago) from Miss Lückes[479] that Miss [Bella] Deyns has an attack of scarlet fever, and though very mild, they have been obliged to send her, as they do all their nurses, to the London Fever Hospital, Liverpool Road, Islington. I am afraid it is a great disappointment to Miss Deyns. She had just completed her month, and very well, in the children's ward. And Miss Lückes says that they always reckon three months before a nurse can resume work. Miss Lückes asks me to "*let the chairman know* what has occurred," and I am afraid I must ask *you* to do this. They *have* communicated with Miss Deyns's relations "in the routine way."

They say they do not know how she caught it, but that is all the old-fashioned idea of infection. They say there was no scarlet fever in the ward. But there is always scarlet fever when the first rains come after the heat. We have one case, at least, among the probationers at St Thomas', but then we have the advantage of a separate block for it.

478 Arthur, duke of Connaught (1850-1942), son of Queen Victoria.
479 Eva C.E. Lückes (1854-1919), matron, London Hospital.

10 October 1895

Don't go to the London Fever Hospital, even to see Miss Deyns—the French call our fever hospitals "foyers d'infection" [places of infection] and they are right.

Source: From a letter to Douglas Galton, Add Mss 45767 ff179-80

26 September 1896

E. London Water Supply. About the cisterns in East London famine—the fight continues: water company and *Times* of course on one side, *Daily Chronicle* and many medical officers of health on the other. I am sorry to say the L.G.B. [Local Government Board] is not sound on the subject, and Dr Barry? is a very formidable opponent.

If you do not remember, I could give you a very brief sketch of the subject, over again, and also of what has happened since I last wrote in the way of M.O.s of health for and against.

Editor: In 1899, H.F. Geltsen, secretary of the Nurses Co-operation, an agency that sent out private nurses, asked to show Nightingale the plans and consult her on several points of a new nurses' home for its staff. Geltsen had been in touch with her for two years on various nursing issues; now she described the site, and offered to wait on Nightingale if she preferred to give her advice verbally: "I am anxious to have the Nurses' Home as nearly perfect as a building can be." Their donor, Lady Howard de Walden, had provided for an exterior of glazed bricks, which gave a "goodly appearance."[480]

Nightingale sought the advice of senior St Thomas' nursing administrators, either the matron, Louisa Gordon (1845-1903), or the home sister, Florence Amelia Haig Brown (1862-1931), on key practical points.

Source: From a letter to the matron or home sister, Add Mss 47737 f246

5 October 1899

Immediate. I am to be consulted this afternoon on the plans (requisites) for a nurses' home. There is a fashion about these things, which is not so absurd as it seems, because think of the difference in the character of the nurses. To save you trouble, I have put down what I think

480 Geltsen letter 3 October 1899, Add Mss 45815 f100. There is correspondence from her to Nightingale 1897-99, but Nightingale's letters to her are not extant.

I have heard you say you want. Please return it to me with your own comments. *Please return.*

Do you want:

1. *Separate* nurses' home, but with covered passage?
2. *Common dining room?*
3. Common sitting room?
4. Garden, if possible?
5. How to make supervision convenient? Probationers not at the top of house. *Where?*
6. Superintendent taking her meals with the others.
7. Bathroom (two baths to each storey). Fireplace? Dressing room. We give up all idea of separating by "pavilions." Thank you for all your kindness.

Source: From a letter to Henry Dyke Acland, Bodleian Library, Oxford University

24 January 1900

I am so thankful to hear of you and almost from you, through Fred Verney. But do you know, I hear from and of you almost every day? in this way—I can remember when pyemia was almost as common a thing in hospitals as any case coming from without—I mean pyemia generated *in* hospital. Now we shout so loud when there is a case that they can hear us all over London. This is an amazing change, and we owe it principally to you and what you have taught us. We do not look upon anything of the kind now as unavoidable, just as there is no such thing as "inevitable infection" now.

I do not see anything to add to your invaluable pamphlet. It is perfect. How much you are doing. You ask after me—I have been a prisoner to my room for above a year—but I have always more to do that I fear I can do properly. I hope to write again. In haste,

ever your affectionate and sympathizing

F. Nightingale

Editor: Nightingale's last documented work on hospitals goes back to her very first position at the Establishment for Gentlewomen during Illness on Harley St., in 1853. By 1901, her old hospital had seriously depleted its capital to pay ongoing expenses and asked Nightingale to assist with fundraising. Her letter to the *Times* is the first item below. It is followed by a note she sent with a receipt to a contributor—exceptionally, she had given her home address on her published letter. The Boer War was still on, the letter explained, which made an appeal for money difficult. The institution in fact survived, to be rebuilt in Lisson Grove in 1909 and, after her death in 1910, named the "Florence Nightingale Hospital for Gentlewomen." In 2000 the name was simplified to the "Florence Nightingale Hospital."

The very last item is an excerpt from a tribute to Nightingale by one of her matrons. These last efforts recall yet another error by F.B. Smith that, after she left for the Crimean War, "there is no evidence that Miss Nightingale ever revisited Harley Street or took any further interest in it."[481]

Source: Published letter, *Times* 12 November 1901:6a

10 South St.

Sir, I write to make an appeal for an institution which is doing good work—work after my own heart, and, I trust, God's work.

It is, everyone says, a bad time for appeals for money. The needs of our soldiers and of the thousands of sufferers in South Africa are still with us, but are not the burdens to be borne that war must inevitably bring, and the sufferers at home yet not be forgotten?

No. 90 Harley Street is an establishment for gentlewomen in temporary illness and has been in existence since 1850 [1853], when, with the help of Lady Canning, I was able to set it on foot and to preside over it until I went to the Crimean War. There is no other institution exactly like this. In it our governesses (who are primarily eligible), the wives and daughters of the clergy, of our naval, military and other professional men receive every possible care, comfort and first-rate advice at the most moderate cost. But this cannot be done without larger contributions.

Look at these few statistics, which I take from the report of 1901, and these may be considered fair averages of past years: ordinary expenses £2,424.9s.1d, ordinary receipts £1,770.19s.6d, deficit in 1900 £653.9s.7d.

This deficit has been met year after year by trenching on the small invested capital or by using legacies instead of investing them, but for 1901 there is no such help forthcoming by legacies.

The number of beds in the home is twenty. The average cost of each patient per week is £3.10s.76d. In 1900, patients treated 164, cured 145, operations performed 123.

All this good work has been done entirely gratuitously by eminent physicians and surgeons. The patients contribute to their board and lodging, and thus meet half the expenses of the establishment.

---

481 Smith, *Florence Nightingale: Reputation and Power* 17.

Everyone connected with this home and haven for the suffering is doing their utmost for it and it is always full. It is conducted on the same lines as from its beginning, by a committee of ladies, of which Mrs Walter is the president, and she will be glad to receive contributions at 90 Harley Street, W.

I ask and pray my friends who still remember me not to let this truly sacred work languish and die for want of a little more money. What is more grievous than suffering which cannot be relieved for want of means?

yours obediently
Florence Nightingale

Source: Letter to Miss Edith Glandie, Florence Nightingale Museum 0545

18 November 1901

Dear Madam, Allow me to thank you for the Postal Order for £1 (one pound) in answer to my appeal for the Ladies' Home, Harley St.

yours truly
Florence Nightingale

Editor: In 1908 nursing matron Flora Masson reported the details of Nightingale's last act in support of her old hospital:

> At her own request the money which would have been spent on a gold casket was devoted to charity, the sum of 100 guineas being given instead to the Hospital for Invalid Gentlewomen, and the casket presented to Miss Nightingale was of oak.[482]

Trends in Hospital Reform since Nightingale's Time

Editor: Before closing this volume and the series, a word about subsequent trends might be in order. The hospitals we see today bear little relation to those Nightingale advocated. Technological advances gradually made many key principles of the pavilion system, including the need for the "Nightingale ward," obsolete. With telephones, bells and, later, a diversity of electronic monitoring devices, the need for the ward sister to be able to observe by eye all her patients was no longer necessary. Improvements in toilets and washing facilities similarly obviated the need for their installation separately from the wards.

---

482 Flora Masson, *Florence Nightingale, O.M., By One Who Knew Her* 20.

A letter by an anonymous surgeon in *The Builder* in 1896 showed the desire by some members of the medical community to escape the constraints of the pavilion model. The writer mistakenly credited the impetus for the pavilion system to the "terrible mortality in the crowded huts on the Crimean battlefields," when the great killers in the Crimean War were not the huts but the great hospitals. He (correctly) cited improvements from Lister, along with improved equipment for warming and ventilation, such that artificial ventilation could be relied on for an adequate "continuous supply of fresh air." A hospital ward could thus "be constructed of any width or shape, provided always that there be sufficient light."[483] A debate among architects ensued.

One architect promptly related the "great joy" architects would feel at "their emancipation from the incubus and terrible tyranny of the pavilion system of construction."[484] He noted technological improvements in ventilation. Two architects wrote the following week with further considerations. One, William A. Pite, was critical of the supposed technological improvements in ventilation cited by the initial surgeon, and stressed the advantages of the pavilion system for both ventilation and light: the "health-giving constituents of sunlight" should not be overlooked.[485]

The rise of antibiotics by the midpoint of the twentieth century was at least as influential in ending the need for pavilions. Effective antibiotics changed medical practice, drastically cutting deaths from fever and shortening hospital stays. Instead of nurses being needed to monitor patients in crisis, drugs combatted the disease directly, reduced the fever and ended the crisis. The nurse's room at the end of the ward, with its observation window, was no longer needed. The rising standard of living postwar was another factor, resulting in a greater demand for privacy. Wards became small rooms and hospitals built or rebuilt after World War II went highrise.

Social change over the years changed the nature of nursing itself and the type of person who entered the profession. The notion of a ward sister being on duty so many hours of the day and sleeping with

---

483 FRCS [Fellow of the Royal College of Surgeons], "On the Plan of Construction of Hospitals and Infirmaries," *The Builder* 70,2786 (27 June 1896):561.

484 An Architect, "The Construction of Hospitals and Infirmaries," *The Builder* 71,2791 (1 August 1896):102.

485 Letter, "On the Plan and Construction of Hospitals and Infirmaries, *The Builder* 71,2792 (8 August 1896):122.

an observation window into her ward(s) is unthinkable today. With improvements in education and advances in birth control and women's rights, family size declined and large numbers of nurses were married women, albeit with family responsibilities. Men began to enter the profession while many women became doctors.

Upon ending this volume and the *Collected Works*, we might briefly consider how relevant Nightingale's work on hospital reform might be for today's hospitals. While the specifics of pavilion design, ward size, separate laundries, nurses' homes and nurses' rooms off wards for observation all became obsolete over time, Nightingale's basic principles arguably still hold. Indeed, with the rise of drug-resistant pathogens, and high death rates from hospital-acquired infections, one might even urge that they be revisited. The Centers of Disease Control estimated that 2 million patients in the United States in 2008 were infected, of whom an estimated 90,000 died.[486] For Canada the estimate for the year was 220,000 patients who fell ill, of whom about 8000 died.[487] The population of Canada is roughly a tenth that of the United States, and half that of Great Britain.

The need for better infection control has led to the provision of many more single rooms in hospitals. However, the same pressure of land costs that led to three- and four-storey buildings in Nightingale's day—too high, in her opinion—have continued to push hospitals much higher in the twentieth and twenty-first centuries.

American architect Stephen Verderber updated Nightingale's famous preface warning at the beginning of his 2010 book, *Innovations in Hospital Architecture*: The very first requirement of a hospital is that it shall cause neither human nor ecological harm."[488] Verderber saw continuities and an ongoing Nightingale influence from her role in the late nineteenth century, when she "set the standard for sustainability against which the performance—functionally or otherwise—of all hospitals would be judged to a greater extent until the outbreak of World War II" (22). She was "the most widely quoted hospital reformer of her era" (24). Instead of a sharp break, he saw "a new generation of skyscraper Nightingale hospitals," built in the period after her death in 1910 to World War II (1940 is his date). Certainly some of the "skyscraper" hospitals had narrow, well-lit wards, in accordance with Nightingale's principles.

---

486 Atul Gawande, *Better: A Surgeon's Notes on Performance*, Part 1 Diligence.
487 "Hospitals Face Hand-washing Crackdown," *Globe and Mail* 20 May 2008 A1.
488 Stephen Verderber, *Innovations in Hospital Architecture* v.

The eco-humanist work of Florence Nightingale centred on the provision of clean, well-lit and ventilated hospitals affording the patient a meaningful view of the outdoor natural landscape from within an open ward (43). In contrast with the "unsustainable megahospital 1945-2000," Verderber continued, which he faulted for suburban sprawl, "Nightingale hospitals were characterized by their low profile, relatively narrow open wards with interspersed landscaped courtyard," the nursing station located on the inward end of each ward, "adjacent to a circulation artery" (43). This architect in effect brings together the advances in hospital design possible with innovations in medical treatment and equipment for heating and air conditioning, with a more patient friendly, less obviously utilitarian ambience, with fresh air and sunlight, and a variety of scene, qualities advocated by the "eco-humanist" Nightingale.

An announcement of a major hospital renovation in Toronto in 2012 refers to a major focus on infection control (increasing the number of single rooms), but intriguingly also to "more natural light," "large gardens and lawn areas" and a "roof garden," features said to be linked to "shorter hospital stays and improved patient outcomes."[489]

Nightingale's core principles would seem to make sense today as much as if not more than ever:

* Measures for prevention (good nutrition, housing, clean air and water) preferred to treatment after the fact;

* Intervention at the minimal level possible (hospital stays the last resort, home visits and out-patient visits preferred);

* Safe design and site for hospitals when required;

* In hospitals, high standards of cleanliness, in accordance with the best knowledge available, set out in tested protocols appropriate to the staff concerned;

* Hospital space to be allocated to minimize exposure to disease sources;

* Considerations for efficient nursing (patients come first, both for safety and convenience);

* Reliance on the healing properties of natural sunlight, fresh air, outdoor balconies and gardens for recovery;

* Careful monitoring of treatment, especially new modes, with timely reporting of results (evidence-based health care);

---

489 Carly Weeks, "Thomsons Donate $5-Million for Patient-Care Centre at Toronto East General," *Globe and Mail* 22 February 2012 A6.

* The collection of uniform hospital statistics to permit comparisons; particular monitoring of nurse deaths as a key indicator of hospital safety.

The sunlight, fresh air, balconies and gardens Nightingale advocated as early as 1858 appear now as elements of an "environmental" approach to patient care. These are considerations not only for acute-care hospitals but the growing number of care facilities for the aged.

Finally, it is worth remembering how consistent Nightingale was in setting out her core principles, how she integrated the goal of nurse welfare with that of patient care, continued to stress prevention over cure after the fact, and always saw the key role of knowledge, gained through rigorous statistical analysis, as essential to achieving good health care. She crafted her message clearly and forcefully, as these last examples—a final summary—demonstrate:

The principles of hospital construction which we have now laid before our readers are a tacit condemnation of the majority of hospitals in the three kingdoms (16:304) – 1858.

If disease ever appears to spread anywhere, in hospital or out of hospital, by infection or "contagion," no stronger proof of bad construction or of neglect of hygiene could be adduced (6:354) – 1859.

It may seem a strange principal to enunciate as the very first requirement in a hospital, that it should do the sick no harm (16:88) – 1863.

In all hospitals (in children's hospitals much more than in others) the patient must not stay a day longer than is absolutely necessary (6:528) – 1860.

The building and organization of a convalescent hospital should be, in nearly every respect, almost the very reverse of those of a hospital for acute medical and surgical cases (16:926) – 1891.

To make the people's dwellings . . . such as will not make sickness . . . is of course our first duty (12:769) – 1872.

Nothing gives such a really good criterion of the sanitary (or non-sanitary) construction of hospitals . . . [as] the mortality of nurses (16:516) – 1858.

A nurse must not be a scrubber. And a scrubber cannot be a nurse (16:123) – 1863.

APPENDIX

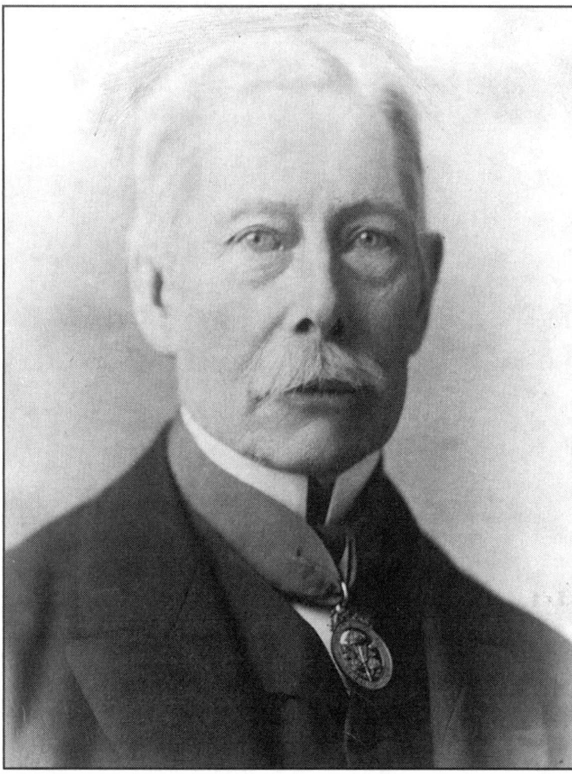

Douglas Galton, Royal Engineer, Nightingale's most trusted expert on hospital design. Photograph courtesy of NPL.

Appendix A: Biographical Sketches

(Sir) Douglas Galton (1822-99)

Douglas Strutt Galton,[1] a relative by marriage to Nightingale cousin, Marianne Nicholson (1821-1909), was an esteemed Royal Engineer and a favourite colleague. Nightingale worked mightily behind the scenes to get him appointed as assistant under secretary at the War Office, in 1862, as the best chance to get the planned army health measures actually implemented. After he left that position in 1868, he became director of Public Works and Buildings, 1869-74. During the Franco-Prussian War he served on the National Aid Society. Nightingale also greatly appreciated his contributions as a member of the Cubic Space Committee and the Metropolitan Asylums Board. He was made a fellow of the Royal Society in 1859 and knighted in 1887.

Galton was a member of a wealthy family, with a fine country establishment at Droitwich, near Worcester, purchased by his father, John Howard Galton. Francis Galton and Charles Darwin were both cousins. The Galtons' religious affiliations were complicated, with Quakers on his father's side, and Plymouth Brethren on his mother's, the Strutt family of Derbyshire. The family became Church of England at Droitwich, where Douglas was baptized. His older brother with his wife later converted to Roman Catholicism and two of their sons became Jesuits. Galton himself remained a faithful member of the Church of England.

The Galtons had two daughters, whom Nightingale knew and to whom she left legacies. Nightingale was godmother to their only son, named with such hope Herbert Nightingale Douglas Galton, who was born in 1861 and died the following year.

---

1 On Galton see the entry in the *Oxford Dictionary of National Biography.*

Galton and Nightingale held similar views on public health and its importance. Each brought their own professional knowledge and particular skills. She set the goals and the broad principles, which he shared, and he contributed his considerable technical expertise as a trained army engineer. The correspondence shows enormous deference on his part. He incorporated her views on all matters of nursing and the basic precepts on hospital construction. In turn, she deferred to him on all technical matters. Each asked the other to vet their writing. He was assiduous in answering questions for her and rose to the challenge when she wanted more detail. She frequently asked him to go over her critiques of hospital plans before sending them in to the hospital committee or architect in question. The two obviously liked each other enormously—he was a rare visitor who was urged to stay for coffee when he brought her information. Much of their correspondence has survived, in ADD MSS 45759-67, including numerous letters designated "BURN." Nightingale left him £300 in her will, but he predeceased her.

Galton is remembered in the restoration of a Warwickshire church: "The 15th century glass in this window was restored and dedicated to the glory of God by the parishioners of Himbleton in dear memory of Captain Sir Douglas Galton, KCB, an earnest and true-hearted seeker after God. A.D. 1901."

(Sir) Robert Rawlinson (1810-98)

Robert Rawlinson (1810-98),[2] son of a builder, became a government public health inspector in 1848, and later headed the department. In 1855 he went with the sanitary commission, headed by Dr Sutherland, to clean up the British Army hospitals of the Crimean War. He and Nightingale became friends there and, after the war, he became a member of her inner circle of collaborators. He assisted in the work for the first royal commission, and was a member of the Indian royal commission and the War Office's Army Sanitary Commission. For over forty years he was Nightingale's major consultant on civil engineering and water issues. Each consulted the other on their respective projects. Rawlinson was one of the "wise old men" Nightingale's sister described as being not too proud to learn from Nightingale, "so profoundly convinced of her knowledge."[3]

---

2 On Rawlinson see the entry in the *Oxford Dictionary of National Biography*.

3 Cited in Cook, *The Life of Florence Nightingale* 1:353.

Nightingale liked him enormously and worried that her father would not treat her friend correctly when he went to Embley, at her request, to supervise some sanitary engineering. She wrote detailed instructions as to how he should be received: "as a gentleman," although he was being paid a professional fee. He was knighted in 1883.

A volume of correspondence from him in Add Mss 45769 shows their close working association.

Hospital Architects (in Alphabetical Order)

* Denotes that Nightingale met with the architect on plans.

Bellamy,* Thomas (1798-1876): King's College Hospital (advice not taken).

Brandon, David (1813-97), Queen Victoria's favourite architect: Buckinghamshire County Infirmary, Aylesbury 1859-69 correspondence available to and from him.

Bryce, David (1803-76), leading Scottish architect: Edinburgh Royal Infirmary; no correspondence either way.

Brydon, John McKean (1840-1901): Women's Hospital, Euston Road 1888; no correspondence available either way.

Butterfield,* William (1814-1900), renowned for church restorations: Hampshire County Hospital, Winchester 1858-65; Gordon Boys' Home 1885-90; correspondence available from him.

Currey, Henry (1820-1900), leading hospital architect: St Thomas' Hospital 1859-74, correspondence available from him.

Giles, John (d. 1900): St Pancras Workhouse Infirmary 1868, correspondence available from him.

Graham,* Alex (1847-1922): Swansea Infirmary 1864-65; Yoxall Cottage Hospital 1872-74; Montreal General Hospital 1874-76 (not built); Lincoln Hospital 1879; correspondence available to and from him.

Gropius, Martin (1824-80): Städtisches Krankenhaus im Friedrichshain, Berlin; no correspondence either way.

Humbert, Albert Jenkins (1822-77), Lisbon Children's Hospital 1859-60: correspondence available to and from him.

Hume, James (1796-1868): Sydney Infirmary, Macquarie St.; no correspondence either way.

Hunt, John Horbury (1838-1904): Australian architect, Catherine Hayes Hospital, Sydney (children's), no correspondence either way.

Mennie, R.O., surveyor: architect of Netley Hospital; brief correspondence to.

Norman, Alfred (1823-93), Gothic Revival architect, Devonport, Stonehouse and Cornwall Hospital; no correspondence either way.

Pite, William Alfred (1860-1949), FRIBA, architect of London Homeopathic; correspondence from him.

Scott, George Gilbert (1811-78), Gothic Revival architect, head of the largest English firm of architects: Leeds Infirmary 1861-69; no correspondence either way.

Snell, Henry Saxon (c1831-1904), leading workhouse infirmary architect: St Marylebone Infirmary Nurses' Home 1882-83; Royal Victoria Hospital, Montreal 1888-39; correspondence available to and from him.

Stevens, Isaac Henry (c1807-73), church architect: Nightingale Wing of Derbyshire General Infirmary; no correspondence either way.

Waterhouse,* Alfred (1830-1905), Gothic Revival architect: Liverpool Royal Infirmary; correspondence available to him.

Weinbrenner, Pofessor architect of Carlsruhe Clinique; correspondence regarding him.

Worthington, Thomas (1826-1909), architect of first pavilion workhouse infirmary: Chorlton Union Workhouse 1865-66; Prestwich Union Workhouse Infirmary, Crumpsall, 1868; Liverpool Convalescent Home; correspondence available to and from him.

Wyatt, Thomas Henry (1807-80), an architect Nightingale recommended: Herbert Memorial Convalescent Home, Bournemouth 1865-67; Norfolk and Norwich Hospital 1875; Montreal General Hospital 1874-76 (not built); Malta General Hospital and Asylum 1863; correspondence available to and from him

Young,* Keith Downes (1848-1929): architect of the first circular hospital in England (Miller Memorial Hospital, Greenwich), and of the Derbyshire Royal Infirmary Nurses' Home 1891-94; correspondence available about his plans and meeting with him.

Bibliography

Bibliography

Abel-Smith, Brian. *The Hospitals 1800-1948: A Study in Social Administration in England and Wales.* London: Heinemann 1964.

Adams, Annmarie. *Medicine by Design: The Architect and the Modern Hospital 1893-1947.* Minneapolis: University of Minnesota Press 2008.

Adams, Francis, trans. *The Seven Books of Paulus Aegineta.* 3 vols. London: Sydenham Society 1844-47.

Anning, Stephen Towers. *The General Infirmary at Leeds.* 2 vols. London: E. & S. Livingstone 1963 and 1966.

A Record of Sixty Years' Work: St John's House Queen Square. St John's House 1909.

Ayers, Gwendoline M. *England's First State Hospitals and the Metropolitan Asylums Board 1867-1930.* London: Wellcome Institute of the History of Medicine 1971.

Baudens, Lucien. *On Military and Camp Hospitals, and the Health of Troops in the Field, Being the Results of a Commission to Inspect the Sanitary Arrangements of the French Army, and Incidentally of Other Armies in the Crimean War,* trans. Franklin B. Hough. London and Paris: J.B. Baillière et Fils 1862.

Billings, John S. *Description of the Johns Hopkins Hospital.* Baltimore: Johns Hopkins Hospital 1890.

Bishop, W.J., and Sue Goldie, comps., *A Bio-Bibliography of Florence Nightingale.* London: Dawsons 1962.

Borg, Malcolm. *British Colonial Architecture: Malta (1800-1900).* San Gwann, Malta: Publishers Enterprise Group 2001.

Burdett, Henry Charles. *The Cottage Hospital: Its Origin, Progress, Management and Work.* London: J. & A. Churchill 1877.

Burke, Brian. *The Historic Lands of England.* London: E. Churton 1849.

Calwell, H.G. *The Life and Times of a Voluntary Hospital: The History of the Royal Belfast Hospital for Sick Children 1873-1948.* Belfast: Brough, Cox & Dunn 1973.

Chenu, Jean Charles. *De la mortalité dans l'armée et des moyens d'économiser la vie humaine, extraits des statistiques médico-chirurgicales.* Paris: Hachette 1870.

Chesney, Alan M. *The Johns Hopkins Hospital and the Johns Hopkins University School of Medicine.* Baltimore: Johns Hopkins Press 1943.

Chevers, Norman. *A Brief Review of the Means of Preserving the Health of European Soldiers in India.* Calcutta: Cranenburg 1858.

Combe, Dr. *The Army in Its Medico-Sanitary Relations.* London: Simpkin, Marshall 1859.

Cook, Edward T. *The Life of Florence Nightingale.* 2 vols. London: Macmillan 1913.

Cook, G.C. *Victorian Incurables: A History of the Royal Hospital for Neuro-Disability, Putney.* Spennymoor Durham: Memoir Club 2004.

Cope, Zachary. *A Hundred Years of Nursing at St Mary's Hospital, Paddington.* London: Heinemann 1955.

Cotton, Elizabeth Reid. *Our Coffee Room.* 3rd ed. London: James Nisbet 1876.

———. *More About Our Coffee Room.* London: James Nisbet 1878.

Croft, John. *Notes of Lectures at St Thomas' Hospital.* London: St Thomas/ Blades, East & Blades 1873.

Cunningham, Colin, and Prudence Waterhouse. *Alfred Waterhouse 1830-1905: Biography of a Practice.* Oxford: Clarendon 1992.

Davies, T.G. *Deeds Not Words: A History of the Swansea General and Eye Hospital 1817-1948.* Cardiff: University of Wales 1988.

Douglas, George, and George Dalhousie Ramsay, eds. *The Panmure Papers, Being a Selection from the Correspondence of Fox-Maule, Second Baron Panmure, Afterwards Eleventh Earl of Dalhousie.* 2 vols. London: Hodder & Stoughton 1908.

Emrys-Roberts, Meyrick. *The Cottage Hospitals 1869-1990: Arrival, Survival and Revival.* Motcombe: Tern 1991.

Galton, Douglas. *Report to the Right Hon the Earl de Grey and Ripon, Secretary of State for War, Descriptive of the Herbert Hospital at Woolwich.* London: Eyre & Spottiswoode 1865.

———. *An Address on the General Principles which Should Be Observed in the Construction of Hospitals.* London: Macmillan 1869.

———. *Observations on the Construction of Healthy Dwellings, Namely, Houses, Hospitals, Barracks, Asylums, etc.* Oxford: Clarendon 1880.

Gawande, Atul. *Better: A Surgeon's Notes on Performance.* New York: Metropolitan 2007.

General Board of Health. *Papers Relating to the Sanitary State of the People of England.* London: Eyre & Spottiswoode 1858.

Gibbs, Robert. *A History of Aylesbury.* Aylesbury 1885.

Gibson, Charles Bernard. *Life among Convicts.* 2 vols. London 1863.

Goldie, Sue M., comp. *A Calendar of the Letters of Florence Nightingale.* Oxford Microform 1983.

Goodman, Margaret. *Experiences of an English Sister of Mercy.* London: Smith, Elder 1862.

———. *Sisterhoods in the Church of England.* London: Smith, Elder 1863.

Greenhow, Edward Headlam. *On the Different Prevalence of Certain Diseases in Different Districts in England and Wales* (1858). Reprinted Westmead, Farnborough, Hants: Gregg 1973.

Hordley, R.A. *A Concise History of the Rise and Progress of the North Staffordshire Infirmary and Eye Hospital.* Newcastle: Staffs 1902.

Howard, John. *The State of the Prisons in England and Wales, with Preliminary Observations and an Account of Some Foreign Prisons and Hospitals.* Warrington: W. Eyres 1784.

———. *An Account of the Principal Lazarettos in Europe, with Various Papers Relative to the Plague, Together with Some Further Observations on Some Foreign Prisons and Hospitals.* London: T. Cadell 1789.

Husson, Armand. *Etude sur les hôpitaux, considérés sous le rapport de leur construction, de la distribution et de leurs batiments.* Paris: Paul Dumont 1862.

———. *Statistique médicale des hôpitaux de Paris.* Paris: Administration Générale de l'Assistance Publique 1867.

Jebb, Joshua. *Modern Prisons: Their Construction and Ventilation.* London 1844.

Judd, Catherine. *Bedside Seductions: Nursing and the Victorian Imagination, 1830-1880.* New York: St Martin's 1998.

Lardner, Dionysius. *Steam and Its Uses, Including the Steam Engine.* London: Museum of Science and Art 1856.

Leach, Arthur Francis. *A History of Bradfield College.* London: H. Frowde 1900.

Le Marchant, Denis. *Memoir of John Charles Viscount Althorp, Third Earl Spencer.* London: Bentley 1876.

Leveaux, V.M. *History of the Derbyshire General Infirmary.* Cromford: Scarthin 1999.

Lyons, Robert D. *Report on the Pathology, Therapeutics and General Aitiology of the Epidemic of Yellow Fever which Prevailed at Lisbon, During the Latter Half of the Year 1857.* London: Eyre & Spottiswoode 1859.

MacDermot, H.E. *A History of the Montreal General Hospital.* Montreal: Montreal General Hospital 1950.

Marberry, Sara O., ed., *Innovations in Healthcare Design.* New York: Van Nostrand Reinhard 1990.

Masson, Flora. *Florence Nightingale, O.M., By One Who Knew Her.* London: Scientific Press 1910.

McGrigor, James. *Autobiography and Services: With Notes and Original Correspondence.* London 1861.

———. *Sir James McGrigor—The Scalpel and the Sword: The Autobiography of the Father of Army Medicine,* ed. Mary McGrigor. Dalkeith: Scottish Cultural Press 2000.

McIlraith, John. *The Life of Sir John Richardson.* London: Longmans, Green 1868.

McInnes, E.M. *St Thomas' Hospital.* London: Allen & Unwin 1963.

Mitton, Lavinia. *The Victorian Hospital.* Princes Risborough: Shire Publications 2008.

Moxley, Cyril. *Cathedral College and Hospital: An Account of the Chaplaincy of the Royal Hampshire County Hospital 1736-1986.* Winchester: Self-published 1986.

Murchison, Charles. *A Treatise on the Continued Fevers of Great Britain.* London: Parker 1862.

Oldfield, Sybil. *Jeanie, an "Army of One," Mrs Nassau Senior 1828-1877: The First Woman in Whitehall.* Brighton: Sussex Academic Press 2009.

Papers and Discussions in the International Congress of Charities, Correction and Philanthropy (Section 3, Chicago June 12 to 17th 1893), ed. John S. Billings and Henry Hurd. New York: McGraw-Hill 1949 [1893].

Parsons, F.G. *The History of St Thomas's Hospital.* 3 vols. London: Methuen 1936.

Pass, Anthony J. *Thomas Worthington: Victorian Architecture and Social Purpose.* Manchester: Manchester Literary & Philosophical Publications 1988.

Pickstone, John V. *Medicine and Industrial Society: A History of Hospital Development in Manchester and Its Region, 1752-1946.* Manchester: Manchester University Press 1985.

Poynter, F.N.L., ed. *The Evolution of Hospitals in Britain.* London: Pitman 1964.

Prasad, Sunand, ed. *Changing Hospital Architecture.* London: RBA 2008.

Pringle, John. *Observations on the Diseases of the Army in Camp and Garrison.* 3rd ed. London: Millar 1761 [1752].

Rathbone, William. *The Organization of Nursing in a Large Town.* With an Introduction by Florence Nightingale. Liverpool: Holden 1865.

Rennie, David Field. *Bhotan and the Story of the Dooar War.* London: John Murray 1866.

Richardson, Harriet, ed. *English Hospitals 1660-1948: A Survey of Their Architecture and Design.* Royal Commission on the Historical Monuments of England, Swindon 1998.

Rivett, Geoffrey. *The Development of the London Hospital System 1823-1982.* London: King Edward's Hospital Fund for London 1986.

Rosenberg, C.E., ed. *Healing and History: Essays for George Rosen.* New York: Science History 1979.

———, ed. *Florence Nightingale on Hospital Reform.* New York: Garland 1989.

Roundell, Mrs. *Agnes Jones, or She Hath Done What She Could.* London: Bickers & Son 1896.

Saunders, Hilary St George. *The Middlesex Hospital 1745-1948.* London: Max Parrish 1949.

Scrive, Gaspard M., *Relation médico-chirurgicale de la Campagne d'Orient du 31 mars 1854, occupation de Gallipoli, au 6 juillet 1856, évacuation de la Crimée.* Paris: Victor Masson 1857.

Ser, Louis. *Rapport sur les hôpitaux civils de la ville de Londres au point de vue de la comparaison de ces établissements avec les hôpitaux de la ville de Paris.* Paris: P. Dupont 1862.

Simpson, James Y. *Hospitalism: Its Effects on the Results of Surgical Operations.* Edinburgh 1869.

Small, Hugh. *Florence Nightingale: Avenging Angel.* London: Constable 1998.

Smith, Andrew. *Medical and Surgical History of the British Army which Served in Turkey and the Crimea.* 2 vols. London: Harrison 1858.

Smith, Edward. *Practical Dietaries for Families, Schools and the Working Classes.* London: 1864.

Smith, F.B. *Florence Nightingale: Reputation and Power.* London: Croom Helm 1982.

Snell, Henry Saxon. *Charitable and Parochial Establishments.* London: B.T. Batsford 1881.

Stevenson, Christine. *Medicine and Magnificence: British Hospital and Asylum Architecture, 1660-1815.* New Haven: Yale University Press 2000.

Sympson, Thomas. *A Short Account of the Old and of the New Lincoln County Hospitals.* Lincoln: James Williamson 1878.

Taylor, Jeremy. *Hospital and Asylum Architecture in England 1840-1914: Building for Health Care.* London: Mansell 1991.

———. *The Architect and the Pavilion Hospital: Dialogue and Design Creativity in England 1850-1914.* Leicester: Leicester University Press 1997.

———. *The Rebirth of the Norfolk and Norwich Hospital 1874-1883: An Architectural Exploration.* London: Wellcome Unit for the History of Medicine 2000.

Tenon, Jacques. *Mémoires sur les hopitaux de Paris.* English translation and with an Introduction by Dora B. Weiner, ed., *Memoirs on Paris Hospitals.* Canton MA: Science History 1996 [1788].

The Organization of Nursing in a Large Town. With Introduction by Florence Nightingale. Liverpool: Holden 1865.

Thompson, John D., and Grace Goldin. *The Hospital: A Social and Architectural History.* New Haven: Yale University Press 1975.

Topinard, Paul. *Quelques aperçus sur la chirurgie anglaise.* Paris 1860.

Turner, Barbara Carpenter. *A History of the Royal Hampshire County Hospital.* Chichester: Phillimore 1986.

United Kingdom. *Report of the Commissioners Appointed to Inquire into the Regulations Affecting the Sanitary Condition of the Army and the Treatment of the Sick and Wounded.* 2 vols. London: HMSO 1858.

Verderber, Stephen. *Innovations in Hospital Architecture.* New York: Routledge 2010.

Wagenaar, Cor, ed., *The Architecture of Hospitals.* Belgium: NAI 2006.

Waring, Edward John. *The Hospital Prayer Book.* London 1872.

Wells, Thomas Spencer. *Diseases of the Ovaries: Their Diagnosis and Treatment.* London: 1865.

West, Charles. *How to Nurse Sick Children, Intended Especially as a Help to the Nurses at the Hospital for Sick Children.* London: Longman, Brown 1854.

Woodward, J.H. *"To Do the Sick No Harm": A Study of the British Voluntary Hospital System until 1875.* London: Routledge & Kegan Paul 1974.

Worboys, Michael. *Spreading Germs: Disease Theories and Medical Practice in Britain, 1865-1900.* Cambridge University Press 2000.

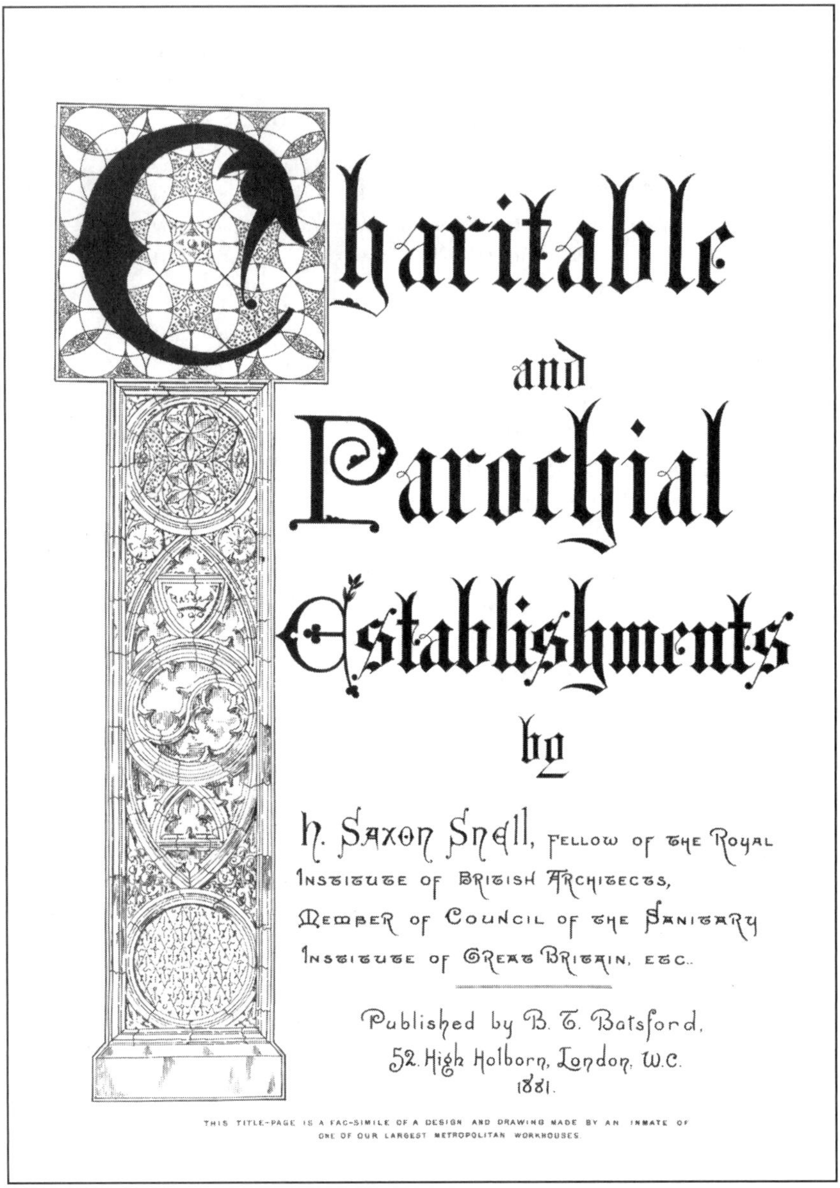

Charitable and Parochial Establishments by H. Saxon Snell, Fellow of the Royal Institute of British Architects, Member of Council of the Sanitary Institute of Great Britain, etc.

Published by B. T. Batsford, 52. High Holborn, London, W.C. 1881.

THIS TITLE-PAGE IS A FAC-SIMILE OF A DESIGN AND DRAWING MADE BY AN INMATE OF ONE OF OUR LARGEST METROPOLITAN WORKHOUSES.

Title page of architect Henry Saxon Snell's *Charitable and Parochial Establishments.* He sent a copy to Nightingale in 1882.

Index

INDEX

Space limitations required some compromises in the index. Proper names are included wherever known. Entries with identifying information are italicized. Persons known by more than one name are indexed under the name most frequently appearing in the text, cross-referenced to any other appearing. British Army hospitals (peacetime) are listed by name under army hospitals; Crimean War hospitals are listed by name under Crimean War.

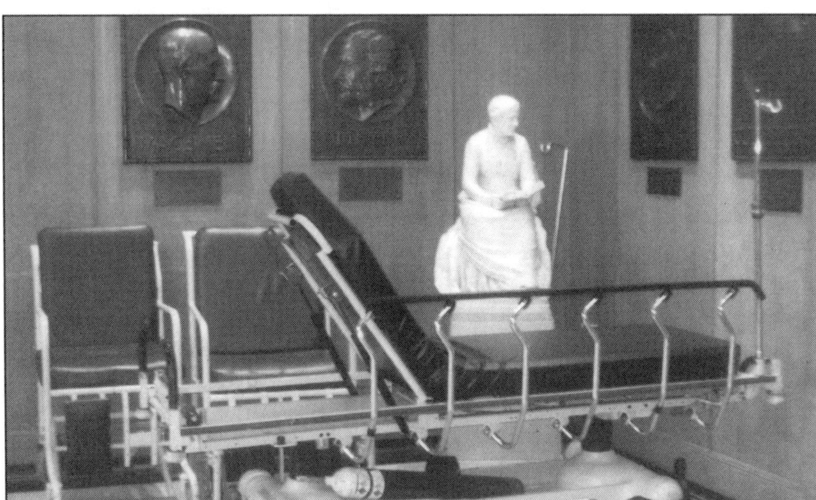

Nightingale statue surrounded by hospital equipment in the main lobby of the Glasgow Royal Infirmary. Photograph courtesy of Sandra Hunter.